HUMAN MOTOR DEVELOPME...

Human Motor Development: A Lifespan Approach, 10th Edition, offers an overview to the study of changes in human movement across the lifespan. The book uses a holistic approach and emphasizes the importance of intellectual, social, and physical development and their impact on human motor development at all ages.

The tenth edition has been completely revised and updated to reflect the most recent research and technology in human motor development. Organized into five parts, the book examines key topics in motor development including the relationship between cognitive and social development and motor development, factors affecting development, changes across the lifespan, and assessment in motor development.

Highly illustrated and written for student accessibility, *Human Motor Development: A Lifespan Approach* is essential reading for students of motor control and development, kinesiology, human performance, and students interested in physical therapy, physical education, and exercise science. The book also provides access to a fully updated companion website, which includes laboratory exercises, an instructors' manual, a test bank, and lecture slides.

V. Gregory Payne is a Professor Emeritus in the Department of Kinesiology at San Jose State University, USA. He formerly served as the Associate Dean for Research in the College of Applied Sciences and Arts and as Chair of the Department of Kinesiology. Payne has produced over 170 publications, including numerous refereed articles and 19 editions of five books, and has made nearly 300 presentations. He is an elected Fellow of the National Academy of Kinesiology and was a member of the task force that developed the NASPE National Physical Education Standards. Payne's awards include being selected International Professor of the Year at SJSU, receiving the Distinguished Service Award from the California Governor's Council on Physical Fitness and Sports and the prestigious Research Quarterly for Exercise and Sport Research Writing Award. He has held offices in several organizations including President of NASPE and Chair of the Motor Development Academy. He is an elected Fellow of the National Academy of Kinesiology and the Research Consortium of AAHPERD (SHAPE America), and has chaired two editorial boards.

Larry D. Isaacs is Professor Emeritus and former Director of the Exercise Physiology Program, Department of Biological Sciences, College of Science and Mathematics at Wright State University, USA. He has published numerous scholarly articles and has authored, co-authored, and contributed to 21 textbooks. He is certified with the American College of Sports Medicine (Certified Exercise Physiologist) and was awarded Research Fellow status by AAHPERD/SHAPE. In addition, he has received the Wright State University Presidential Recognition award for research. Isaacs continues to work part-time as a clinical exercise physiologist at Hilton Head Hospital, Hilton Head Island, South Carolina, where he works with both cardiac and pulmonary patients.

Human Motor Development: A Lifespan Approach takes an applied approach to examining fundamental movement skill acquisition leading up to childhood and provides relatable examples on how all domains of human development impact further development and/or inhibit development of movement skills across the lifespan. The textbook provides a foundation of understanding that can be utilized by undergraduate students pursuing professions in physical therapy, occupational, physical education, applied behaviour analysis, etc.

Marquell Johnson,
University of Wisconsin-Eau Claire

Human Motor Development: A Lifespan Approach explores motor development as it relates to the other domains of human development – and it is the only book to do that! It is key to understanding how humans learn how to move in the context of their general development, and the importance of movement across the lifespan.

Priscila Caçola,
University of Texas at Arlington

Human Motor Development

A Lifespan Approach

10th Edition

V. GREGORY PAYNE • LARRY D. ISAACS

Routledge
Taylor & Francis Group
NEW YORK AND LONDON

Tenth edition published 2020
by Routledge
52 Vanderbilt Avenue, New York, NY 10017

and by Routledge
2 Park Square, Milton Park, Abingdon, Oxon, OX14 4RN

Routledge is an imprint of the Taylor & Francis Group, an informa business

Ninth edition published by Holcomb Hathaway 2016

Library of Congress Cataloging-in-Publication Data
Names: Payne, V. Gregory, 1950- author. | Isaacs, Larry D. (Larry David), 1949- author.
Title: Human motor development : a lifespan approach / V. Gregory Payne, Larry D. Isaacs.
Description: 10th edition. | New York, NY : Routledge, 2020. | Includes bibliographical references and index.
Identifiers: LCCN 2019039091 (print) | LCCN 2019039092 (ebook) | ISBN 9780367347369 (hardback) | ISBN 9780367347376 (paperback) | ISBN 9780429327568 (ebook)
Subjects: LCSH: Motor ability in children. | Physical fitness for children.
Classification: LCC RJ133 .P39 2020 (print) | LCC RJ133 (ebook) | DDC 613.7/042--dc23
LC record available at https://lccn.loc.gov/2019039091
LC ebook record available at https://lccn.loc.gov/2019039092

ISBN: 978-0-367-34736-9 (hbk)
ISBN: 978-0-367-34737-6 (pbk)
ISBN: 978-0-429-32756-8 (ebk)

Typeset in Sabon, Helvetica Neue and Humanist 777
by Servis Filmsetting Ltd, Stockport, Cheshire

Visit the companion website: www.routledge.com/cw/Payne

Dedicated to my family and several decades of wonderful students, colleagues, and mentors at San Jose State University and beyond.

V.G.P.

To my wife, Joy, grandson, Liam Finnerty; and the loving memory of my parents, Linwood and Gracie Isaacs. And to all of my feline companions (past and present), whose movements are truly a study in motor skill development: Lucy, Bert and Ernie, Elmo, Ginger, and Ollie.

L.D.I.

Note: The authors' names appear side by side on the title page to denote an equal contribution to the production of this textbook.

CONTENTS

PREFACE

In this tenth edition of *Human Motor Development: A Lifespan Approach* we were delighted to establish a new relationship with Routledge. Through this partnership, and in the creation of this tenth edition, we have maintained our long-standing emphasis on appropriate, research-based, undergraduate-level information related to the study of human motor development. Our primary mission has been, and continues to be, presenting this information in the most understandable and student-oriented way.

SPECIAL FEATURES AND ORGANIZATION

Historically, human motor development has been studied and presented as a process that focused exclusively on children and adolescence. Our book approaches the topic as a lifespan proposition, recognizing the dramatic changes to our population's demographics (rapidly increasing numbers of older people) and the pressing need to engage in what has become a popular and important area of research: studying people of all ages, including those in early, middle, and late adulthood.

We also adhere to the philosophy that human movement is integral to cognitive, social-emotional, and physical development. We believe that these areas of development have similarly powerful effects on motor development. Therefore, separate chapters are allocated to each of these areas of development and how they interrelate with human movement. We believe this is one of many unique features of our book.

This latest edition of *Human Motor Development: A Lifespan Approach* retains the straightforward organization of earlier editions. Part I provides an overview of human development and includes chapters on the relationship between motor development and cognitive, social-emotional, and moral development. Part II covers factors affecting development, including effects of early stimulation and deprivation. Part III, "Physical Changes Across the Lifespan," and Part IV, "Movement Across the Lifespan," present the book's core concepts. Part V covers the all-important topic of assessing motor development.

KEY CHANGES TO THE TENTH EDITION

This tenth edition of *Human Motor Development: A Lifespan Approach* has undergone thorough revision and updating. All the chapters have been substantially modified to reflect contemporary thought and theory while maintaining the book's readability for students. Numerous photos, figures, and tables are provided to allow a greater depth of understanding. In addition, to enhance the book's aesthetics and readability, it is now presented in full color. We have also streamlined where possible to enable a more concise and time-sensitive coverage of the material. The focus on adult development, however, has been expanded as demographic changes worldwide are dictating that all areas of development more closely consider the importance of studying adulthood and older adulthood. Nevertheless, the comprehensive and detailed attention to the all-important developmental years of childhood and adolescence has been maintained. Another key change in this new edition is a more focused examination to motor development as an international proposition. More than ever, remarkable research is evolving from all parts of the world to give us a greater understanding of this field of study in the United States and around the world. We believe this is another unique feature of this book.

SUPPLEMENTS

Chapters in this tenth edition conclude with a list of key terms, questions for reflection, and complete references. Most chapters also conclude with a list of related websites for additional relevant reading. A comprehensive package of supplementary materials designed to enhance teaching and learning is also available on the Companion Website of the tenth edition of *Human Motor Development: A Lifespan Approach*, available at: www.routledge.com/cw/Payne

PEDAGOGICAL AIDS FOR STUDENTS AND INSTRUCTORS

Our book's Companion Website (www.routledge.com/cw/Payne) has been extensively updated and revamped for the tenth edition. It includes, for students and instructors:

- chapter-by-chapter PowerPoint presentations
- lists of valuable related online resources
- lists of relevant videos for most chapters
- a glossary of all key terms from the book. The key terms are shown in bold in the text.

Specifically for students, we have included:

- matching, true-false questions
- fill in the blank quizzes for self-assessments of learning.

Specifically for instructors, we have prepared:

- approximately 500 multiple choice questions
- a sample course syllabus
- numerous expanded course assignments with suggestions for expected length, criteria for evaluation, and problems the students may encounter in completing the assignment. These assignments are in a ready-to-use format and are easily adapted to the instructor's preferences
- creative and useful **laboratory activities** for each chapter, complete with answer sheets specifically designed for each lab.

ACKNOWLEDGMENTS

We extend special thanks to the staff at Routledge. Their guidance through this revision process was detailed and professional. Most impressively, their careful consideration of our work was collegial, professional, and friendly. This made the process especially gratifying. We thoroughly enjoyed creating this tenth edition. We would specifically like to thank David Varley, our Senior Editor; Megan Smith, Editorial Assistant; Edward Gibbons, the Senior Production Editor; and Susan Dunsmore, who copyedited our book.

We are also grateful to several anonymous reviewers who graciously and expertly offered input regarding our proposal for this tenth edition. Their insights were thoughtful, informed, and integral to our work.

Lastly, but certainly no less important, we would like to express our gratitude to Kim Komenich of San Francisco State University. A Pulitzer Prize-winning photographer, Kim provided the photos of the infants in Chapter 9: Infant Reflexes and Stereotypies.

TO THE STUDENT

www.routledge.com/cw/payne

Visit the Human Motor Development website designed to accompany your textbook for study aids and additional resources. To help you prepare for exams and extend your learning, the companion website provides a variety of tools, including:

- Short answer, true-false, and matching quizzes for review and test preparation.
- An interactive key concept review and glossary.
- Lab activities.
- Links to YouTube videos that demonstrate key movement concepts.
- Links to key motor development online resources.

TO INSTRUCTORS

INSTRUCTOR'S MANUAL AND TESTBANK

The updated manual includes a sample syllabus; a testbank with approximately 500 multiple-choice and short essay questions; suggested assignments for each chapter; and a group of extended assignments. For the instructor, the extended assignments include such details as expected length, criteria for evaluation, and challenges the student may encounter in completing the assignment. These assignments are in a ready-to-use format or are easily adaptable to the instructor's own course or preferences.

The testbank is also available via the Respondus platform, allowing you to create and manage exams that can be printed out or integrated with Blackboard, D2L, Moodle, and other learning systems.

POWERPOINT SLIDES

A complete set of PowerPoint slides is available for download. Keyed to the major points in each chapter, these slide sets can be modified or expanded to better fit your lectures.

PART I

An Overview of Development

1 INTRODUCTION TO MOTOR DEVELOPMENT

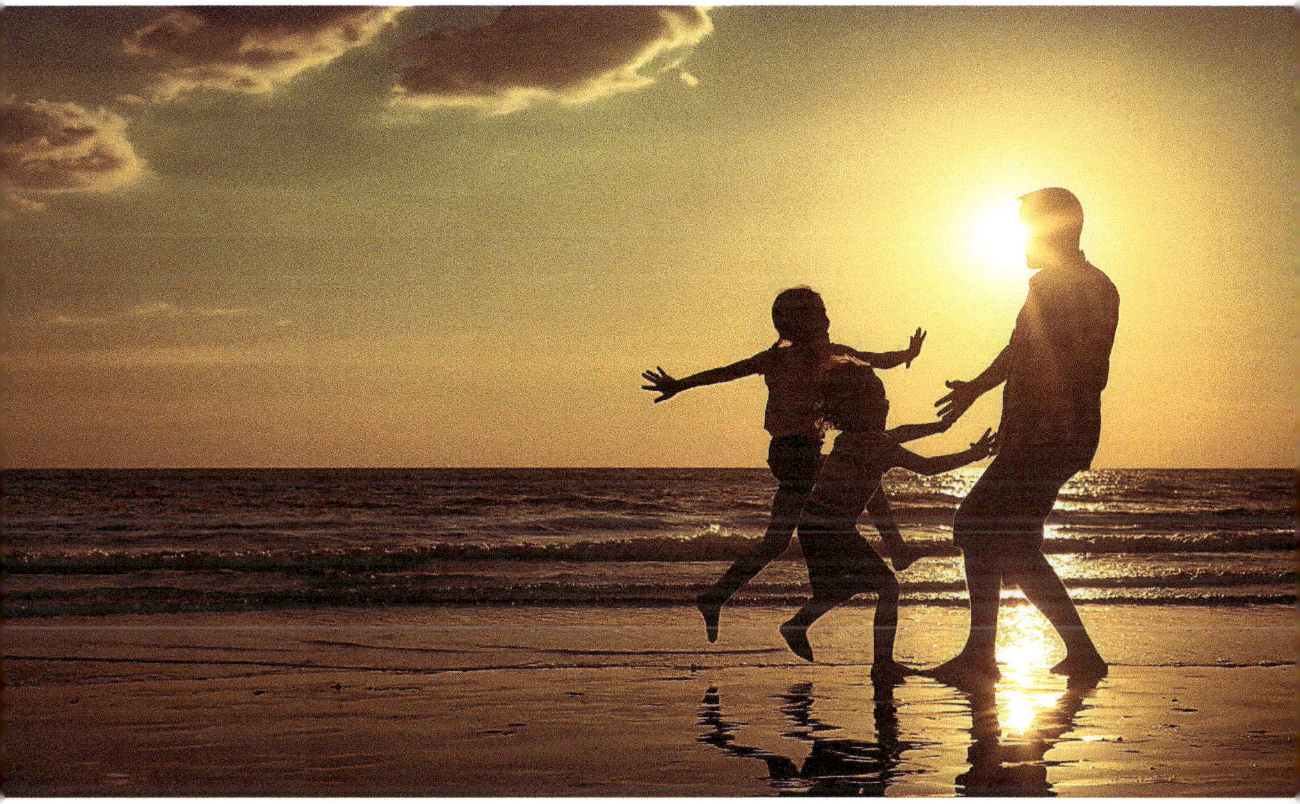

Chapter Objectives

From the information presented in this chapter, you will be able to

- Define human development and human motor development
- Explain why the study of human motor development is important
- Describe the four domains of human development and explain how they interact
- Explain the concepts of development, maturation, and growth, and describe the elements of developmental change
- Define common terms in the study of human motor development
- Describe the process-product controversy and how it relates to human motor development
- Define various terms for age periods throughout the lifespan
- Describe and explain the "Mountain of Motor Development." Why is it important?
- List the periods and describe the history of the field of motor development

HUMAN MOTOR DEVELOPMENT

Human motor development is both a process through which we pass during the course of life and an academic field of study. As a human process, motor development refers to the changes that occur in our ability to move and our movement in general as we proceed through the lifespan. As a field of study, it is the "study of changes in human movement across the lifespan and the processes that affect those changes" (Clark & Whitall, 1989, p. 194). Or, to paraphrase Whitall (2009), as a field of study, motor development seeks to determine what changes we see in human movement and when, how, and why change occurs. Motor development research is often interdisciplinary; we team with experts from other areas of study to do our research. However, what makes motor development researchers unique in the field of human movement is that we do not stop with understanding the present motor behavior; our primary interest in change drives us to understand what the movement was, what it will be, and how and why it was and will be. We refer to this approach as a **developmental perspective.**

THE IMPORTANCE OF MOTOR DEVELOPMENT

Human development is a diverse, complex area of study in which we cannot consider ourselves completely educated until we understand all aspects of the changes that occur throughout the lifespan. We must strive to understand the movement changes that we commonly experience with age and their accompanying intellectual, social, and emotional changes. Too often descriptions and explanations of motor development are isolated in single chapters, or even brief sections of development texts, despite the fact that changes in human movement can initiate and contribute significantly to important developmental change in areas such as human perception, intellect, and social interaction. To date, most research on motor development has been generated by researchers from Western countries studying relatively traditional Western people. Thus, our current understanding of human development may be somewhat biased by this phenomenon and represents a need for much more cross-cultural research (Adolph & Robinson, 2015). Nevertheless, our knowledge of all aspects of human development is integral to a full understanding of ourselves, our development, and the world we live in. Although knowledge gained purely for the sake of knowledge is important, knowledge gained from the study of motor development can be very practical and potentially life-enhancing.

For easy communication and efficient organization, in this book, we divide the study of human development into the cognitive, affective (socioemotional), motor, and physical domains. These domains of human behavior are constantly interacting, and a complete understanding of any one domain requires knowledge of the domains with which it interacts. Full understanding of motor development, therefore, requires knowledge of the cognitive, affective, and physical domains because they so profoundly affect movement behavior. Conversely, full understanding of human development in the cognitive, affective, and physical domains requires knowledge of motor development. As discussed in the upcoming chapters, motor development has profound effects on the development of cognitive, social, and physical behaviors throughout the lifespan.

Knowledge of motor development has other applications, as well. For example, understanding the way people typically develop movement skills throughout the lifespan enables us to diagnose problems in those individuals who may be developing atypically. Consider an infant who does not exhibit a particular reflex at the expected time of appearance. As discussed in greater detail in Chapter 9, certain reflexive movements typically occur at certain ages. Any significant deviations from the expected time line may indicate the need for special treatment.

Understanding human motor development is also important for helping people improve their movement performance, which can yield many benefits. For example, an improved self-concept often accompanies improved movement and enables a person to become more emotionally stable and satisfied. Enhancing one's movement ability can also be extremely motivating, leading to a more physically active lifestyle and ultimately improved health and wellness. Also, because there are links among all domains of behavior, improvement in the motor domain may indirectly lead to improvements in intellectual or social development. Activities can be devised to assist in the development of movement potential. To create such a movement curriculum with accuracy, we must know about typically developing motor development. With that knowledge and the subsequent structuring of developmentally appropriate movement tasks, we can challenge individuals relative to their levels of achievement. Developmentally appropriate (appropriate for the individual and for his or her age) movement curricula lead to more effective learning of motor tasks because the participants seldom become frustrated or bored by tasks that are too difficult or too easy.

For all of these reasons, knowledge of motor development is important for movement specialists working with typically developing children. This same knowledge can often be applied in work with individuals with special needs. Although many atypical conditions lead to a developmental lag in an individual's movement performance, the sequence or pattern of development is generally similar to the movement patterns of typically developing individuals, though an individual with special needs may not ultimately achieve as much maturity in their movement. For example, autism spectrum disorder (ASD) is the fastest growing developmental disorder in the United States (Liu, Hamilton, Davis, & ElGarhy, 2014). In research conducted by MacDonald, Lord, and Ulrich (2014), children with ASD were found to often have deficits in motor skill starting at a very young age. Specifically, gait, control of posture, general fine and gross motor skill, and the ability to plan motor strategies were found to be affected. In addition, the severity of the deficit was highly correlated with the severity of the children's ASD symptomology. Understanding the nature of these delays, according to these authors, may be integral to effective preliminary diagnosis of this condition. These authors also suggest that children with ASD may benefit from early intervention programs designed to enhance motor skills and note a "need for well-controlled motor skill based early interventions for young children with ASD" (p. 101). In short, understanding the pattern of motor skill development in children with ASD may be integral in predicting the severity of ASD and to developing intervention and rehabilitation strategies, techniques, and programs for young children with ASD (MacDonald, Lord, & Ulrich, 2014).

Similar findings were generated in work conducted by Liu and associates (2014), where children with ASD were tested on their gross motor development and compared to typically developing children of a similar age. All children were approximately 8 years old. For both locomotor and object control skills, approximately two-thirds of the children with ASD generated "poor" scores with approximately one-third generating "very poor" scores. For "overall gross motor scores" three-fourths of the ASD children received a "very poor" score while a significant difference was found in the performance of the children with ASD when compared to the typically

Table 1.1 Why should we study motor development?

1.	Human development is multifaceted. In addition to changes in human movement, intellectual, social, and emotional changes occur. Because these domains of human development are in constant interaction, we can never fully understand ourselves until we fully understand each of these domains, including the motor domain.
2.	Knowledge of the way most people develop in their movement enables us to diagnose cases that are sufficiently atypical to warrant intervention and remediation.
3.	Knowledge of human motor development allows the establishment of developmentally appropriate activities that enable optimal teaching/learning of movement skills for people of all ages and all ability levels.

developing group. Thus, the authors concluded that a therapeutic intervention may be especially beneficial, even necessary, for children with ASD (Liu et al., 2014). Clearly, the study of motor development and knowledge of expected trajectories in motor development offers many benefits. See Table 1.1 for a summary of the importance of such research and knowledge.

THE DOMAINS OF HUMAN DEVELOPMENT

Over 60 years ago, Benjamin Bloom (1956) devised a taxonomy (method of classification or organization) to categorize educational objectives. In his taxonomy, he created three categories of educational objectives and deemed each a "domain." These domains were the cognitive, the affective, and the psychomotor. Though our focus in this book is not educational objectives, Bloom's domains, with one significant change, work nicely in categorizing the study of human development. The significant change is to add one more domain, the physical domain.

These four domains provide a neat framework for organizing our study of human development. The cognitive domain, which concerns human intellectual development, has been the main focus of developmentalists throughout history. Jean Piaget, the most prominent developmentalist of all time, emphasized intellectual development. His work in relationship to motor development is examined in Chapter 2. To understand cognitive development in a practical way, imagine a third-grade girl sitting at her desk at school. If our focus is on her cognitive development, we would be most concerned with her reading, problem solving in math, pondering facts in social studies, and other similar activities.

The affective domain is primarily concerned with the social and emotional aspects of human development. Thus, we often refer to this domain as the socioemotional domain, a term recognizable to most. In considering our third-grader, we would focus on aspects such as her feelings of self-worth, her ability to interact with her peers in the classroom, and how she feels about their interactions with her (see Figure 1.1).

The **psychomotor**, or motor, domain is the main focus of this book. Here, we emphasize the development of human movement and the factors that affect that development. In this domain, for our third-grader, focus shifts to

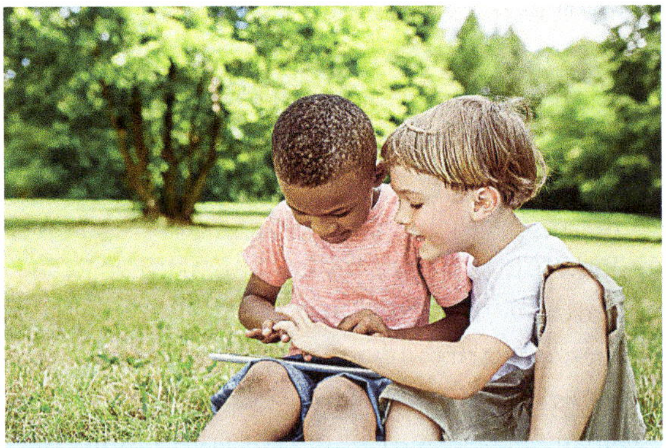

Figure 1.1 The affective domain includes the social and emotional aspects of human development

examinations of her handwriting ability; her movement technique and level of maturity in running, throwing, and jumping; and her rhythmic ability in dance activities.

As mentioned, the fourth domain involves physical change. We believe that this domain, too often merged with the motor domain, deserves separate recognition. Here, we include all types of bodily change. With regard to our third-grader, we are concerned with bodily types of change, such as her increases in height and weight. Has body fat increased or decreased? What is her range of motion around joints or her cardiorespiratory endurance? Though these factors all affect the other domains, they can also be clearly distinguished.

Finally, though these four domains are extremely useful in organizing our study of human development, we must remember that this organizational schema is also a bit artificial. When we think in terms of discrete categories of development, we imagine our third-grader switching into and out of domains of development based on whether she has been given a math worksheet or has just heard the recess bell. In fact, these domains constantly interact with one another. Each influences all of the others and, in turn, is influenced by all of the others (see Figure 1.2). For example, has your performance on a written exam (cognitive domain) ever been influenced by your emotional state (affective domain)? Does your muscular strength (physical domain) affect your athletic performance (motor domain)? Or, have you ever been affected emotionally (affective domain) by measures of your own body fat or muscle mass (physical domain)?

Because the interaction of domains is so prevalent in human development, isolating any one area of development can be difficult. Thus, though our primary intent is to emphasize changes in human movement throughout the lifespan, we often examine the interactions just described, with special focus on human movement. Specific examples include

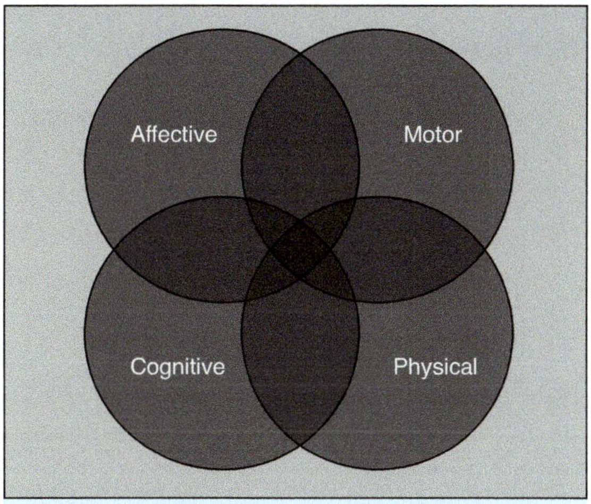

Figure 1.2 The four domains of human development are useful for categorizing our study of such areas as motor development. However, we must remember that these domains are not discrete; they are in constant interaction with one another.

Chapters 2 and 3, where we examine motor development in relationship to cognitive and affective (socioemotional) development. In Chapters 6 and 7, the emphasis will be on the interrelationship between the physical and motor domains.

DEVELOPMENT, MATURATION, AND GROWTH

Development

The term **development**, as it applies to human beings, refers to changes we experience as we pass through life. Though this book focuses on human movement, people obviously develop intellectually, socially, emotionally, and physically as well. The term *development* has increased in popularity, especially in educational circles, since the publication by the National Association for the Education of Young Children (NAEYC) of a 1997 position statement and guidelines on developmentally appropriate practice for early childhood programs. An updated statement was published in 2009 (NAEYC, 2009). The 1997 document

PSYCHOMOTOR OR MOTOR?

For this book we deliberately chose to use *motor* as a general term to refer to any form of human movement behavior, rather than using the narrower term psychomotor used by Bloom in his taxonomy. *Psychomotor* is particularly useful for referring to the domain of human development that involves human movement though it is very specific, as it refers to those movements initiated by an electrical impulse from the higher brain centers, for example, the motor cortex. Most human movement is the result of such stimulation. However, because there is a form of movement behavior—reflexive movement—that is initiated in the lower brain centers or the central nervous system, we use the more general term *motor* so as not to exclude the reflexes from the movement-related domain, the motor domain.

Nevertheless, the term *psychomotor* deserves special attention. This word was coined in recognition of the interaction between the mind (psycho) and human movement (motor). The mind is a critical component in the production of almost all human movement. This interactive relationship is thoroughly examined in Chapter 2. We also study the equally important effects of human movement on mental or cognitive development.

was meant to "describe developmentally appropriate practice in early childhood programs for administrators, teachers, parents, policy makers, and others who make decisions about care and education for young children" (Bredekamp & Copple, 1997, p. 1). Its authors believed that many programs for very young children failed to consider the "basic developmental needs of young children." They noted, "Programs should be tailored to meet the needs of children, rather than expecting children to adjust to the demands of a specific program" (p. 1). In other words, programs should be **developmentally appropriate**. According to the NAEYC, this term has two dimensions: age appropriateness and individual appropriateness. *Age appropriateness* refers to the predictable sequences of growth and development through which most children pass. Knowledge of these sequences provides a basis upon which we can build to provide optimal instructional experiences for children. Professional decisions based on these sequences should be "grounded in the research . . . and promote young children's optimal learning and development" (p. 1). *Individual appropriateness* refers to the uniqueness of each child. Though predictable developmental sequences exist, children have individual patterns and rates of growth, as well as unique personalities, approaches to learning, and home experiences. Educators must consider all such matters when composing learning activities for children, in any domain.

According to the NAEYC's position statement (2009), "intentionality" is integral to the concept of developmental appropriateness. Thus, child development practitioners should purposefully use current research and knowledge of children's development when making decisions and establishing goals for a child's education and achievement. The position statement continues by describing what informed practitioners are able to do; they are

> able to make broad predictions about what children of a particular age group typically will be like, what they typically will and will not be capable of, and what strategies and approaches will most likely promote their optimal learning and development.
>
> (p. 9)

To be most effective in working with children, we should start by "thinking about what we know from theory and practice about children of the age and developmental status represented. This knowledge provides a general idea of the activities, routines, interactions, and curriculum that will be effective with that group" (p. 10). However, we must simultaneously consider who the child is as an individual within the scope of their own environment and social situation. These kinds of considerations will form the basis for the selection of developmentally appropriate educational experiences.

As a result of the increase in their popularity, terms such as *development* and *developmentally appropriate* have come to be frequently misused or abused, taking on many meanings according to individual agendas. The term *development* must be clearly defined and understood if the concept is to be optimally integrated into programs for children and youth. In this book, the term refers to the changes that all human beings face across their lifespan. Such changes result from increasing age, as well as from one's experiences in life, one's genetic potential, and the interactions of all three factors at any given time. Therefore, development is "an interactional process that leads to changes in behavior over the life-span" (Motor Development Task Force, 1995, p. 2).

Table 1.2 Elements of developmental change

Development is	
• Qualitative	• Directional
• Sequential	• Multifactorial
• Cumulative	• Individual
Understanding the elements of developmental change is essential to attaining a developmental perspective: looking at current behaviors with an interest in what preceded them and what will follow, and understanding that development is "age related but not completely age determined" (Motor Development Task Force, 1995, p. 5).	

Source: Position statement of the National Association of Sport and Physical Education (NASPE), prepared by the Motor Development Task Force (1995).

Elements of Developmental Change

According to a position statement prepared by the Motor Development Task Force, six elements or components comprise developmental change: it is qualitative, sequential, cumulative, directional, multifactorial, and individual (see Table 1.2).

1. *Qualitative* implies that developmental change is not just "more of something." It also implies that developmental change may not always be a progressive or positive. As we discuss in more detail in Chapter 11, handwriting development in the later stages of life qualitatively changes. The technique, or process, employed in writing may subtly evolve, as well as the product (output) of the handwriting. Of interest, the task force that created these elements of developmental change did not include "quantitative." Of course development can also be quantitative, or measurable. With maturity, children can learn to throw farther, run faster, and jump higher. Perhaps because of the obvious nature of this type of change, or because of the excess emphasis once placed on only quantitiative kinds of changes, the task force did not include what would seem like another clear element of developmental change.
2. *Sequential.* The sequential element of change implies that certain motor patterns precede others and that the patterns are orderly in their appearance. According to the NAEYC position statement (2009), "Many aspects of children's learning and development follow well documented sequences with later abilities, skills, and knowledge building on those already acquired" (p. 11). Nevertheless, development often proceeds at

different rates for different children, though the sequence may remain unaltered. For example, we leap (e.g., making an extended running stride to cross a small stream) before we run, or we reach before we grasp. Sequences of development have been identified in motor development, and knowledge of these sequences is crucial for optimal teaching and interventions related to movement skills.

3. *Cumulative* suggests that behaviors are additive. Current behaviors are built on previous ones. The early behaviors are, therefore, stepping stones to more mature movements. For example, unassisted standing evolves from the ability to stand with a minimum of support or a handhold from a caregiver.
4. *Directional*. The directional element suggests that development has an ultimate goal. We generally tend to think of development as progressive, but it can also be regressive. In other words, skills can become less mature. This can happen as a result of ceasing training or practice or through the long-term effects of aging or disease.
5. *Multifactorial*. Developmental change is also multifactorial. This means that no one factor directs such change. Factors that can influence developmental change include genetics, physical characteristics, such as strength, flexibility, and endurance, and emotional factors, such as motivation. The environment also affects change and the rate of change. As we enter the later stage of life, environmental factors such as exercise, practice, and therapy play critical roles in the maintenance of our movement abilities.
6. *Individual* implies that the rate of developmental change varies for all people, though the general sequence of development remains relatively similar. One child may exhibit a relatively mature pattern for running at 4 years of age, and another's running pattern may remain quite immature at the same age. Change is the result of many factors that interact in unique ways. Factors that make development individual include the individual characteristics of each body and the equally unique environmental circumstances surrounding each person (Motor Development Task Force, 1995).

Developmental Perspective

Understanding these elements of developmental change is critical to gaining a developmental perspective in which we consider not just today's behavior but what preceded the behavior and what will evolve from it. For example, when we take this perspective, we will not consider age alone when we assess development. Though age is important, development is "age related but not completely age determined" (Motor Development Task Force, 1995, p. 5). In other words, most 7-year-olds use a mature technique in handwriting. However, the fact that a child is 7 does not ensure this level of development. Furthermore, when a 4-year-old does not take a step in batting a ball, this pattern is not incorrect. It may be quite appropriate for the developmental status of the child. Though this batting technique would not indicate a mature performance, the child may be well on his or her way to a mature pattern of batting.

Maturation and Growth

So, development for our purposes is a relatively general term that refers to changes in the human being across time. It includes two other terms, or processes, important to our understanding of human development: **maturation** and **growth**.

Although it is acceptable in casual conversation to use all three of these terms, *development*, *maturation*, and *growth*, somewhat synonymously, for the purposes of our study and research in motor development we use them more specifically and differently, according to exact definitions for each. In this textbook, *development* includes both maturation and growth. It is the umbrella term for the other two. The qualitative functional changes that occur with age are collectively known as maturation. Growth refers to the quantitative structural changes that occur with age. It is "an increase in size by the addition of material from cell multiplication or increase in cell size" (Dye, 2017, p. 141). Although both terms indicate specific aspects of a metamorphosis from childhood to adulthood, *maturation* refers to organizational changes in the function of the organs and tissues. The individual's behavior is subsequently modified as a result of these qualitative changes. An example of maturation is the neurological organization of the brain during childhood. Virtually all anatomical parts of the brain are present from very early in childhood, but qualitative change in brain function occurs throughout childhood, enabling children to achieve ever higher levels of cognitive and motor ability.

Growth, as mentioned, is simply an increase in physical size. This physical transformation primarily involves hyperplasia—"an increase in the size of tissue resulting from an increase in the number of cells" (Dye, 2017, p. 165) or hypertrophy—an increase in cell size; and accretion—an increase in intercellular matter (Malina, Bouchard, & Bar-Or, 2004). Although these processes are gradual, generally imperceptible phenomena, they become increasingly evident when a human being is observed over a long period of time. One of the most noticeable examples of growth occurs at the onset of adolescence: both male and female individuals experience a growth spurt. During that time, an increase in height of several inches over a single year is not unusual. That increase in height, independent of any simultaneous changes, is growth.

Maturation and growth should be separately defined for facilitating our understanding of development, but they are related aspects of the developmental process. Growth and maturation are intertwined because functions change as the body grows. However, most people's rate of growth (other than increase in body fat) slows greatly when they are about 20 years old. In contrast, maturation proceeds until the end of the lifespan.

TRENDS IN GROWTH AND MOTOR DEVELOPMENT

As discussed earlier, there are important reasons why we need a general understanding of human motor development. Although many of us pride ourselves on the characteristics that make us unique, the general motor development of all human beings is remarkably similar. Motor development researchers use several terms to describe the general growth and maturation trends that occur throughout the population.

Developmental Direction

Cephalocaudal and *proximodistal* are frequently referred to as the developmental directions because they indicate the direction in which growth and movement maturation proceeds. **Cephalocaudal** literally means "from the head to the tail." Specifically, this term refers to the development of the human being from the top of the body, the head, downward toward the "tail" or the feet (Venes, 2017). This phenomenon is especially noticeable as it applies to growth. The head of a human fetus or infant is much larger than the head of an older child, adolescent, or adult relative to the body. The head experiences greater growth earlier than the rest of the body.

The cephalocaudal concept can also be applied to the maturation of human movement. The development of walking is an excellent example. When children first learn to walk, their legs are stiff and their feet flat. This awkward but typical walking technique is partly caused by cephalocaudal development. Control over the muscles that govern the hip joint enables the infant to swing the entire leg, but the child has not yet achieved similar ability at the knee or the ankle. With time, the child will gain comparable control at the knee and then the ankle, eventually achieving the mature walking technique.

Proximodistal, the second developmental direction, means from those points close to the body's center to those points close to the periphery, or farthest from the body's center (Venes, 2017). This phenomenon is evidenced by human prenatal growth. The human evolves from the neural groove, a tiny elongated mass of cells that eventually forms the central portion of the body, the spinal column. From that central portion of the body, all else will evolve until the fingers and toes have been completed.

A similar process occurs in the acquisition of movement skill, such as an infant's early attempts at reaching and grasping (prehension). Initially, the infant's arm is controlled by the muscles that are predominantly responsible for shoulder movement. Gradually, dominance over the elbow also evolves, which allows much greater accuracy of movement. Finally, control over the wrist and then the fingers concludes the typical progression in prehension.

Interestingly, as a person ages and movement ability begins to regress, the cephalocaudal and proximodistal processes reverse. The most currently acquired movements of the lower body or periphery will be the first to exhibit signs of regression. The process of movement regression slowly evolves in a "tail to head" and "outside-in" direction. However, as discussed in upcoming chapters, people can slow such regression throughout most of their lives.

The cephalocaudal and proximodistal concepts are useful tools in our efforts to gain a general understanding of motor development. These processes generally apply to human growth and motor development, but there are a few exceptions. For example, in the case of prehension, a child typically acquires control of the fingers before control of the thumb. Some may consider this an exception to the proximodistal rule because the thumb is generally closer to the body's center than are the fingers (though not in the anatomical position).

Differentiation and Integration

Two other terms useful for describing general motor development are *differentiation* and *integration*. **Differentiation** is the progression from gross, immature movement to precise, well-controlled, intentional movement. Walking illustrates differentiation. Whereas early in the development of the walking pattern the leg swing is predominantly under the control of the large muscles surrounding the hip joint, eventually each segment of the leg becomes differentiated. That is, each segment of the leg develops a unique duty or specialization in the walking pattern, and, thus, the stiff, inconsistent gait that characterizes immature walking evolves into a more efficient movement pattern as the segments of the leg begin to function as individual units rather than as a unified block.

Integration is a related, similar change that occurs as an individual's movement ability gradually progresses. As just described, various muscle systems develop or change duties as movement skill improves. As the muscle systems become differentiated, they also "come together to become capable of functioning as a harmonious whole." (Venes, 2017). For example, a young child who is handed a toy may hold on to it with only the hand closest to the toy. If the child is immediately handed a second toy on the same side, she will place the first toy in her other hand for safekeeping, if

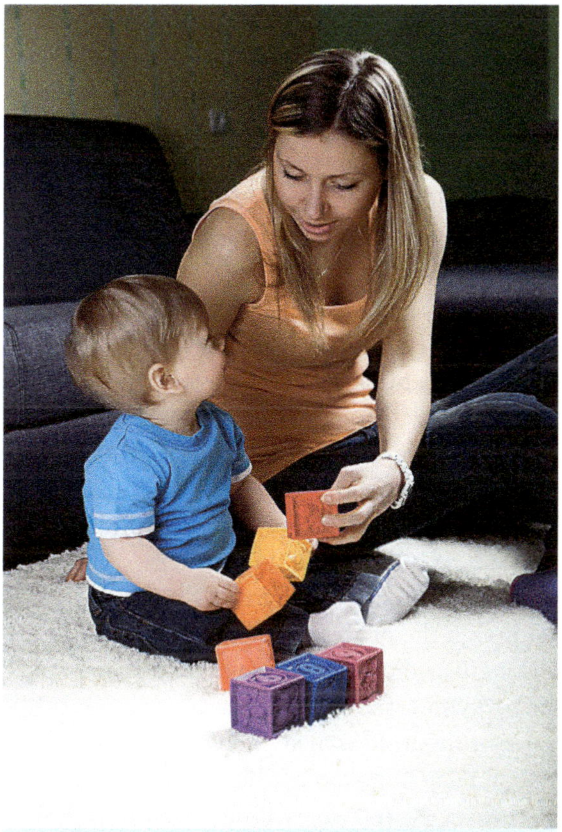

Figure 1.3 A young child receiving a succession of toys may exhibit integration of the hands and arms by acquiring a toy in one hand and storing it in the other. This storage process frees the receiving hand for additional receptions.

she is capable of integrating the use of one hand with the other. The child who is incapable of such integration or coordination will simply discard the first toy in favor of the second one, freeing the receiving hand to take the new toy (see Figure 1.3). This movement may represent the hands' or arms' lack of integrative ability for this particular task.

Like the cephalocaudal and proximodistal processes, differentiation and integration reverse when movement regression occurs later in life. In other words, the improved motor ability acquired as a result of differentiation and integration is gradually lost. The coordination achieved between body parts and the parts' ability to perform highly specific duties during movement activity return to a lower level of functioning. Individuals can allay such regression, however, by maintaining certain habits and attitudes throughout life. Adulthood and movement regression are discussed in Chapter 15.

Gross Movement and Fine Movement

The terms *gross movement* and *fine movement* are generally used to categorize types of movements; however, they can also generally describe motor development. **Gross movements** are primarily controlled by the large muscles or muscle groups. One relatively large muscle group, for example, is in the upper leg. These muscles are integral in producing an array of movements, such as walking, running, and skipping. Such movements, primarily a function of large muscle groups, are considered gross movements.

Fine movements are primarily governed by the small muscles or muscle groups. Many movements performed with the hands are considered fine movements because the smaller muscles of the fingers, hand, and forearm are critical to the production of finger and hand movement. Therefore, such movements as drawing, sewing, typing, or playing a musical instrument are considered fine movements.

Although movements are frequently categorized as gross or fine, very few are completely governed by either the small or the large muscle groups. For example, handwriting is typically considered a fine movement, but, as in most fine movements, there is a gross motor component: the large muscles of the shoulder are necessary for positioning the arm before the more subtle movements that the smaller muscles create can be effective.

A combination of the large and small muscle groups is often responsible for the production of gross movements, as well. Throwing, for example, is considered a gross movement, a logical categorization because upon casual observation the most significant muscle involvement appears to emanate from the shoulder and the legs. A throw, however, is typically initiated with the intention of a certain degree of accuracy. The large muscles of the shoulder and the legs contribute greatly to the desired accuracy, but minute, subtle adjustments of the wrist and fingers are imperative for optimal precision. Therefore, although throwing is considered a gross movement, a fine motor component is critical to perfection in throwing. In fact, the degree of fine motor control is a reasonably accurate indication of movement perfection. An individual may be capable of performing the necessary gross motor aspects of a movement, but the skill may not be honed until the person acquires the fine motor components.

We can use the terms *gross motor* and *fine motor* either to categorize movement or to describe general progression or regression in motor development. As a person matures in a particular movement, the fine components of the skill become increasingly significant; the person becomes increasingly adept at both fine and gross motor aspects of the movement. During movement regression, which often occurs from lack of activity in later life, the reverse occurs: the performer initially loses the ability to incorporate the fine motor aspect of the movement. After extreme regression, even the gross motor components of a movement begin to diminish.

THE PROCESS-PRODUCT CONTROVERSY

As described in the previous section, we can observe and usefully categorize movements by simple and general means. Often, however, movement specialists require more specific measurement. Depending on the objective of their investigation and their philosophical stance, researchers generally use a **product** or a **process approach.**

In the product, or task-oriented, approach to measuring movement, the end result—the outcome—of the movement is the focus. For example, for a child's catching performance, the product-oriented approach analyzes the child's control of the ball.

The process-oriented approach emphasizes the movement itself, with little attention to the movement's outcome. In the example of catching, a researcher who is taking the process-oriented approach focuses on the technique the child uses to attempt to receive the ball accurately rather than the child's amount of ball control. In some cases, the movement product and process are the same. Although the process and product can easily be distinguished in a movement like catching, in many gymnastics-related movements the process involved is also the product. For example, in a movement like a forward roll, the process is the *technique* used to perform the movement. However, in the forward roll, the *technique* can also be the desired product because in competitive situations such movements are judged on their level of perfection.

The process orientation has grown more popular over the years because researchers believe that process, compared with outcome, reveals more information about the underlying factors critical to understanding human movement. However, the product orientation, criticized for its lack of concern for the underlying movement processes, can be valuable in movement research designed to have educational implications. For example, considerable research has attempted to determine the factors that most significantly affect the outcome of certain movement skills. Children's success in movement outcome is widely accepted as an important factor in keeping children interested in and motivated by the activity. Product-oriented research can determine that certain variables negatively or positively affect movement outcome, potentially hampering or enhancing the child's likelihood of further pursuing the movement activity. Although the process approach was derived from dissatisfaction with the product approach, both means of analyzing movement have potential value in motor development.

TERMS FOR AGE PERIODS THROUGHOUT THE LIFESPAN

As depicted in Figure 1.4, specific terms are applied to the various age periods throughout the lifespan. These terms vary slightly from source to source in the ages specified but otherwise are generally accepted for use in the study of human development. These terms are *not* intended to suggest that everyone in a particular age range will possess the same movement characteristics. The terms are helpful in organizing our discussion and communicating statements about persons at a particular time of life. Because these terms are frequently used throughout this book, we now briefly discuss them in the order of their occurrence.

CHILDHOOD

Prenatal

The first age period is the prenatal period, which spans the time from conception to birth. This period was once considered insignificant for human development but is now believed to be one of the most influential periods in the entire lifespan, particularly during the first 8 weeks of the prenatal period, the embryonic period. Movement begins to occur within weeks after conception once synapses are functionally capable of innervating muscle fibers. Prenatal movements includes a vast repertoire of activity with examples including twitching, movements of the head and limbs, kicks, sucking fingers, and grasping the umbilicus to name a few (Adolph & Robinson, 2015). During the embryonic period, the developing human is known as an embryo. At the conclusion of the first 8 weeks of gestation, the fetal period begins. The onset of the fetal period is often described as the point at which the individual has become recognizable as a human being. *Organogenesis*, the formation or development of the vital organs (Cunha et al., 2015), has occurred, although considerable growth and maturation have yet to take place. The individual is referred to as a fetus until the fetal period culminates at birth.

Infancy and Toddlerhood

The first 28 days following birth make up the neonatal period (Venes, 2017). These 28 days are included in the period known as infancy. Therefore, a baby younger than 28 days can be called an infant or, more specifically, a neonate. Infancy lasts from birth throughout the first year of life (Venes, 2017), to the onset of independent walking.

Once children have begun to walk alone, they are considered toddlers. The approximate mean age for this landmark occurrence is 1 year; toddlerhood culminates at 4 years.

Childhood

Somewhat arbitrary limits have been established to distinguish early childhood, which follows toddlerhood, from middle childhood. Early childhood begins at approximately age 4 and ends when the child is 7 years old. Middle childhood ceases at 9 years and precedes preadolescence or late childhood. Late childhood spans approximately 3 years and, as with all the periods discussed here, does not necessarily indicate an abrupt transformation to a new mode of behavior. An individual in the late childhood period is typically quite different in

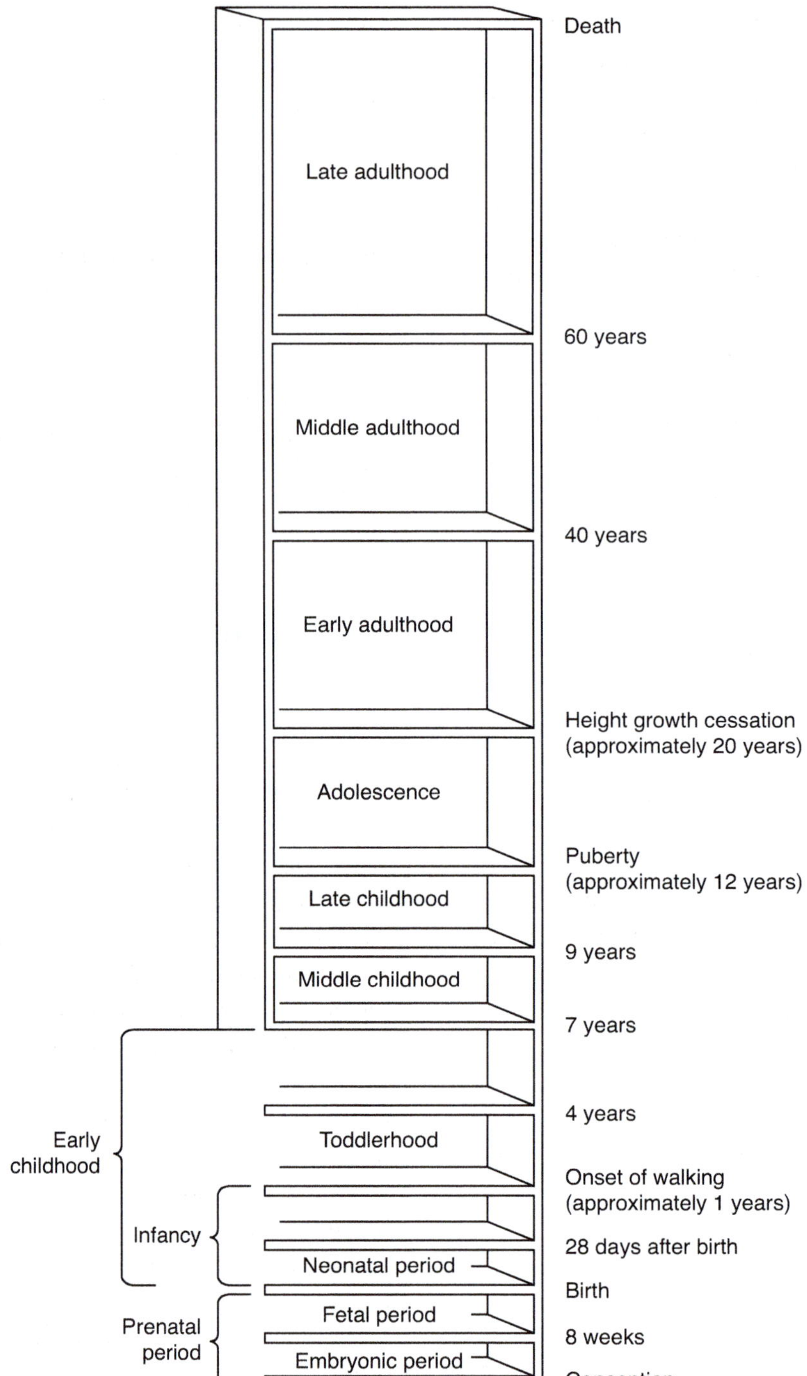

Figure 1.4 Age periods across the lifespan

many respects from a person in middle childhood. However, the transformation is gradual, with the newly emerging behaviors often imperceptible. In fact, the transition from the first to the second year of late childhood may involve behavioral change as profound as that in the transition from the last year of middle childhood to the first year of late childhood.

Though this terminology is somewhat arbitrary, dividing the childhood stage into these age periods helps organize our study, facilitates our communication, and promotes efficiency in examining the entire lifespan.

Adolescence

The next age period, adolescence, is marked by a significant landmark of life. According to most developmentalists, the process known as puberty begins adolescence. *Puberty* is a time of radical hormonal releases that are directly and indirectly associated with many of the behavioral changes accompanying adolescence. This phenomenon is more thoroughly discussed in later chapters dealing with human physical changes and their effects on motor development. This important developmental landmark commonly occurs in girls around age 11 and in boys around age 13. For this reason we should declare separate times of onset for adolescence based on gender. Although the onset of adolescence is signaled by puberty, its termination is sometimes determined by sociocultural factors such as graduating from high school or reaching voting age. Some simply assume that completion of the teen years indicates attainment of adulthood. The most commonly referenced indicator, however, is physical—the achievement of maximal height. According to this measure, adulthood is typically achieved by young women at around age 19; young men usually require two additional years (Malina et al., 2004).

Adulthood

Adulthood typically spans a much greater time than any of the preceding periods of life. In fact, adulthood commonly encompasses more than 60 years. To organize our discussion, we divide this lengthy block of time into early, middle, and late adulthood. Early adulthood begins at age 20 and continues until age 40. Middle adulthood encompasses the subsequent 20 years, ending at age 60. Finally, late adulthood begins at 60 and ends at death. With people gradually living longer lives, the term "old-old" has come into common use to describe adults over the age of 80 years. It is the last age period and precedes death.

STAGES OF DEVELOPMENT

The age periods we discussed in the previous section could all be termed **stages**, or age stages. *Stage* is one of the most frequently encountered words in the study of human development, often used interchangeably with *period*, *phase*, *time*, or even *level*. The term stage implies that there are particular times in the life of a human being that are characterized by certain behaviors. These behaviors are not evident prior to the onset of the stage and may not remain evident in the same form when the stage ends. The premise of the "terrible twos" stage, for example, is that it is common for children at or about 2 years to exhibit disruptive behavior. Furthermore, this behavior was not present before age 2 and will cease or become modified before the child passes into the next stage of behavior.

Do stages such as the terrible twos really exist? There is a major controversy among developmentalists as to whether such abrupt beginnings and ends of behavioral states really occur. The continuity versus discontinuity debate poses the questions: Does life proceed smoothly and continuously from birth to death with occasional "peaks and valleys?" Or is life discontinuous, with relatively abrupt behavior changes occurring throughout?

Most of us find it difficult to accept the possibility that stages do not exist. The popularity of such terms as *terrible twos* and *teenager* has led us to believe that stages of unique behavior are a fact of life. Nevertheless, the existence versus nonexistence of stages remains an ongoing controversy among developmentalists. There is no absolute evidence to substantiate either viewpoint conclusively.

This controversy also prevails in the field of motor development. If stages do exist, certain assumptions may be presumed. For example, a hierarchical, qualitative change must occur in human movement behavior. In other words, one stage of behavior flows into a subsequent, qualitatively different stage. Furthermore, each stage would be distinct from all others but would necessarily possess traits linking it to the preceding stage. The ordering of these behavior states would be constant and universal. That is, a person would not progress through the stages in reverse or mixed order, and everyone would experience these stages. Researchers have tested these and other criteria to determine whether stages are present in motor development. However, the research remains inconclusive regarding the existence or nonexistence of stages in human motor development.

Even though this controversy remains unresolved, it is useful to organize the study of human development into stages. Compartmentalizing aspects of human development into stages or manageable portions of information facilitates our attempts to study and communicate. Therefore, despite a lack of definitive documentation for the existence of stages, we refer throughout this book to stages, phases, or periods. We do not intend, however, to suggest that these stages or periods are absolute times of unique, hierarchical, or universal behaviors.

MODELS OF LIFESPAN MOTOR DEVELOPMENT

Several human motor development experts have proposed models of motor development to explain our movement behavior as we pass from prebirth to death. A model of motor development is simply a visual depiction of a theory, conjecture, or speculation regarding our movement. Like theories, models help us understand complex concepts, and ultimately, testing the model or theory can further enhance our knowledge and understanding of our own behavior. The scope of models has ranged from merely describing the expected movements or changes in movements at various times of life, to attempting to explain why movement develops the way it does. Gallahue, Ozmun, and Goodway (2012) portrayed motor development in an hourglass model: as time passes, the stages or phases of development move up the hourglass. Heredity and environment affect this development and are pictured as grains of sand trickling through the hourglass. The top part of the hourglass corresponds to adult motor development.

Other Models of Motor Development

Another model was created by Newell (1986). Newell based his model on constraints that affect movement throughout life. **Constraints** are factors that limit, contain, or help shape the development of movement. Newell's model emphasized the interactive roles of a person's structure and function, a particular task (for instance, striking a tennis ball with a racket, climbing a mountain), and environmental constraints (such as the speed of the ball, wind conditions, temperature on the mountain, the slope of the mountain). In short, his model is a visual reminder that human structural characteristics (height, weight, length of arms and legs, and so on) and human functional characteristics (such as motivation, past experiences, and confidence) are important to a full understanding of motor development.

It is especially important to note these qualities as they interact with the movement task being performed and the environment in which the task is being performed. Imagine, for example, a young child who is attempting to hit a target by throwing a ball. Clearly, the child's arm length, past experience in throwing, confidence in the task, and motivation to try (to name a few) are all important variables that help to determine the outcome. So, too, are the task constraints. How heavy or light is the ball, and how is it shaped? Is the target moving or stationary, and how big is it? How far away is it? In addition, we cannot forget the environmental constraints. How visible is the target? Is there adequate lighting? How much breeze is present? Are people watching, and, if so, are they cheering supportively or jeering critically?

Newell's model provides a useful reminder of the many constraints that affect our motor development and how the interactions between these constraints are dynamic or constantly changing. Understanding the constraints involved in a particular human skill can be important to professionals for creating viable educational or therapeutic approaches for their students or clients.

In this text, we will focus more closely on a "metaphor" of human motor development proposed by Clark and Metcalfe (2002) than on the other model. According to Clark and Metcalfe, "a metaphor is often the first approximation of a representation and is therefore less formal and more speculative [than a model]" (p. 164). Despite these modest differences, the purposes of a metaphor and a model are similar in that they both seek to explain while offering the possibility of advancing understanding and knowledge. We have chosen Clark and Metcalfe's **Mountain of Motor Development** (see Figure 1.5) as our representation of human motor development because it combines a description of the expected changes in motor development across

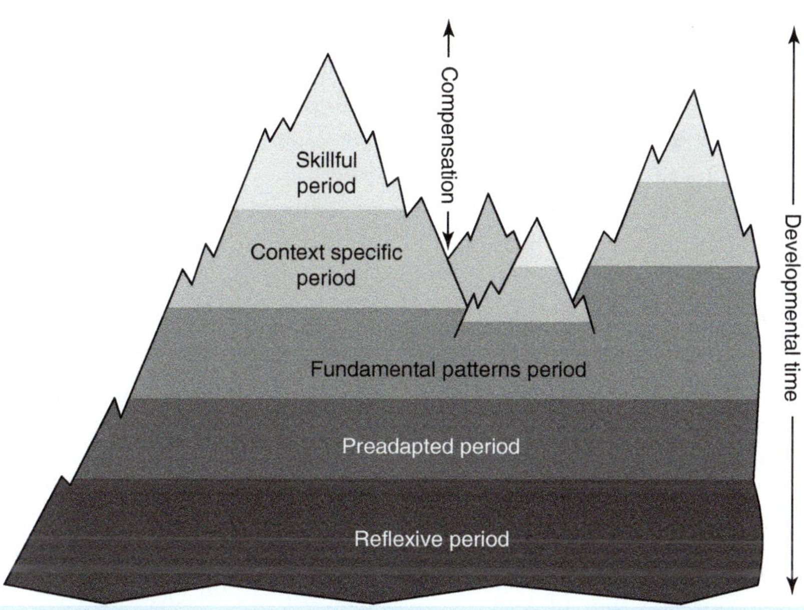

Figure 1.5 Clark and Metcalfe's Mountain of Motor Development

Source: Adapted from Figure 1, in Clark & Metcalfe (2002). Reprinted with permission of SHAPE America, www.shape america.org. The Mountain of Motor Development.

the lifespan with explanations for how these changes may ensue. In addition, Clark and Metcalfe believe the metaphor applies to everyone, including those individuals who experience some form of atypical development.

In this metaphor, motor development is compared to learning to climb a mountain: the process takes years, it is a sequential and cumulative process, and it is strongly affected by the personal skills and traits of the individual climber. It is also a nonlinear process. Like climbing a mountain, human motor development is characterized by progression, sometimes followed by regression, which often yields to further progress later in life. The elevation one achieves on the mountain can be compared to the acquisition of higher levels of motor skill. The image of the mountain also conveys the continuously changing limits or constraints placed on us as we pass through life and suggests that we must adapt to those changes to ascend successfully to the next level. More mature levels of motor development result from a continuous interaction between the climber (the individual), his or her skills, and the mountain (the constantly changing environmental conditions we encounter as we pass through life). Note the similarity between Newell's emphasis on constraints, as described earlier, and the emphasis that Clark and Metcalfe (2002) place on these factors that impact our development (our progression up the mountain). The time (often years) required to learn many human movements is reflected in the arduous ascent up the mountain, as is the sequential and cumulative nature of the acquisition of human movement skills across the lifespan. Arriving at the top of the mountain can be construed as the ultimate attainment of proficiency in movement. In short, the mountain portrays the "lifelong, cumulative, and progressive adaptation" that we see in our own motor development (p. 181).

The ascent up the mountain includes the passage through six periods of human motor development: the reflexive period, the preadapted period, the fundamental patterns period, the context-specific period, the skillful period, and the compensation period. Each period contributes to the acquisition of the skills necessary for the next. And given that development is related to age but is not strictly dependent on the age of the individual, the time spent in each period of development varies for each individual, being highly dependent on factors that govern motor skill acquisition, such as the individual's amount of experience or instruction, the quality of instruction, and inherent individual qualities (such as height, strength, and movement speed). Development is a function of adaptations throughout life as we learn to integrate our personal structural and functional characteristics with our environment (Clark & Metcalfe, 2002).

Clark and Metcalfe explain that the ascent of the developmental mountain begins long before we arrive at its base. Considerable preparation and preplanning precede the ascent of a mountain. This, they say, is analogous to the role of prenatal development (see Chapter 4). Even the behaviors (nutrition, drug use, stress levels, and so on) and genetic structure of the parents and grandparents ultimately affect their offspring. Though these factors do not fully determine a child's future development, they certainly play a role through the interaction of genetic (nature) and environmental (nurture) factors. For some individuals, this initial ascent is gradual and relatively uneventful; others encounter a much more difficult beginning to their climb.

Reflexive Period

The **reflexive period** is the first of Clark and Metcalfe's six periods of the Mountain of Motor Development. This period is characterized by the individual's beginning to learn the ways of the world. It includes the last third (approximately 3 months) of the prenatal state, as well as the initial weeks following birth, even though many infant reflexes will continue to flourish throughout the first year or more of life. During that time, the infant reflexes, described in detail in Chapter 9, are critical to the child's survival (protection, nourishment, and so on) and serve as a necessary stepping stone to both cognitive (intellectual) and motor development.

Reflexes are involuntary responses to stimuli (for example, when you touch a baby's palm, the hand closes). They are subcortical (below the level of the cortex of the brain). In other words, they are a function of reactions in the lower brain centers or even in the central nervous system. In a way, they happen to us rather than we making them happen. Many of the infant reflexes (the crawling reflex and stepping reflex, for instance) experienced during this period are necessary components to the development of future voluntary movements. Although these reflexes initiate and facilitate the infant's interactions with the world, they can impede future development if they endure too long. In typically developing, healthy infants these reactions gradually "disappear" across the first year of life. In children with developmental delays, these reflexes can persevere, slowing the child's rate of development.

Preadapted Period

As the infant reflexes, described above, begin to disappear or become inhibited, voluntary movement emerges. In voluntary movement we produce movement via an impulse from the higher brain centers, including the cerebral cortex. Chapter 10 is dedicated to a comprehensive discussion of these voluntary movements of infancy and early childhood. These movements are often conscious and the product of an intent to move. Voluntary reaching and grasping are an example.

Clark and Metcalfe explain that the term *preadapted* reflects the emergence of motor skill as we overcome early constraints (such as genetic limitations, gravitational forces, and environmental limitations) on our movement and learn to function in our gravity-bound environment. As part of this process, we gradually gain increasingly independent function, including an ability to move somewhat selectively through the space that surrounds us. Through a progression of movement behaviors that often begins with maintaining control of our own head and neck, we gain greater control of the upper body, hips, legs, and feet until we can sit, stand, and walk independently. Similarly, during the **preadapted period**, reaching and grasping behaviors emerge as part of an intricate interaction between our developing postural ability, our arm and hand actions (which themselves are engaged in an evolving interaction), and our visual control.

Clark and Metcalfe state that the preadapted period ends once the child can feed himself and begin walking. Obviously, self-feeding is greatly dependent on emerging eye-hand coordination, just as walking depends on the child's evolving postural control.

Fundamental Patterns Period

The **fundamental patterns period** builds on the skills learned in the previous period. The young child now begins to establish a fundamental framework for future movements. Particularly noteworthy in this period is the establishment of an array of movements that enable a quantity and quality of movement skill in later life. These fundamental movements begin during infancy but will endure throughout childhood. As in all periods of the Mountain of Motor Development, many factors affect the rate and breadth of an individual's acquisition of movement skills. Some children, for example, may have ample opportunity to experience a variety of movements, including the luxury of high-quality instruction and practice. Others may have limited access to such activities, and for these children the ascent up the mountain may be more arduous.

This period of development includes the emergence of fundamental locomotor skills, such as those discussed in much greater detail in Chapter 12, and fundamental object-control skills, such as those detailed in Chapter 13. Throughout this period, with the appropriate interaction of inherent genetic properties and environmental constraints, we typically see locomotion evolving from shaky, assisted first steps in walking, for example, to a controlled, balanced, and effectively functional form of upright locomotion. A few months thereafter, a number of more advanced forms of locomotion, such as running, galloping, hopping, and skipping, will emerge. These fundamental locomotor skills are integral to the level and breadth of movement the individual may one day undertake.

Clark and Metcalfe subdivide the fundamental object-control skills into object projection skills (such as throwing and kicking) and object interception skills (such as catching and trapping). Both types of movement require increasing levels of interaction between the individual and the environment.

This period also includes the development of fine motor manipulation, described in great detail in Chapter 11. Examples of these movements, which are characterized by the dominance of the small muscles or muscle groups of the body, include using scissors, handwriting, drawing, eating (for instance, use of a spoon or chopsticks), and playing certain musical instruments. Achievement is affected by the child's experiences and accomplishments earlier on the mountain, in the reflexive and preadapted periods.

The importance of the fundamental patterns period of development cannot be overstated, as it establishes the basis for future movement endeavors. Movement choices made later in life will hinge on skills developed during this critical time. Whether an individual ultimately decides to engage in exercise, physical games, sports, or even artistic pursuits, such as playing a musical instrument, painting, or sculpting, will be a function of the skill developed at this juncture. Hence, this point of the journey up the mountain can be considered "base camp," to which the performer may want or need to return from time to time to refine skills or develop new ones (Clark & Metcalfe, 2002).

Context-Specific Period

Once the individual has arrived at this "base camp" of movement and has established a solid repertoire of fundamental movement skills, opportunities arise for expanding the movement repertoire into more varied and advanced movements by combining and varying the fundamental movement patterns to adapt to new and different movement situations. Because movement can take on so many new and different forms at this time of life, the Mountain of Motor Development (refer back to Figure 1.5) begins to split into several different peaks, with each leading to an apex of development for different movement skills. Individuals may begin to branch off onto other peaks or even seek to climb several, as they "experiment" with different kinds of movement. They have not yet decided which ones, if any, they will want to pursue on a longer-term basis, or whether they would like to try to develop further skill, even to excel. For example, a middle school-aged child might decide to join the school's track team, only to drop that sport a year or so later in favor of another activity. Perhaps the child will decide not to play sports at all.

Thus, in the illustration of the Mountain of Motor Development, each peak rising from the context-specific period reaches a different height, indicating that the individual might not attain full proficiency in the movement symbolized by that peak. Note, too, that the varying heights of the peaks could indicate the varying degrees of difficulty an individual might encounter in seeking proficiency in one movement versus another. For example, a young adolescent might have developed considerable skill in throwing and catching while being a fast runner. She is experienced enough to have developed skill in these areas but is not experienced enough to know where she might like to apply these skills. She may decide to play baseball, basketball, and soccer. She may continue these activities for several years, thus ascending several different peaks on the mountain, until she decides that one of these sports is her favorite and where she wants to dedicate her time and effort. Thus, she will descend one or more of the peaks as she continues to ascend another.

Skillful Period

According to Clark and Metcalfe (2002), the attainment of the **skillful period** of development requires both experience and practice. This level of motor development is influenced by the previous period, in that a broad-based and well-developed supply of movement skills will assist the individual in the development of higher levels of skill in this period. The skillful period is not achieved by all, and it is intentional, the result of months or years of dedication to achieving proficiency.

The person who achieves this period has developed some degree of proficiency in a specific movement skill or skills. It may be the level of proficiency seen in a middle-school athlete of average or above-average ability. It could also be the level of skill we observe in a classical guitarist who has risen to concert stature. Clearly, only through years of instruction, practice, and dedication can such skill be attained.

Attainment of this higher level of proficiency or expertise is often determined by the individual's ability to perform the movements with less concentration, enabling the performer to attend to strategies or adaptations of the movement during the performance. This ability is ultimately important for success in many higher-level movement endeavors. For example, a jazz pianist playing an intricate piece may want to improvise or adapt the piece spontaneously, based on factors such as how he feels, what the accompanying musicians are playing, or how the audience reacts. In this improvisation, the pianist continues the intricate fingering on the keyboard, but his high level of skill on the piano enables him to ponder many other factors simultaneously, enabling him to adapt or improvise as he plays. The same phenomenon is common in sports, where performers who have developed this level of skill will certainly have a competitive edge. The ability to adapt while performing with increasing levels of confidence or "maximum certainty" (Clark and Metcalfe, 2002, p. 180) across a broad range of movement situations is an indication of the attainment of a higher level of skill.

These high levels of proficiency in movement are attained through the individual's high motivation to excel. This motivation may come from the person's family, the childhood neighborhood, or the individual's cultural background. It may also arise out of geographic factors, peer pressure, or external incentives that ultimately affect the performer's interest level, the amount and quality of coaching or instruction that is available, and the individual's dedication to practice. For example, children who live near a neighborhood swimming pool may develop an interest in taking lessons and, later, swim competitively and receive coaching as members of a team. Thus, they may be more likely to become skillful swimmers than basketball players; they ascend one peak (swimming) instead of another (basketball). A child whose parents are expert martial artists might be more motivated to practice martial arts relative to other activities, having a "built-in" opportunity for instruction right at home, along with parental encouragement. Another factor affecting the ability to become a skillful mover is physiology (e.g., height, weight, strength, endurance, and flexibility).

We can improve some of these factors through physical training. However, regardless of motivation, opportunity, instruction, and practice, some individuals will simply never attain the levels attained by others, or it may take them longer and require more work. Thus, their ascent up the peak may be more arduous. In addition, there is a limit to the number of skills in which any one person can become skillful. Rarely does an individual participate at an elite or professional level in more than one sport. There are many different skills to develop—different peaks to ascend—and most of us will attempt to ascend fewer peaks, and will ascend them to lower levels, than the multisport professional athlete.

In short, the development of skill is the result of gradual, sequential, progressive refinement of movement ability over a relatively long period of time (Clark & Metcalfe, 2002). When a high level of skill is attained, it must be maintained with effort and cannot be maintained forever.

Compensation Period

The sixth and last period on the Mountain of Motor Development involves **compensation.** Compensation is generally considered to be a nullifying of or adaptation to the effects of some type of negative influence. Clark and Metcalfe (2002) note two types of compensation: one arises from injury, and the other arises from the declines that come with aging in middle to late adulthood.

Injury can occur at any time throughout life. The effects of injury can be permanent and can affect an individual's ability to continue climbing to higher plateaus. In fact, injury often results in a regression to a previous period of development or "level" on the mountain. Nevertheless, we humans often overcome the adversity experienced with injury and resume the climb, frequently attaining higher levels than ever. Imagine an elite athlete who suffers a severe knee injury. Initially the athlete ceases all participation in the sport and may undergo surgery, followed by physical therapy. Slowly, she may return to play, achieve her former skill level, and even surpass that level—achieving full and successful compensation. However, the injury may be so severe that she cannot regain her former ability or even resume playing at all.

As will be discussed in Chapter 15, much can be done to overcome the typical declines in movement and physical performance (such as slowing speed and reductions in strength, endurance, and flexibility) that accompany aging. In fact, growing older becomes a much more optimistic proposition when we learn the beneficial effects of exercise, practice, and education on the aging process and the associated physiological and motor declines associated with that time of life. Nevertheless, some decline with aging appears to be inevitable. We can, however, adapt to these declines, and often we can overcome them for a period of time. Just as with injury in earlier periods of life, we can adapt to the changes that come with aging, redirect our efforts, and, often, regain a very functional status.

In short, our motor development during later adulthood does not have to be a slow and systematic decline. It can be replete with periods of progression. Imagine an older adult who has allowed years to pass without participating in any form of vigorous activity. Following a less than positive medical checkup, he decides to begin exercising by walking. After a period of time he decides to start jogging. As described throughout this book, that physical activity will likely yield widespread benefits physically, socially, emotionally, and even intellectually. After gaining initial improvements in fitness, the jogger might decide to stop jogging and take up softball with a local league for older adults. Thus, he resumed his climb up one peak, came back down, and started up another—a common and expected pattern that is accounted for by the Mountain of Motor Development.

THE HISTORY OF THE FIELD OF MOTOR DEVELOPMENT

Compared to other areas of human development, few research studies have focused exclusively on motor development in the last few decades. According to Adolph and Robinson (2015), this was not the case in the early part of last century when many of the early developmentalists like Myrtle McGraw, Arnold Gesell, and Mary Shirley emphasized motor development in their research. The apparent decline in interest in motor development may be related to the heavy reliance early investigators placed on building developmental norms or milestones. These descriptions of what movements to expect at what times of life are important, but fell short of explaining the processes related to why and how these changes unfolded. For example, though motor developmentalists have long been aware of the importance of bodily change on motor development, little attention was initially paid to the role of environmental impacts. In addition, at about this same time, curiosity in the area of cognitive development began to thrive and possibly attracted some researchers away from motor development. Motor development has regained some popularity in recent years, but still pales in comparison to most other areas of developmental research (e.g., cognitive, social, perceptual). This is somewhat perplexing in that motor development is a vast and influential domain of study that offers the advantage of being directly observable; we can see it. Thus it holds the potential of being a model for interpreting other domains of behavior (Adolph & Robinson, 2015) while having profound effects on them. Those interactions will be more closely examined in later chapters (e.g., 2, 3, and 6), especially those relating to cognitive, social, and physiological change.

Many brief histories of motor development have been published over the years (Clark & Whitall, 1989; Keogh, 1977; Roberton, 1988, 1989; Smoll, 1982; Thelen, 1987; Thomas & Thomas, 1984). Keogh (1977) and Thomas and Thomas (1984) suggested that the study of motor development began around 1920 to 1930 when physicians created scales to note the developmental progress of infants. Roberton (1988, 1989) indicated a much earlier starting point. She believes the study of motor development may have begun with the work of the "baby biographers" of the late 1800s through the early 1900s. Included in this group were Darwin (1877) and Shinn (1900), who wrote "A Biographical Sketch of an Infant" and *The Biography of a Baby*, respectively. Clark and Whitall (1989) cited an even earlier starting point. They agreed that Darwin and Shinn were influential but felt that Tiedemann's (1787, as cited by Borstelmann, 1983) observations of his son's first 2.5 years marked the beginning of what Clark and Whitall (1989) and Whitall (2009) named the **precursor period** of the field of motor development, the first of five historical periods of motor development research. Table 1.3 summarizes the historical periods of the study of motor development.

Clearly, the history of motor development did not cease in the year 2000 at the end of the **dynamic systems period**. However, Whitall (2009) indicates that although we are undergoing a sixth period in the history of motor development, we are not yet ready to characterize it. Any attempt to do so too early would likely lead to considerable disagreement among contemporary experts. One notable

Table 1.3 Clark and Whitall's periods in the history of the field of motor development

Period	Description
1787–1928 Precursor Period	Descriptive observation was established as a method for studying human development. The most significant influence was Darwin's (1877) "A Biographical Sketch of an Infant." Early researchers were most interested in the function of the mind, though their research benefited the motor developmentalists who followed.
1928–1946 Maturational Period	Motor development as a primary interest began to emerge, and the maturational philosophy predominated. This philosophy held that the biological processes were the main influence shaping human development. Work by Gesell (1928) and McGraw (1935) yielded valuable product- and process-oriented information concerning human movement. Bayley's scales of motor development, still used today, were a product of this period. These norm-referenced scales charted motor behavior across the first 3 years of life.
1946–1970 Normative/ Descriptive Period	In the mid-1940s, interest in motor development became "dormant" (Keogh, 1977). In the early 1960s, however, a revival began. This revival was led by physical educators who were interested in children's movement and developed norm-referenced standardized tests for measuring motor performance. Kephart's publication of *The Slow Learner in the Classroom* (1960) was also an influence. Kephart maintained that certain movement activities enhanced academic performance. Though never well supported by the research, Kephart's theory still influences professional practice today.
1970–1982 Process-Oriented Period	This period is characterized by a return to studying the processes underlying motor development rather than simply describing change. Interest grew in information-processing theory, which suggested that the human mind functions much like a computer. This theory may have contributed to many psychologists' return to the study of motor development.
1982–2000 Dynamic Systems Period	**Dynamic systems theory**, or perspective, deviated substantially from information-processing theory, positing that developmental systems are complex, coordinated, and self-organizing. Motor development is thought to be impacted by constraints that are internal (e.g., the mover's limb length), external (e.g., environmental, such as the slope or condition of a walking surface), and task-related. Of course, like the motor skill in question, these constraints are dynamic—constantly changing in relationship to one another. This interaction facilitates the emergence of a relatively stable movement skill, even though the movement pattern was never "coded" in the central nervous system. In dynamic systems perspective, reduced emphasis is placed on more traditional elements (such as the performer's age or genetics) and increased value is placed on environmental interaction.

Sources: Clark & Whitall (1989), Whitall (2009).

characteristic of the current historical period is the rapid advance of state-of-the-art, noninvasive technology that researchers can use in investigating developmental change, especially brain and central nervous system physiology during movement performance. Examples of technological methods that could be employed for this purpose include magnetic resonance imaging (MRI), electroencephalography (EEG), functional magnetic resonance imaging (fMRI), magnetoencephalography (MEG), and transcranial magnetic stimulation (TMS). Through a variety of techniques, all of these technologies enable us to examine and map brain activity for the purposes of research and medical diagnosis (Whitall, 2009).

SUMMARY

- Motor development is the study of changes in human movement over the lifespan, the processes underlying these changes, and the factors affecting them. It is an important area of study because it helps us understand all aspects of human development. Practical applications from this field of study include detection of atypical movement, which facilitates early intervention and remediation, educationally and therapeutically. Knowledge of motor development permits the creation of valid, efficient, and science-based programs for teaching movement skills and the development of effective interventions or rehabilitative strategies for people of all ages.

- Human development is often categorized into motor, cognitive, affective, and physical domains. The motor domain refers to human movement. The cognitive domain refers to intellectual change; the affective domain refers to socioemotional change. The physical domain refers to actual bodily changes, such as height or weight. All domains are in constant interaction. Motor development (including physical development) strongly influences—and is strongly influenced by—cognitive and affective development. Human development encompasses the progressions and regressions that occur within human beings as they age.
- Developmental change is characterized by six components or elements. It is qualitative, sequential, cumulative, directional, multifactorial, and individual. Understanding these elements is essential to attaining a developmental perspective: looking at current behaviors with an interest in what preceded them and what will follow and understanding that development is "age related but not completely age determined" (Motor Development Task Force, 1995, p. 5).
- Maturation is a specific aspect of development involving the qualitative, functional changes that occur with aging. Growth, another aspect of development, concerns increases in physical size—that is, quantitative, structural increases that occur with aging.
- The terms *cephalocaudal*, *proximodistal*, *differentiation*, and *integration* describe general motor development trends. In their development all individuals follow the general progression that these terms describe, but they vary considerably in their rates of change.
- The terms *gross motor* and *fine motor* refer to movements created by the large and small muscle groups, respectively. These terms help us generally categorize movements and describe movement progressions and regressions throughout the lifespan.
- We use process- and product-oriented approaches to evaluate or measure movement performances. The process approach emphasizes the technique of the movement; the product approach examines the outcome or end product of the movement.
- An age-period approach can facilitate the study of motor development throughout the lifespan. We use common terms to refer to various age periods, such as infancy, toddlerhood, and early adulthood. This approach is particularly useful, but we do not suggest that these age periods are uniformly characterized by specific behavioral traits of the individuals included within the periods.
- Many models of human motor development have been created over the years; for example, Newell's (1986) model is based on the constraints that affect movement throughout life. The Mountain of Motor Development, devised by Clark and Metcalfe (2002), is a model-like metaphor defining six periods of developmental change: the reflexive period, the preadapted period, the fundamental patterns period, the context-specific period, the skillful period, and the compensation period. This metaphor can help us understand the process of motor development and the factors that affect it as individuals pass through life.

- The history of the study of motor development, according to Clark and Whitall (1989), can be divided into five periods: the precursor period, 1787 to 1928; the maturational period, 1928 to 1946; the normative/descriptive period, 1946 to 1970; the process-oriented period, 1970 to 1982; and the dynamic systems period, 1982 to 2000. The field is now in its sixth historical period. Although this period is yet to be characterized, one notable characteristic is the advance of noninvasive technology to investigate developmental change.

key concept review

cephalocaudal
compensation period
constraints
context-specific period
development
developmental perspective
developmentally appropriate
differentiation
dynamic systems period
dynamic systems theory
fine movement
fundamental patterns period
gross movement
growth
human motor development
integration
maturation
maturational period
Mountain of Motor Development
normative/descriptive period
preadapted period
precursor period
process approach
process-oriented period
product approach
proximodistal
psychomotor
reflexive period
skillful period
stage

questions for reflection

1. Why is our knowledge of motor development important? Give at least three specific examples of how this information can be practically employed.
2. What do we mean by *developmentally appropriate?* What are the two dimensions of the term as discussed in this chapter? Can you define each?
3. What does it mean to have a developmental perspective? Why is that important?
4. List and describe the six components of developmental change.
5. Explain the terms *differentiation* and *integration*. provide an example of each.
6. Some controversy exists as to whether stages really exist in motor development. Take a stand. What do you think? Provide some rationale for your position.
7. What is the Mountain of Motor Development and how is it relevant to the study of human motor development?
8. According to Clark and Whitall, what are the historical periods in the field of motor development and what characterized each?

online resources

American Academy of Pediatrics, www.aap.org
American College of Sports Medicine, www.acsm.org
Centers for Disease Control and Prevention, www.cdc.gov
Centers for Disease Control and Prevention, Morbidity and Mortality Weekly report, www.cdc.gov/mmwr/mmwr_wk.html
National Association for the Education of Young Children, www.naeyc.org/
North American Society for the Psychology of Sport and Physical Activity, www.naspspa.com
Society of Health and Physical Educators (SHAPE), www.shapeamerica.org

REFERENCES

Adolph, K.E., & Robinson, S.R. (2015). Motor development. In R. M. Lerner (Ed.), *Handbook of child psychology and developmental science*, vol. 2, 7th ed. New York: Wiley.

Bloom, B. S. (1956). *Taxonomy of educational objectives: Handbook I. Cognitive domain*. New York: McKay.

Borstelmann, L. J. (1983). Children before psychology. In W. Kessen (Ed.), *Handbook of child psychology*. Vol. 1: *History, theory, and methods*. 4th ed. New York: Wiley.

Bredekamp, S., & Copple, C. (1997). *Developmentally appropriate practice in early childhood programs*. Rev. ed. Washington, DC: National Association for the Education of Young Children.

Clark, J. E., & Metcalfe, J. S. (2002). The mountain of motor development: A metaphor. In J. E. Clark & J. Humphrey (Eds.), *Motor development: Research and reviews*. Reston, VA: NASPE Publications.

Clark, J. E., & Whitall, J. (1989). What is motor development?: The lessons of history. *Quest*, *41*, 183–202.

Cunha, G., Overland, M., Li, Y., Cao, M., Shen, J., et al. (2015). Methods of studying human organogenesis. *Differentiation*, *91*, 10–14.

Darwin, C. (1877). A biographical sketch of an infant. *Mind*, *2*, 285–294.

Dye, F. J. (2017). *Dictionary of stem cells, regenerative medicine and translational medicine*. Hoboken, NJ: Wiley Blackwell.

Gallahue, D. L., Ozmun, J. C., & Goodway, J. (2012). *Understanding motor development*. 7th ed. New York: McGraw-Hill.

Gesell, A. (1928). *Infancy and human growth*. New York: Macmillan.

Keogh, J. F. (1977). The study of movement skill development. *Quest*, *28*, 76–88.

Kephart, N. C. (1960). *The slow learner in the classroom*. Columbus, OH: Merrill.

Liu, T., Hamilton, M., Davis, L., & ElGarhy, S. (2014). Gross motor development by children with Autism Spectrum Disorder and typi ally developing children on TGMD-2. *Child and Adolescent Behavior*, 2, dx.doi.org/10.4172/jacalb.1000123.

MacDonald, M., Lord, C., & Ulrich, D. (2014). Motor skills and calibrated autism severity in young children with autism spectrum disorder. *Adapted Physical Activity Quarterly*, *31*, 95–105.

Malina, R. M., Bouchard, C., & Bar-Or, O. (2004). *Growth, maturation, and physical activity*. 2nd ed. Champaign, IL: Human Kinetics.

McGraw, M. (1935). *Growth: A study of Johnny and Jimmy*. New York: Appleton-Century-Crofts.

Motor Development Task Force (1995). *Looking at physical education from a developmental perspective: A guide to teaching*. Reston, VA: National Association for Sports and Physical Education.

NAEYC (National Association for the Education of Young Children) (2009). *Developmentally appropriate practice in early childhood programs serving children from birth through age 8: Position statement, 1–32*. Retrieved from www.naeyc.org/files/naeyc/file/positions/PSDAP.pdf.

Newell, K. M. (1986). Constraints on the development of coordination. In M. G. Wade & H. T. A. Whiting (Eds.), *Motor development in children: Aspects of coordination and control* (pp. 341–361). Amsterdam: Nijhoff.

Roberton, M. A. (1988). The weaver's loom: A developmental metaphor. In J. E. Clark & J. H. Humphrey (Eds.), *Advances in motor development research 2*. New York: AMS Press.

Roberton, M. A. (1989). Motor development: Recognizing our roots, charting our future. *Quest*, *41*, 213–223.

Shinn, M. (1900). *The biography of a baby*. Boston: Houghton Mifflin.

Smoll, F. L. (1982). Developmental kinesiology: Toward a subdiscipline focusing on motor development. In J. S. Kelso & J. E. Clark (Eds.), *The development of movement control and coordination*. New York: Wiley.

Thelen, E. (1987). The role of motor development in developmental psychology: A view of the past and an agenda for the future. In N. Eisenberg (Ed.), *Contemporary topics in developmental psychology*. New York: Wiley.

Thomas, J. R., & Thomas, K. (1984). Planning kiddie research: Little kids but big problems. In J. R. Thomas (Ed.), *Motor development during childhood and adolescence*. Minneapolis, MN: Burgess.

Venes, D. (Ed.) (2017). *Taber's cyclopedic medical dictionary*. Philadelphia, PA: F.A. Davis.

Whitall, J. (2009). Research on children: New approaches to answer old questions, but is this sufficient? *Quest*, *61*, 93–107.

2 COGNITIVE AND MOTOR DEVELOPMENT

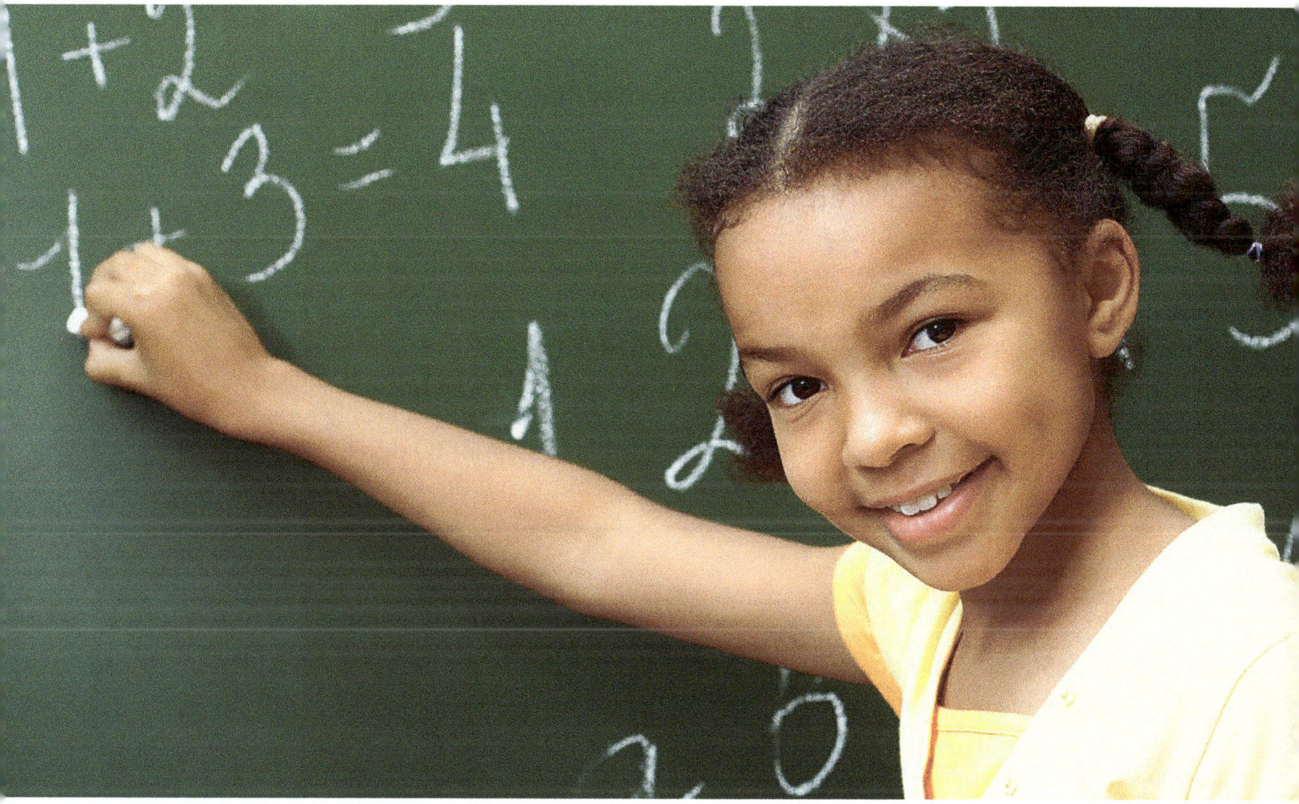

Chapter Objectives

From the information presented in this chapter, you will be able to

- Explain the work of Jean Piaget on cognitive development
- Describe Piaget's theory of cognitive development and its relationship to motor development
- Describe Piaget's sensorimotor stage and related motor development
- Describe Piaget's preoperations stage and related motor development
- Describe cognitive and motor development in later childhood and adolescence
- Describe Piaget's concrete operational stage and related motor development
- Describe Piaget's formal operational stage and related motor development
- Describe postformal operations and cognitive development in adulthood
- Explain the relationship between movement skill/expertise and cognitive development
- Explain the relationship between physical activity and cognitive development

As mentioned in Chapter 1, the four domains of human development are the affective, cognitive, motor, and physical. This system of categorizing human behavior into domains evolved because it is useful for organizing and simplifying the study of human development. Although these domains of development are usually studied as individual units, we must remember that they are in constant interaction with one another (refer back to Figure 1.2). Everything we do in the motor domain is affected by our emotions, social interactions, and cognitive development. Furthermore, all of our behavior in the affective and cognitive domains is strongly influenced by our motor behavior (see Figure 2.1). Can our emotional state affect weight gain? Does our physical state (percent body fat, muscle mass) affect self-esteem? Of course! All domains affect all others.

One example of the types of interrelationships referred to here is the work of Piek, Dawson, Smith, and Gasson (2008). These researchers examined the connection between early movement ability, movement ability in later childhood, and intellectual development in later childhood. Specifically, they sought to determine whether movement ability during the first four years of life predicts motor and cognitive abilities later in childhood. To understand this relationship, the researchers studied 33 boys and girls who had been tested for intellectual, fine motor, and gross motor ability from 4 months to 4 years of age. They were assessed again from 6 to just over 11 years of age. Interestingly, but not surprisingly, the children's social economic status was found to affect their intellectual status and fine motor performance, with intellectual status being the more profoundly related. However, gross motor performance was not found to be predicted by social economic status. In addition, though early fine motor performance was not found to hold a strong relationship with later cognitive development, gross motor performance was. In fact, Piek and colleagues stated that early gross movement ability may be a better predictor of later cognitive development than early fine movement or intellectual ability itself. Gross movement was specifically found to impact several areas of IQ development, working memory, and the speed at which information is processed intellectually.

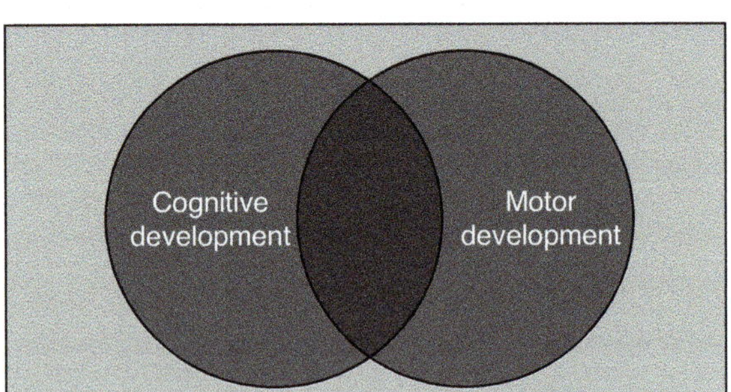

Figure 2.1 Cognitive and motor development interact continually throughout the lifespan as they reciprocally inhibit or facilitate each other

Similarly, in a paper on developmental coordination disorder (DCD), Deng, Li, Ding, and associates (2014) sought to understand the relationship between DCD and the associated cognitive impairments. According to these authors, DCD is characterized by impaired motor coordination that interferes with academic achievement and general activities of daily living. For a diagnosis of DCD, no other medical condition (e.g., muscular dystrophy, cerebral palsy) can be attributed to causation. The condition is much more common in boys than girls and has been noted in approximately 2 percent to nearly 19 percent of school children in various countries throughout the world. Research suggests that DCD may be related to central nervous system dysfunctions, but the disorder—particularly the motor deficits associated with the condition—can be somewhat ameliorated by therapeutic interventions. Deng and associates (2014) believe that DCD is an example of the "dynamic interplay between sensorimotor and cognition systems" (p. 210).

Imamizu (2015) specifically examined the changes in brain networks caused by motor and cognitive learning. In a sophisticated resting state functional magnetic resonance image of the brain, Imamizu observed adaptations of brain connections, networking, and spontaneous activity related to motor skill learning. He also found that motor learning affected both neural firing sequences and the brain's ability to encode information for use in future activities. Imamizu further indicated that these "intrinsic architectural" changes in the brain can lead to positive behavioral and cognitive changes, with implications for the development of movement programs—for example, the design of physical rehabilitation programs. In general, Imamizu believed that experience, including movement activities, affects large-scale brain networks and that a full understanding of this relationship is useful for devising specific tasks that will most positively affect the brain's structure and function.

Thus, based on the work of Piek and associates (2008), Deng's team of researchers (2014), and the work of Imamizu (2015), a strong relationship exists between motor skill learning and performance and cognitive function. Knowledge of this important relationship is integral to our complete understanding of human development. It can be influential in the establishment of intervention strategies to enhance people's gross motor or intellectual performance.

Like the work of Piek and associates, this chapter examines several important specific interrelationships between the cognitive and motor domains. *Cognitive* refers to our reasoning, our intellect, our thought processes, or simply the acquisition of knowledge. How does our gradually changing motor ability affect our cognitive development? How does our evolving cognitive development affect our motor development? What are some significant areas of integration?

JEAN PIAGET'S THEORY OF COGNITIVE DEVELOPMENT

Unquestionably, developmentalists have paid more attention to cognitive development than to any other domain of human behavior. And no one wrote more about cognitive development than the most famous developmentalist, Jean Piaget. Piaget is generally accepted as one of the most innovative, accurate, informative, and prolific developmentalists (Sigelman & Rider, 2018). He wrote more than 40 internationally acclaimed books and was labeled a genius by Albert Einstein.

Piaget's interest in human intellectual development emerged after years of study in related fields of interest. When he was 10 years old, he published his first biology-oriented article, and his interest in biology gradually increased throughout his childhood, adolescence, and early adulthood.

Eventually, Piaget became interested in examining how we "know"—that is, the process of thinking. According to Piaget, this process is a critical function in life that enables us to adapt to our environment. Of particular interest to Piaget were children's incorrect responses to questions or problem-solving situations. By observing these responses, Piaget found that children demonstrated varying impressions of the world relative to one another and to adults. This system of inquiry evolved into what is now known as Piaget's **clinical method**, a system of collecting data in question-and-answer sessions to understand more fully the process of thinking (Newman & Newman, 2018). Piaget questioned children and carefully noted their mode of approaching problems and issues. By including children from several age groups in his interviews, Piaget was able to categorize similar behaviors into the four stages of development that constitute his famous theory of cognitive development.

Between 1925 and 1931, Piaget's wife gave birth to three children. The births were a particularly important impetus for Piaget to understand the changing cognitive processes of children. During those years, he developed the basis of what is still the most widely accepted theory of cognitive development. In fact, Piaget's theory of cognitive development is the most detailed, systematic interpretation of any aspect of human development. This theory, although largely based on Piaget's observations of his own children rather than on formal scientific inquiry, provides a guideline for understanding the changing thought process throughout childhood and adolescence. Furthermore, this theory has given cognitive developmentalists a specific basis from which to begin their own investigations. Because cognitive and motor development constantly interact, an awareness of Piaget's theory is critical to a thorough understanding of motor development. Cognitive development strongly depends on the movement capabilities the individual has acquired; similarly, motor development depends on intellectual capabilities. This interactive process is apparent in Piaget's theory.

The Process of Adaptation

According to Piaget, cognitive development occurs through a process he called adaptation (see Table 2.1). **Adaptation** is adjusting to the demands of the environment and the intellectualization of that adjustment through two complementary acts, assimilation and accommodation. **Assimilation** is a process by which children attempt to interpret new experiences based on their present interpretation of the world (Shaffer & Kipp, 2014). This process of perceiving experiences relative to a past mode of thinking is exemplified by an infant who, with one hand, attempts to grasp a ball that is slightly too large for the child's small hand (Figure 2.2). The one-handed "plan" to grasp the ball is in the child's cognitive repertoire as a result of previous experiences with rattles or other smaller objects. Thus, the infant tries to incorporate the ball, the new experience, into the cognitive repertoire by using an already established mode of thinking.

In **accommodation**, the second facet of adaptation, the individual attempts to adjust

Table 2.1 Components of the process of adaptation

Component	Process
Assimilation	Children attempt to interpret new experiences based on their present interpretation of the world.
Accommodation	Children attempt to adjust existing thought structures to account for, or accommodate, new experiences.

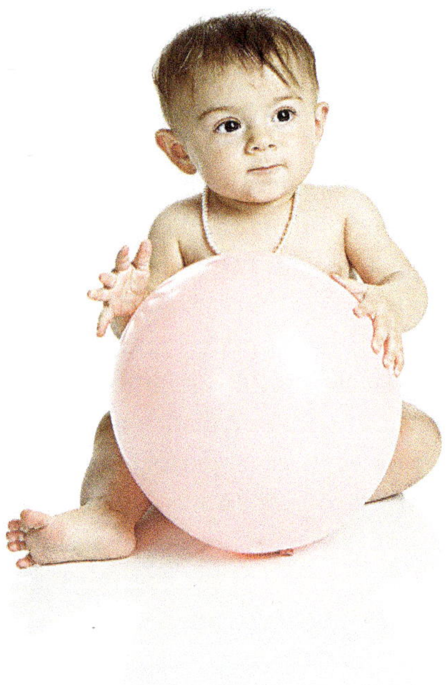

Figure 2.2 An example of assimilation. The infant is trying to grasp a large ball. This new experience is being incorporated into the child's cognitive repertoire by using an existing mode of thinking.

existing thought structures to account for, or accommodate, new experiences. In the case of the infant trying to obtain the large ball, accommodation could occur when the child recognizes that the ball is larger than the more familiar rattle. The infant then modifies the approach to obtaining the ball by either adapting the one-handed grasp or by using the other hand to help. In some way, the child makes an adjustment to accommodate the ball. A new experience or environmental event has altered the child's behavior and understanding or interpretation of the event.

According to Piaget, assimilation and accommodation always work together. The concept of assimilation suggests that an individual always experiences new events according to what is already known; the concept of accommodation implies that the environment always challenges the individual to modify actions relative to the specific situation (Sigelman & Rider, 2018). As the example of the infant trying to grasp a large ball illustrates, both components of adaptation are highly dependent on the individual's movement, especially during Piaget's first stage of cognitive development, the sensorimotor stage. Adaptation and its two facets, assimilation and accommodation, are basic to Piaget's theory of cognitive development and reflect the importance he placed on the role of the environment in human development.

Piaget's Stages of Cognitive Development

The four major stages in Piaget's theory of cognitive development are the sensorimotor, preoperational, concrete operational, and formal operational stages (see Table 2.2). The ages Piaget cited for each stage are only guidelines. Individual variation is expected, although it is believed that most children approximate the course of development Piaget suggested. Furthermore, not everyone achieves

Table 2.2 Major stages of Piaget's theory of cognitive development and approximate ages or periods of occurrence

Stage	Age/period of occurrence
Sensorimotor	Birth to 2 years
Preoperational	2 to 7 years
Concrete operational	7 to 11 years
Formal operational	Early to mid-adolescence (11 to 12 years)

Piaget's highest level of cognitive development, formal thought. However, children do follow the same sequence through the stages, regardless of the level of cognitive ability they eventually attain. In other words, the stages are always experienced in the same order, and no stage is ever skipped, although the rate of progress and degree of completion vary with each child. Each stage is increasingly more complex than its predecessor and builds on the cognitive abilities gained in the previous stage.

Sensorimotor Stage and Motor Development

The interaction between motor and cognitive development, although a lifelong process, is particularly evident during a child's first two years. This is acknowledged in Piaget's theory and his decision to call the first stage of cognitive development sensorimotor. In the **sensorimotor stage**, intelligence develops as a result of movement actions and their consequences. According to Piaget, movement is critical to the thought process.

The sensorimotor stage, which typically lasts throughout the first 24 months of life, is the time of creating a foundation for all subsequent understanding that hinges on a child's ability to perform bodily movement. An infant's experience of being able to grasp and hold with certainty simultaneously influences the development of cognition. In the sensorimotor

Table 2.3 Substages of the sensorimotor stage of development and their approximate ages of occurrence

Substage	Age of occurrence
Exercise of reflexes	Birth to 1 month
Primary circular reactions	1 to 4 months
Secondary circular reactions	4 to 8 months
Secondary schemata	8 to 12 months
Tertiary circular reactions	12 to 18 months
Invention of new means through mental combinations	18 to 24 months

stage, knowing and thinking emerge as a result of action that occurs via bodily movement. Of particular importance in this stage are the environment and motor development. The sensorimotor stage is subdivided into six substages (see Table 2.3), making this stage the most detailed of Piaget's four major stages.

Exercise of reflexes. The first substage lasts from birth through the first month of life. This substage is characterized by the earliest form of movement behavior: the reflexes and their repetition (Figure 2.3), which

- enable the child to explore the world, forming the foundation for cognitive understanding;

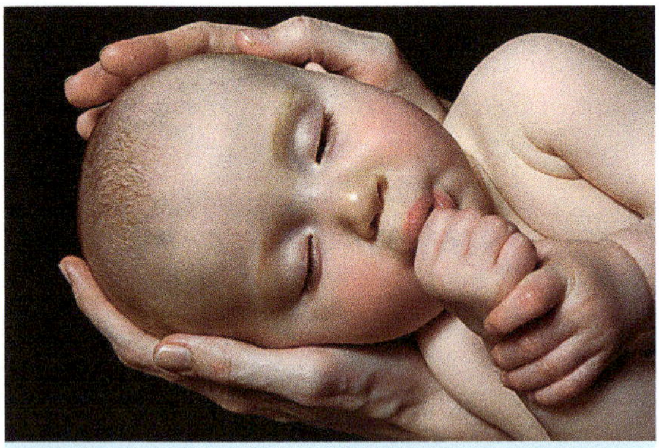

Figure 2.3 The first substage of Piaget's sensorimotor stage of development, exercise of reflexes, is characterized by the repetition of reflexive movements such as sucking

- are the impetus for all future motor and intellectual development;
- help the infant adapt and modify behaviors through experience to form completely new behaviors.

Primary circular reactions. The second sensorimotor substage, lasting from the end of the first month until approximately 4 months, is characterized by the onset of increased voluntary movement, which enables the child:

- to create certain movement behaviors consciously and gradually more capably;
- to repeat desired acts consciously;
- to realize that certain stimuli allow the child to repeat an activity voluntarily when the same stimuli are presented in the future;
- to engage in repeated actions, known as circular reactions, that are considered primary because they occur close to the infant;
- to improve cognitive abilities to facilitate movements such as reaching and grasping.

In this substage, movement plays an integral role in the development of thought processes.

Secondary circular reactions. The third substage, lasting from about 4 to 8 months of age, is a continuation of the primary circular reactions stage but incorporates more enduring behaviors: movement behavior is intended to make an event lasting (see Figure 2.4). The infant repeats the primary circular reactions. Examples of behaviors common in this substage are persistent shaking of a rattle and banging of a toy to make noise. Such behavior familiarizes the infant with the environment and its forces.

Also in this substage:

- The child experiences a gradually expanding interaction with the environment.
- The child learns to combine two or more movement forms to enable even more

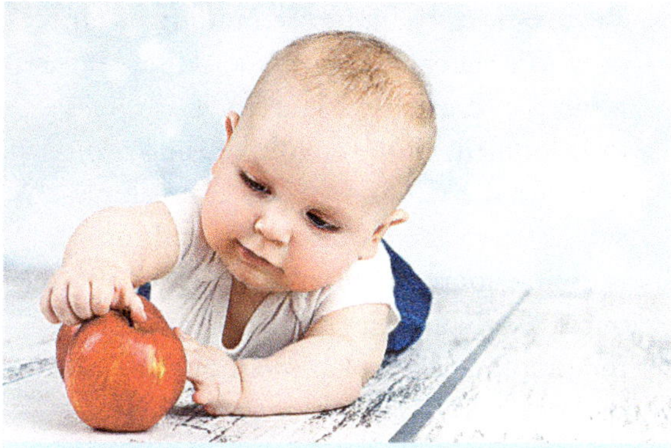

Figure 2.4 Secondary circular reactions is Piaget's third substage of the sensorimotor stage of cognitive development. The infant's interaction with the environment gradually expands to enable more thorough investigation of the environment.

interaction with and manipulation of the environment (e.g., seeing a rattle and wanting to shake it).

- The infant learns, via his or her own movement and the resulting interaction with the environment, the stimuli and actions necessary to initiate certain behaviors at certain times.
- Once the child can integrate vision, hearing, grasping, and certain movement behaviors, imitation—a major characteristic of secondary circular reactions—becomes possible.
- The infant still has not yet developed a sense of permanence: objects "exist" only as long as they are viewed. In the infant's understanding, a rattle that is removed from view no longer exists.
- Imitation is performed only as long as the object of imitation is immediately present.

Secondary schemata. From approximately 8 to 12 months, the fourth substage of the sensorimotor stage takes place. Movement continues to play a critical role in the continuing development of the intellect. Past modes of movement, designed to interact with the environment, are now applied to new situations, enabling many new behaviors to emerge. Other characteristics of this substage include:

- New behaviors are facilitated by increasing movement capabilities (such as crawling and creeping), which allow greater exploration and more contact with new objects and situations.
- Repetition of experimentation increases, and trial-and-error exploration continues.
- The child develops an ability to anticipate actions or situations.
- The child learns to predict potential occurrences beyond the immediate activity. This constitutes the actual onset of intellectual reasoning, according to Piaget.
- The child learns to pair objects with their related activities and act on the basis of that connection. For example, when a ball is rolled to an infant 8 to 12 months old, the child can return it. More importantly, children in this substage prepare for their turn at receiving the ball as they realize it will again be returned to them.

Tertiary circular reactions. The fifth substage of Piaget's sensorimotor stage, which occurs in the first half of the second year, is characterized by the discovery through active experimentation of new ways to produce desired results. In fact, active experimentation now consumes a major portion of the infant's time. Other characteristics of this substage include the following:

- The results of experimentation are incorporated into existing intellectual frameworks to create entirely new knowledge.
- Reasoning becomes fairly well developed in this substage and necessary for the cyclical repetition of activities.
- The infant's interest in the surrounding environment intensifies, and the child makes constant attempts to understand it.

- The sensory modalities, especially vision, become extremely important in furnishing environmental information.
- The child realizes that the discovery of a new object and the actual use of that object are separate entities. For example, a child recognizes that a ball can be thrown but knows she does not have to toss the ball at that time; she can delay the act until later, and the ball will not lose its property of being able to be thrown.
- The child becomes capable of visualizing an object beyond its immediate use.
- Immediate relationships are the only relationships that are clearly understood.
- The infant improves in the ability to recognize that other people are different from the self. This helps create action through others, as in the next point.
- Other people become increasingly important as potential sources of resolution of the child's "problems." That is, children will seek solutions to problems from parents or older siblings—a critical social skill, important to the establishment of emotion, competition, and rivalry.

Invention of new means through mental combinations. The last of Piaget's substages in the sensorimotor stage, this substage lasts from 18 to 24 months. It is a period of metamorphosis from active involvement in movement interactions with the environment to increased reflection about these movements. This substage is often considered the climax of the sensorimotor stage and a transitional phase into the preoperational stage.

Characteristics of this substage include:

- Clearly recognizing objects as independent from the self.
- Recognizing oneself as one object among the many existing in the environment.
- Continuing interactions with environmental objects via movement activities, enabling the child to develop an understanding of object properties such as size, shape, color, texture, weight, and use (see Figure 2.5).
- Development of the cognitive ability to consider the self and an object in simple situations in the past, present, and future, enabling contemplation of activities and the onset of what Piaget termed semimental functioning: the replacement of "thinking with the body" by thinking with the mind.
- Development of new skills, as the child can now recall an event without physically reenacting what happened and, therefore, can ponder alternatives and predict outcomes to situations without first performing the acts.

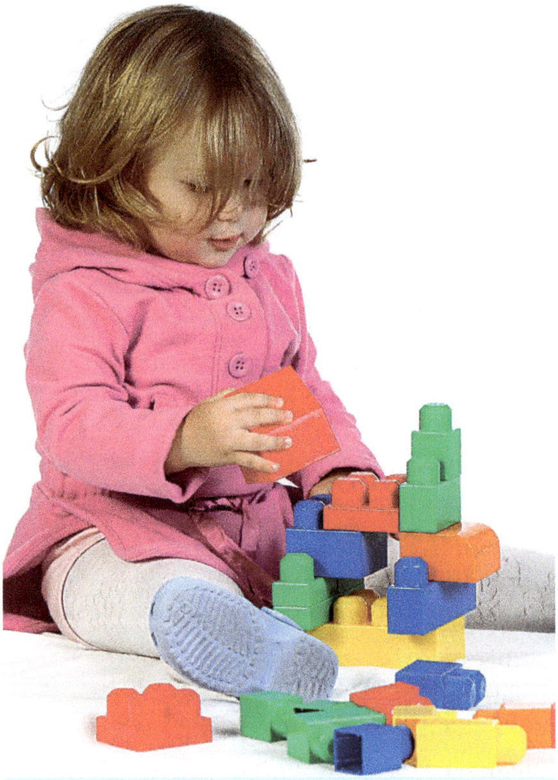

Figure 2.5 In the last substage of Piaget's sensorimotor stage of cognitive development, children recognize objects as clearly independent from themselves as they begin to understand properties such as size, shape, color, texture, weight, and use

Preoperational Stage and Motor Development

Piaget's second major stage, the preoperational, begins at around 2 years and spans the next five years. This stage builds on the skills learned earlier in life as the child becomes more imaginative in play and recognizes that everyone views the world from a slightly different perspective. Furthermore, the child improves in the ability to use symbols to represent objects in the environment. This capability enables the emergence of one of the most important of all cognitive skills: verbal communication.

Language development is the most important characteristic of the preoperational stage and is strongly linked to the onset of walking (Walle & Campos, 2014). The child becomes particularly adept at verbal communication very soon after learning to walk upright unassisted. Walking enables the child to explore and, therefore, understand the environment more thoroughly, and the rapidly expanding repertoire of new concepts that the child gains from this increased exploration facilitates language development. By the middle of the preoperational stage, most children possess a highly efficient ability to communicate verbally as a result of this important interaction between motor and cognitive development.

Although Piaget generally focused on the cognitive attributes gained in each of his stages of cognitive development, in the preoperational stage he emphasized the child's limitations. In fact, he coined the term *preoperational* because at this stage children still do not have the ability to think logically or operationally. This second major stage in Piaget's theory is subdivided into two substages: preconceptual (from 2 to 4 years) and intuitive (4 to 7 years).

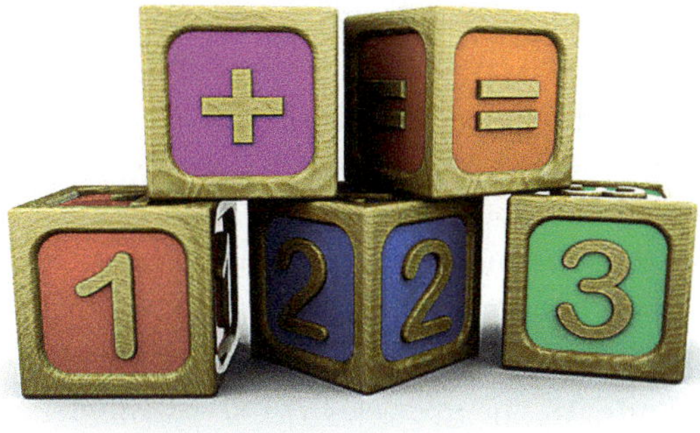

Figure 2.6 In the preconceptual substage of the preoperations stage in Piaget's theory of cognitive development, children improve in their ability to use symbols to represent objects in their environment

Preconceptual. During the preconceptual substage, an ability to use symbols to represent objects in the environment emerges—for example, using a rock to represent a turtle or the word *Dad* to represent a certain person (see Figure 2.6). Obviously, this new skill is critical to language development, but it also helps the child to reconstruct past events and facilitates pretend play. During pretend play, children role play; they pretend they are other individuals and use props to symbolize objects to supplement their play. This play often focuses on various movement activities and contributes significantly to all areas of the child's development, including motor development. It is believed that movement is enhanced by a child's pretend play, which may include the imitation of a parent or other role model engaged in a favorite movement activity.

Piaget believed that the preconceptual substage was characterized by a level of cognitive ability that is primitive relative to adult capabilities. Piaget said that during this stage children's thinking is flawed by their tendency to animate inanimate objects. For example, a child might refer to the emotional state of a drooping flower by saying, "The flower is sad!" This is a fun and interesting way to perceive the world, but it is also unrealistic and usually erroneous.

Transductive reasoning is another characteristic of the preconceptual substage. In this form of flawed reasoning, the child assumes that a cause-and-effect relationship exists between two events occurring simultaneously. For example, a child who has missed breakfast might declare that it cannot be morning because breakfast has not been prepared; obviously, the preparation of breakfast does not cause morning to occur. Transductive reasoning often leads to incorrect assumptions.

Perhaps the most serious deficiency of this substage of preoperational thought is egocentrism. Children aged 2–4 years old view the world from a very narrow perspective. They have difficulty visualizing the perspective of others and do not adapt their rapidly developing language skills to facilitate the listener's understanding. Motor activities help in this regard because they increase a child's capability to interact socially by providing means of locomoting to other children, thereby creating opportunities for social activity and enhanced social awareness. Increased social interaction expands the child's sensitivity to the needs and feelings of others and generally reduces the egocentrism characteristic of this stage of cognitive development.

Intuitive. The intuitive substage, an extension of the preconceptual substage, is characterized by a reduction in egocentrism and continuing improvement in the use of symbols. Piaget called this substage "intuitive" because the child's understanding of the ways of the world is based on the appearance of objects and events that may not accurately reflect reality.

As in the first substage of the preoperational stage, in the intuitive substage Piaget continued to characterize cognitive development in terms of the child's limitations. In both substages, the child continues to lack an ability Piaget called **conservation**. Conservation allows a person to understand that certain characteristics of an object may remain the same when the object's appearance is rearranged (Shaffer & Kipp, 2014). The concept of conservation is exemplified by Piaget's classic test involving a ball of clay. When the ball is manually transformed into an elongated sausage, the child incapable of conservation responds that the elongated clay weighs more. The child capable of conservation knows that the spatial transformation of the clay has no effect on the weight of the clay.

The inability to conserve comes from the child's difficulty in attending to more than one aspect of a problem-solving situation at one time. Children in the preoperational stage cannot "decenter" their attention from one particular component of a problem. Once they attain this ability, they can concentrate on more than one aspect of a problem simultaneously. In the example with the ball of clay, the child with conservation ability can ponder the weight, length, and even the width of the clay rather than being restricted to one aspect of the clay.

Inability to decenter attention can also have significant implications in motor development. By this time, children have become involved in many new motor activities, such as games. The inability to consider multiple aspects of a problem simultaneously inhibits a child's efforts in games or activities that involve complex strategies or multiple movements. Consider young children playing soccer: their attention often becomes so focused on the objective of scoring a goal that they are impervious to the possibility of passing off to a teammate.

Concrete Operational Stage and Motor Development

Piaget's third major stage of cognitive development, the **concrete operational stage**, generally spans ages 7–11. Many experts believe that children attain concrete operations once they have gained the ability to conserve. Thus, a major characteristic of this stage is the enhanced ability to decenter attention from one variable in a problem-solving situation. As mentioned earlier, this ability to decenter attention can have important implications for motor development.

Also in this stage of development, children and young adolescents gradually attain the mental ability to modify, organize, or even reverse their thought processes. A characteristic such as reversibility can be demonstrated by rolling three balls (A, B, and C) through a small tube (Figure 2.7). We ask the child, "What order will the balls be in as they exit the other end of the tube?" In both the preoperational and the concrete operational stages, the child can correctly answer "A, B, and C." However, if we immediately roll the balls back through the tube without altering the order in which they exited, and ask, "What will the order of exit be this time?" only the child who has achieved concrete operations can correctly respond "C, B, and A."

Piaget used the term *concrete operational* because the child at this level of cognitive development faces a major limitation. Although this stage is a major advance over the preoperational stage, the child is still limited to pondering objects, events, or situations that are real or based on experience. This, of course, impedes mental efforts to examine hypothetical or abstract situations.

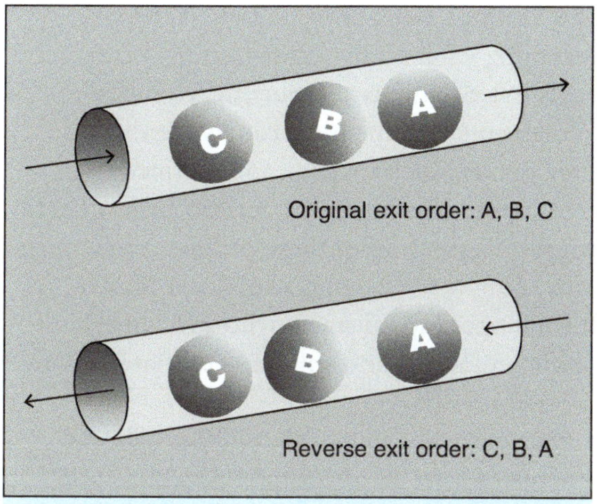

Figure 2.7 Demonstration of reversibility. The child who has achieved concrete operations can predict the sequence of balls A, B, and C as they exit the tube in both the original and the reverse order.

On the positive side, the child who has attained this level of cognitive ability is now capable of mentally representing objects, actions, or events. This mental capability has obvious implications for motor development. For example, the child can facilitate many movement activities by formulating strategies for or expectations about an opposing player's or team's possible intent. With the ability to ponder probable events or actions, the child can anticipate the opponent's tactics and has a chance to counter them with success.

Piaget considered *seriation* another characteristic common to children at this level of development. **Seriation** is the ability to arrange a set of items by a certain characteristic. For example, teammates can be arranged by height, and the relative relationships among these individuals can then be discerned. In other words, if a group of children at the concrete operational stage are informed that the basketball team's center is taller than the forward and that the forward is taller than the guard, they are able to determine that the center is also taller than the guard.

As emphasized throughout this chapter, there is a constant, reciprocal, mutually beneficial relationship between cognitive development and motor development. Piaget indirectly referred to this phenomenon throughout his theory; the concrete operational stage is no exception. In this stage (as well as others), Piaget stressed that learning can be facilitated by doing or by actions. That is, such cognitive skills as seriation can best be taught by having children manipulate objects of various lengths and widths into series. Piaget suggested that one of the best modes of teaching such concepts as space and distance was to have children "do": instructing the children to move through the space or the distance under consideration. In Piaget's mind, movement in the form of doing, or action, was a critical component in the development of cognitive ability.

Formal Operational Stage and Motor Development

According to Piaget, the highest level of cognitive ability, which begins at about age 11 to 12, is often known as the **formal operational stage** or, simply, formal operations. The main accomplishment in this final stage is the ability to consider ideas that are not based on reality; that is, the individual is no longer confined to observable objects or experience-based thoughts. Abstract ideas are possible, and this enables young people to resolve problems that violate their concepts about reality. Children in the concrete operational stage may be completely baffled by questions concerning abstract or nonexistent events or objects. In fact, these children may respond that no response is possible because the concept being asked about does not exist. In the formal operational stage, however, individuals are challenged and enjoy the opportunity to ponder a new concept. According to Piaget, many individuals never achieve this stage of development. In fact, people who score below average on intelligence tests most likely have not achieved formal operations (Shaffer & Kipp, 2014).

Individuals who reach this stage are also capable of performing what Piaget called **interpropositional thought**. This enhanced level of cognitive ability allows children to relate one or more parts of a proposition or a situation to another part to arrive at a solution to a problem. To illustrate, a child in the concrete operational stage who is confronted with the statement "The ball is in my left hand or it isn't in my left hand" may need to inspect his or her hands visually before responding. The young adolescent in formal operations, however, can determine that the statement, although somewhat unusual, is correct. By simultaneously considering the two propositions within the statement, the formal operator determines that the ball either is in the hand or is somewhere else; hence, the statement is correct.

The ability to perform interpropositional thought can be useful in many situations. In complex movement situations, this capability could enhance an individual's success strategically. In many team activities, the positioning of two or more players—each a "movement proposition"—may indicate that a particular play is about to occur. A defender who can "read" the interrelationship between these movement propositions can prepare accordingly and help the team counter the play.

An additional product of formal thought is what Piaget referred to as **hypothetical-deductive reasoning**. This term indicates a problem-solving style in which the individual generates and systematically considers possible solutions to a problem. This rational, systematic, and abstract form of reasoning facilitates the selection of the correct solution. Piaget believed that this new form of reasoning, which allows consideration of the abstract, has dramatic effects on a child's emotional development, including the development of new feelings, behaviors, and goals. Newly emerging values may result from this enhanced cognitive capability. Frequently, young adolescents become increasingly idealistic as they ponder such magnanimous concepts as world peace or the search for the perfect energy source. Resolution of these problems may seem fairly simple to a young adolescent in the formal operational stage, who can now think about situations and solutions that are beyond current reality.

The changing values that Piaget believed emerge as a result of formal operations may also affect the young adolescent's decisions concerning participation in movement endeavors. Because of increased idealism, the adolescent may decide that the competition that is prevalent in adolescent movement activities is not mutually beneficial to all involved and, therefore, might choose not to participate. Or the adolescent may begin to become aware of the potential benefits of participation and learn to cherish the possibility of being exceptionally fit or successful in a movement endeavor. The extent and direction of the individual's new values are influenced by current trends among peers and society; this topic is discussed in Chapter 3.

Criticisms of Piaget's Theory

Jean Piaget's theory has been well accepted by experts throughout the world and has profoundly influenced theory and practice. As a result, it has also been the subject of considerable examination, scrutiny, and criticism. Some aspects of these criticisms are worth consideration (see Table 2.4). First, although Piaget became adept at his clinical method of gathering data concerning children's thought processes, this method has been criticized for lacking scientific control during the collection process. In addition, much of Piaget's observation centered on his own children, which, of course, leads to concerns about his potential bias in interpreting the thought processes of people so dear to him. Nevertheless, Piaget's theory of cognitive development has withstood considerable scrutiny for many years and continues to be the most significant guide in our efforts to understand human development more fully.

Table 2.4 Criticisms of Piaget's work on cognitive development

1.	Piaget's clinical method lacked sufficient scientific control.
2.	Much of Piaget's work was conducted with his own children as subjects.
3.	Piaget's examination of cognitive change did not have a lifespan orientation.
4.	Piaget may have underestimated children's capabilities.
5.	Piaget did not discern well between competency and performance.
6.	Piaget placed too little emphasis on the influence of motivation and emotions.
7.	Piaget's stages of development were too broad.
8.	Piaget described but did not clearly explain development.

Perhaps the most strongly contested aspect of Piaget's theory is his proposal that the highest level of intellectual development is formal operational, a stage he claims is often achieved by children as young as 11 years of age. Although Piaget stated that some children may never achieve formal operations and some may not achieve them until as late as age 20, a significant portion of the lifespan remains unaccounted for. Strong proponents of Piagetian theory support his notion, but subsequent research in adult development has led to the supposition that development continues beyond adolescence (Sigelman & Rider, 2018). Undoubtedly, cognitive behavior continues to develop long after early adolescence, despite Piaget's omission of this time of life. Several of the important cognitive changes that occur during adulthood and their relationship to motor development are discussed in the next section.

Piaget has also been criticized for his underestimation of the true capabilities of children. Furthermore, Piaget may not have fully recognized the distinction between competency and performance. In other words, if a child performed poorly on one of Piaget's tasks, the assumption was that the child lacked intellectual competence. In fact, the child may have been competent but may have performed poorly as a result of the child's emotional state, lack of motivation, degree of verbal ability, memory, or lack of familiarity with the task, or because of the nature of social influences from parents, peers, teachers, and siblings. The assumption that the cause of poor performance was lack of intellectual competence could have affected the age guidelines that Piaget provided for each of his stages (Sigelman & Rider, 2018).

Other critics have noted that Piaget's stages of development may be too encompassing or broad. This criticism arises out of recent research indicating that intellect may be mainly content-specific rather than existing in a certain mode across a wide range of problem-solving areas, as Piaget suggested. Still other critics have noted how well Piaget described development but have lamented his apparent inattention to explaining the process. Piaget failed to address questions such as, for example, how do specific intellectual changes evolve anatomically, and how do life experiences contribute to this whole process (Sigelman & Rider, 2018)?

ADULTHOOD: GENERAL THEORIES OF INTELLECTUAL DEVELOPMENT

As stated earlier, like his predecessors in development and the developmentalists of his day, Piaget did not specifically consider adulthood in his theory of cognitive development. We now clearly recognize that development is a lifelong process and seek to understand all age groups. Therefore, cognitive developmentalists have speculated as to the nature of intellectual change throughout the adult years. Some have proposed adding a fifth stage to Piaget's work, called postformal operations, to indicate this stage of continuing cognitive development during adulthood. Others among the expert community assert that certain forms of intellectual decline occur with age. Regardless, an "intellectual tension" exists among theorists in the area of aging and cognitive function. Some purport that aging has pervasive effects throughout the information-processing system with some aspects of cognition showing more notable declines than others (Poon & Harrington, 2006).

Postformal Operations

Even among healthy individuals, reduced function in motor and cognitive areas may occur later in life, though the speed and extent of the decline are dependent on many factors. For example, as we discuss later in the chapter, physical activity levels can improve or, at least, offset the rate and intensity of cognitive declines (Gajewski & Falkenstein, 2016). Studies involving thousands of people from throughout the world have found that as many as 15–20 percent of adults over the age of 60 years may experience some degree of mild cognitve impairment. However, this number increases as one ages and devolves into dementia in as many as one in ten people. Thus, seeking effective interventions at an early age is critical (Peterson, 2016).

To further ponder the development of cognitive abilities later in life and beyond the extent of Piaget's theory, Arlin once proposed adding a so-called fifth stage to Piaget's work. This fifth stage was considered a higher level of ability because it involved larger quantities of information. Berger (2017) suggested that **postformal operations** (i.e., what happens after Piaget's last stage of cognitive development) may involve more than dealing with larger quantities of information. This stage would be characterized by a more flexible, logical, and complex form of thought. In Piaget's formal operations stage we can become consumed by our newfound logical capabilities and assume that logical answers exist for all problems. As we continue to develop beyond formal operations, we come to see answers as more relative and less absolute. In advanced levels of thinking, we enjoy detecting paradoxes and inconsistencies in ideas and attempting to reconcile them. We develop the ability to think logically about abstract concepts and can manipulate whole systems of ideas. These advanced capabilities, however, are thought to exist only in a minority of adults, mostly among those with advanced education who reside in a culture that embraces new ideas and freethinking. This observation reinforces the idea that cognitive development, like other aspects of human development, does not depend on age. Rather, it is tied to life experiences and challenges to think at home, at work, and throughout our communities (Sigelman & Rider, 2018).

Currently, the most widely accepted view on aging and intellect posits that cognitive decline occurs in some intellectual areas but not others. Salthouse (2012), for example, notes that, though cognitive declines may occur with older age, in the area of job performance a strong correlation exists between age and cognition up to the age of 65 years or older. In addition, he says, older age is rarely associated with "lower levels of real-world functioning" (p. 201), though strict laboratory testing can be more "pessimistic" (p. 201). Thus, "age related declines can . . . occur in important cognitive abilities without major consequences for functioning in society" (p. 202). The explanation for this is unclear. Salthouse posits that it may be related to the fact that life situations rarely require a maximal cognitive effort and the important role of increased knowledge, often gained through age and experience.

Also, societal stigmas regarding old age and "senility" are often criticized for being self-fulfilling prophecies; that is, if we think it will happen, it will. For example, a person who has negative thoughts about his own memory will probably lose confidence in it. This, in turn, hampers the individual's performance (see Figure 2.8). Studies on Chinese elders, who receive much more respect for their wisdom and experience and, therefore, are less likely to encounter negative stereotypes than their American counterparts, have demonstrated less intellectual decline when compared with younger Chinese adults.

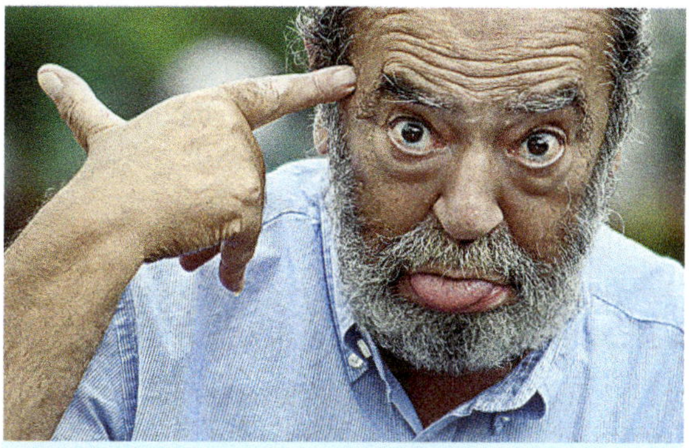

Figure 2.8 Negative thoughts about memory can hamper confidence and ultimately affect memory in older adulthood

Clearly, aside from age, many other factors can contribute to a decline or the lack of a decline in cognitive performance. An individual's knowledge base has also been found to be a factor. A greater base of information may help offset losses in processing efficiency (Sigelman & Rider, 2018). Knowledge really is power! In researching several hundred Swedish elders with an average age of just under 85 years, Bendayan and colleagues (2017) noted an overall significant age-related cognitive decline with those with dementia generating the fastest declines and the poorest cognitive performances. Individuals who were better educated performed better on cognitive tasks overall, though the greater education did not slow the rate of decline compared to those participants who were not so well educated (Bendayan et al., 2017).

The recognition of factors other than age and their effects on intellectual change across time is often referred to as a **contextual perspective**. This simply means recognizing that learning and memory depend in part on factors such as culture, as we saw in the studies of Chinese elders. Noncognitive, situational factors can strongly affect the degree to which any decline occurs (Zacks, Hasher, & Li, 2000). Factors such as a person's goals, motivation, social activities, modifications of daily routines, changes in emotions, and ability related to the task in question can also affect performance. Even an individual's own optimistic or pessimistic self-appraisal can affect performance. Thus, the decline we often see in intellectual abilities is not convincingly universal and not completely a function of inevitable biological decline (Sigelman & Rider, 2018).

However, biological effects are clearly involved (Chang, Pan, Chen, et al., 2012). Changes such as declining neural systems, slowing neural activation, and loss of efficiency in vascular or circulatory processes are thought to contribute. The brain tends to decrease in size with age; however, this effect is highly variable. Neuronal losses are gradual in typical aging, and the greatest loss of neurons occurs during the prenatal period. The overall longevity and adaptive capacity of the human nervous system are generally remarkable, with most neurons maintaining strong adaptive capacity throughout life.

There appear to be "no simple rules about when age differences in memory will and will not occur, and if they do, whether differences will be small, modest, or large" (Zacks et al., 2000, p. 342), but considerable recent research has centered on **implicit** and **explicit memory** and learning. Some researchers have concluded that "nowhere is there a trend more salient than in research on implicit memory" (p. 305). Implicit memory is unintentional, automatic, or without awareness. It is memory where we have no recollection of the source of the memory, but it still affects our behavior. Perhaps the best example of implicit memory is riding a bicycle. Once a person has learned this skill, it becomes somewhat fixed. In other words, we do not have to ponder consciously how to ride a bike in order to ride it (Howe, 2015). The same applies to everyday tasks such as washing one's face or shaving, or even reciting the alphabet. Therefore, implicit memory can be tested without the subject's being aware of being tested. Explicit memory is deliberate and effortful and is tested by traditional tests of recall or recognition. These two types of memory are believed to follow quite different developmental paths. Explicit memory improves from infancy to adulthood and then shows decline. Implicit memory also improves from infancy but does not change much at all during adulthood, with elders performing no worse than young adults (Sigelman & Rider, 2018).

Many other trends have been noted in research on aging and intellect. For example, memory for information learned earlier, rather than later, in life is superior in older adulthood. If information is well established early in life, it will be easier to retrieve than information learned later. An age-related decline for "new learning" relative to "old learning" appears to be clear cut (Prull et al., 2000; Zacks et al., 2000).

Another clear trend is that older adults tend to respond more slowly than younger individuals. When time restrictions are placed on intellectual tasks, the performance of older adults is more likely to be negatively affected (Sigelman & Rider, 2018). In fact, the decline in speed of processing may be the most obvious, well-established decline with age. It contributes significantly to age-related declines on many cognitive tasks (Zacks et al., 2000). Obviously, this decline in speed of mental processing has clear ramifications for motor development. Many movement activities require fast, even split-second decision making. Thus, motor ability may decline with increasing age. We will thoroughly discuss this phenomenon in Chapter 15.

THE ROLE OF MOVEMENT SKILL IN FACILITATING COGNITIVE PERFORMANCE

As discussed, declines in intellect are often noted during later adulthood. Nevertheless,

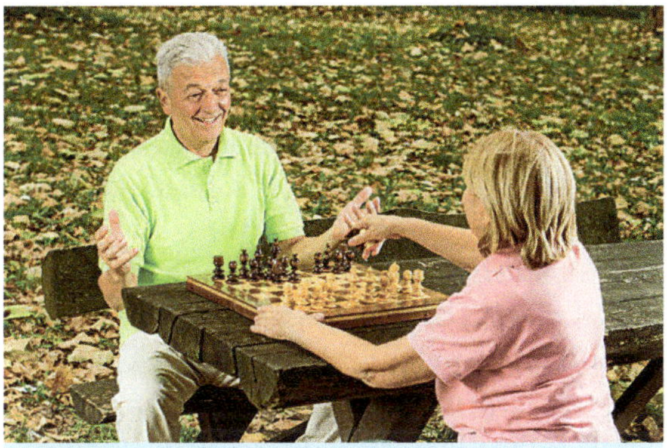

Figure 2.9 Practicing cognitive abilities during older adulthood can delay or even prevent declines that might otherwise occur

research indicates that much can be done to allay their onset. A lifestyle can be designed that optimizes cognitive attributes. When cognitive abilities are practiced, declines are often delayed or avoided altogether (Sigelman & Rider, 2018) (see Figure 2.9), and cognitive training has been shown to be effective in enhancing the capabilities of older adults. In a meta-analysis (a powerful statistical review of literature) on the effects of extended practice on cognitive outcomes, Hindin and Zelinski (2012) found that extended practice of cognitive tasks resulted in significant positive outcomes in older adults. The effects of such factors across the lifespan have been extensively studied. In this section, the focus is on the specific effects of improvements in motor abilities on various forms of cognitive status.

For example, Cameron and associates (2016) studied motor skill development and school performance. They proclaimed that children's success in school is incumbent upon a range of incoming skills, including movement skill. More specifically, these researchers indicate that specific cognitive measures like motor coordination, executive function, and visuospatial skill (understanding visual representations and their spatial relationships) are strongly related to motor behavior and ultimately affect the ability to accurately perform academic skills. Examples of academic skills referenced here include decoding letters and words for reading and writing, solving quantitative problems encountered in subjects like math, and even interacting effectively in social situations. This, these authors believe, is a function of motor skills being more than movement. Movement abilities require cognitive aptitude during their performance as they integrate various perceptual abilities with the movement systems required to perform the skill in question. Thus, motor skill development impacts physical, social, and cognitive well-being. Development of fine movement skill is even more strongly related to academic achievement, they say. This finding was based on research on young children (5 years of age) where those with stronger motor skills performed better than those with poorer skills on math and reading performance one, three, and five years later. In general, these experts also proclaimed that motor skill development, both gross and fine, was also integral to self-regulation in the classroom and academic ability in reading, writing, and quantitative problem solving (Cameron, Cottone, Murrah, & Grissmer, 2016).

In a similar study to examine the relationship between motor development, specifically motor coordination, cognitive ability, and academic achievement, individuals from 8–14 years of age were tested on both a motor coordination test and a test to determine their shuttle run speed. School achievement scores and sub-tests of the Wechsler Intelligence Scale were then correlated with the outcomes of the motor tests. Stroop Test scores that assessed selective attention, concentration, cognitive flexibility, and inhibitory control were also correlated with the motor scores. Findings led the researchers to conclude that motor coordination, though not so much agility, was well correlated with academic achievement and cognitive function (Fernandes et al., 2016).

Roca and Williams (2016) focused their research on athletes (experts in the motor domain) from many different sports who, they say, often demonstrate superior perceptual-cognitive skills. This is especially true regarding one's ability to note and attend to early environmental cues and recognizing ongoing task-related patterns that are critical to successful problem solving. They also demonstrate more accurate prediction capabilities to assure success in specific situations. According to these authors, improved understanding of these relationships is important to the potential development of programs to facilitate intellectual function in people of all ages, especially older folks who may be facing some degree of intellectual decline.

Neumann, Lotze, and Eickhoff (2016) conducted a meta-analysis to compare individuals with and without expertise in a variety of activities (e.g., mental calculations, language, chess, memory feats, and musical performance). Specifically, they sought to compare brain activation patterns of the young adult experts to the non-experts. In their review of literature, they located twenty-six studies on their topic. The majority of these studies found an increase in activation patterns in the experts in a number of brain areas including the premotor cortex that exerts control over the performance of voluntary movement. Overall, the experts' brain activation patterns were found to be enhanced. In other words, they experienced additional brain activity over the non-expert participants.

Interestingly, involvement in elite-level sport participation combines exercise and motor skill development with cognitive training, especially in specific kinds of activities like interactive sports. An example would be a soccer player upon receiving the ball and dribbling toward his own goal. Based on the positioning of the defenders, he is faced with a number of decisions. He may choose to pass or continue dribbling toward the goal. To be most successful, his decision must be instantaneous and based on the memory he has amassed from previous similar experiences. Cognitive demands of this type are common in many sports and demand keen perceptual and decision-making skill (Heppe, Kohler, Fleddermann, & Zentgraf, 2016).

In a powerful meta-analysis on this topic, Voss et al. (2010) found that athletes perform better than non-elite athletes on some cognitive measures, especially those involving processing speed. These same researchers also determined that cognitive skills derived and employed in a sporting situation can be transferred to a more general non-sport context. Sports that involved interception skills like soccer, tennis, or volleyball were found to be most effective in this relationship between sport performance and cognitive ability. Sports involving clear strategies were next in effectiveness followed by static sports (e.g., running, swimming) where the relationship was least pronounced. Experts believe that the greater aerobic demands of some sports are also beneficial to cognitive function as well as the complex requirements to rapidly coordinate movement while facing continual decision-making demands (Voss et al., 2010).

In similar research, a group of top division soccer players were contrasted with lower division players and a control (norm) group on a series of tests designed to measure areas of executive function such as response inhibition and cognitive flexibility. Participants included males and females and all groups averaged in age from their early to mid-twenties. Both groups of soccer players performed better on these measures than the norm group while the top division players performed better than the lower division players. These researchers believed these types of cognitive tests could be useful in predicting success in various ball sports. These outcomes could be a function of sport success often being dependent on physical skill, motor coordination, and one's ability to process complex information in rapidly varying contexts. According to the researchers, these findings suggest that elite athletes often have superior cognitive ability, especially when it comes to problems that are similar to game-like situations (Vestberg, Gustafson, Maurex, Martin, & Petrovic, 2012).

In research strictly involving adult participants, three treatment groups were formed. Overall, nearly seventy male and female subjects, averaging approximately 30 years of age, were studied. Participants were involved in aerobic training, novel cognitive training, or a combination of the two which the researchers referred to as a "designed sport." Participants were involved in their specific activity for eight weeks whereby the cognitive training group focused on improving working memory. The designed sport was a novel physical activity that included problem solving, specifically working memory and problem-solving requirements during the actual physical activity. The aerobic training group engaged in physical activities designed to enhance their aerobic capacity.

Results indicated that the designed sport condition enhanced cognitive abilities (e.g., spatial ability and working memory) while also improving health-related factors like blood pressure and heart rate. The researchers concluded that the complex motor activities that combined physical and cognitive demands offered considerable promise as a training approach. The working memory group was also found to improve intellectually, though they did not demonstrate the same beneficial physical health effects. The authors clearly indicated that their designed sport program is only one of many ways that cognitive and physiological improvement may be attained. Using such cognitively based physical activities as dance or orienteering might result in similar positive outcomes. The research team expressed optimism that their research found that cognitive ability can be improved and that it can be achieved by means that are interesting, potentially exciting, and physically health-enhancing (Moreau, Morrison, & Conway, 2015). (See Figure 2.10.)

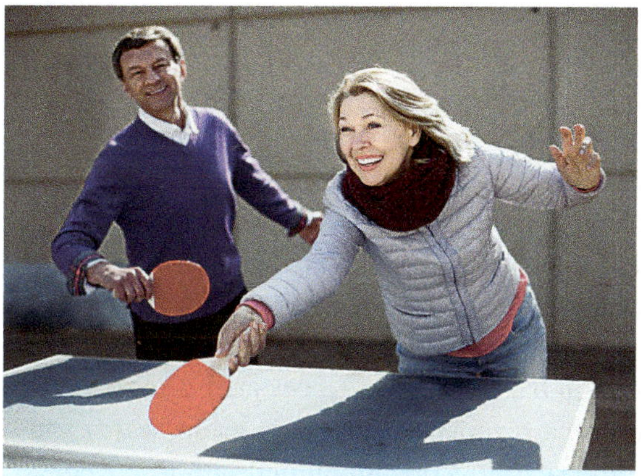

Figure 2.10 Research has determined that cognitive ability can be enhanced in ways that are fun, interesting, and beneficial to physical health

In another study on the effects of motor skill on cognition, Müller and associates (2016) studied the fine motor skill of piano playing and intelligence on procedural learning and typical age-related decrements. Well over a hundred participants were tested on memory tasks, learning speed, and a finger-tapping movement task. Male and female participants ranged in age from 18 to 69 years of age and included those who had minimal experience in playing the piano or other musical instruments and those who had, at least, 500 hours of playing experience. Thus, the researchers were able to examine the effects of piano experience, age, and gender on procedural learning and memory consolidation. Results revealed that previous piano players were faster learners and remembered better in the finger-tapping task. This was especially notable in the older adult participants, leading the research team to conclude that, for that group, related motor experience would improve learning speed and memory. The researchers indicated that previous piano playing experience provided some degree of protection against memory decrements that are often common in older age. In other words, training in some motor skills may help maintain cognitive function (Müller et al., 2016).

As discussed earlier in the chapter, as we age, brain structures may show a degree of degradation. These declines can affect a number of functional attributes like balance and cognitive performance. However, the aging brain maintains its ability to adapt, a phenomenon referred to as neuroplasticity. This notion has led experts to consider a number of training regimens to maintain brain health and the related functional abilities with age. Rehfeld and colleagues (2017) specifically examined dance in elderly participants as one avenue of preserving brain health and cognition. They chose dance because it combined considerable cognitive demands with an aerobic component and motor skill. To determine the effectiveness of a dance training intervention, the researchers contrasted a year and a half dance training program with a more traditional health fitness training program on balance and anatomical brain changes determined from MRIs. Both groups showed positive changes in brain anatomy (e.g., increase in the volume of the hippocampus) with the dancers demonstrating additional increases (e.g., increases in left dentate gyrus and right subiculum). The dancers also generated significantly better balance scores, leading these researchers to conclude that dance is a viable means to offset physical and mental declines often seen in older individuals (Rehfeld et al., 2017). These conclusions paralleled many of the findings of Mann, Williams, Ward, and Janelle (2007), who conducted a similar meta-analysis on movement expertise and perceptual-cognitive ability. In an examination of participants of varying levels of ability, experts were found to perform better than non-experts in their ability to ascertain pertinent visual cues. They also generated better response times and response accuracy, and they visually fixated less frequently, but for longer periods of time. Mann and his colleagues stated that, in general, movement experts possess "greater procedural (how to do something) and **declarative knowledge** that enables them to extrapolate important information from the environment to anticipate and predict future events" (p. 458). More specifically, declarative knowledge is factual information or an awareness of something (an event, an object, or even an idea). However, despite having this awareness, an individual may be unable to employ the knowledge functionally, and the awareness of something does not necessarily imply an understanding of it. **Procedural knowledge** is understanding a procedure, or how to do something, that is, "knowing how." Specific examples of the application of procedural knowledge include developing plans, solving a problem, or developing and delivering an argument (Barrouillet, Corbin, Dagry, & Camos, 2014). Clearly, both types of knowledge play a role in human movement, and both are affected by changes in cognitive and motor development. In most cases, when a person is learning a sport, both declarative knowledge and procedural knowledge are important. In tennis, for example, declarative knowledge would include the rules of the game, the etiquette, where to strike the ball on the racket face, and how to grip the racket properly. Procedural knowledge would be illustrated by a player's ability to employ that declarative knowledge in the execution of a technically correct serve, volley, or ground stroke. The player must know what is required (declarative knowledge) and be able to apply it (procedural knowledge) to achieve a technically sound movement.

THE ROLE OF PHYSICAL ACTIVITY IN FACILITATING COGNITIVE PERFORMANCE

In addition to the extensive research on motor skill development and cognition, many scientific claims have been made regarding the positive impact of greater amounts of physical activity on various aspects of cognition, especially executive function or control, managing and regulating the cognitive processes to perform goal-directed tasks. Older adulthood, where cognitive impairment is of increasing concern, has garnered much of this research attention. Claims touting the benefits of physical activity on cognition have spawned an array of investigations seeking to better understand this relationship and the true effects of exercise or physical activity on cognitive function across the lifespan. So many investigations have now been undertaken that researchers have, in many cases, been able to conduct powerful meta-analyses, large-scale, objective, and quantitative reviews of the literature that merge many studies to yield conclusions based on an entire body of literature rather than any one study. Considerable research on this topic now exists for both genders, most age groups, and even individuals with varying maladies like Parkinson's and Alzheimer's diseases.

For example, a study of preschool-aged children (3–5-year-olds) was designed to examine active versus sedentary time and their effects on short-term executive function. Here, researchers studied short-term executive function following sedentary and active situations. Over seventy children wore accelerometers to determine the quantity of physical activity. Aspects of executive control that were studied included inhibitory control, working memory, and some iPad-based cognitive tasks. Despite strong beliefs that physical activity improves cognitive performance in early childhood, participants actually had better inhibitory control following sedentary periods. More active times generated no apparent short-term impact on executive function. Still, given all other benefits of physical activity, the researchers encouraged promoting physical activity within this age group and concluded that longer-term effects still need to be examined (Tandon et al., 2018).

Willoughby and colleagues (2018) cross-sectionally examined the association between physical activity (sedentary, light, moderate to vigorous) and children's executive control. Participants were 3–5-year-olds from center-based pre-schools (n = 85). Accelerometer data were again used to assess the magnitude of physical activity. These children were found to be sedentary 60 percent of the time while spending just over 30 percent of their time in light physical activity (PA). Just over 10 percent of their time was spent in moderate to vigorous PA. A poor relationship was found between sedentary or light physical activity and executive function. Interestingly, vigorous activity was inversely related to performance on executive function tasks. In other words, increased levels of PA were found to decrease performance on executive function tasks, a somewhat surprising finding (Willoughby, Wylie, & Catellier, 2018).

Researchers have also studied slightly older children. For example, one study assessed the effects of a large school-based physical activity intervention on children's level of distraction and their ability to maintain focus, both aspects of executive function. More than a thousand 7–12-year-olds from two primary schools were engaged in 45 minutes of physical activity for six to eight months in addition to a regular physical education class once a week. Both the control group, that did not participate in the physical activity intervention, and the active group improved on measures of executive control. However, no significant differences were noted on executive control between the groups, leading the researchers to conclude that the intervention did not generally affect executive control (Konijnenberg & Fredricksen, 2018).

Despite the findings of the previous individual studies cited, Álvarez-Bueno and her colleagues performed two large-scale systematic reviews with meta-analyses (2017a;

2017b). In the first meta-analysis, the aim was to examine the effect of physical activity on cognitive ability of 4–18-year-olds and to determine the nature of the programs that were most effective. Thirty-six total studies were located on this topic and were included in the analysis. Physical activity was found to be an overall positive factor for cognition. School physical education programs and efforts to increase amounts of daily physical activity were among the most positive interventions for an array of cognitive functions (Álvarez-Bueno et al., 2017a).

The second meta-analysis performed by these researchers was specifically designed to measure the effects of physical activity on classroom behavior and academic achievement while determining the characteristics of the most effective programs. The authors state that academic achievement is strongly related to executive function. As in their previous meta-analysis, this study examined children and adolescents. Specific academic areas included were language, math, reading, and an overall or composite academic score. Twenty-six studies were included in this analysis, leading the researchers to conclude that physical activity, especially from in-school physical education, enhances both classroom behavior and performance. Math, reading, and the composite academic score were most positively affected. Thus, physical activity promotion, according to these authors, is an effective academic tool and is worthy of promotion as such (Álvarez-Bueno et al., 2017b).

These findings were similar to those from research examining the effects of a physical activity program on the executive functioning of 11–14-year-old middle school girls. Researchers here indicated that the participants were at-risk for reduced self-esteem, general physical inactivity, and related health outcomes. The treatment group of girls was engaged in a five-month long triathlon training program while a comparable control group did not exercise. Upon completion of the program, a significant improvement was noted in several aspects of executive function as well as the girls' achievement in an academic science program (Gatz, Kelly, & Clark, 2018).

Similarly, another meta-analytic study was designed to systematically review thirty-one previous studies examining the relationship between physical activity and executive function, attention, and academic performance in preadolescent children ranging in age from 6 to 12 years. The thirty-one studies located on this topic were objectively and quantitatively examined for their effects. Specifically, inhibition, working memory, cognitive flexibility, and planning were the cognitive variables while math, spelling, and reading were examined in the area of academic performance. The various types of physical activity (aerobic or cognitively engaging) were also considered. Results indicated that physical activity had a positive effect on executive function with particularly positive effects on attention and academic performance. The most significant effects were generated for regular physical activity lasting for several weeks (De Greef, Bosker, Oosterlan, Visscher, & Hartman, 2018).

Raine and colleagues (2018) also re-examined several sets of data on the association between aerobic fitness and cognition on preadolescent boys and girls from 8–11 years of age. Specifically, these researchers examined the relation of aerobic activity to factors including inhibitory control, response accuracy, reaction time, response variability, and cognitive strategies. Aerobic fitness was associated positively with response accuracy, but not reaction time, though reaction time variability was reduced while discriminatory accuracy was better among those with higher levels of fitness. Overall, these researchers believed that involvement in aerobic activity enhances cognition and specific related behaviors. This, they say, has important implications for public health as it may indicate that certain types of physical activity during childhood may impact school performance and function through life (Raine et al., 2018).

The research on adults and older adults generally generated an even more compelling and consistent relationship between physical activity and cognitive function. In a recent review examining the association between physical activity/exercise and cognitive vitality, researchers found that physical activity was related to a "modest" decrease in cognitive decrements while assisting in the maintenance and enhancement of cognition. For older adults, they said, this was most likely a result of positive effects on the neural circuitry in the prefrontal cortex and the hippocampus of the brain. More specifically, these researchers concluded that physical activity was linked to positive outcomes in general cognitive function, speed of mental processing, episodic memory (i.e., remembering events in one's life), and executive control (using sophisticated mental processes to perform goal-directed tasks) while promoting neural plasticity (keeping the brain adapting and learning). The research was prompted, in part, by the interest in physical inactivity across the population in today's culture. They further stated that physical activity contributes to improved overall health, reduces the occurrence of many diseases, and extends mortality. Though most studies have focused on these associations later in life, modest support has also been established for positive associations between physical activity and cognitive function in children and young adults. Associated areas of cognitive improvement included attention, inhibitory control (overriding natural responses when appropriate), and relational memory (connecting elements of past experiences) (Prakash, Voss, Erickson, & Kramer, 2015).

Kramer and Colcombe (2018) reflected on a meta-analysis they conducted to examine if, and how much, physical activity can assist in avoiding cognitive decline with age. In this article, the authors focused on participants over the age of 55 years as, they say, so much of the previous adult research had examined much older individuals. According to these researchers, and their simultaneous examination of eighteen studies, a clear relationship was found between exercise and cognition with, at least, a modest effect. The effect was found to be broad-based with particularly large effects found for executive control processes like planning, scheduling, working memory, and multitasking. Most of the studies they examined used aerobic exercise as the treatment, though they also examined resistance training studies in their research. All forms of exercise were found to have beneficial effects with aerobic and combined (i.e., aerobic and resistance training) exercise having the most substantial effect. Of particular interest, the oldest subjects experienced the greatest positive effect in this research. These researchers indicate that exercise can have a positive effect on cognition across the lifespan as a result of such factors as increasing cerebral blood flow, increased volume of the hippocampus as well as the frontal and temporal gray matter, and white matter integrity. Nevertheless, these researchers also indicated that most research, to date, has been cross-sectional and designed to only examine relationships, not causation. Thus, more studies designed to establish true causation are needed (Kramer & Colcombe, 2018).

Noting that the specific amount of activity needed to enhance brain health is unknown and not well understood, Peven and associates (2018) examined the relationship between moderate to vigorous physical activity lasting less than ten minutes to similar intensities lasting longer than 10 minutes in just under a hundred community-dwelling adults averaging just over 65 years of age. Sensor arm bands were employed to objectively determine quantities of physical activity. Executive function was measured using a series of cognitive performance tasks. Their results suggest that the total accumulated minutes of moderate to vigorous physical activity, independent of the duration of the individual bout, may be most important in relation to cognitive performance in older adults. These researchers further noted that their results are important when establishing activity guidelines and recommendations for older adults. And, in short, bouts of moderate to vigorous physical activity exceeding ten minutes may yield significant cognitive benefits (Peven, Grove, Jakicic, Alessi, & Erikson, 2018).

Northey and associates (2018) also sought to determine if physical exercise improves cognitive function. Specifically, they studied community-dwelling adults over the age of 50 years. In yet another systematic meta-analytic review of the literature (thirty-nine studies included), overall results indicated that exercise improved cognitive function. Exercise interventions included aerobic exercise, resistance training, "multicomponent" training, and tai chi. All were found to be positive contributors to improved cognitive performance. Exercise duration was also examined with exercise bouts of 45–60 minutes at a minimum of moderate intensity showing positive associations with cognition, regardless of the initial cognitive status of the individual. Thus, physical exercise was deemed a viable means for clinicians or practitioners to assist clients in maintaining or improving cognitive abilities. These researchers further advised that both aerobic and resistance training, as many days per week as possible, and at a minimum of moderate intensity, are included in exercise prescriptions (Northey, Cherbuin, Pumpa, Smee, & Rattray, 2018).

Acknowledging that "physical activity is known to improve cognitive function at older age," Gheysen's team of researchers took a slightly different approach to their research. They sought to determine if cognitive gains can be improved by incorporating cognitive components into the physical activity. Thus, they compared the effects of physical activity programs alone, cognitive activity alone, and programs that include both physical activity and cognitive enhancements. Participants in these studies were older adults with a mean age of 65 years with and without cognitive impairments. Over forty individual studies were included in the investigation. Significant benefits were noted for the groups receiving both physical and cognitive activities compared to control groups who did not participate in any of these activities. Benefits were slightly greater when activities were combined, though physical activity alone also improved cognitive performance. Regarding the effect of the various activities, no significant differences were found between older adults who were and were not cognitively impaired. These findings led the researchers to conclude that integrating challenging cognitive activities into the physical activity program should be implemented and promoted for prevention and treatment of cognitive decline in older adults (Gheysen, Poppe, DeSmet, et al., 2018).

In a similar investigation, Hamer, Terrera, and Demakakos (2018) conducted a ten-year longitudinal study of English men and women averaging 65 years of age. Their aim was to examine the association between physical activity and decline in cognitive function. Involving over 10,000 community-dwelling males and females (average age of 65 years), the researchers used self-reports to determine physical activity levels and a variety of neurophysiological and memory tests to assess executive function. At the onset, very little difference existed in cognitive function between the men and women in the study. However, across the ten years, the inactive women in the study experienced more severe decrements in memory and executive function. For the male participants, memory was unaffected though the active participants performed slightly better on executive function tasks. The general conclusion of the research indicated that physical activity was associated with positive cognitive outcomes, especially in female participants (Hamer, Terrera, & Demakakos, 2018).

Similar research has also been conducted on older participants with specific maladies like Parkinson's disease. In a review of literature, Loprinzi and Frith (2018) studied if and how exercise might reduce the risk of contracting Parkinson's disease as well as the effect of exercise on the magnitude of symptoms among those with the disease. They concluded that exercise does appear to offer some protection against Parkinson's disease and this may be a function of the role of exercise in altering such factors as dopamine levels and inflammation. It was also determined that exercise enhanced memory, motor function, and psychological function while those who exercised also lived longer (Loprinzi & Frith, 2018).

Loprinzi and colleagues also conducted a systematic review of research to examine the overall effects of exercise on memory among adults who were mildly cognitively impaired. All studies employed experimental designs, and involved short- or long-term bouts of exercise. Eleven studies were included in the review with most showing a small to moderate effect on both short-term and long-term memory with exercise. These findings led the researchers to conclude that exercise can help improve memory in mildly cognitively impaired individuals. Thus, exercise is recommended and should be promoted among such patients (Loprinzi, Blough, Ryu, & Kang, 2018).

In general, considerable recent research indicates that physical activity enhances general well-being and life quality though some individual studies on very young children have not found that to be the case. Powerful meta-analytic studies, however, provide strong evidence that factors like self-esteem, self-efficacy, depression and cognitive factors like executive function and working memory in older adults are strongly linked to physical activity levels (Ehlers, Salerno, Aguiñaga, & McCauley, 2018). As we have seen in the research cited above, that relationship appears to be particularly stronger among older participants. Though recent research has substantially increased the understanding of the relationship between physical activity and cognitive function, much remains to be known regarding exact doses and types of activity required for these positive responses.

SUMMARY

- As motor and cognitive abilities develop, they uniquely facilitate or inhibit all other aspects of development. These abilities reciprocally interact at all times throughout the lifespan, significantly affecting motor and cognitive behavior.
- Jean Piaget was the most famous and prolific of all developmentalists. His theory concerning cognitive development—the most widely accepted theory in that area—proposes the sensorimotor, preoperational, concrete operational, and formal operational stages.
- The interaction between motor and cognitive development is particularly evident in the sensorimotor stage, which spans the first two years of life. This stage is characterized by "thinking by bodily movement," which suggests that actions created by the body enhance the cognitive process.
- Major accomplishments during the sensorimotor stage include the ability to differentiate between the self and others and

to recognize that objects continue to exist even though they are no longer in the visual field. Also, the child becomes capable of producing mental images that allow contemplation of the past and future, as well as the present.

- The main cognitive achievement during the preoperational stage is acquisition of language. This process is facilitated by rapidly improving manipulation and locomotor skills. These skills aid the child in exploring and understanding the environment, contributing to the child's ability to express related concepts verbally.
- The concrete operational stage is reached when the child develops the ability to decenter attention from one to two or more aspects of a problem-solving situation. This decentering skill is important in accurately planning and executing many movement activities.
- Piaget believed that the formal operational stage was the highest level of cognitive ability. In formal operations, the major cognitive landmark is the acquisition of the ability to think hypothetically—that is, to ponder the unreal. New cognitive abilities, such as interpropositional thought, may continue to enhance an individual's ability in strategic movement situations.
- Many experts disagree with Piaget's view that formal operations are the highest level of cognitive ability. These experts believe that cognitive development continues throughout adulthood, although they debate the specific nature of the change. Adulthood (postformal operations) is traditionally and stereotypically viewed as a time of cognitive decline; however, current evidence suggests that cognitive development depends not only on age but also on life experiences and demands.
- The typical age-related decline in split-second decision making seriously impairs performance in many movement activities. However, maintenance of an active, movement-oriented lifestyle may delay the onset and slow the rate of cognitive decline because movement activity increases cerebral blood flow and brings about other helpful physiological effects. Numerous studies on the relationship between motor skill development, movement expertise, and physical activity suggest a strong relationship between these factors and cognitive development across the lifespan. This relationship is so prevalent that many experts recommend these kinds of programs to enhance cognitive development through life, or at least, decrease the decrements that are particularly noticeable in later life.

key concept review

accommodation
adaptation
assimilation
clinical method
concrete operational stage
conservation
contextual perspective
declarative knowledge
exercise of reflexes
explicit memory
formal operational stage
hypothetical-deductive reasoning
implicit memory
interpropositional thought
intuitive
invention of new means through mental combinations
postformal operations
preconceptual
preoperational stage
primary circular reactions
procedural knowledge
secondary circular reactions
secondary schemata
sensorimotor stage
seriation
tertiary circular reactions
transductive reasoning

questions for reflection

1. What do we mean by the terms *adaptation, assimilation*, and *accommodation*? Define each and distinguish the differences among them.
2. Though Piaget's theory has been widely accepted, explain three criticisms one might raise against it.
3. In order, what are the substages of Piaget's sensorimotor stage of development? Characterize each.
4. What are the major developments of the sensorimotor stage of development?
5. What does Piaget mean by "thinking with the body"?
6. What are some potential relationships between motor development and children's cognitive ability in the preoperational stage of development?
7. What does Piaget mean by "interpropositional thought," and how is this concept important to development? How might it be important for motor development?
8. Name two theories that attempt to explain cognitive change throughout adulthood. What are the major characteristics of each? Which would you subscribe to and why?
9. What are the differences between explicit and implicit memory?
10. What are some differences between declarative knowledge and procedural knowledge, and how do they relate to sport performance?
11. How can improving motor skill development or physical activity levels help prevent age-related cognitive decline? What evidence exists to support this?

REFERENCES

Álvarez-Bueno, C., Pesce, C., Cavero-Redondo, I., Sánchez-López, M., Martínez-Hortelano, J.A., & Martínez-Vizcaíno, V. (2017a). The effect of physical activity interventions on children's cognition and metacognition: a systematic review and meta-analysis, *Journal of the American Academy of Child and Adolescent Psychiatry, 56*, 729–738.

Álvarez-Bueno, C., Pesce, C., Cavero-Redondo, I., Sánchez-López, M., Garrido-Miguel, M., & Martínez-Vizcaíno, V. (2017b). Academic achievement and physical activity: A meta-analysis. *Pediatrics*, doi: 10.1542/peds. 2017-1498.

Arlin, P. K. (1975). Cognitive development in adulthood: A fifth stage? *Developmental Psychology, 11*, 602–606.

Barrouillet, P., Corbin, L., Dagry, I., & Camos, V. (2014). An empirical test of the independence between declarative and procedural working memory in Oberauer's (2009) theory. *Psychonomic Bulletin and Review*, 1302–1317.

Bendayan, R., Piccinin, A. M., Hofer, S. M., Cadar, D., Johansson, B., & Muniz-Terrera, G. (2017). Decline in memory, visuospatial ability, and crystalized cognitive abilities in older adults: Normative aging or terminal decline? *Journal of Aging Research*, doi.org/10.1155/2017/6210105.

Berger, K. S. (2017). *Developing person through the lifespan*. 10th ed. New York: Worth.

Cameron, C. E., Cottone, E. A., Murrah, W. M., & Grissmer, D. W. (2016). How are motor skills linked to children's school performance and academic achievement? *Child Development Perspectives*, doi.org/10.1111/cdep.12168.

Chang, Y., Pan, C., Chen, F., Tsai, C., & Huang, C. (2012). Effect of resistance-exercise training on cognitive function in healthy older adults: A review. *Journal of Aging and Physical Activity*, doi.org/10.1123/japa.20.4.497.

De Greef, J. W., Bosker, R. J., Oosterlan, J., Visscher, C., & Hartman, E. (2018). Effects of physical activity on executive functions, attention and academic performance in preadolescent children: A meta-analysis. *Journal of Science and Medicine in Sport, 21*, 501–507.

Deng, S., Li, W., Ding, J., Wu, J., Zhang, Y., Li, F., et al. (2014). Understanding the mechanisms of cognitive impairments in developmental coordination disorder. *Pediatric Research, 75*, 210–216.

Ehlers, D. K., Salerno, E. A., Aguiñaga, S., & McCauley, E. (2018). Physical activity interventions: Effects on well-being outcomes in older adults. In E. Diener, S. Oishi, & L. Tay (Eds.), *Handbook of well-being*. Salt Lake City, UT: DEF Publishers. doi:nobashcolar.com.

Fernandes, V. R., Scipião Ribeiro, M. L., Melo, T., de Tarso Maciel-Pinheiro, P., Guimarães, T. T., Araújo, N.B., et al. (2016). Motor coordination correlates with academic achievement and cognitive function in children. *Frontiers in Psychology*, doi.org/10.3389/fpsyg.2016.00318.

Gajewski, P. D., & Falkenstein, M. (2016). Physical activity and neurocognitive functioning in aging: A condensed updated review. *European Review of Aging and Physical Activity*, doi.org/10.1186/s11556-016-0161-3.

Gatz, J., Kelly, A. M., & Clark, S. L. (2018). Improved executive function and science achievement for at-risk middle school girls in an aerobic fitness program. *The Journal of Early Adolescence*, doi.org/10.1177/02724316187707862018.

Gheysen, F., Poppe, L., DeSmet, A., Swinnen, S., Cardon, G., De Bourdeaudhuij, I., et al. (2018). Physical activity to improve cognition in older adults: can physical activity programs enriched with cognitive challenges enhance the effects? A systematic review and meta-analysis. *International Journal of Behavioral Nutrition and Physical Activity*, doi.org/10.1186/s12966-018-0697-x.

Hamer, M., Terrera, G., & Demakakos, P. (2018). Physical activity and trajectories in cognitive function: English Longitudinal Study of Ageing. *Journal of Epidemiology and Community Health*, doi.org/10.1136/jech-2017-210228.

Heppe, H., Kohler, A., Fleddermann, M.T., & Zentgraf, D. (2016). The relationship between expertise in sports, visuospatial, and basic cognitive skills. *Frontiers of Psychology*, doi.org/10.3389/fpsyg.2016.00904.

Hindin, S. B., & Zelinski, E. M. (2012). Extended practice and aerobic exercise interventions benefit untrained cognitive outcomes in older adults: A meta-analysis. *Journal of American Geriatrics Society*, 60, 136–141.

Howe, M. L. (2015). Memory development. In R. M. Lerner (Ed.), *Handbook of child psychology and developmental science*, 7th ed. New York: Wiley.

Imamizu, H. (2015). Changes in human brain networks caused by motor and cognitive learning. In K. Kansaku, L. G. Cohen, & N. Birbaumer (Eds.), *Clinical systems neuroscience*. New York: Springer.

Konijnenberg, C. & Fredriksen, P. (2018). The effects of a school-based physical activity intervention programme on children's executive control: The Health Oriented Pedagogical Project (HOPP). *Scandinavian Journal of Public Health*, doi.org/10.1177/1403494818767823.

Kramer, A.F., & Colcombe, S. (2018). Effects on the cognitive function of older adults: A meta-analytic study—Revisited. *Perspectives on Psychological Science*, doi.org/10.1177/1745691617707316.

Loprinzi, P. D., Blough, J., Ryu, S., & Kang, M. (2018). Experimental effects of exercise on memory function among mild cognitive impairment: Systematic review and meta-analysis. *The Physician and Sportsmedicine*, doi.org/10.1080/00913847.2018.1527647.

Loprinzi, P. D., & Frith, E. (2018). Memorcise in the context of Parkinson's disease. *Journal of Cognitive Enhancement*. doi.org/10.1007/s41465-018-0075-2.

Mann, D. T. Y., Williams, A. M., Ward, P., & Janelle, C. M. (2007). Perceptual-cognitive expertise in sport: A meta-analysis. *Journal of Sport and Exercise Psychology, 29*, 457–478.

Moreau, D., Morrison, A. B., & Conway, A. R. A. (2015). An ecological approach to cognitive enhancement: Complex motor training. *Acta Psychologica, 157*, 44–55, doi.org/10.1016/j.actpsy.2015.02.007.

Müller, N. C. J., Genzel, L., Konrad, B. N., Pawlowski, M., Neville, D., Fernández, G., et al. (2016). Motor skills enhance procedural memory formation and protect against age-related decline. *PLOS*, doi.org/10.1371/journal.pone.0157770.

Neumann, N., Lotze, M., & Eickhoff, S. B. (2016). Cognitive expertise: An ALE meta-analysis. *Human Brain Mapping*, 37, doi: 10.1002/hbm.23028.

Newman, B. M., & Newman, P. R. (2018). *Development through life: A psychosocial approach*. 13th ed. Boston: Cengage.

Northey, J. M., Cherbuin, N., Pumpa, K. L., Smee, D. J., & Rattray, B. (2018). Exercise interventions for cognitive function in adults older than 50: A systematic review with meta-analysis. *British Journal of Sports Medicine*, doi.org/10.1136/bjsports-2016-096587.

Peterson, K., Hahn, H., Lee, A. J., Madison, C. A., & Atri, A. (2016). In the Information Age, do dementia caregivers get the information they need? Semi-structured interviews to determine informal caregivers' education needs, barriers, and preferences. *BMC Geriatrics*, doi.org/10.1186/s12877-016-0338-7.

Peven, J.C., Grove, G. A., Jakicic, J. M., Alessi, M. G., & Erickson, K. I. (2018). Associations between short and long bouts of physical activity with executive function in older adults. *Journal of Cognitive Enhancement*, *2*, 137–145.

Piek, J. P., Dawson, L., Smith, L. M., & Gasson, N. (2008). The role of early fine and gross motor development on later motor and cognitive ability. *Human Movement Science*, *27*, 668–681.

Poon, L. W., & Harrington, C. A. (2006). Commonalities in aging and fitness-related impact on cognition. In L. W. Poon, W. Chodzko-Zajko, & P. D. Tomporowski (Eds.), *Active living, cognitive functioning and aging*. Champaign, IL: Human Kinetics.

Prakash, R. S., Voss, M. W., Erickson, K. I., & Kramer, A. F. (2015). Physical activity and cognitive vitality. *Annual Review of Psychology*, *66*, 769–797.

Prull, M. W., Gabrieli, J. D. E., & Bunge, S. A. (2000). Age-related changes in memory: A cognitive neuroscience perspective. In F. I. M. Craik & T. A. Salthouse (Eds.), *The handbook of aging and cognition*. Mahwah, NJ: Erlbaum.

Raine, L. B., Kao, S. C., Pindus, D., Westfall, D. R., Shigeta, T. T., Logan, N., et al. (2018). A large-scale reanalysis of childhood fitness and inhibitory control. *Journal of Cognitive Enhancement*, doi.org/10.1007/s41465-018-0070-7.

Rehfeld, K., Müller, P., Aye, N., Schmicker, M., Dordevic, M., Kaufmann, J., Hökelmann, A., & Müller, N.G. (2017). Dancing or fitness sport? The effects of two training programs on hippocampal plasticity and balance abilities in healthy seniors. *Frontiers in Human Neuroscience*, doi.org/10.3389/fnhum.2017.00305.

Roca, A., & Williams, A. M. (2016). Expertise and the interaction between different perceptual-cognitive skills: Implications for testing and training. *Frontiers of Psychology*, doi.org/10.3389/fpsyg.2016.00792.

Salthouse, T. (2012). Consequences of age-related cognitive declines. *Annual Review of Psychology*, *63*, 201–226.

Shaffer, D. R., & Kipp, K. (2014). *Developmental psychology: Childhood and adolescence*. 9th ed. Boston: Cengage.

Sigelman, C. K., & Rider, E. A. (2018). *Life-span human development*. 9th ed. Boston: Cengage.

Spirduso, W. W., Poon, L. W., & Chodzko-Zajko, W. (2008). Using resources and reserves in an exercise-cognition model. In W. W. Spirduso, L. W. Poon, & W. Chodzko-Zajko (Eds.), *Exercise and its mediating effects on cognition*. Champaign, IL: Human Kinetics.

Tandon, P. S., Klein, M., Saelens, B. E., Christakis, D. A., Marchese, A .J., & Lengua, L. (2018). Short term impact of physical activity vs. sedentary behavior on preschoolers' cognitive functions. *Mental Health and Physical Activity*, *15*, 17–21.

Vestberg, T., Gustafson, R., Maurex, L., Martin, I., & Petrovic, P. (2012). Executive functions predict the success of top-soccer players. *PLoS One*, doi:10.1371/journal.pone.0034731.

Voss, M. W., Kramer, A. F., Basak, C., Prakash, R. S., & Roberts, B. (2010). Are expert athletes "expert" in the cognitive laboratory? A meta-analytic review of cognition and sport expertise. *Applied Cognitive Psychology*, *24*, 812–826.

Walle, E. A., & Campos, J. J. (2014). Infant language is related to acquisition of walking. *Developmental Psychology*, *50*, 336–348.

Willoughby, M.T., Wylie, A.C., & Catellier, D.J. (2018). Testing the association between physical activity and executive function skills in early childhood. *Early Childhood Research Quarterly*, *44*, 82–89.

Zacks, R. T., Hasher, L., & Li, K. Z. H. (2000). Human memory. In F. I. M. Craik & T. A. Salthouse (Eds.), *The handbook of aging and cognition*. Mahwah, NJ: Erlbaum.

3 SOCIAL AND MOTOR DEVELOPMENT

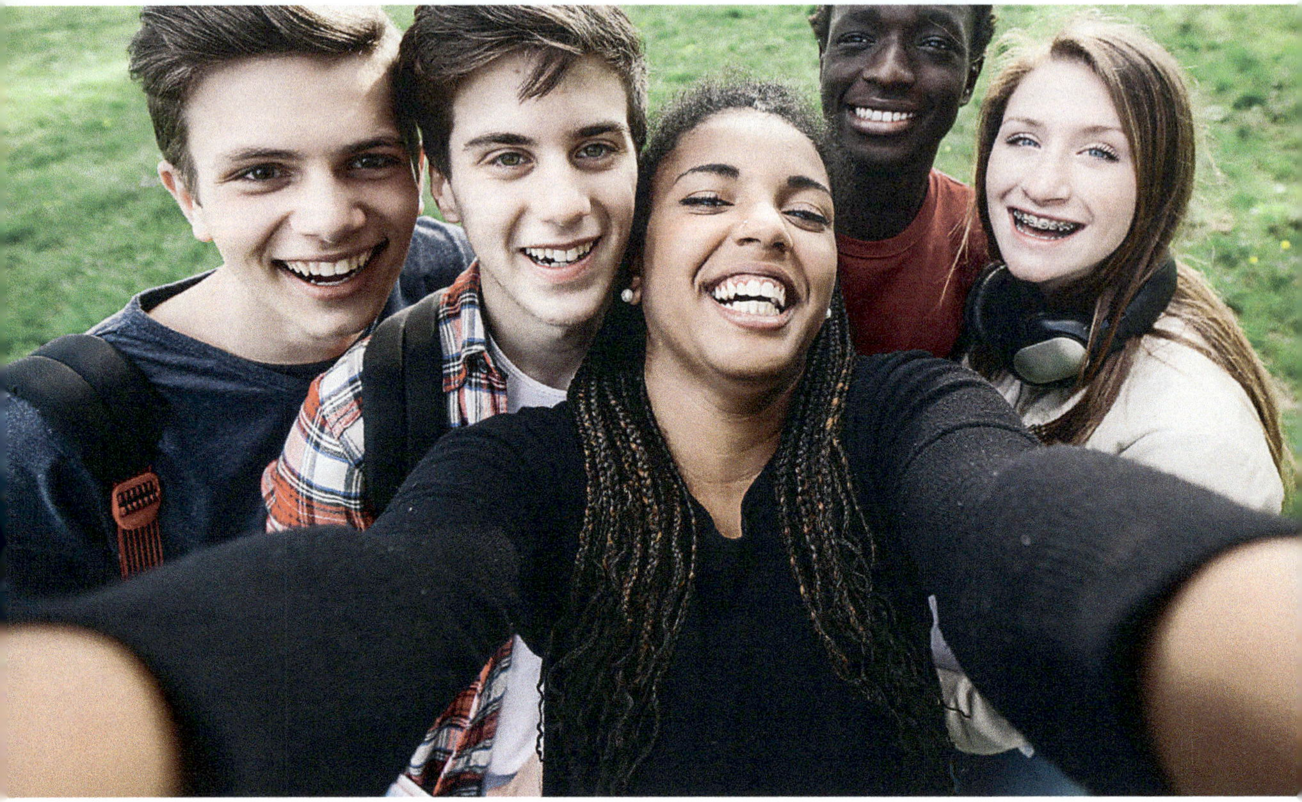

Chapter Objectives

From the information presented in this chapter, you will be able to

- Define socialization
- Explain self-esteem development and its relationship to physical activity and motor development
- Describe the main social influences affecting motor development during infancy
- Describe the main social influences affecting motor development during childhood
- Describe the main social influences affecting motor development during older childhood and adolescence
- Describe the main social factors affecting motor development in adulthood
- Draw a diagram and explain the exercise-aging cycle
- Explain how to delay the exercise-aging cycle

Although the somewhat arbitrary classification of human functioning into the cognitive, affective, motor, and physical domains facilitates discussion of human development, it does not produce a realistic portrayal of the person. Human behavior is *not* compartmentalized; there is a complex system of constant, reciprocal exchange among an individual's cognitive, affective, motor, and physical aspects. That which affects an individual in one domain is bound to have a subsequent effect in all other domains, as well. For example, Chapter 2 emphasized the strong relationship between human intellectual function and movement: intellectual change is often accompanied by changes in motor function. In addition, memory can be considered, in part, a social process because it involves the construction of knowledge through social interaction as well as interaction of past actions in communications with others. Thus, memory, a cognitive function is closely intertwined with social interaction (Carpendale & Lewis, 2015) as well as motor development. Through socialization we experience interactions and acquire tools to help us organize and refine our thinking. Many of these changes are so subtle that they are of no obvious consequence in a person's life, but other changes produce tremendous effects and may have lifelong implications for human movement, as well as for social, emotional, and physical well-being.

This chapter examines another reciprocal relationship of particular importance to human motor development: social behavior and movement. Social behavior affects a person's movement behavior; conversely, motor behavior equally affects an individual's social development.

SOCIALIZATION

According to Coakley (2017):

> Socialization is a process of learning and social development, which occurs as we interact with one another and become familiar with social worlds. It involves forming ideas about who we are and what is important in our lives. We are *not* simply passive learners in this process. We actively participate in our own socialization as we form relationships and are influenced by others at the same time as we influence them. We actively interpret what we see and hear, and we accept, resist, and revise messages that we receive from others about who we are and how we are connected with social worlds. Therefore, socialization is not simply a one-way process of being molded and shaped by our social environment. Instead, it is an interactive process through which we make decisions about our relationships, our interpretation of information that comes to us through interaction, and what we will say and do.
>
> (p. 52)

Socialization is an active process of forming relationships and learning from those with whom we interact as we teach them. It is a process of engagement with others in our society that requires the synthesis of the new information gained, decision making about those ideas, and use of that information to shape our lives and, subsequently, the lives of others (see Figure 3.1). Though socialization is generally associated with learning that occurs through social interactions, it can include any means by which a person gathers information about society, and it generally includes the entire process of becoming a human being. Common means of socialization include observation, inference, modeling, and trial and error, but the most important is social interaction.

The influence of others around us is extremely important in determining how and when we acquire certain movement abilities. Our social circle is also an integral part in

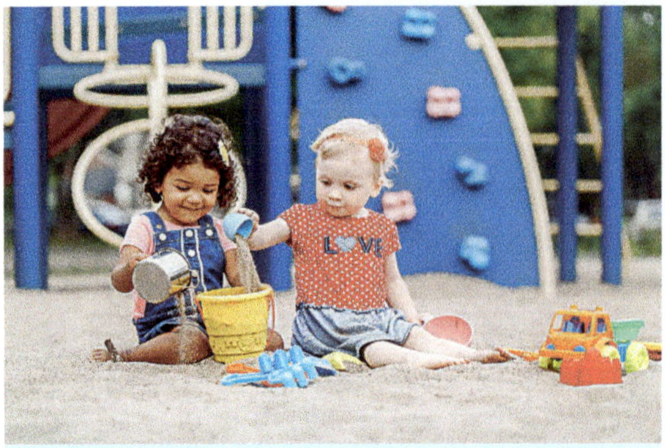

Figure 3.1 Socialization helps us learn who we are and how we are connected to our world

determining which movement activities we choose. The amount of social support supplied by significant others in our lives is positively associated with the extent of our participation in physical activity. Researchers have determined that parents, caregivers in general, siblings, teachers, coaches, and friends can all have varying amounts of influence on the choices we make concerning physical activity. In turn, the movement activities we choose affect our ability to "fit in" socially, depending on the compatibility of our choices with dominant social values. Our movement choices also affect our self-identity, social mobility, educational achievement, attitudes concerning masculinity and femininity, and even moral development (e.g., attitudes about cheating and fair play).

Although often associated with development during childhood, socialization is a lifelong process, facilitating a person's functioning within society throughout childhood, adolescence, and adulthood. Furthermore, as mentioned earlier, even though the term is commonly associated with the learning that occurs through social interaction, socialization can include any means by which a person gathers information about society. Nevertheless, the most important means of learning societal rules and expectations is through social interaction, which is also true for learning human movement. The influence of others is extremely important in determining how and when an individual acquires certain movements, as well as which movements are acquired.

The process of socialization teaches the members of society their social roles. A **social role** is "a special position an individual possesses within a network, which indicates his or her behaviours, expectations, and responsibilities" (Abnar, Takaffoli, Rabbany, & Zafane, 2014, p. 289). There are many social roles in any society. The occupational role of, say, a professor, healthcare provider, or police officer is defined by specific expected behaviors. Family roles can be illustrated by a mother or a father, who is expected to exhibit certain behaviors relative to the rest of the family and society. Society's role expectations tremendously influence human motor development. A particular movement may or may not be acquired, depending on whether individuals believe that movement to be role appropriate. In other words, is it a movement that individuals assume to be appropriate for what they consider their role in society?

The set of expectations about behavior is formally called a **norm**. Norms are shared and stable perceptions held by a society regarding appropriate or inappropriate behaviors within a specific context (Popa, Phillips, & Robertson, 2014). Societal norms can facilitate or inhibit an individual's movement development, depending on the person's perspective on the norms. For example, in many areas of the United States, the norm is to expect less of older adults, so many older adults indeed do expect less of themselves. They are inhibited or constrained by the societal norm concerning their age group. As another example, the norm for male adolescents regarding physical activity is vigorous involvement in movement pursuits, to the extent that a young male's social success may depend on his athletic prowess. Both of these examples are examined more thoroughly later in this chapter.

SELF-ESTEEM DEVELOPMENT AND PHYSICAL ACTIVITY

One extremely important human characteristic affected by social interaction and physical activity is **self-esteem**, how much we believe ourselves to be competent, successful, significant, and worthy, or how much we like ourselves. Other terms often used interchangeably with self-esteem include *self-concept, self-worth, self-schema, self-perception, self-acceptance, self-like, self-love, self-respect*, and *self-regard* (Pestana, 2015). Simply stated, self-esteem is the value we place on ourselves as individuals. It is one of the most important aspects of self-development and generally begins to emerge in early childhood (Berk, 2018). It is influenced by factors such as age, maturity, interactions with other people, the context of a situation, and, of course, our culture in general.

According to Pestana (2015), self-esteem is learned and can be modified. In fact, though somewhat consistent, it is constantly evolving. Furthermore, Pestana believes it can consist of "subselves" based on different aspects of a person's life. For example, a child can also be a brother or sister, a cousin, and even an aunt or uncle all at one time. Later, that same person can become a parent. Similarly, a teacher may also be a coach, a parent, an aunt or uncle, and even a grandparent. Together, all these selves and the individual's perception of each contribute to the person's global, or overall, self-esteem. Global self-esteem is strongly tied to our feelings of closeness to or acceptance by those who are significant in our lives, such as our peers, our siblings, and our primary caregivers. Peer acceptance, in particular, is critical during adolescence and early adulthood, when attachment to caregivers may wane (Birkeland, Breivik, & Wold, 2014).

Research on Self-Esteem and Physical Activity

Self-esteem has been widely studied, with most researchers finding it to be affected significantly by involvement in physical activity. So much research has been conducted on this subject over the years that Gruber (1985) was able to conduct a classic meta-analysis. He found 84 articles, 27 of which offered sufficient data for use in his meta-analysis. Of those 27 studies, 18 found physical activity to affect self-concept or self-esteem significantly. Overall, Gruber determined that, in the studies he examined, 66 percent of the children who participated in physical education or directed-play situations exceeded the self-concept or self-esteem scores of the children in non-physical activity settings. Physical activity programs with physical fitness objectives were found to be particularly beneficial for the children studied.

Gruber also determined that children with emotional disturbances, certain types of intellectual disability, perceptual disabilities, or economic disadvantages and who were physically active exhibited a mean self-concept score much higher than the scores of similar groups of children who were physically inactive. Gruber suggested that active children, in particular, begin to feel important when they are allowed opportunities for involvement in programs of motor enrichment that are conducted by trained and supportive professionals. The greatest gains in self-esteem were, therefore, found in those children who most needed it, though typically developing children also exhibited an improvement.

In conclusion, Gruber stated that involvement in directed play or physical education can enhance self-esteem in children, though it is not clear why. Perhaps the distraction itself is sufficient to increase self-esteem. Some researchers have hypothesized a physiological change. The physical activity could affect endorphins or monoamine (a brain neurotransmitter), which, in turn, would alter a child's affective state. In general, Gruber believed these findings to be critical because improvements in self-image greatly affect future behavior.

In similar research, Piek, Baynam, and Barrett (2006) examined the relationship between self-perceptions and both fine and gross motor development in children (7.5 to 11 years) and adolescents (12 to 15.5 years). This research was prompted by the findings of previous research examining individuals who had exhibited problems in motor coordination. In these individuals, difficulties were noted in the performance of routine gross movements such as running and jumping, as well as common fine movements such as buttoning clothing and brushing hair. Movement difficulties like these can affect the way children are perceived socially and greatly diminish their feelings of self-worth. Children who have these movement difficulties tend to avoid activities where the difficulties can be observed. As we will discuss later in this chapter, most people gravitate toward movements where they experience success and shy away from those where their ability is limited. This can create a negative cycle of inactivity, where a person's aversion leads to nonparticipation. In turn, the nonparticipation reduces opportunities for experience and practice and further impairs movement ability, even affecting a person's physique or body image. Evidence indicates that children as young as 5 years old may gauge their level of performance against that of their peers, potentially leading to loss of confidence and subsequent performance decrements at an early age (Piek et al., 2006).

Piek and colleagues (2006) specifically examined some of these phenomena in their study of children with and without developmental coordination disorder (DCD), by using a scale designed to measure fine and gross motor development. The items measured included jumping and balance skills, as well as skills more related to fine movement, such as placing beads in a box or on a rod. The researchers also measured self-perception through a scale involving items such as scholastic competence, physical appearance, athletic competence, and behavioral conduct. Results indicated that children with DCD performed more poorly on the motor tasks than their age-matched counterparts. They were also found to achieve lower scores on measures of scholastic and athletic competence, as well as on their perceptions of their own appearance and behavior. According to the authors, these findings are similar to those of previous research where children and adolescents with relatively low levels of motor development were found to be at risk for behavioral, emotional, and even social problems (Piek et al., 2006).

According to these authors, these findings were expected. The expectation that poor motor ability will correspond to a variety of negative outcomes is especially true in the area of scholastic competence, where fine movements such as handwriting play an important role. By comparison, gross motor performance was not found to affect scholastic competence, though it affected athletic competence. Interestingly, older participants (adolescents) in the study were more likely to score low on perceptions of their athletic ability, a very important component of social status, especially among boys. Self-worth was found to be affected by both scholastic and athletic competence, though boys were much more impacted by athletic competence than by scholastic competence. Athletic competence was found to be similarly important for boys with and without DCD, indicating how important this disorder can be in affecting the development of self-worth and the social and emotional development of boys.

Girls demonstrated a stronger link between scholastic competence and fine motor development; however, for girls with DCD, their (low) perceptions of athletic competence were found to contribute significantly to their feelings of self-worth. In short, movement ability seems to be an important factor related to social and emotional development (Piek et al., 2006).

Development of Self-Esteem

Harter (1988) determined that self-esteem evolves developmentally in a series of somewhat predictable steps.

Early Childhood

Harter (1988) found that young children are incapable of making meaningful and consistent judgments about their **global self-worth**, the overall value that a person places on himself or herself as a person. They can, however, make reliable judgments about such elements of self-worth as cognitive and social competence and their own behavioral conduct, though they cannot accurately distinguish between them. Harter contends that young children also cannot distinguish between their competency in cognitive and in physical skills. This does not mean that young children do not have a sense of self-worth. Rather, they simply have difficulty expressing it verbally because of their limited cognitive capabilities.

Mid- to Late Childhood

Harter (1988) believes the ability of children to express their sense of self-worth improves at mid-childhood because their cognitive capabilities increase. Around 8 years of age, children can begin to verbalize their feelings of self-worth and make judgments about their own self-esteem. Furthermore, between the ages of 8 and 12, children develop the ability to distinguish among scholastic and athletic competence, peer social acceptance, physical appearance, and their own behavioral conduct.

Adolescence and Young Adulthood

Harter (1988) notes that adolescents are capable of even greater articulation and discrimination concerning the elements of self-worth. They can distinguish all the same elements as before, with the addition of close friendships, romantic appeal, and job competence. This process of development continues with college students, in whom more distinctions are exhibited. In addition to global self-worth, Harter believed the college-age individual can differentiate and articulate twelve elements of self-worth: scholastic competence, intellectual ability, creativity, job competence, athletic competence, physical appearance, romantic appeal, peer social acceptance, close friendships, parent relationships, sense of humor, and morality. Interestingly, Harter indicated that individuals in this age group clearly distinguish between scholastic competence, intellectual ability, and creativity. For college students, self-worth was a function of their perceived competence in the areas that had become most important to them personally.

As in all other groups, young adults' global self-worth was most affected by their self-appraisal of their own physical appearance and social acceptance. These elements were followed in importance by intimate relations and sociability. Intelligence and adequacy as a provider were also found to be important contributors in young adults. The two least important elements of self-worth for young adults were household management and athletic ability (Harter, 1988).

Adulthood

The adult has developed a need to distinguish additional elements of self-esteem or self-worth. Specifically, these include intimate relationships, nurturance, adequacy as a provider, and household management. The elements mentioned for younger age groups continue to be significant. This need for new elements among each additional age group implies a developmental change in individuals' self-esteem as they mature (Harter, 1988).

Harter also noted that, for each age group, certain elements of self-esteem contribute more or less than others to global self-worth. Physical appearance and social acceptance were the most important elements contributing to the global self-worth of elementary school children. In fact, surprisingly, these two elements of self-worth were the two most important for all age groups. For adolescents, parent and classmate support were also major contributors to global self-worth, followed by friend and teacher support. Harter expressed some surprise at the contribution of parent support for adolescents, who are generally believed to be gradually increasing their reliance on peers and decreasing their reliance on parents.

Like Gruber, Harter (1988) believed findings relative to self-worth or self-esteem are significant. She specifically noted the pervasive effect of self-worth on an individual's mood or affective state. Individuals with higher levels of self-worth are more cheerful and exude higher levels of energy, whereas low self-esteem has a depressing effect on behavior. No doubt, these mood alterations could have at least an indirect effect on motor development. The depressing effect of low self-esteem could translate to a lack of desire to participate in physical activity, which would, in turn, inhibit the practice necessary to develop certain movement skills. Conversely, successful attainment of certain levels of motor development likely has a reciprocal effect on self-concept. The feeling of accomplishment in movement or the simple act of participation, as illustrated by Gruber's research, can positively affect a person's self-concept.

SOCIAL INFLUENCES ON MOTOR DEVELOPMENT

As we discussed in Chapter 2 and earlier in this chapter, motor development is in constant interaction with other aspects of our development. Chapter 2 specifically examined how cognitive development affects motor development, and, importantly, how motor development affects cognitive development. A similar reciprocal relationship exists between motor development and social development. As we will see in the following discussion, the nature of that relationship evolves with an individual's age.

Infancy

The first year of life is often considered egocentric or asocial (Berk, 2018). Although the infant becomes increasingly social during that first year and on into adulthood, the baby's first few months of life involve relatively limited social interaction (see Figure 3.2). Because the baby relies on the caregiver, any social interactions at this time depend largely on the caregiver's whims. If an interaction occurs, it is generally a result of the caregiver's initiation. However, some social ties do form early in infancy. During this period infants attempt to maintain some form of contact with their objects of attachment, such as by visual exchange or through reciprocal touch, and will often express distress when the object of attachment leaves or is absent. Early social attachment is also seen in the fact that infants distinguish and differentially respond to their caregivers. Something as simple as a gesture, like pointing with the index finger, is a relatively simple, but important, motor skill developed through socialization as an initial step to communicating an idea. Interestngly, this is an area that has received considerable research attention as it indicates that infants now know to expect certain responses in

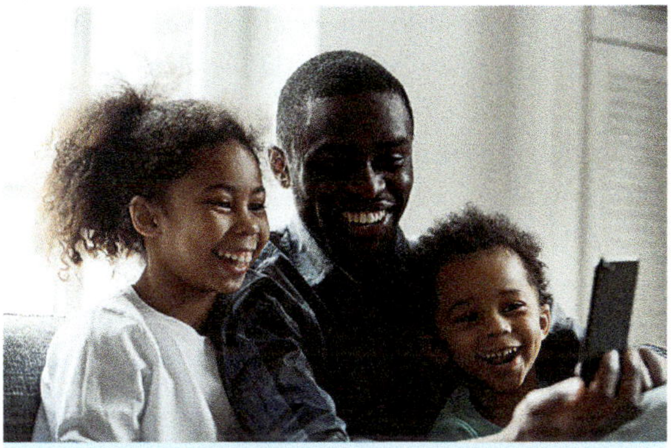

Figure 3.2 Infants have very few social ties, but the strong family relationship created during infancy can significantly affect their motor development

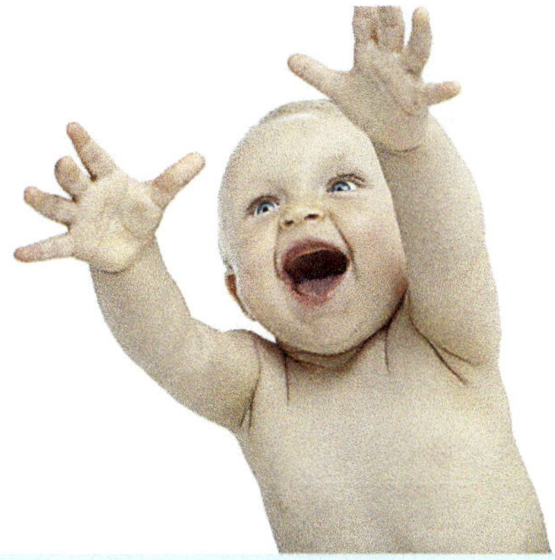

Figure 3.3 Gaining control of the arms and hands enables infants to respond manually to social touches

certain situations. They realize a point can indicate a nearby object or a direction. Though pointing is pervasive in western cultures, it is not a world-wide phenomenon as it is considered impolite in some cultures where using the lips or a head nod would be similarly learned at this time of life (Carpendale & Lewis, 2015).

According to Newman and Newman (2018), the formation of social attachment during infancy occurs in four stages. These stages are particularly worthy of our examination because of movement's apparent role in facilitating social attachment. According to these researchers, initially the infant grasps, sucks, roots, and performs numerous other infant reflexes. The infant also visually tracks, gazes, cries, and smiles in an effort to initiate and maintain close social contact with the object of attachment. These behaviors are all prominently involved in the social attachment process up to the age of approximately 3 months and are critical elements in the formation of the bond between the child and the caregiver.

During the next three months, the baby rapidly progresses in distinguishing between strangers and familiar human figures. In the third stage, from around 7 months to 2 years, the baby becomes increasingly adept at locomotion; this newfound ability enables the baby actively to seek close physical proximity with the object(s) of attachment. In the fourth stage (see Figure 3.3), the baby gradually gains control of the arms and hands, allowing him or her to pursue and manually respond to social touches.

Thus, the infant's newly developing movement activities facilitate and expand social interaction, and the child's increasing social sophistication promotes and stimulates greater motor activity. The expanded social repertoire allows the baby to be more actively involved with the environment, further enhancing her or his motor abilities, as well as the infant's intellectual and emotional behaviors.

Childhood

Although social interrelationships are limited during infancy because babies lack social, intellectual, and motor abilities, the social influences expand throughout childhood. Many specific forces contribute to a child's social development and, therefore, motor development. The family, specifically the parents or primary caregivers, is the primary socializing agency during childhood. Although the magnitude of the family's effect may be diminishing because of present cultural trends,

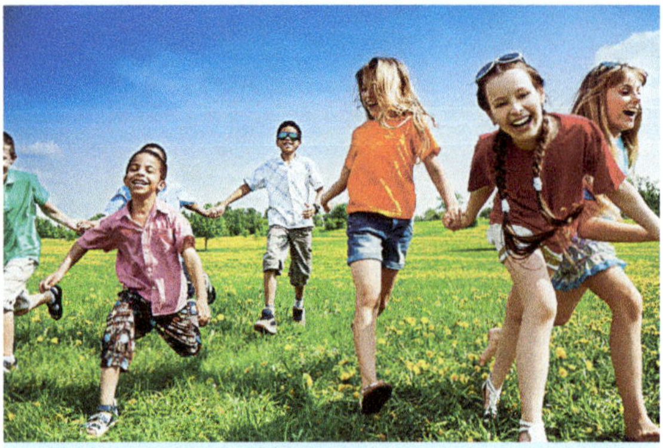

Figure 3.4 Play is crucial to learning the rules of society and many skills critical to functioning in that society

the family still exerts more influence on a child than does any other force. Play, whether the child engages in it alone or in the presence of others, is another major socializing force during childhood (see Figure 3.4). Pleasurable activity is considered important to the development of such skills as problem solving, creativity, and language, and of many movements in general. In addition, teachers, coaches, siblings, peer groups, and even the media are other important socializing agents as we grow up (Grusec & Davidov, 2015).

Influence of Family

As mentioned, the family is the most important socializing force in the lives of most children (see Figure 3.5). The family is also the earliest and, in most cases, greatest determinant of a child's movement choices and movement success because it strongly influences the child's attitudes and expectations about movement. Parents have even been described as being "biologically prepared" to be socializing forces as they are inherently attracted to remain close to the child (Grusec & Davidov, 2015, p. 159). Most societies tacitly assign this caregiving role to parents or guardians, in addition to the role of controlling important elements of a child's early life (e.g., financial resources, transportation, environment). Furthermore, the family is largely responsible for the role that children envision for themselves. Depending on the family's views concerning physical activity, for example, a child may or may not assume a role that is movement-related. In fact, a child can even acquire many movement characteristics that are reminiscent of those of the caregivers. When a caregiver is of the same sex as the child the influence on such movement acquisition is increased, although caregivers of both genders exert remarkable influence in shaping the child's movement idiosyncrasies involving, for example, gesture, gait, or posture (see Figure 3.6). The child can acquire these movement habits from long-term observation of the caregiver.

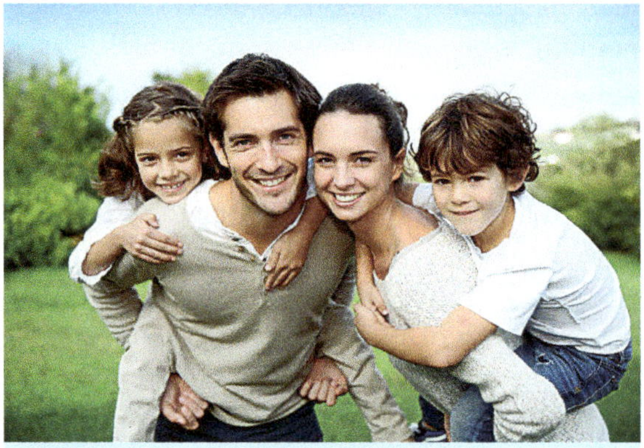

Figure 3.5 Family is the most important socializing force in the lives of most children

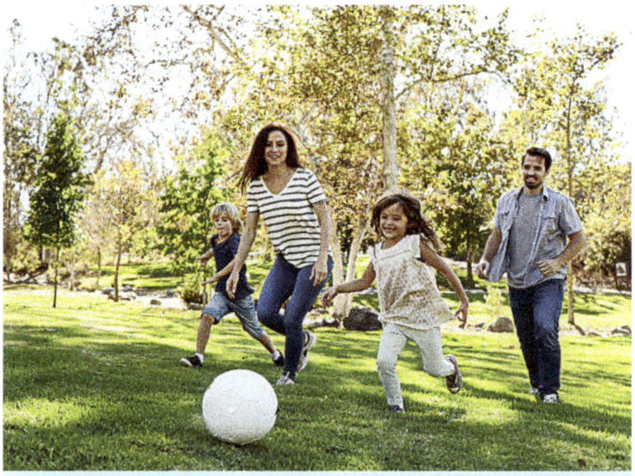

Figure 3.6 Although all caregivers help shape a child's movement repertoire, a caregiver of the same sex is often most influential

In a powerful review of the factors that affect involvement in physical activity in childhood through adulthood, researchers analyzed numerous studies on this topic, including the influence of the family. They determined that the social environment, family included, clearly contributes to the level of an individual's physical activity. For children, gender was a factor, especially for children from 4 to 9 years of age, when boys were likely to be more active than girls. This trend continued in later childhood, though it was less powerful, and gender was even less a factor among adolescents, though still well correlated. Ethnicity was also a factor, with the "white ethnic" group being most active. Importantly, individuals' confidence in their own ability was strongly tied to their likelihood of being active, as was their previous experience in physical activity. Clearly, both of these factors can be influenced within the family structure. Thus, for both children and adolescents, family support was found to be important to their likelihood of being active (Bauman, Reis, Sallis, et al., 2012).

In the same study, for adults, strong correlates with physical activity were individuals' confidence in their own ability, their health, and their personal history in physical activity. Age, gender, education level, and overall social support were also found to affect an individual's likelihood of leading an active lifestyle: a wealthy, young adult male would have the highest likelihood of being physically active. Adults were found to be less active if they experienced stress, job strain, or were working long hours. As with children, having social support, especially from the family, was consistently important for maintaining a physically active lifestyle. Among environmental factors, transportation and access to recreational facilities were critical. According to the authors of this research, knowing and understanding all the correlates are important in determining proper interventions to increase overall physical activity in our society (Bauman et al., 2012).

In a similar though more specific study on the effect of parenting on children's sport participation in the United Kingdom, Downward, Hallmann, and Pawlowski (2014) found parental influence to have substantial effects on children's decisions to participate in sports. This was especially notable for the male parent and his effect on male children. Mothers were also found to have an effect on male children, though less than the father's. Female children were influenced by their mother's attitude, but the effect was relatively mild compared to parental effects on male children. In general, the authors concluded that parental promotion of sport activity is effective in developing a positive attitude toward sport participation in children and would even increase the children's likelihood of participating later in life.

The family's approval or disapproval of a child's movement endeavors is also crucial in determining the child's future movement habits. If a child is rewarded, either overtly or subtly, for motoric behavior, he or she is likely to reproduce that behavior. However, behavior that is ignored or that receives negative responses may subside. Therefore, the family can consciously or subconsciously shape children's movement behavior and become one of the most potent of socializing institutions.

Recognizing the important role parents play in the development of their children, Erkelenz, and colleagues (2014) studied the relationship between the level of a parent's physical activity and the child's physical activity level, body mass index, and likelihood of participating in an organized youth sports program. Over 1600 boys and girls, averaging approximately 7 years of age, were included in the study in Germany. Though little association was determined between parental and child physical activity levels, children were more likely to be involved in youth sports programs, if their parents were more active. In addition, offspring of more active parents tended to have lower BMI and were not as prone to being overweight or obese. The child's incidence of being overweight was reduced even more, if both parents were physically active. Contrary to previous studies, the association between parental and child physical activity was not significant. This led the researchers to presume that the parents' support for physical activity during childhood may be more important than the parent actually modeling the active lifestyle. Of interest, the activity level of the mothers in the study had a particularly strong association with their children's likelihood of participation in youth sports programs. The research team posited that this may be a function of mothers being generally responsible for organizing their children's sports (e.g., knowing the schedules, providing transportation, assuring that they arrive on time) and providing overall logistical support. Another interesting finding from this research was that the children of active parents were more likely to be involved in organized sports, but were not necessarily more physically active. This, of course, could call into question the physical activity levels of the sports practices. Perhaps they failed to achieve levels advised from published physical activity guidelines. Nevertheless, the strong association between parental physical activity levels, lower BMI, and greater youth sports participation in their children emphasizes the importance of parental activity and how it might be used in future intervention programs (Erkelenz et al., 2014).

The Influence of Play

People of all ages, especially children, engage in **play**. The word evokes images of individuals engaged in some pleasurable, generally movement-oriented activity. The American Academy of Pediatrics, in a postion statement on toys and play, indicate that play is broadly beneficial to a child's development being essential to cognitive, physical, social, and emotional well-being (Healey & Mendelsohn, 2019). It can also be important in reducing toxic stress that can interfere with typical development while having a positive influence on social skill, listening and attending abilities, self-regulation, and ability to solve verbal disputes. In addition, it is important for school readiness and broadening the imagination. Through play, health can also be enhanced a number of ways. For example, the increased physical activity incurred through play can help in weight maintenance, improve endurance and immune function, decrease fatigue, reduce the incidence of injury, and improve coordination, agility, balance, strength and flexibility. It also offers wonderful opportunities for parents to interact with their children (Yogman et al., 2018). It has such a profound developmental effect that play is often considered essential for optimal development.

Though experts disagree and struggle to define play, several criteria characterize the activity. It is generally believed to be repetitive, spontaneous, voluntary, and fun. Furthermore, the motivation to play is intrinsic and often involves active participation by the player.

Play obviously varies by culture and is believed to be evolving with time with many children today engaging in more structured play than in years past. Examples here would include playing with LEGO, that may come with pre-established plans for construction, as opposed to simple wooden building blocks. Similarly, pre-schools were once more oriented toward play and social skill development, whereas many contemporary parents seek programs that are geared toward academics like reading and math readiness. Finally, so much more play today is driven by electronic devices whereby the physical aspect, or gross motor component, of play would be greatly reduced. Researchers have yet to fully determine how these kinds of changes affect development (Lillard, 2015).

Play can be categorized in many ways. General categories, however, may include object, rough and tumble (or physical), outdoor, and guided play. **Object play** is where the child explores or interacts with an object and often learns from this interaction. Rough and tumble play is more action or physically oriented and facilitates gross motor development, communication, negotiating skill, emotional stability, cooperation, and generally promotes a healthy active lifestyle. Similarly, outdoor play is important for many of these same characteristics as well as cognitive and language skills. Guided play is an activity that is shaped by an adult or older supervisor like a teacher or sibling. Guided play can generate opportunities for the child to interact positively with older individuals while more self-directed or free play is useful in helping the child determine their own personal preferences and interests as well as exploration skills (Yogman, Garner, Hutchinson, Hirsh-Pasek, & Michnick Golinkoff, 2018).

Other types of play include **interpersonal play** where the child plays with another individual. In **exploratory play**, children often examine and explore the detailed characteristics (such as size, shape, texture, and color) of objects, such as toys, in their environment. **Pretend play** finds the child creating imaginary representations with objects in the environment. For example, a round toy may be imagined as a rock or a turtle. Later the child may think of a small end table as a cabin or a cave. Play becomes increasingly sophisticated as children progress in their intellectual, social, and motor skills. Improvements in language ability will enhance children's play opportunities, especially interpersonal play with family members or friends. Choices regarding types of play, toys, or even play partners are highly individual and often determined by the child's gender or cultural background (Sumaroka & Bornstein, 2008).

The importance of play. Although play is often seen as an insignificant act, in reality, it is a crucial part of learning the rules of society, as well as many skills critical to functioning in that society. According to Henricks (2015), play is an important "vehicle for personal development" (p. 2) that allows the participant to experience new roles, distinguish the self from others, restore energy, and expand the imagination. It is a valuable tool for language development and is characterized by the positive emotions attached to it. Burghardt (2015) describes play as generally nonserious, rewarding, and done in a relaxed setting where the participants feel safe psychologically. It is seemingly nonfunctional, though, as mentioned above, it is integral to language, as well as social, motor, and overall cognitive development. Play clearly is important for us to learn our place in the social order, and it fosters cooperation among members of society. Importantly, because play is so often movement-oriented, it also enhances physical fitness (Burghardt, 2015) and is a key component in developing important motor skills.

In a study on the topic of play, Greve, Thomsen, and Dehio (2014) noted that the cognitive and emotional benefits of play during childhood have been well established over the years. In their research, they tested the long-term effects of childhood play on developmental "success" later in life. Adult participants were asked to recollect their play experiences during childhood, and these were compared to the subjects' current developmental status, mostly in terms of social success. The findings indicated that free play during childhood was a strong indicator of adaptability in adulthood and led to flexibility in adult goal setting. Generally, childhood play provided "developmental resources" for an individual to succeed as an adult.

The importance of play was further supported by a recent report from the American Academy of Pediatrics. This report proclaimed that play is an "essential" element in a child's learning. Generally, parents and other caregivers are the ones who create or mold the play experiences for very young children. Often, this is done with the help of toys. According to Healey et al. and the American Academy of Pediatrics (2019), toys should be carefully selected because they can be instrumental in a child's development. This is particularly important given that electronic media and various technological toys have replaced more traditional and personal interactions between the child and the caregiver. This holds the potential for impacting social, cognitive, language, and motor development of the child. Though toys can provide a supplement to the parent-child interaction leading up to or within play, they should never substitute for warm, caring, loving attention from the parent or caregiver. The right toy, however, can enhance the bond between the child and the caregiver by creating a means for additional social interaction. Child-caregiver relationships involving play are instrumental in early brain development, mastery of play activities, self-esteem, and the development of play-related skills. Toys employed during gross motor play (e.g., balls) can enhance gross motor development, social interrelationships, and social skills like the negotiations involving rules of game. In short, the AAP indicates that the "best" toys are ones that are most conducive to the child's developmental status while encouraging the acquisition of new skills (Yogman et al., 2018).

Obviously, play is often movement-oriented. When movement, such as running, jumping, or even clapping or laughing, is involved, the pleasurable aspects of play are most clearly visible. In fact, one of the first forms of amusement for a child may involve being jostled or hoisted by a caregiver. Gradually, children become more involved with other children and expand their play experiences. Play appears to evolve through a series of increasingly social stages until it reaches a point of group involvement. Group play becomes particularly evident at early school age.

Development of play. The first signs of play are seen during infancy as early as six weeks of age with babies socially smiling and mimicking sounds. Initially, it involves various reciprocal interactions with parents and other family members. It can include babbling and peek-a-boo games and eventually evolves into more gross motor play involving hopping, skipping, running. The early reciprocal actions with caregivers contribute to important developmental qualities like self-regulation, impulse control, and general understanding of social exchanges. It is essential for language development, both verbal and non-verbal (Yogman et al., 2018).

Historically, a number of experts have described the changes in play behavior that take place across childhood. Piaget, discussed in detail in Chapter 2, described what he called "practice play" as being most common during infancy and toddlerhood. In this type of play, similar actions are repeated with toys or other objects. The repetition evolves and becomes more complex as new components are added. For children between 4 and 7 years of age, Piaget described "pretence play," in which interaction with peers, or even adults, becomes more common. Pretence play often involves fantasy play, where children focus their play on creating a world that is more sensible and meaningful to them than the "real" world (e.g., a large box becomes a spaceship, or a blanket draped over furniture becomes a fortress). Pretence play often evolves into the use of toy figures, dolls, or other toys that are integrated into the child's pretend world. From here, according to Piaget, play gradually evolves into increasingly complex games that may involve multiple peers, even adults, and have complicated rules. In contrast, early games tend to involve few participants and few rules (e.g., patty cake, peek-a-boo). In the latter stage of childhood play, children often modify the rules to accommodate their situation or simply to make the game more fun. Modifying rules provides opportunities for discussion, social interaction, and problem solving to ensure that the new version of the game is fair and equitable (Bergen, 2014).

A slightly different account of the development of play was provided by Cratty (1986), who maintained that for children at an early age, play remains rather unsocial even when social opportunities exist. When children are between 24 and 30 months old, their most common type of play is solitary (see Figure 3.7). Two children playing side by side pay little attention to each other and make few, if any, attempts at social interaction. They are generally engrossed in their own activity, and their companion's activity is minimally important. This behavior soon evolves into what is known as **parallel play** (see Figure 3.8). By the time children are 2.5 to 3.5 years old, they will still make few attempts to interact socially, but they may begin to display an awareness of each other and may even subtly copy each other's play behavior through observation and imitation. Nevertheless, the children are not likely to interact to any greater extent.

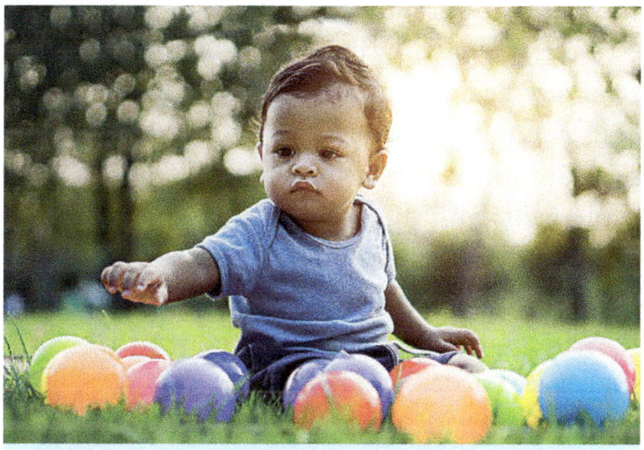

Figure 3.7 Solitary play characterizes most children up to about 30 months of age. During this time, they are focused on their own activity rather than on any nearby children.

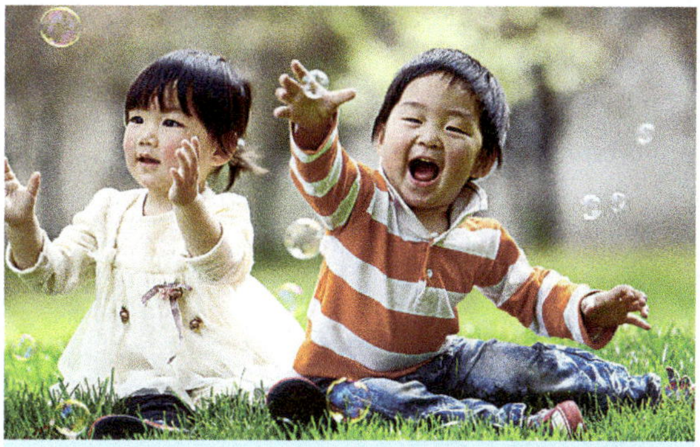

Figure 3.8 From 2.5 to 3.5 years of age children often exhibit characteristics of parallel play, interacting very little but showing occasional awareness of each other

Approximately one year later, when they are 3.5 to 4.5 years old, children begin to display the interaction that was missing in their previous levels of play behavior. In **associative play**, two or more children exhibit an awareness of each other and begin to exchange toys; however, there is no group goal. This is a major difference between associative play and the final level of play during early childhood, cooperative play. Cooperative play generally begins when children are around 4.5 to 5 years old and is evidenced by purposeful, group-oriented play activities involving games and even group leaders. During cooperative play, children form social units. The movement activities selected for use within the larger group enable children to develop leadership skills, as well as to learn to compete, cooperate, and value social recognition. As children's social skills develop, group activities become more attractive to them and are more commonly sought out. Increased participation in popular group movement activities facilitates children's motor development. Thus, a positive, reciprocal relationship can develop between social and motor development; in fact, to a surprising extent, one form of development may depend on the other. Even at the young age of 5 or 6 years, group leaders are likely to be those children who are superior in performing such physical activities as running, throwing, and balancing (Cratty, 1986). This is an expected phenomenon during early to late adolescence, but to observe such a relationship between movement and social success for children at such a young age is surprising.

School

Another major socializing agent, although generally not a factor until a child is 4 or 5, is school, where teachers and coaches play immediate roles in children's cultural education. In fact, the school can overtake the family as the major socializing agency as children approach adolescence and teachers and coaches become increasingly important in exposing children to life's tendencies. Some experts have even referred to the important "hidden curriculum" (Grusec & Davidov, 2015, p. 172) of school, where intentionally and unintentionally socializing messages are transmitted through casual or structured group activities; formal and informal language; and modeling by teachers, coaches, and even other students. Importantly, it is often at school where children begin to develop peer groups, which can be a tremendous influence on their socialization process. Children's relationships with peer groups become increasingly important as they approach their adolescent years.

Older Childhood and Adolescence

As the child approaches adolescence, the family's influence generally begins to diminish and the peer group, one's closest non-family age-mates, becomes an increasingly important social force. The parent, teacher, and other adults in the child's life slowly lose their power of persuasion over the child, and a need for peer approval becomes particularly powerful. This new social force, the older child/adolescent's **peer group**, is less structured than adult social groups but considerably more structured than the peer groups in the child's previous social environment (see Figure 3.9). The peer group is also characterized by its transitory nature; it may vary from the neighborhood to the school, as well as from day to day. It has the power to shape the mode of older children's dress, speech, and actions, including their decisions concerning participation in movement activities. For example, members of the same peer group often share similar gait and speech patterns. Furthermore, the relationships created in the peer group give the older child or young adolescent styles of friendship, support, companionship, and fun that are not available from the family. Peers strongly influence one another by interacting as equals, a situation very different from the family structure, which generally has a primary authority figure. The peer group, therefore, often exerts a strong general influence on older children or adolescents and the decisions they make, including choices regarding exercise and sport activities. Peers are often selected on the basis of "gender, race, ethnicity, or behavioral style (e.g., more or less aggressive or socially withdrawn), and academic achievement" (p. 19). Level of popularity, religious values, body weight, and interest in physical activity can also draw teens together. In any event, peers are a strong developmental force and are

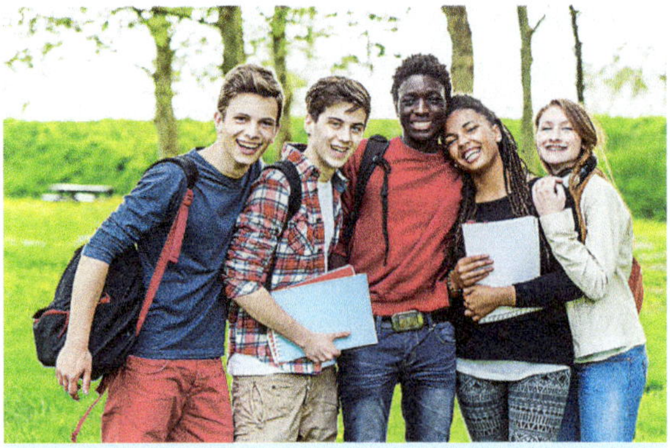

Figure 3.9 Approaching and in adolescence, the peer group usually emerges as a powerful force in their lives

often the group with which teens spend the majority of their waking hours. Technological advances have made this even more conceivable as more rapid and extensive contact is possible via the internet and social media (Rubin, Bukowski, & Bowker, 2015).

This gradually evolving independence from the family enables older children to shed the egocentrism so common during earlier childhood. A person's daily interaction with peers also provides considerable learning experiences. For example, youth develop an increasing appreciation of many points of view because members of the same peer group often express diverse opinions, even disagree, and feel free to do so because of their equal status (Grusec & Davidov, 2015). Additionally, young adolescents become increasingly aware of social norms and pressures. In fact, their social acceptability may depend on how they conform to the expectations of their social group. Two of the most common determinants of social acceptability, particularly for boys, are athletic ability and willingness to become involved in athletically oriented activities. Other determinants of social acceptability, as defined by the peer group, may include appearance, academic achievement, career expectations, in-group or out-group status, and special talents. Many of these characteristics, such as appearance and special talents, may, again, reflect the extent to which an individual participates in movement activities. These characteristics are not generally announced overtly as qualifiers for status in a particular peer group, but consistent standards such as these are frequently used to include and exclude members.

As mentioned earlier, an individual's movement ability partly determines her or his peer group association, but this ability can also be molded within the group. Associating with others who hold new and diverse opinions may lead a person to participate in new versions of old games or attempt previously untried movement endeavors. Gaining respect and approval can become increasingly important to members of a peer group, and respect and approval depend on adherence to the group's expectations. In this way the peer group applies pressure toward conformity, but the type of conformity varies tremendously from one peer group to another. If participation in movement activities is an accepted norm for a group, members will feel pressure to be active. Hence, a peer group can guide an individual into or away from participation, and perhaps achievement, in athletic activities.

Silva, Lott, Mota, and Welk (2014) studied the effects of social support, especially from peers and parents, on youth involvement in physical activity. They noted that this social support is instrumental in youth participation in physical activity. It impacts the level of enjoyment that a person experiences in an activity, and it enhances participants' self-efficacy, or confidence in one's own ability to achieve, in the activity. Interestingly, though support from both parents and peers was found to be important for older children and adolescents, the *magnitude* of the peer support was substantially more influential than the magnitude of parental support in young people's level of involvement. While parental support is generally more important for younger children, peer support was the most important and most consistently related variable to physical activity for children and youth from grade 1 to grade 12. Friendship, and the influence of friends, were also found to be a motivating factor. Although parental influence was also an important variable, the influence of peer support was stronger. This supports the notion that parental influence is often gradually replaced by peer influence, especially as a child approaches and enters adolescence. Other factors that were particularly important, especially for girls, were their self-efficacy related to the activity in question and the convenience of the activity's location. These authors indicate that, in general, children and youth with higher self-efficacy and a generally positive attitude were more likely to be physically active. Finally, the authors also indicated that the participant's enjoyment in the activity was also an important reason for involvement (Silva, Lott, Mota, & Welk, 2014).

Team Play

During later childhood and adolescence, youth encounter an increasing sense of team or club participation. This factor is particularly important for influencing the types of movement activities older children or young adolescents may select. Whereas during earlier childhood youngsters are content to play alone or in a small group, the emphasis changes as children approach adolescence. Because of increasing social capabilities and their developing relationship with the peer group, adolescents often actively seek group or team activities. Those who decide to participate in a team movement experience frequently devote much energy to trying to ensure the team's success (Newman & Newman, 2018).

Movement participation through team membership can greatly affect a child's or adolescent's development. Through team participation, youth learn to work toward achieving group or team goals while subordinating personal goals—a major developmental stride for those who may still be overcoming the egocentrism so prevalent earlier in their lives (see Figure 3.10). Team participation also teaches children the importance of the division of labor. Gradually, youth learn that every member of the team has a duty and a responsibility and that the team's goals are most likely to be accomplished when the members share these duties and responsibilities. Also, team membership often makes greater intellectual demands on children than do the unstructured group or individual

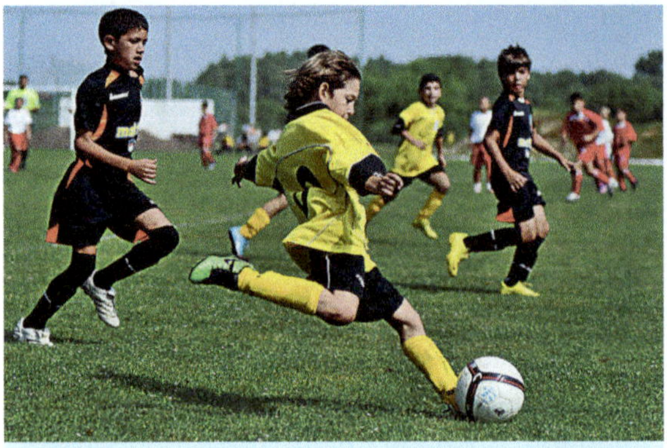

Figure 3.10 Team play teaches the value of cooperative efforts to achieve group goals, an important lesson for children who may still be overcoming their childhood egocentrism

activities of young childhood. More rules, strategies, and responsibilities tend to occur in team activities than in childhood group play.

In team play, the players also assume greater social responsibilities than are associated with earlier forms of play. If players do not carry out their assigned duties, they may be ostracized or ridiculed. On the other hand, tremendous individual recognition is possible for those who are particularly successful in carrying out their duty to the team. Ideally, the more proficient participants should, and often do, assist the less capable, which is to the team's advantage. However, too frequently the less capable are scorned, and their inability to perform is blamed for the team's failure.

Although it is unpleasant to think of a child or young adolescent being scorned or ostracized in team play, in many ways the team is a model for life in general. In one respect, team participation teaches youth about failure and success, as well as such common emotions as shame and embarrassment. For more successful participants, team play is an avenue for learning to show humility or modesty. Experiencing these emotions personally and witnessing them in others provide important lessons that may help older children and adolescents deal with more difficult situations later in life.

Gender Role Identification and Movement Activity

In addition to all the functions discussed previously, the peer group serves another critical developmental purpose: it facilitates awareness of gender roles and interaction with others on the basis of gender. Adolescence is when dating generally begins and gender roles become increasingly apparent. The degree to which adolescents identify with the role ascribed to their gender depends on several factors. The peer group influences the degree to which young adolescents may identify with their gender, but **gender role identity** begins much earlier in life. Social expectations for behavior based on gender begin to be imposed early in childhood, and whether and how a child conforms to them often depend on the quality of the child's relationship with the same-sex parent.

Even though many behaviors once commonly accepted for only one gender are now acceptable for both, many human characteristics are still considered masculine or feminine. For example, aggressive behavior is often more acceptable in boys and men than in women and girls. Boys and men may be scorned if they are excessively dependent, whereas the opposite can be true for girls and women. This gender typing often reflects rigid concepts regarding abilities and behaviors, and it no doubt affects individuals' decisions concerning their involvement in movement activity. Gender role conflict is often experienced by girls who seek to participate in movement activity and boys who do not. Unfortunately, in both cases, the result can be emotional distress and the failure to achieve personal potential because the development of self-selected talents and skills has been inhibited.

Heinze, Heinze, Davis, and their colleagues (2014) studied gender role beliefs and their effects on parental support for children's athletic participation. These researchers noted that many people hold traditional gender role beliefs, based on socialization at home and in society in general. Individuals who hold these traditional gender role beliefs view certain sports as more masculine; these masculine sports are generally more widely supported by society than the "feminine" sports, and boys are generally able to achieve more status than girls through participation or attaining athletic ability. According to Heinze and colleagues (2014), the traditionally male roles are perceived as competitive, dangerous, and fast, while the traditionally female roles stress "aesthetics and femininity" (p. 6). Social "punishments" (p. 3) can exist for children seen as violating the traditional gendered roles in sports. Thus, boys and girls who make choices that violate these societal norms may be ostracized or discriminated against, or they may simply receive less adulation when they excel. Further, the threat of these societal punishments can be sufficient to shape choices made by both parents and their children in their selection of sporting options. The threat can even cause some individuals, especially girls, to avoid participation altogether. Sport participation is as beneficial for girls as for boys (e.g., greater physical activity, reduced body mass index, reduced obesity, greater fitness levels), so understanding the social forces that affect participation is important.

In general, Heinze and associates (2014) found that parents were influential in the sport participation of their children. Both boys and girls were more likely to participate in vigorous physical activity when their parents valued participation, believed that such activities were important, and believed their children were capable. Still, parents generally valued sport participation more highly for their male children. This was true both ideologically and financially. Parents' traditional gender role beliefs led them to spend more money for their sons' sporting activities and influenced the types of activities they sought for their male versus female children.

Clearly, gender stereotypes can have major implications in an adolescent's decision to participate in a movement activity. An activity may seem enticing, but the gender role associated with that activity may conflict with the role that the adolescent deems appropriate for himself or herself. If he or she decides to participate anyway, a **role conflict** may be created. That is, an emotional trauma may develop out of the mismatch between the gender role that the adolescent considers appropriate and the gender role that the relevant society views as appropriate.

Research on 10- to 11-year-olds and the psychosocial factors affecting their physical activity found that girls were less active than boys, and boys had better overall social support for their movement choices. Boys also had more positive perceptions of the perceived benefits of their physical activity and their own ability to be successful in physical activity. The authors concluded that more research is necessary to prevent a further decline in physical activity levels, especially among the girls, during the transition from childhood to adolescence (Cardon, Philippaerts, Lefevre, et al., 2005).

Perceptions concerning the role of women and girls in sport have been changing. Sport participation for high-school boys has a long and significant history from which girls were long excluded. However, girls' participation increased markedly following the 1972 passage of Title IX, the federal law that stipulates that no one can be excluded or denied benefits from educational programs that receive federal funding and prohibits sexual discrimination within these programs. Soon after Title IX's enactment, the number of girls participating in high-school sports increased from less than 4 percent to nearly a third. In fact, the change was so dramatic it has been referred to as "revolutionizing mass sports participation in the United States" (Stevenson, 2007, p. 1). Cooky and Lavoi (2012) observe that "Title IX has dramatically increased the number of sport opportunities for girls and women," especially in educational institutions (p. 43). From 1971 to 2010, the number of girls participating in high-school sports increased more than tenfold, with a sixfold increase seen at the college level (Acosta & Carpenter, 2014). According to Stevenson (2007), these are indications that Title IX has made a difference.

Stevenson (2007) speculates that the potential value of sport participation may go well beyond sport itself, as a positive correlation exists between involvement in school sports and educational attainment. Athletes frequently have higher academic aspirations and ultimately achieve more education than non-athletes. Stevenson (2007) speculates that this may be related to the positive opportunities that athletics provide for appropriate peer pressure and involvement with positively influential adults. Athletic participation may even enhance the preparation of girls and women as they enter the workforce and may influence the types of careers they choose (Stevenson, 2006).

Early Adulthood

Early adulthood begins when adolescence ends. Experts disagree about the actual time of the onset of adulthood; as discussed in Chapter 1, we are assuming that it begins at age 20. Unfortunately, as many people age, their involvement in movement activities or sports begins to decline. In fact, age is a prime determinant of sport or physical activity involvement, and participation is clearly moderated by a number of social circumstances and landmarks of early adulthood. According to Engberg, Alen, Kukkonen-Harjula, and colleagues (2012), certain life events can significantly affect an individual's engagement in physical activity by increasing emotional distress or simply by altering the person's life routine. Factors such as transitioning to college, getting a job, marrying or changing one's relationship status, having children, and the death of a spouse, along with many others, can cause physical activity levels to change dramatically. In various stages of adulthood, that change is often a reduction.

In early adulthood, three major social factors affecting human movement often have their greatest negative impact on adult motor behavior, significantly affecting individuals' lifestyles and generally contributing to a tendency toward decreased participation in movement activity. These social forces are (1) taking a companion with the intent of cohabitation for life; (2) having children; and (3) leaving school/going to work.

Brown and Trost (2003) studied this phenomenon in more than 7,000 young adult women (late teens and early 20s) to determine the effects of key events in their lives on their physical activity levels. The participants self-reported their physical activity and life events during the study period, their body mass index, and their sociodemographic information. For most of these young women, no change was found in physical activity levels across the 4 years of their participation in the study. However, 20 percent of the participants moved from being physically active to physically inactive. These participants were more likely than their counterparts to have reported getting married, having a first or subsequent child, or beginning paid work. The researchers concluded that these life events are associated with decreased levels of physical activity in young women. Thus, programs and ideas are needed to promote physical activity during the time of life when women most often experience such important life events (Brown & Trost, 2003).

Many people experience all of these key factors early in adulthood. Once an individual begins regular employment, marries or cohabits, and/or has children, the tendency for physiological regression and an ensuing decline in motor performance increases greatly. For example, strength, cardiorespiratory endurance, and flexibility may all begin to decrease. This decline is much more difficult to predict than many of the motor changes that occur in children and adolescents because there is much greater individual variability among adults. Thus, although a decline in motor performance often occurs when a person experiences the three social factors listed above, some individuals' performance may actually improve. Those who overcome the prevailing social forces by staying involved in movement activities can reduce the rate of the regression. In fact, adults can progress in movement endeavors until late in life if they continue to participate in those activities regularly. Unfortunately, though, for many people, these social factors mark the onset of a regression in motor development that will extend throughout the remainder of their lifespan.

In slightly more recent research, Althoff and colleagues (2017) studied physical activity trends in 111 countries. A key finding was related to a city's "walkability." Greater walkability increased activity across age groups and genders with the greatest increase for women. In general, physical activity was found to decline with age and with increasing body mass index. It was also generally lower among females than males as has been consistently determined in previous research. Both developed and developing countries were included in the study (e.g., the US, France, Germany, the UK, Saudi Arabia, Malaysia, Indonesia, the Philippines) (Althoff et al., 2017).

Influence of Marriage and Parenthood

Marriage and having children also have important effects of physical activity levels and motor development in young adulthood. In a large-scale longitudinal study on the effects of

RESEARCH ON PHYSICAL ACTIVITY TRENDS

In a study of physical activity throughout the world, involving 122 countries, researchers found that a third of adolescents and nearly 80 percent of adults did not achieve recommended levels of physical activity (Hallal, Andersen, Bull, et al., 2012). The percentages tended to be higher for women than men and higher in older versus younger adults. Though some increases with age were noted in leisure-time physical activity, overall occupational activity (work-related physical activity) was found to decrease with age. Some regional differences were noted; for example, Southeast Asians over the age of 60 were found to be considerably more active than older adults in other regions of the world. Somewhat surprisingly, activity levels were found to be higher in countries with lower social economic levels, but this was assumed to be a result of higher levels of occupational activity in the lower social economic areas and may change if the incidence of occupational activity decreases in those countries. Interestingly, levels of participation in one of the most common forms of physical activity, walking, were found to be somewhat similar between men and women, in different regions of the world, and across age groups.

These researchers also found that for all age groups from adolescents through older adults, men were more likely to be vigorously physically active than women, and participation at vigorous levels generally decreased with age. Similarly, sedentary behavior (time spent sitting) varied by worldwide region but was similar for men and women and increased with age across adulthood. This was thought to be related to a number of social factors, including the increasing use of motor vehicles, overall mechanization, urbanization, and continuing technological advances (e.g. cell phones, video-streaming, intelligent personal assistants) throughout the world. In the United States, work-related physical activity was found to have decreased over the past half century by over 100 kilocalories/day. Again, social trends were thought to be the cause (Hallal et al., 2012).

one's relationship (single, dating, married or living together), Rapp and Schneider (2013) studied German participants over the age of 17 years across nearly two decades. Over 30,000 participants were interviewed to determine their relationship status and physical activity levels during leisure time. Reduced physical activity with increasing age was determined for each of the relationship types, for both men and women. However, the magnitude of decline in physical activity was greatest for those who were married and least for dating couples. Having young children at home was also found to reduce the amount of physical activity per week. According to the researchers, for men, these findings were partly a function of age as declines in physical activity attributed to marriage and living together lessened with time. Eventually, marriage and living together actually became positive factors. This was not the case for women where the apparent effect of marriage resulted in reduced physical activity and was maintained into old age (Rapp & Schneider, 2013).

Similarly, Syrda (2017) studied the effects of marriage and parenthood on men and found that married men have higher body mass index (BMI) than their unmarried counterparts. Of interest, the BMI of men was significantly correlated to the BMI of their wives. Though the BMI for the husbands increased after marriage, it decreased before and after divorce. Husbands, who were also fathers and married, or partnered, were also found to have greater adiposity (i.e., fatness) and BMI as opposed to unmarried men without offspring. This could be a function of activity levels as as negative correlation was also determined between parenthood and physical activity. This was true for both mothers and fathers as mothers also had higher BMIs than women without children. This was presumed to be because married couples and parents had less time to pursue physical activity interests than their unmarried counterparts with no children (Syrda, 2017).

Influence of Leaving School and Employment

For most people, leaving school and beginning full-time employment, depending on the type of employment, produces long-term effects similar to those of marriage and parenthood (see Figure 3.11). Work ordinarily creates a relatively permanent lifestyle change by structuring or limiting the time a person has for participation in activities that were once a regular source of recreational pleasure. Furthermore, workers typically have few coworkers with similar movement interests. Unless a worker participates alone in a physical activity or has friends with the same interest outside the workplace, he or she may decrease or discontinue an activity. This situation contrasts considerably with attending school, where the person was surrounded by same-age peers who likely had similar interests. Leaving school, therefore, often results in a decrease in the number of people with whom a person can interact socially in a movement activity. A high-school student can easily locate nine friends for a basketball game, but an adult may have a difficult time finding one partner for racquetball.

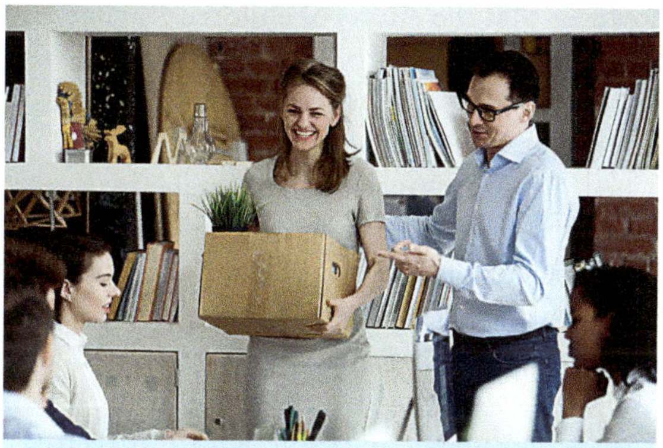

Figure 3.11 Beginning regular employment early in adulthood can lead to a decrease in physical activity unless an active effort is made to stay engaged in movement

Middle and Late Adulthood

Conditions that usually occur in middle to late adulthood can also contribute to a relatively permanent change in movement behavior. This change is typically a regression, but in less typical cases, an individual may revive an interest in a movement, which could lead to an improvement of movement status. Three of the most important of these situations are (1) the children leaving home; (2) retirement; and (3) the death of a spouse. Other factors that can cause a change in movement status, more general in nature, are the influence of social activities with friends and family; society's negative view of aging; and the common tendency to experience a downward spiral of reduced physical activity, reduced physical capacity, and poorer health, followed by further reductions in physical activity (the exercise-aging cycle).

Influence of Children Leaving Home

When children leave home, the quality of life for aging parents or caregivers can be negatively affected. Many people think the parents are now "liberated" to pursue their personal interests and activities, which they may have set aside in favor of their children's interests. Researchers have determined, however, that the effects of children leaving the home can contribute to depression and, in more serious cases, can even undermine the parents' or caregivers' overall quality of life (Chen, Yang, & Aagard, 2012). Individuals with depressive symptoms often fail to achieve recommended doses of daily physical activity (Da Silva, Singh-Manouz, Brunner, et al., 2012). Children's presence at home may have had a somewhat positive effect on their parents' movement, in that it helped to keep them at least minimally active. When a child departs, however, the parents may view it as a milestone indicating that they are no longer youthful as they once were. This, coupled with the potential emotional toll of a child leaving home, can increase the likelihood of a more sedentary lifestyle. Although some parents may rediscover movement activity, which of course benefits their movement in general, the "empty-nest" syndrome can contribute to a less active lifestyle.

To further understand this phenomenon, Zhang and fellow researchers examined 250 empty-nest (children had left home) elderly parents in China using a questionnaire to determine their level of resilience. Resilience was considered to be the participants' ability to positively respond when confronted with obstacles in life. These experts considered this population to be potentially vulnerable as they appeared to experience a decline in physical and psychological health that included conditions like depression, anxiety, and loneliness. The most resilient group studied were positively impacted by factors like their educational level, their relationship with their offspring, and the amount of physical activity they experienced. These researchers noted that previous studies had also indicated that the elderly "empty-nesters" were psychologically less healthy than elderly individuals who still had children living at home. Overall, maintaining an active lifestyle was considered to be paramount as it increased the opportunity for social engagement while benefitting physical and psychological health (Zhang et al., 2017).

Also studying empty-nest Chinese elderly, Gao and associates found that the empty nest had a negative impact on cognition on those participants from urban areas. However, among those from urban areas, younger elders, men, and those with a self-generated source of income performed better intellectually. Having a supportive spouse and an active lifestyle also enhanced cognition. Nevertheless, the empty nest had a negative effect on many participants from both urban and rural areas. This was particularly true for those who were older, single, had recently experienced illness, and did not exercise. When studying activities of daily living in the urban dwellers, females performed more poorly as males activities of daily living seemed to be unaffected by the empty-nest phenomenon. For all participants, the researchers found that physical and social activities were particularly important as they were related to improved health and a reduction in cognitive issues. In conclusion, the empty nest was thought to have a generally adverse effect on the elders studied, especially those who were physically inactive, female, and over 75 years of age (Gao et al., 2017).

Influence of Retirement

Today more people are living and working past age 65 than ever before, which means that many retirees will undergo a major shift in their life pattern even later in life. Retirement begins a period of leisure that has the potential for giving the retiree time to pursue movement endeavors (see Figure 3.12). Nevertheless, some studies show that physical activity often declines with age in adulthood even though it is so clearly a factor for maintaining most aspects of good health. So, Feng, Croteau, Kolt, and Astell-Burt (2016) sought to examine physical activity levels before and after retirement when the retiree would have

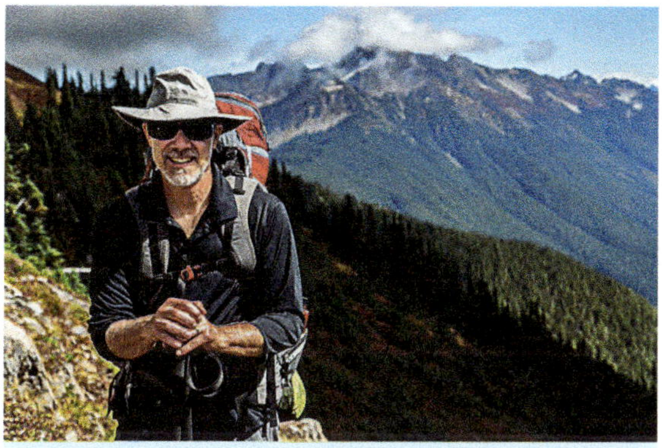

Figure 3.12 Retirement often frees individuals for the active pursuit of movement activities; unfortunately, active movement frequently decreases after retirement

potentially more time for physical activity. To do this, the researchers obtained data from nearly 6,000 males and females ranging in age from 50 to 75 years of age. Most notable in the study was the high number of non-participants in all levels of physical activity among those people leaving employment because of a disability. For people in the study who remained employed, physical activity level changed little with most people in the study claiming to engage in physical activity at least two times per week. For those transitioning into full or semi-retirement some increase in activity level was experienced. In short, these researchers indicated that the relationship between retirement and physical activity is complex and related to factors like age of retirement, whether one transitions into part-time work or no work, and the reason for retirement (e.g., disability) (Feng et al., 2016).

In a similar, significant, and large-scale longitudinal study, Stenholm and associates (2016) studied nearly 10,000 Finnish retirees and their leisure time physical activity for ten years before and ten years after retirement. The average age of retirement was found to be dependent upon the type of retirement. For example, those entering statutory (required) retirement averaged just under 62 years of age. Those entering part-time retirement were just under 60 years, and those retiring because of disability were slightly over 55 years of age. Generally, physical activity tended to increase temporarily upon retirement. More specifically, those entering statutory retirement, on average, increased physical activity for four years, but then decreased thereafter. In addition, retirees who were older at retirement, were retiring from a "higher" work status, and were healthier upon retirement saw a higher correlation with physical activity (Stenholm et al., 2016).

In a study of more than 25,000 English retirees from 45 to 79 years of age, researchers sought to determine a number of life changes associated with retiring from one's occupation (Barnett, van Sluijs, Ogilvie, & Wareham, 2013). Based mostly on self-reports and questionnaires, these researchers found that retirement was a time of declining physical activity. Declines were found to be more common among women than men and among manual social classes (i.e., working classes) than non-manual classes of people. This was probably explained, in part, by the fact that members of the manual social class retired from relatively active work environments. Also, many manual workers may fail to establish physically active recreational habits prior to retirement because of the physical requirements of their jobs. These researchers also found that retirement was associated with a significant increase in television viewing, with, again, more viewing by the manual social class.

An overall decline in physical activity in retirement has been reported in the research, though it may defy the common perception that individuals would become more active as more time becomes available to them in retirement (Barnett et al., 2013). The portion of the population over 60 years of age is less active than any other age group. Retirement is an important transitional period when people are faced with establishing new routines while reconsidering their former ways of life. Because of declining activity levels, it is critical that researchers understand physical activity trends and patterns among retirees and find ways to assist them in maintaining locomotor ability and overall good health. Retirement is an important period for the promotion of programs that enhance household, transport (e.g., walking), occupational, and recreational physical activity.

Unfortunately, retirement too frequently marks a significant decline in standard of living, causing financial, transportation, and even nutritional problems. Certainly, retirement may have a negative impact on retirees' financial status. Whereas they once had a regular income from employment, many retirees have to rely on Social Security and/or limited pension payments. In many cases, the postretirement years can be a struggle for economic survival. Members of minority groups often suffer the consequences of poverty in old age more severely than do nonminority older adults. In any case, poor economic conditions can lead to emotional trauma that, as discussed earlier, may affect an individual's desire or ability to become involved in movement activities. The resultant lack of movement exacerbates the physiological and subsequent motor decline generally associated with aging. In other words, a vicious cycle develops: as older adults become less active, they become less able to be active.

The financial struggle that frequently accompanies retirement is the basis of a series of associated problems. Insufficient finances often impede individuals' ability to acquire transportation. If a retiree has a car, maintaining the automobile in satisfactory condition becomes an additional burden. Other forms of travel, such as taxi or bus, may be too costly or cumbersome for an older person. Many communities provide transportation, but in many others it is unavailable or individuals who could benefit from it are unaware of its availability. In these situations, the likelihood of retirees actively interacting with society decreases. The lack of interaction increases the level of disengagement among retirees and causes some older adults to finish their lives in a sedentary, depressed, and lonely fashion.

Decreased finances and lack of transportation may also affect retirees' nutritional status. Without sufficient money and transportation, older adults may find buying food a significant burden, so rather than shop, they may attempt to go without proper nourishment. A poor diet obviously affects an individual's ability to engage with society, and, in fact, may cause serious health problems that further devastate the older adult's attempts at staying active. The isolation that indirectly results from limited funds, lack of transportation, and poor nutrition also can contribute to an attitude that impedes any desire on the part of the adult to participate in movement activities. In turn, this lack of participation contributes to the gradual decline in overall motor function that begins at the onset of early adulthood.

Influence of Death of a Spouse or Life Partner

Most Americans will experience retirement and its accompanying social implications. Those who are married may also experience the death of their spouse. This tragic experience can be so traumatic that it brings about the death of the remaining spouse. Carey, Shah, DeWilde, and colleagues (2014) found a 41 percent increase in the chance of death of the remaining spouse following the death of a husband or wife. Clearly, the death of a spouse can be one of life's most stressful events. In addition to increasing the liklihood of death for the remaining spouse, it often increases depression and sleep disorders, the chance of suicide, significant health events (e.g., stroke, heart attack, cancer) and can lead to hospitalization or disability. Widowhood can also dramatically impact one's social circle and daily routine.

Research on this topic has indicated that physical activity following widowhood can ease the transition that can otherwise be intense and lengthy (Stahl & Schulz, 2014).

In their study on the effects of widowhood on physical activity, Stahl and Schulz examined just under 400 married control participants and a similar number of widows and widowers. They averaged just under 73 years old. Widowed men were actually found to increase their physical activity levels compared to widowed women or married controls following the death of their wives. However, this increase was not sustained over time. Specifically, six months into widowhood, men's and women's activity levels were similar. However, after a year the men significantly increased their activity levels though it declined the following year. The researchers surmised that this could be due to lower initial levels of physical activity among the women, or that men and women were simply affected differently by the experience (Stahl & Schulz, 2014).

Influence of Relationships with Family and Friends

Huxhold, Miche, and Schüz (2014) studied the importance of informal social activities with friends and family in personal well-being in people from 40 to 85 years of age. social activities led to increased physical activity and life satisfaction, especially in the middle adult group. The older adult group experienced increased positive affect with family activities, but this seemed to have less impact on their overall life satisfaction than interactions with friends, where close social relationships led to greater optimism, improved health, and better subjective well-being. Social activities were generally believed to be integral to successful aging, according to the authors.

Of particular interest were the differing results when older adults' social activities involved family versus friends. Social activities with family sometimes increased negative affect. This was especially true if difficult family circumstances existed, and the effect was heightened among older adults. With friends, social activities improved positive affect regardless of the relationships' quality. The authors attributed this to the fact that family relationships are predetermined, whereas friendships are chosen or voluntary. Friends are generally selected on the basis of being peers, possessing shared characteristics, and having common lifestyles and life experiences. In short, they often can be better sources of companionship than family members (Huxhold et al., 2014).

In general, members of the older age group experienced fewer social activities with family and friends. According to these authors, social activities may have been reduced in the older adults versus the adults of middle age because individuals in the older group were less healthy, were less motivated to be involved, and had reduced cognitive resources at their disposal. Overall, the authors concluded that leisure-time social activities are beneficial to people in middle and older adulthood as they increase feelings of fun, increase interest in life in general, and improve life satisfaction. This, of course, has strong implications for maintaining mental and physical health as we age (Huxhold et al., 2014).

In similar research on over 3,000 participants over 53 years of age, Becofsky and associates studied social support and social network size on all-cause mortality. Participants completed a survey regarding these factors once and then again nearly fourteen years later. Social support from relatives (including spouses), but not friends, was found to reduce mortality risk by nearly 20 percent. Social contact, rather than support, with six to seven friends per week, was associated with a nearly 25 percent decrease in mortality risk. Somewhat strangely, this was not the case with two to five friends or more than eight friends. The research group indicated that this demonstrated the importance of interaction with friends and family and that these findings may be useful in designing interventions to prolongue life (Becofsky et al., 2015).

Ageism

The four factors just discussed critically affect motor development in mid- to late adulthood. These factors, however, are not the only social elements that inhibit adults' level of involvement in active movement over the remainder of their lifespan. Negative stereotypes concerning older adults—**ageism**—can affect these individuals' physical activity levels. Like racism or sexism, ageism can lead to discrimination and the exclusion of older adults from some activities. Ageism may indicate society's aversion to the aging process and subsequent death of older adults. Given the rapidity with which our population is aging, society needs to attend to the ways older adults are perceived.

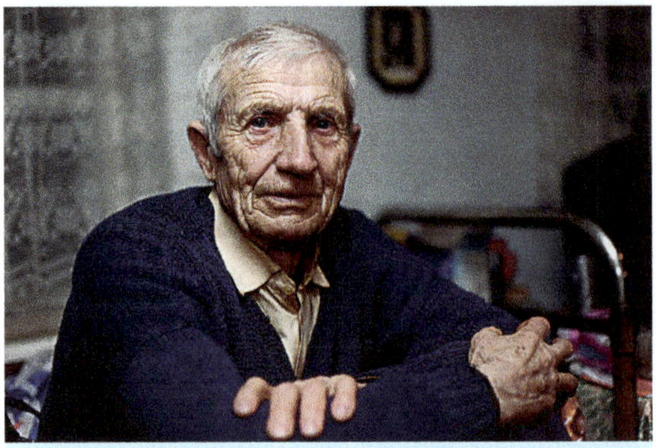

Figure 3.13 Stereotypes concerning older Americans are often negative, a phenomenon known as *ageism*. Ageism can inhibit an older adult's attempts at engaging in society.

Unfortunately, stereotypes about aging are common in the United States and may lead to harmful psychological, physical, and cognitive effects on older members of the population. In fact, the effects of these stereotypes can even impair longevity (Ory, Kinney Hoffman, Hawkins, et al., 2003). This form of discrimination often inhibits the older adult's attempts to become an active participant in society (see Figure 3.13). Some older adults are "forced" into a life of inactivity despite their attempts to interact; as a result, their movement capabilities, as well as many other behaviors, continue to regress.

Research conducted by Hausdorff, Levy, and Wei (1999) examined the effects of ageism on physical function and its reversibility. Looking specifically at walking, or gait patterns, these researchers exposed 63- to 82-year-old participants to subconscious positive or negative stereotypes while they played a computer game. Results indicated significant increases in walking speed when positive stereotypes related to aging were reinforced. This finding led the researchers to conclude that stereotypes about aging appear to have a powerful effect on the walking patterns of older adults, and that interventions designed to overcome these negative stereotypes may prove beneficial in functional movements such as walking. This research is important, as it points to ways society can assist older adults to maintain their independence and continue to thrive. In the future, more positive societal attitudes regarding older adults may reduce the need for such interventions (Hausdorff et al., 1999). This was affirmed in recent controlled trials research conducted by Wolff, Warner, Ziegelmann, and Wurm (2014) that found that typical negative views on aging can be very detrimental to older adults' health behaviors. Wolff and colleagues also found that interventions involving positive views of older adults during physical activity programs were useful in positively changing attitudes and enhancing physical activity.

The Exercise-Aging Cycle

As indicated in the previous sections, a number of sociocultural factors contribute to the declines in physical activity and fitness that often occur across adulthood. Foremost among these is the phenomenon of ageism, which contributes to increasingly undesirable views of people as they age. Too often older individuals are inaccurately labeled as being poor, frail, unhealthy, forgetful, and physically incapable.

The factors discussed earlier combine to create a sense of diminished self-expectancy and a low valuation of exercise among adults. The physical skills of many adults are so poor that these individuals may perceive physical activity as embarrassing. Figures from *Healthy People 2020* (USDHHS, 2014) indicate that more than three-quarters of adults do not meet established guidelines for both aerobic and muscle-strengthening activity. This is critically important as lack of sufficient physical activity is associated with conditions including early death, coronary heart disease, stroke, high blood pressure, type 2 diabetes, breast and colon cancer, the prevalence of falls, and even depression. *Healthy People 2020* reinforces the points we have made in this chapter: that social support from peers, family, and an individual's spouse is integral to achieving adequate levels of physical activity. Among adults and older adults, reasons cited for neglecting physical activity include lack of time, poor motivation, being overweight or obese, having a disability, lack of transportation, the cost of the activity, and fear of becoming injured (USDHHS, 2014).

Though too few adults meet the recommended guidelines for physical activity, some positive trends have been noted. For example, the percentage of adults from 45 to over 75 years of age who participate in *no* leisure-time activity decreased nearly 7 percent from 2007 to 2012. Other favorable trends noted in *Healthy People 2020* are listed in Table 3.1. Despite these trends, one fact remains clear: the older we get, the less active we become.

Table 3.1 Results for select goals related to adults and physical activity from *Healthy People 2020* (%)

Goal	2007	2008	2012
Older adults who have moderate to severe functional limitations	29.3	—	32.2
Older adults with reduced physical or cognitive function who engage in light, moderate, or vigorous leisure-time physical activity	—	33	39
Older adults who engage in no leisure-time physical activity	—	36.2	29.6
Adults who engage in aerobic physical activity of at least moderate intensity for at least 150 minutes/week, activity of vigorous intensity for at least 75 minutes/week, or an equivalent combination	—	43.5	50
Adults who perform muscle-strengthening activities two or more days/week	—	21.9	23.9
Adults who meet objectives for aerobic physical activity and muscle-strengthening activity	—	18	21

Source: USDHHS (2014).

Figure 3.14 illustrates the **exercise-aging cycle**. Early in adulthood, in part because of the factors discussed earlier, people tend to disengage gradually from physical activities. As a result of this disengagement, physical changes become apparent. For example, for many individuals, physical ability declines, percent fat increases, muscular atrophy occurs, and energy levels decline. These individuals may then begin to feel "old." Stress levels and depression may also increase, and self-esteem may decline. All of these factors further decrease these individuals' interest in being physically active. Over time, the cycle becomes

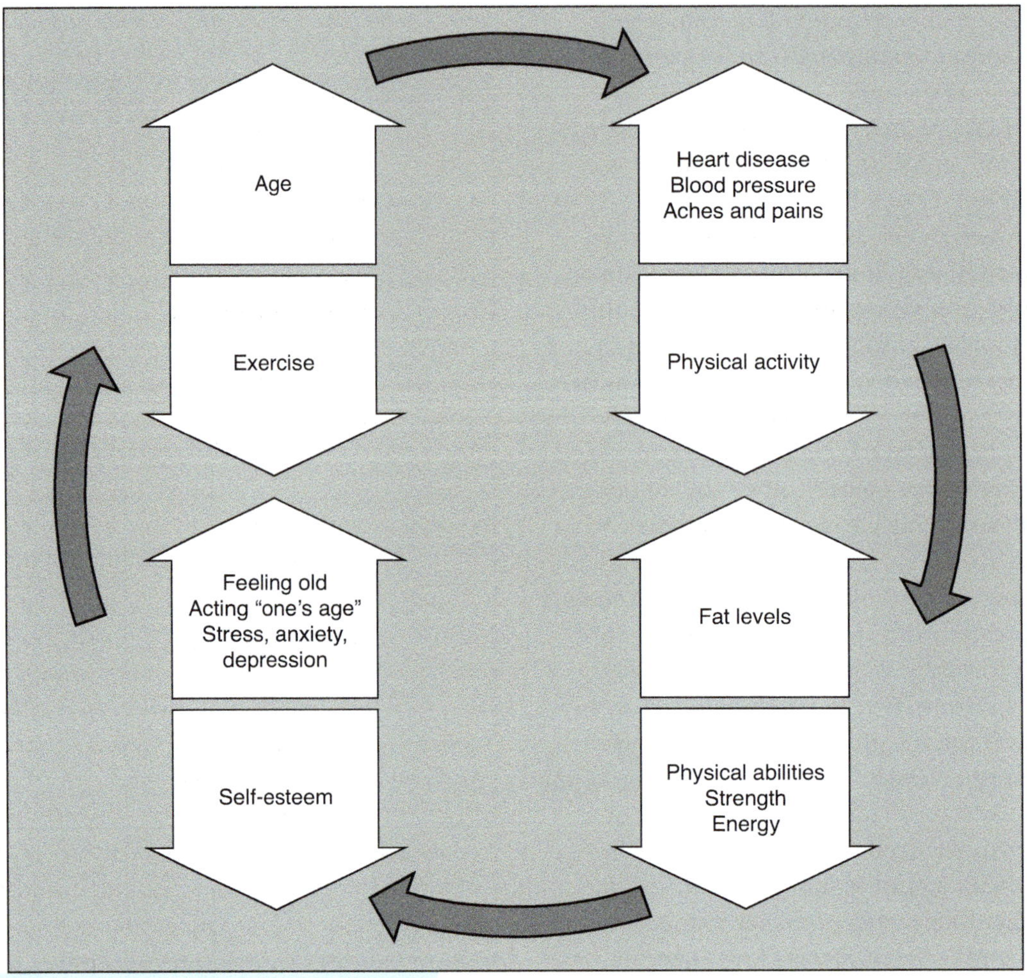

Figure 3.14 The exercise-aging cycle
Source: Adapted from Berger & Hecht (1989).

more severe (Berger & Hecht, 1989; Berger & McInman, 1993).

Sociocultural phenomena are not exclusively responsible for declines in physical ability. According to Berger and McInman (1993), as much as 50 percent of the declines associated with aging may actually be related to a phenomenon known as disuse atrophy, rather than the biological process of aging. **Disuse atrophy** is the wasting away of muscle mass that is the direct result of physical inactivity, occurring when an individual simply does not use the muscles sufficiently. A more general term, **sarcopenia**, describes an "age-related, involuntary loss of skeletal muscle and the corresponding strength" that can occur as a result of disuse but may also occur as a result of typical biological (e.g., hormonal) changes that accompany older age (Walston, 2012, p. 1). A number of causes have been associated with sarcopenia, both environmental and biological. Poor nutrition and lack of physical activity are prime considerations, while hormonal changes, chronic illness, increasing inflammation, and even fatty infiltration from increasing obesity levels are believed to be other contributing factors. Regardless of the causes, loss of strength can certainly contribute to the exercise-aging cycle. Thus, beginning in an individual's forties, muscle mass and strength often begin to decline. By their eighties, many people have lost nearly 50 percent of their muscle mass. This loss contributes to an increased incidence of functional loss, frailty, and disability. Fortunately, interventions—with nutritional and exercise interventions being among the most successful—can help reverse the cycle (Walston, 2012).

Though the effects of aging cannot be completely overcome, individuals who choose to engage in an appropriate level of physical activity can greatly lessen the regression that occurs as a result of the sociocultural effects discussed earlier. Regression does not have to begin so early in adulthood or be so severe. Individuals who are aware of the effects of decreased physical activity through adulthood and are motivated to do something about it can actively improve the quality of the rest of their life (see Figure 3.15).

Although some individuals may believe that, at some point, they may become too old and frail to engage in a physical activity program, research suggests otherwise. Chou, Hwang, and Wu (2012) conducted a meta-analysis of the effect of exercise on the physical function, activities of daily living, and life quality in older adults who are frail. In their review, these authors noted that our rapidly aging society makes understanding exercise and exercise capacity in adulthood and older adulthood critically important.

This meta-analysis showed that, in the studies reviewed, exercise significantly improved gait speed, balance, and performance on activities of daily living in the older adult participants who were frail. Mental health also improved, as did general quality of life. The authors indicated that gait speed is often strongly related to muscle strength, and when gait speed improved, it slowed the progression of deterioration. Similarly, improved balance reduces the fear of falling and enhances older individuals' motivation to walk to maintain independence. Importantly, these researchers found no adverse effects from the exercise interventions while participants maintained high rates of adherence to their programs (i.e., over 70 percent). Clearly, according to these authors, exercise intervention is generally beneficial among older adults who are frail (Chou et al., 2012).

In short, a well-designed training program for any age group in adulthood can increase muscle strength and endurance, increase cardiorespiratory endurance, halt bone decalcification, improve joint flexibility, and

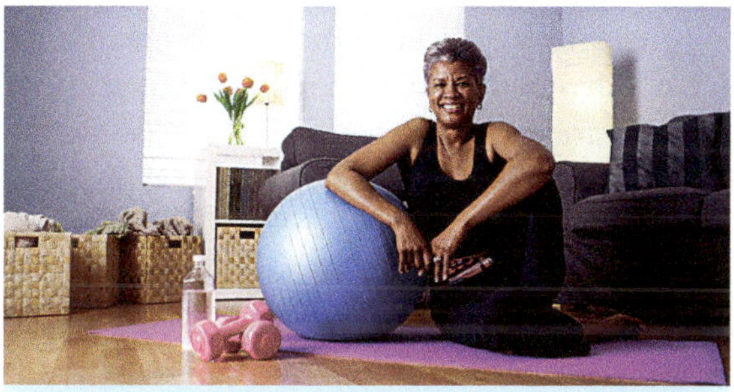

Figure 3.15 Adults who are sufficiently motivated and able can overcome the exercise-aging cycle by continuing physical activity and maintaining their quality of life

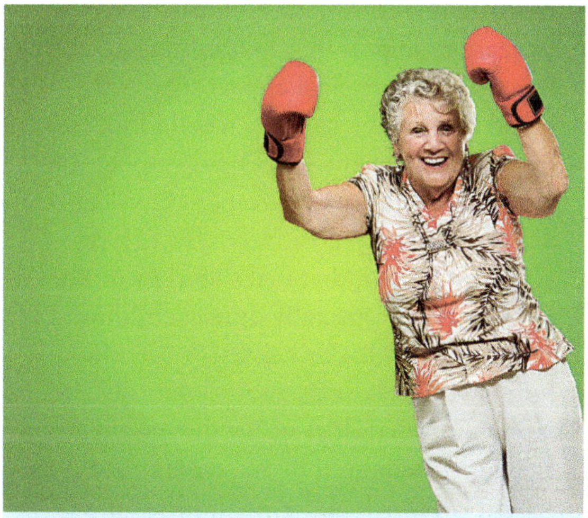

Figure 3.16 The typical regression in movement activity and ability through adulthood can be slowed or delayed

generally improve life satisfaction, enabling individuals to overcome and even temporarily reverse the exercise-aging cycle (see Figure 3.16).

SUMMARY

- Socialization is one of the most dominant facilitators of movement acquisition throughout the lifespan. Because this process of learning society's expected roles, behaviors, rules, and regulations greatly influences an individual's decisions concerning movement participation, it is a major force in human motor development.
- Self-esteem is how much we value ourselves. It is greatly affected by social interactions and has also been found to be significantly influenced by involvement in physical activity. Self-esteem follows a predictable developmental pattern in which individuals increase in their ability to articulate and differentiate its elements. As people age, the nature of their social relationships and the effects of those relationships on self-esteem also change, as elements of self-worth such as peer acceptance and romantic appeal decline in importance.
- Intimate relationships and nurturance increase in importance in adulthood. Interestingly, physical appearance and social acceptance have been found to be important elements influencing global self-worth throughout the lifespan. Physical activity generally positively affects self-esteem, and an individual's level of motor development, especially during childhood, can also affect his or her self-perception.
- Infancy is a relatively asocial period. The interaction that does occur during this time is greatly facilitated by movements such as reciprocal touch and eye contact. These social interactions offer the baby chances to practice movement and expand movement opportunities. The development of locomotor skills, such as crawling, enables a baby to initiate social interactions actively.
- Family, play, and school are important social influences that contribute to motor development throughout childhood. Whereas the family—especially the parents, guardians, or caregivers—is the primary socializing agent during childhood, play is particularly significant because it tends to depend greatly on bodily movement. Once a child begins to attend school, teachers, coaches, and other children become increasingly important social forces.
- Signs of play are seen early in infancy. Play becomes increasingly sophisticated with age and maturity and is an important means of learning the rules of society; play is critical to all aspects of personal development. The quality of play generally evolves in predictable stages, becoming increasingly social as the individual matures through childhood. During later childhood and adolescence, team play becomes common, allowing the child to perfect movement skills and develop new social, cognitive, and emotional behaviors.
- During the latter part of childhood and early adolescence, the peer group increases in social importance as the family gradually becomes less significant. By adolescence, the peer group is generally the dominant social force and is critical to the establishment of an individual's movement-related interests. Peers are greatly influential in a person's decisions about exercise, sport, and physical activity in general. Thus, the peer group can greatly affect motor development. Of particular interest during later childhood and early adolescence is the increasing opportunity to interact with other children of both genders. This interaction assists in understanding one's own gender role.

Personal conflict can arise if the gender role ascribed to an individual does not conform to the gender role associated with the movement activity the individual chooses. Role conflict can lead to emotional trauma or dropping out of an activity.

- In early adulthood, three significant social influences often affect motor development. These are leaving school/going to work, taking a life partner, and having children. All of these factors can decrease a person's physical activity and inhibit the forces that facilitate motor performance. A gradual, consistent decline in motor performance often begins surprisingly early in adulthood and can continue until death. Similar significant life changes can affect motor development in middle and late adulthood. The influence of children leaving home can often lead to a more sedentary lifestyle; the same is true for retirement and the death of a spouse or life partner. Maintaining strong social ties in later life has been shown to be important to maintaining a physically active lifestyle. Ageism, the negative view of aging and of older people, can lead individuals to avoid older adults. This attitude, all too common in the United States, inhibits older adults' attempts to engage in their society and impedes their attempts to maintain an active lifestyle.
- The exercise-aging cycle outlines the changes often observed in adults as their physical performance, levels of activity, self-esteem, and energy decline. The cycle emphasizes the relationship between decreases in physical activity or exercise and other declines across adulthood. Fortunately, despite many common social challenges that occur across adulthood and their effects on motor development, the onset of movement regression can be delayed and the severity allayed if a person maintains an active lifestyle.

key concept review

ageism
associative play
disuse atrophy
exercise-aging cycle
exploratory play
gender role identity
global self-worth
interpersonal play
norm
object play
parallel play
peer group
play
pretend play
role conflict
sarcopenia
self-esteem
social role
socialization

questions for reflection

1. Define socialization. Why and how is it important in human motor development?
2. What is play? List and describe five elements of play.
3. What is self-esteem? Describe some of the relationships between self-esteem and physical activity.
4. What effect does a person's family have on his or her socialization into sports? List some specific examples for each gender, and cite some research discussed in this chapter to support your claims.
5. What are the benefits of team sport participation during adolescence? Provide some examples for each benefit you list.

6. In general, how can participation in team sports resemble life itself?
7. What social factors could contribute to declining fitness levels in early to mid-adulthood? Give specific examples of where you have seen this in real-life situations.
8. What is the general trend regarding physical activity as individuals enter their retirement years, and what could be the effect of this trend?
9. What is the exercise-aging cycle? Do you think this really happens to most people? Is there anything that can be done to offset the effects of this cycle? Does it have to happen to everyone?

online resources

American Academy of Pediatrics, www.aap.org

Healthy People 2020 and 2030, www.healthypeople.gov

REFERENCES

Abnar, A., Takaffoli, M., Rabbany, R., & Zafane, O. R. (2014). SSRM: Structural social role mining for dynamic social networks. *Proceedings from International Conference on Advances in Social Networks Analysis and Mining (ASONAM)*, 2014 IEEE/ACM, Beijing, August 17–20, 289–296. Retrieved from http://ieeexplore. ieee.org/stamp/stamp.jsp?tp=&arnumber=6921599.

Acosta, V. R., & Carpenter, L. S. (2014). An ongoing, longitudinal, national study that tracks athletic participation rates, and coaching and administrative positions, in women's sport. Retrieved from http://acostacarpenter.org.

Althoff, T., Sosic, R., Hicks, J. L., King, A. C., Delp, S. L., & Leskovec, J. (2017). Large-scale physical activity data reveal worldwide activity inequality. *Nature*, *547*, 336–339.

Barnett, I., van Sluijs, E., Ogilvie, D., & Wareham, N. J. (2013). Changes in household, transport and recreational physical activity and television viewing time across the transition to retirement: Longitudinal evidence from the EPIC-Norfolk cohort. *Journal of Epidemiology and Health*, doi: 10.1136/jech-2013–203225.

Bauman, A. E., Reis, R. S., Sallis, J. F., Wells, J. C., Roos, R. J. F., & Martin, B. W. (2012). Correlates of physical activity: Why are some people physically active and others not? *The Lancet*, *380*, 258–271.

Becofsky, K. M., Shook, R. P., Xuemei S., Wilcox, S., Lavie, C. J., & Blair, S.N. (2015). Influence of the source of social support and size of social network on all-cause mortality. *Mayo Clinic Proceedings*, doi.org/10.1016/j.mayocp.2015.04.007.

Bergen, D. (2014). Foundations of play theory. In L. Brooker, M. Blaise, & S. Edwards (Eds.), *The Sage handbook of play and learning in early childhood*. Los Angeles, CA: Sage.

Berger, B. G., & Hecht, L. M. (1989). Exercise, aging, and psychological well-being: The mind-body question. In A. C. Ostrow (Ed.), *Aging and motor behavior.* Indianapolis, IN: Benchmark.

Berger, B. G., & McInman, A. (1993). Exercise and the quality of life. In R. N. Singer, M. Murphey, & L. K. Tennant (Eds.), *Handbook of research on sport psychology.* New York: Macmillan.

Berk, L. E. (2018). *Development through the lifespan*. 7th ed. Boston: Pearson.

Birkeland, M. S., Breivik, K., & Wold, B. (2014). Peer acceptance protects global self-esteem from negative effects of low closeness to parents during adolescence and early adulthood. *Journal of Youth and Adolescence*, *43*, 70–80.

Brown, W. J., & Trost, S. G. (2003). Life transitions and changing physical activity patterns in young women. *American Journal of Preventive Medicine*, *25*(2), 140–143.

Burghardt, G. M. (2015). Integrative approaches to the biological study of play. In J. Johnson, S. G. Eberle, T. S. Henricks, & D. Kuschner (Eds.), *The handbook of the study of play*, vol. 2. New York: Rowman & Littlefield.

Cardon, G., Philippaerts, R., Lefevre, J., Matton, L., Wijndaele, K., Balduck, A. L., et al. (2005). Physical activity levels in 10- to 11-year olds:

Clustering of psychosocial correlates. *Public Health and Nutrition*, *8*(7), 805–807.
Carey, I. M., Shah, S. M., DeWilde, S., Harris, T., Victor, C. R., & Cook, D. G. (2014). Increased risk of acute cardiovascular events after partner bereavement. *Journal of American Medical Association; Internal Medicine*, *174*, 598–605.
Carpendale, J. L., & Lewis, C. (2015). The development of social understanding. In R. M. Lerner (Ed.), *Handbook of child psychology and developmental science*, 7th ed. New York: Wiley and Sons.
Chen, D., Yang, X., & Aagard, S. D. (2012). The empty nest syndrome: Ways to enhance quality of life. *Educational Gerontology*, doi: 10.1080/03601277.595285.
Chou, C., Hwang, C., & Wu, Y. (2012). Effect of exercise on physical function, daily living activities, and quality of life in the frail older adults: A meta-analysis. *Archives of Physical and Medical Rehabilitation*, *93*, 237–244.
Coakley, J. (2017). *Sports in society: Issues and controversies*. 12th ed. New York: McGraw-Hill.
Cooky, C., & Lavoi, N. M. (2012). Women's sports after Title IX: Playing but losing. *Contexts*, *11*, 42–46.
Cratty, B. J. (1986). *Perceptual and motor development in infants and children*. 3rd ed. Englewood Cliffs, NJ: Prentice-Hall.
Da Silva, M. A., Singh-Manouz, A., Brunner, E. J., Kaffashian, S., Shipley, M. J., Kivimaki, M., et al. (2012). Bidirectional association between physical activity and symptoms of anxiety and depression: The Whitehall II Study. *European Journal of Epidemiology*, *27*, 537–546.
Downward, P., Hallmann, K., & Pawlowski, T. (2014). Assessing parental impact on the sports participation of children: A socio-economic analysis of the UK. *European Journal of Sport Sciences*, *14*, 84–90.
Engberg, A., Alen, M., Kukkonen-Harjula, K., Peltonen, J. E., Tikkanen, H. O., & Pekkarinen, H. (2012). Life events and change in leisure time physical activity. *Sports Medicine*, *42*, 433–447.
Erkelenz, N., Kobel, S., Kettner, S., Drenowatz, C., & Steinacker, J. M. (2014). Parental activity as influence on children's BMI percentiles and physical activity. *Journal of Sports Science and Medicine*, *13*, 645–650.
Feng, X., Croteau, K., Kolt, G.S., & Astell-Burt, T. (2016). Does retirement mean more physical activity? A longitudinal study. *BMC Public Health*, doi: 10.1186/s12889-016-3253-0.
Gao, M., Li, Y., Zhang, S., Gu, L., Zhang, J., Zhuojun, L., et al. (2017). Does an empty nest affect elders' health? Empirical evidence from China. *International Journal of Environmental Research and Public Health*, doi: 10.3390/ijerph14050463.
Greve, W., Thomsen, T., & Dehio, C. (2014). Does playing pay? The fitness-effect of free play during childhood. *Evolutionary Psychology*, *12*, 434–447.
Gruber, J. J. (1985). Physical activity and self-esteem development in children: A meta-analysis. *Academy Papers*, *19*, 30–48.
Grusec, J. E., & Davidov, M. (2015). Analyzing socialization from a domain-specific perspective. In J. E. Grusec & P. D. Hastings (Eds.), *Handbook of socialization: Theory and research*. 2nd ed. New York: Guilford Press.
Hallal, P. C., Andersen, L. B., Bull, F. C., Guthold, R., Haskell, W., & Ekelund, U. (2012). Global physical activity levels: Surveillance progress, pitfalls, and prospects. *The Lancet*, *380*, 247–257.
Harter, S. (1988). Causes, correlates, and the functional role of global self-worth: A life-span perspective. In J. Killigian & R. Sternberg (Eds.), *Perceptions of competence and incompetence across the life-span*. New Haven, CT: Yale University Press.
Hausdorff, J. M., Levy, B. R., & Wei, J. Y. (1999). The power of ageism on physical function of older persons: Reversibility of age-related gait changes. *Journal of the American Geriatric Society*, *47*(11), 1346–1349.
Healey, A., Mendelsohn, A., & American Academy of Pediatrics Council on Early Childhood (2019). Selecting appropriate toys for young children in the digital era. *Pediatrics*, doi: 10.1542/peds.2018-3348.
Heinze, J. E., Heinze, K. L., Davis, M. M., Butchart, A. T., Singer, D. C., & Clark, S. J. (2014). Gender role beliefs and parents' support for athletic participation. *Youth & Society*, 1–24. Retrieved from http://yas.sagepub.com/content/early/2014/10/17/004411 8X14553580.full.pdf+html.

Henricks, T. S. (2015). Overview: Play as self-realization: Toward a general theory of play. In J. Johnson, S. G. Eberle, T. S. Henricks, & D. Kuschner (Eds.), *The handbook of the study of play*, vol. 2. New York: Rowman & Littlefield.

Huxhold, O., Miche, M., & Schüz, B. (2014). Benefits of having friends in older ages: Differential effects of informal social activities on wellbeing in middle-aged and older adults. *Gerontology: Psychological and Social Sciences: Series B*, *69*, 366–375.

Lillard, A. S. (2015). The development of play. In R. M. Lerner (Ed.) *Handbook of child psychology and developmental science*, 7th ed., vol. 2. New York: Wiley.

Newman, B. M., & Newman, P. R. (2018). *Development through life: A psychosocial approach*. 13th ed. Boston: Cengage.

Ory, M., Kinney Hoffman, M., Hawkins, M., Sanner, B., & Mockenhaupt, R. (2003). Challenging aging stereotypes: Strategies for creating a more active society. *American Journal of Preventive Medicine*, *25*(3, Supplemental 2), 164–171.

Pestana, C. (2015). Exploring the self-concept of adults with mild learning disabilities. *British Journal of Learning Disabilities*, *43*, 16–23.

Piek, J. P., Baynam, G. B., & Barrett, C. (2006). The relationship between fine and gross motor ability, self-perceptions and self-worth in children and adolescents. *Human Movement Science*, *25*, 65–75.

Popa, M., Phillips, B. J., & Robertson, C. (2014). Positive outcomes of social norm transgressions. *Journal of Consumer Behaviourism*, *13*, 351–362.

Rapp, I., & Schneider, B. (2013). The impacts of marriage, cohabitation and dating relationships on weekly self-reported physical activity in Germany: A 19-year longitudinal study. *Social Science & Medicine*, doi.org/10.1016/j.socscimed.2013.09.024.

Rubin, K. H., Bukowski, W. M., & Bowker, J. C. (2015). Children in peer groups. In R. M. Lerner (Ed.). *Handbook of child psychology and developmental science*, 7th ed. New York: Wiley.

Silva, P., Lott, R., Mota, J., & Welk, G. (2014). Direct and indirect effects of social support on youth physical activity behavior. *Pediatric Exercise Science*, *26*, 86–94.

Stahl, S., & Schulz, R. (2014). The effect of widowhood on husbands' and wives' physical activity: The cardiovascular health study. *Journal of Behavioral Medicine*, *37*(4), 806–817.

Stenholm, S., Pulakka, A., Kawachi, I., Oksanen, T., Halonen, J., Aalto, V., et al. (2016). Changes in physical activity during transition to retirement: A cohort study. *International Journal of Behavioral Nutritionand Physical Activity*, doi 10.1186/s12966-016-0375-9.

Stevenson, B. (2006). Beyond the classroom: Using Title IX to measure the return to high school sports. Retrieved from http://lawbepress.com/cgi/viewcontent.cgi?article= 1859&context=alea.

Stevenson, B. (2007). Title IX and the evolution of high school sports. Retrieved from http://papers.ssrn.com/sol3/papers.cfm?abstract_id=1070682.

Sumaroka, M., & Bornstein, M. H. (2008). Play. In M. Haith & J. Benson (Eds.), *Encyclopedia of infant and early childhood development*. New York: Elsevier.

Syrda, J. (2017). The impact of marriage and parenthood on male body mass index: Static and dynamic effects. *Social Science and Medicine, 186*, 148–155.

USDHHS (U.S. Department of Health and Human Services), Office of Disease Prevention and Health Promotion (2014). *Healthy People 2020*. Retrieved from www.healthypeople.gov/2020/topics-objectives/topic/physical-activity.

Walston, J. D. (2012). Sarcopenia in older adults. *Current Opinion in Rheumatology*, *24*, 623–627.

Wolff, J. R., Warner, L. M., Ziegelmann, J. P., & Wurm, S. (2014). What do targeting positive views on ageing add to physical activity interventions in older adults? Results from a randomized controlled trial. *Psychology and Health*, *29*, 915–932.

Yogman, M., Garner, A., Hutchinson, J., Hirsh-Pasek, K., & Michnick Golinkoff, R. American Academy of Pediatrics Committee on Psychosocial Aspects of Play and Family Health (2018). The power of play: A pediatric role in enhancing development in young children. *Pediatrics*, doi: 10.1542/peds.2018-2058.

Zhang, J., Zhang, J-P., Cheng, Q., Huang, F., Li, S., Wang, A., et al. (2017). The resilience status of empty-nest elderly in a community: A latent class analysis. *Archives of Gerontology and Geriatrics*. doi.org/10.1016/j.archger.2016.10.011.

PART II

Factors that Affect Development

4 PRENATAL DEVELOPMENT FACTORS

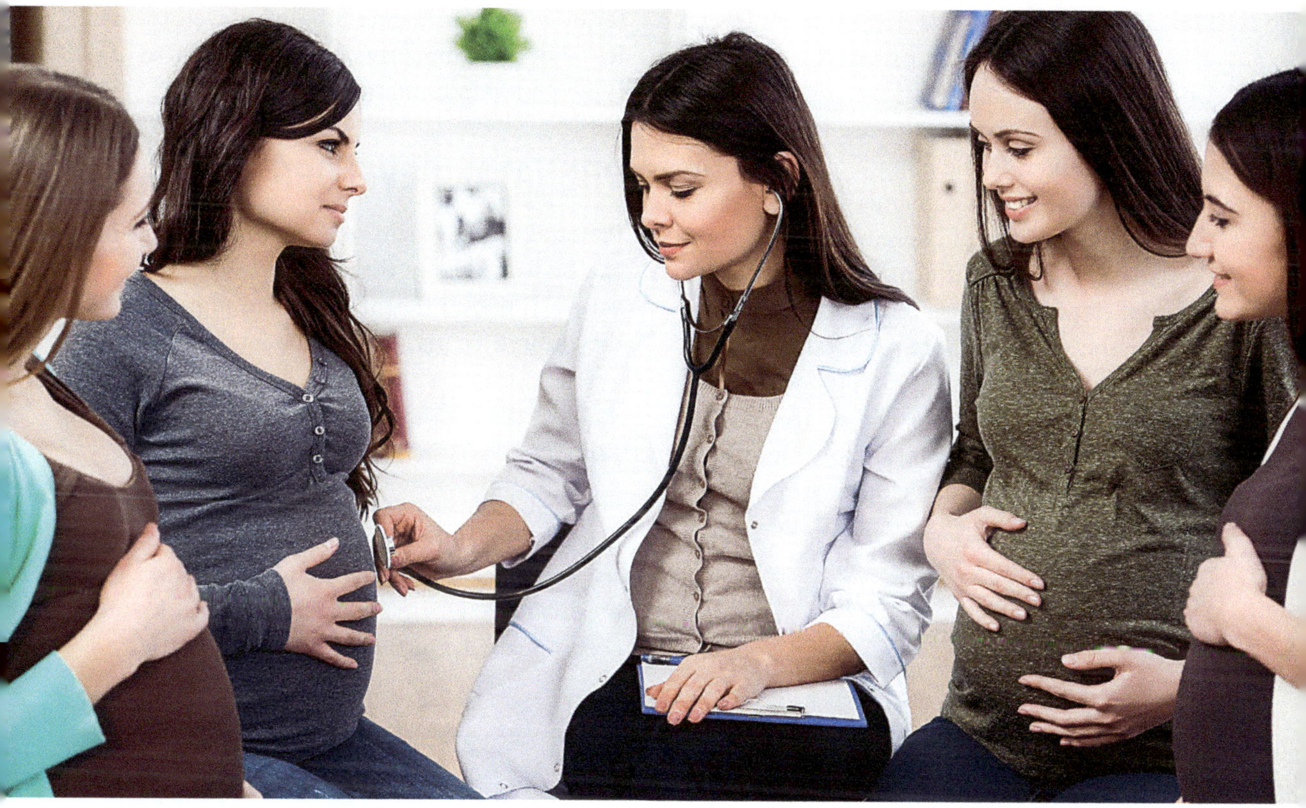

Chapter Objectives

From the information presented in this chapter, you will be able to

- Describe the three major phases of prenatal development
- Describe the possible effects of drugs and medications on both the mother and the developing fetus
- Identify the possible effects of maternal diseases on the developing fetus
- Describe the most common genetic factors known to affect prenatal growth and development
- Identify five prenatal diagnostic procedures and describe the advantages and disadvantages of each
- Describe adequate prenatal nutrition
- Define the three major birth weight categories
- Explain both the ACOG and the U.S. Department of Health and Human Services guidelines concerning exercise during pregnancy and the postpartum period

All human beings are unique, varying in appearance, personality, and movement abilities, but the typical growth and development process is predictable. Although typically everyone attains the same mature human behaviors, the *rate* and ultimate *level* of achievement may vary considerably. Unfortunately, uncontrolled factors occasionally negatively influence the growth and development of the human organism. The effects of such factors can emerge at any time throughout the lifespan; here, we discuss those that are particularly influential during the prenatal stage of growth and development. Because there are far more prenatal factors than we can discuss in this chapter, we have limited our coverage to those that are particularly timely, devastating, or important for the study of motor development.

The factors influencing prenatal life are believed to result from genetic or environmental influences, and they have either a positive or negative effect. An environmental agent that causes harm to the embryo or fetus is known as a **teratogen**. The extent of damage caused by a teratogen is a function of such factors as the amount of exposure, the baby's genetic makeup, and the time of exposure. To understand better how time of exposure to a teratogen can influence a baby's development, let us first examine the anticipated course of typical human prenatal development.

PRENATAL DEVELOPMENT

Prenatal development of the human organism can be described in three major phases: the germinal period (fertilization and implantation), the embryonic period, and the fetal period.

The First 2 Weeks: Germinal Period

Figure 4.1 illustrates the first 2 weeks of prenatal development, which begins with the release of the oocyte from the ovary into the uterine tube, where fertilization is accomplished. During the next 3 days the

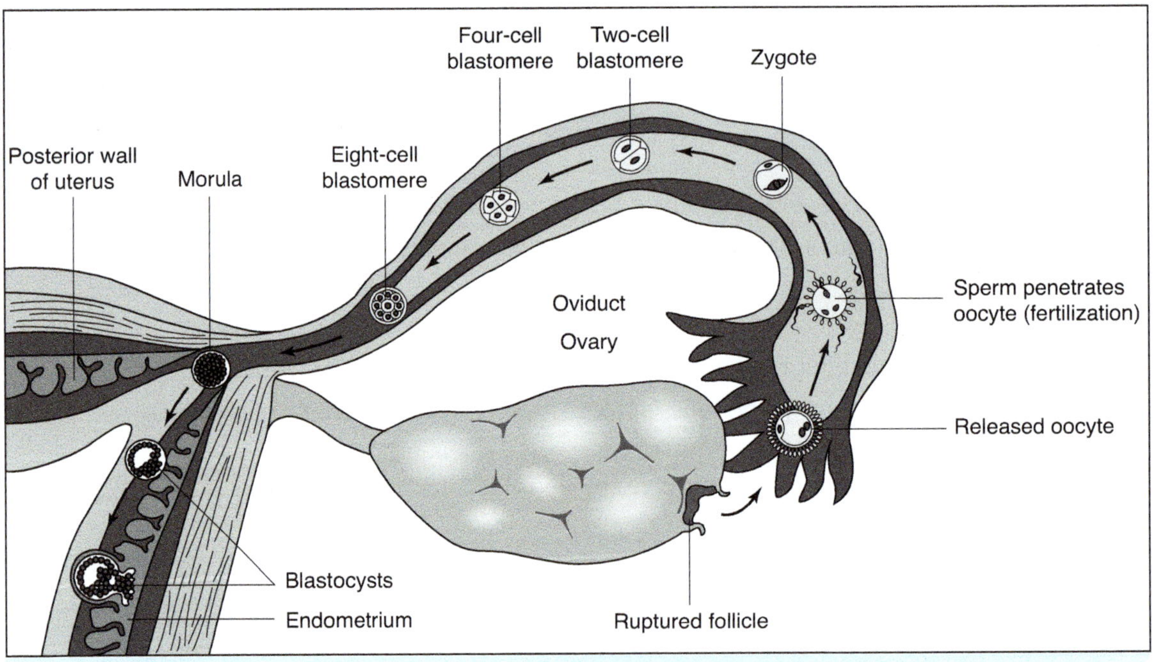

Figure 4.1 Course of development from fertilization to implantation—the germinal period

zygote will divide continuously, forming a blastomere (group of cells) as it proceeds toward the uterus. When cleavage (mitotic division) reaches approximately 12 to 15 blastomeres (Moore, Persaud, & Torchia, 2016), the zygote is termed a *morula*, The term *morula* derives from the Latin word *morus*, meaning mulberry: at this state the blastomere resembles the fruit of a mulberry tree. After the morula enters the uterus, it becomes a blastocyst. Approximately 6 days after fertilization, the blastocyst attaches to the endometrium, usually at the posterior wall of the uterus. During the second week, the blastocyst sinks beneath the endometrium, thus completing implantation.

If a teratogen is introduced during the preembryonic stage, death of the embryo is possible because during this stage the substance is likely to damage all or most of the developing cells. If the teratogen damages only a few cells, the conceptus (early-stage embryo in the uterus) might recover and develop typically.

Weeks 3 to 8: Embryonic Period

The third through the eighth week of prenatal development is referred to as the main embryonic period. During this time, the organ systems and support systems begin to form. More specifically, the zygote forms an inner layer of cells called the **endoderm** and an outer layer of cells that subdivide to form the **ectoderm** and the **mesoderm**. At this point the organism is referred to as an embryo. The endoderm provides the groundwork for the development of both the digestive system and the respiratory system. The ectoderm becomes the basis for the development of the nervous system, sensory receptors (eyes, ears, etc.), and skin features including nails and hair. The circulatory system, muscles, bones, excretory system, and reproductive system are all outgrowths of the mesoderm. Also during the embryonic period, the placenta (where the blood vessels of the mother and embryo intertwine), the umbilical cord (which connects the embryo to the placenta), and the amnion (the clear fluid sac that protects the embryo) develop.

It is during the embryonic period that the embryo is most susceptible to the influences of a teratogen. Recall that this period of development is characterized by the development of the tissue and organ systems. Furthermore, it is during this time that the placenta forms, so the mother's blood supply is now being shared with the embryo. In fact, it was discovered that **thalidomide**, a drug prescribed to treat pregnancy-related morning sickness, was the agent responsible for more than 10,000 malformed births throughout Europe, Australia, and some South American countries. This finding dispelled the myth that the maternal environment was a completely protective shelter for the developing embryo (Dana-Farber Cancer Institute, 2018). The thalidomide tragedy illustrates how the timing of teratogen exposure affects development. Thalidomide had diverse effects on babies, with some babies developing malformed arms, others failing to achieve typical development of the outer ear, and others missing a small bone in the hand. Still others were fortunate to experience no ill effects. Clearly, thalidomide affected the tissue or organ system that was growing and developing the fastest at the time of exposure. Logically, most major congenital anomalies occur in the embryonic stage of development. Figure 4.2 presents a detailed illustration of critical periods in human development. Pay particular attention to the dark shaded areas in Figure 4.2, as they indicate the times of greatest susceptibility.

Week 9 to Birth: Fetal Period

The fetal period begins at about 9 weeks after fertilization and continues until birth. During this period the fetus experiences rapid body

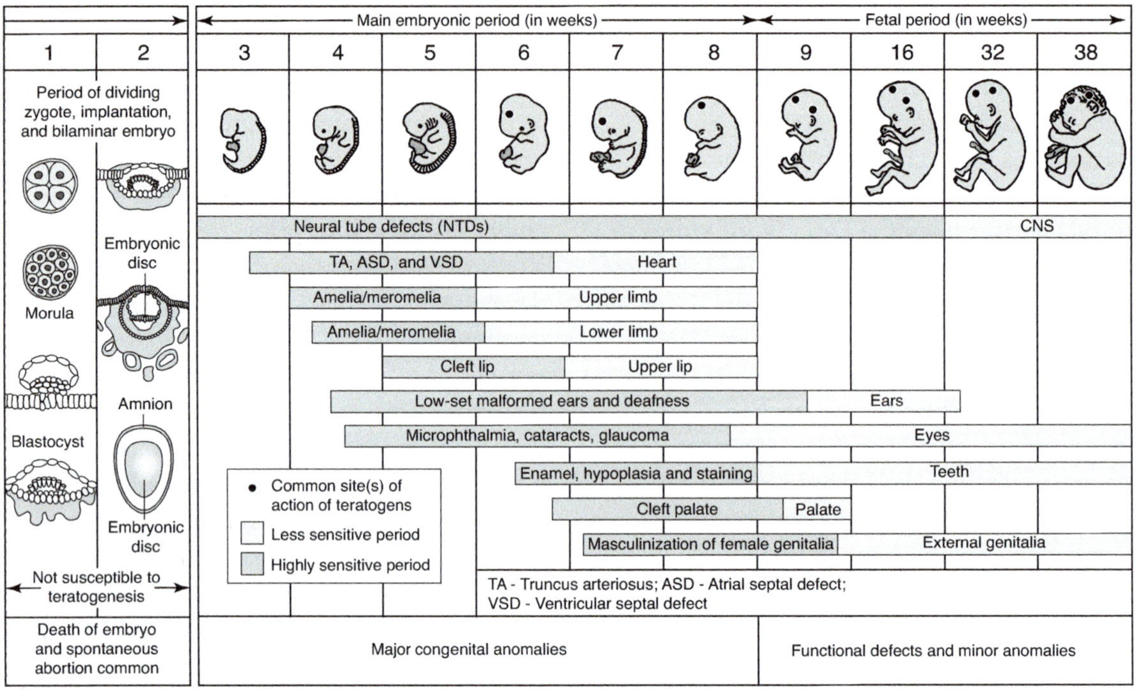

During the first 2 weeks of development, the embryo is not usually susceptible to teratogenesis. During these preembryonic stages, either a substance damages all or most of the cells of the embryo, resulting in death, or it damages only a few cells, allowing the conceptus to recover and the embryo to develop without birth defects. Dark shading denotes highly sensitive periods when major defects may be produced (e.g., limb deficiencies). Lighter shading indicates stages that are less sensitive to teratogens, when minor defects may be induced (e.g., hypoplastic thumbs).

Figure 4.2 Schematic illustration of the critical periods in human development

Source: Reprinted from Moore, Persaud, & Torchia (2016). Copyright ©, 2016 with permission from Elsevier.

growth, as well as differentiation of organ systems. For example, 9 weeks after fertilization the fetus is only about 3 inches long and weighs only 1 ounce. However, by birth the average baby born in the United States will be about 20 in (50.8 cm) long and will weigh about 7 lb (3.175 kg).

Teratogens introduced during the fetal period generally result in relatively minor anomalies and functional defects. This is because the initial development of the tissues and organ systems has occurred and the period is mainly devoted to building up tissues and preparing systems involved in the transition from intrauterine to extrauterine environments, primarily the respiratory and cardiorespiratory systems (Moore, Persaud, & Torchia, 2016).

DRUGS AND MEDICATIONS

Certain drugs and medications can enter fetal circulation; therefore, pregnant women should take them only as advised by a physician. Recreational drugs, prescription drugs, nonprescription drugs, and obstetrical medications are all chemicals that can affect both the mother and the developing fetus.

Recreational Drugs

Recreational drugs are drugs that generally serve no medical purpose. The four most widely used recreational drugs are alcohol, narcotics, cocaine, and tobacco.

Alcohol

According to the CDC's (Centers for Disease Control and Prevention) Behavioral Risk Factor Surveillance System, approximately 1 in 10 (10.2 percent) pregnant women report drinking alcohol during pregnancy (CDC, 2003). More important, however, are findings indicating that the prevalence of any alcohol use among pregnant women is about 1 in 8. Perhaps of even greater concern is that one-third of these pregnant women reported binge drinking (four or more drinks on any one occasion) during pregnancy (CDC, 2015a). Thus, a significant number of women in the United States consume alcohol during pregnancy at levels known to increase the risk of giving birth to a baby having signs or symptoms associated with uterine alcohol exposure.

Women frequently ask, "How much alcohol can I safely drink during pregnancy?" In the opinion of the American Academy of Pediatrics (AAP, 2000a) Committee on Substance Abuse and the Committee on Children with Disabilities, no safe dose of alcohol for pregnant women has been found. Because of the potential damage that drinking alcohol during pregnancy can cause to the developing baby, the AAP recommends a greater societal effort to educate women of all ages about the potential dangers of drinking alcohol during pregnancy.

Strong recommendations are necessary because the incidence of newborns with symptoms associated with maternal alcohol consumption is high. **Fetal alcohol spectrum disorders (FASDs)** is an umbrella term that includes the range of possible effects associated with alcohol consumption during pregnancy. FASDs include **fetal alcohol syndrome (FAS)**, **alcohol-related neurodevelopmental disorders (ARND)**, and **alcohol-related birth defects (ARBD)**. The latter two categories are reserved for newborns who exhibit some but not all of the clinical signs of FAS. The clinical signs associated with FAS include altered facial features, mental retardation, attention deficit disorder with hyperactivity, and retarded physical growth in stature, weight, and head circumference. Because of poor brain growth, children with FAS on average attain an IQ of only 67. The incidence of FAS ranges from 0.2 to 1.5 cases per 1,000 live births (CDC, 2009).

During the neonatal period, a child may even exhibit withdrawal symptoms, known as **neonatal abstinence syndrome (NAS)**. The onset of NAS will generally appear within 7 days following birth (Women's Royal Hospital, 2017). Symptoms generally include tremulousness, hyperactivity, poor appetite, poor weight gain, irritability, and seizures.

In short, few organ tissues or body systems are unaffected by alcohol consumption during the prenatal period. Table 4.1 highlights selected outcomes of FAS, ARND, and ARBD. Note that the atypical outcomes associated with FASDs fall into three categories: growth deficiency, central nervous system dysfunctions, and craniofacial anomalies.

Narcotics

Narcotics are a class of drugs frequently used to treat acute and chronic pain. However, this class of drug can also produce a feeling of relaxation, as well as producing a "high." It is for that reason that some chose to use this as a recreational drug. The use of narcotics, particularly opioids and heroin, has reached epidemic proportions in the United States. These drugs include: codeine, fentanyl, hydrocodone, methadone, oxycodone, tramadol, just to name a few. The 2018 Annual Surveillance Report of Drug-Related Risks and Outcomes (CDC, 2018c) finds that between 1999 and 2016, more than 630,000 people in the United States died from an overdose. According to this CDC report, it appears that this epidemic has escalated in three phases. In the 1990s, the overdoses were driven by prescription opioids that were mainly prescribed to manage chronic pain. In 2010, the increase continued and was driven by the use of

Table 4.1 Selected outcomes of FAS, ARND, and ARBD

Growth Deficiency
Weight and length below 10th percentile corrected for gestational age
Microcephaly
Increased risk of congenital anomalies
Decreased adipose tissue
Central Nervous System Dysfunctions
Poor motor coordination in 50% of infants
Weak sucking reflex
IQ generally less than 70
Increased reaction time
Myopia
Sensorineural hearing loss
Irritability (infancy)
Attention deficit hyperactivity disorder
Hypotonia
Increased risk for seizures
Delayed language development
Fine motor impairment
Craniofacial Anomalies
Epicanthic folds around eyes
Obstruction of upper airway passages
Cleft palate

heroin. The third and final wave started in 2013 with the illicitly manufactured synthetic opioid, fentanyl. It is no wonder that so many overdoses have occurred since this drug has been overprescribed. For example, in 2006, 72.4 opioid prescriptions per 100 persons were prescribed and this overuse continued to increase at a rate of 3 percent per year from 2006 to 2010. Fortunately, since 2010, the number of prescriptions written for an opioid has decreased to 58.5 prescriptions per 100 persons. All said, in 2017, 17.4 percent of the United States population received at least one or more opioid prescriptions, with the average person receiving 3.4 prescriptions (CDC, 2018c). Unfortunately, while there has been a downward trend in the number of legal prescriptions written, there has been a sharp increase in deaths attributed to the increased illicitly manufactured synthetic opioid, fentanyl (CDC, 2018d). In fact, in 2016 there were 19,413 deaths attributed to overdosing on synthetic opioids alone (Center for Behavioral Health Statistics and Quality, 2017).

Like most medications, opioids are also prescribed during pregnancy, especially for the treatment of pregnancy-related pain, such as low back and pelvic pain. Currently, the Food and Drug Administration classify most prescription opioid drugs used in pregnancy as "Category C." Category C denotes drugs where there is evidence of potential harm to a fetus from animal studies but there continues to be an absence of well-controlled human studies (Yazdy, Desai, & Brogly, 2015).

Cocaine

The use of cocaine, usually as a recreational drug, is also a major concern. Because cocaine is one of the most dangerous drugs to the unborn baby, the March of Dimes has strongly advised that women stop use before pregnancy or delay pregnancy until the drug can be avoided. It also advises any woman who is pregnant and uses cocaine to disclose her cocaine use immediately to her physician so that she can receive treatment to help her stop using the drug and so that early prenatal care can begin. Women who use cocaine during pregnancy also have a 25 percent higher incidence of preterm birth (ACOG, 2002).

One potentially devastating effect of cocaine use during pregnancy is fetal brain damage. This damage is believed to result from blood vessel constriction causing oxygen deprivation to the brain. This may explain why cocaine-exposed babies exhibit mental retardation at a rate nearly five times greater than that observed in the general population (Singer, Arendt, Minnes, et al., 2002). Additionally, because of brain and central nervous system damage, "cocaine babies" often score low on tests of responsiveness. For example, they perform poorly on measures of infant reflexes, often having poor sucking ability. Their attention span is also reduced considerably, making them relatively unresponsive to voices or faces. In addition, they are often "jittery" and extremely irritable and cry with minimal provocation. This lack of responsiveness and increase in irritability impede the bonding process and make the task of child rearing especially difficult for the mother, which, in turn, likely contributes to later incidence of child abuse or neglect.

Other effects from maternal cocaine use include increased occurrence of miscarriage. Miscarriage is often caused by uterine contractions late in pregnancy, which can result in premature labor. Cocaine also causes extreme fluctuations in the heart rate and blood pressure of the mother and the fetus. These rapid fluctuations in blood pressure can result in ruptured blood vessels of the brain, leading to stroke and contributing to the fetal brain damage mentioned earlier. Occasionally, the blood vessels to the placenta are also affected. They can be constricted to the point that the passage of nutrients to the fetus is impeded. This causes poor prenatal nutrition and increases the likelihood of a low birth weight baby who is shorter than typical and has a smaller than typical head circumference (Singer et al., 2002). Poor blood supply to the placenta can also cause the placenta to pull away from the uterine wall prematurely, causing extensive bleeding and potentially the death of the mother and baby.

Of particular interest to readers of this text is the influence of cocaine exposure during pregnancy on the child's future motor development. Arendt, Angelopoulos, Salvator, and Singer (1999) reported that 98 cocaine-exposed children performed significantly less well than 101 controls on both fine motor and gross motor indices as measured by the Peabody Developmental Motor Scales (see Chapter 16) during a 2-year follow-up examination. Cocaine exposure independently predicted fine motor deficiencies involving eye-hand coordination and general hand usage. Significant differences in both balance and object reception and propulsion skills were noted within the gross motor scales. Thus, deficiencies in motor development of prenatally cocaine-exposed children remain detectable beyond 2 years of age.

Tobacco

The damaging effects of smoking tobacco during pregnancy were first recognized in 1935. However, intensive studies investigating the effects of smoking on prenatal development did not begin until the 1950s. By 1964, the adverse effects of smoking were so well documented that the Surgeon General's Report led to warning labels being placed on cigarette packages.

More than 7,000 different ingredients have been found in tobacco and tobacco smoke (CDC, 2019). Many of these ingredients are believed to have deleterious effects on the developing fetus (Figure 4.3). The major defects established include low birth weight (Pereira, Da Mata, Figueiredo, et al., 2017), higher rate of mortality at or around the time of birth, increased occurrence of miscarriage, decreased mental functioning in surviving offspring, and a threefold increase in the risk of sudden infant death syndrome (SIDS; AAP, 2000b). Postnatally, nicotine poisoning is a danger for the children of mothers who choose to breast-feed. In fact, Gold stated that "a nursing mother is, in effect, giving her baby a cigarette if she smokes while nursing" (1995, p. 182).

Today, the most studied pharmacological byproducts of tobacco smoke are carbon

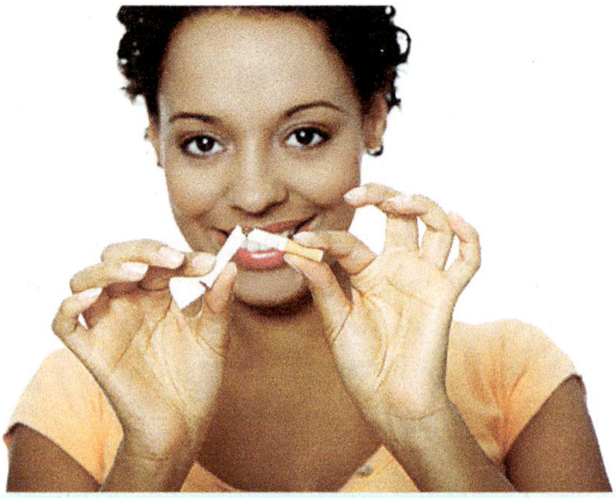

Figure 4.3 Birth defects from maternal smoking are 100 percent preventable

monoxide and nicotine. Carbon monoxide is known to interfere with hemoglobin's oxygen-carrying and oxygen-releasing capabilities and, therefore, to increase the risk of fetal hypoxia (lack of oxygen to body tissues). Nicotine also contributes to fetal hypoxia by causing the adrenals to release epinephrine, a hormone capable of constricting the placenta's blood vessels.

According to the Centers for Disease Control and Prevention, 1 in 14 (7.2 percent) of all women who gave birth in 2016 smoked during their pregnancy (Drake, Driscoll, & Mathews, 2018). The highest rate (10.7 percent) of smoking during pregnancy occurred in women between 20 to 24 years of age. Of most concern to health professionals is the rapid increase in the use of e-cigarettes (Gentzke, Creamer, Cullen, et al., 2019). This increase is the result of marketing that portrays e-cigarettes as being less harmful than smoking tobacco (Rodu & Plurphanswat, 2018). Unfortunately, this is not the case since nicotine exposure is similar in both (Whittington, Simmons, Phillips, et al., 2018).

Also of interest are findings that indicate that breathing second-hand smoke can also lead to maternal complications. Studies have found that children who live in homes where smoking is prevalent exhibit more episodes of respiratory diseases such as bronchiolitis, pneumonia, and asthma (USDHHS, 2007). In addition, there is preliminary evidence that third-hand smoke could also be contributing to the overall tobacco smoking experience, especially for children (Mahabee-Gittens, Merianos, & Matt, 2018). **Third-hand smoke** refers to the pollutants left behind during tobacco smoking, which can be deposited, on environmental surfaces. Children who live in this smoking environment have been found to have these pollutants on their hands and clothing. Table 4.2 summarizes the short- and

Table 4.2 Risk factors associated with maternal tobacco use

Prenatal Complications
Premature rupture of membranes
Placenta previa (placenta covers opening to uterus)
Placenta abruption (placenta peels away from uterine wall prior to delivery)
Increased chance of spontaneous abortion
Higher rates of stillbirth
Intrauterine growth retardation
Postnatal Complications
Congenital heart defects
Lower average birth weight
Small for gestational age
Sudden infant death syndrome (SIDS)
Long-term retardation of growth (weight, stature, and head circumference)
Respiratory disorders (pneumonia, bronchitis, asthma)
Ear infections
Behavioral Effects
Reduced mental alertness
Reduced visual alertness
Mother less likely to breast-feed

long-term risk factors associated with maternal tobacco product use.

Prescription Drugs

Many women have some chronic disease that must be controlled by the continuous use of prescription medications, even during pregnancy. In fact, about 7 in 10 women take at least one prescriptive medication during their pregnancy (CDC, 2018a). These women tend to give birth to malformed infants at a greater rate than do women who do not use prescription medications. There is controversy, however, as to whether the real cause of the reported malformations is the drugs or the mother's general ill health.

Prescription drugs are believed to affect the fetus in two general ways. First, they may, like thalidomide, damage the body part that is growing and developing the fastest during the time of drug use. Second, they may adversely affect in the fetus the system or organ that was intended to be positively affected in the mother. For example, a mother who is taking prescription thyroid medication expects a positive effect on her thyroid gland. Though she may reap such benefits, the thyroid of the fetus may be damaged by the mother's prescription drug use. Table 4.3 lists popular

Table 4.3 Selected prescription medications and their possible effects on the developing fetus

Medication	Use of medication	Possible teratogenic effect
Anticoagulants:	Blood clots	Central nervous system defects
Warfarin		Miscarriage Eye defects
Lithium	Bipolar disorder	Congenital heart defects
Antibiotics:	Infections	Underdevelopment of tooth enamel and tooth yellowing
Tetracycline		
Streptomycin		
Anticonvulsants:	Seizure disorders	Mental retardation
Dilantin		Neural tube defects Hand and face defects
Antithyroids:	Overactive thyroid	Thyroid gland defects
Propylthiouracil, iodide, and methimazole		
Opioids:	Pain relief	Ventricular septal defect
Codeine		Atrial septal defect
Oxycodone		
Hydrocodone		
Morphine		

prescription drugs and their possible side effects if taken during pregnancy.

Nonprescription Drugs

Nonprescription, or over-the-counter, medications are generally assumed to be safe because no prescription is required for them to be dispensed. Although this is generally true, many nonprescription drugs can also have dramatic teratogenic effects on an unborn baby. For that reason, many physicians recommend not treating such illnesses as colds with nonprescription drugs unless absolutely necessary. If a pregnant woman feels she needs to take such a medication, she should consult her physician before doing so.

The most commonly used over-the-counter medications used during pregnancy include aspirin, ibuprofen (Advil, Motrin), and acetaminophen (Tylenol). Aspirin interferes with the blood's ability to clot and may contribute to maternal and fetal bleeding. In general, mothers reporting nonsteroidal anti-inflammatory drug use during pregnancy were significantly more likely to give birth to offspring with gastroschisis, cleft palate, cleft lip, spina bifida, pulmonary valve and other birth defects (Interrante, Ailes, Lind, et al., 2017). Additionally, both aspirin and ibuprofen have been linked to prolonged labor and fetal pulmonary hypertension (Harms, 2012). Acetaminophen (e.g., Tylenol), once thought to be a safe substitute for aspirin, has now been linked to an increased risk of developing attention deficit hyperactivity disorder (Liew, Ritz, Rebordosa, et al., 2014).

A problem with many over-the-counter medications is that they have been designed to treat an array of maladies. Such nonprescription medications should always be avoided if possible during pregnancy because the variety of chemicals they contain increases the risk of prenatal harm. This is the case with many cold medications, whose alcohol content can also be damaging.

Obstetrical Medications

Physicians prescribe and administer many drugs during pregnancy and delivery. The preanesthetic medications most frequently administered to laboring women are oxytocin (to initiate and aid labor), meperidine (to relieve pain), and phenergan (to relieve anxiety). Other forms of anesthetic agents include those for general anesthesia (loss of sensation throughout the entire body—that is, sleep) and regional anesthesia (loss of sensation in a selected area of the body).

Since many of these medications cross the placenta and enter fetal circulation, the drug may exhibit its effect on the baby, as well as the mother. For example, opioids administered to control labor and delivery pain are known to depress fetal respiration. The use of these pain management medications has increased 40 percent over the last decade (Malek & Mattison, 2011).

The ingestion of any drug, whether prescribed or purchased over the counter, carries with it both potential risks and benefits. This is especially true during pregnancy since many medications are capable of affecting not only the mother but the developing fetus, as well. For this reason, pregnant women should consult with their physician about the use of any drugs, including obstetrical medications, so that both risks and benefits can be addressed and an appropriate decision made.

MATERNAL DISEASES

A host of maternal diseases can potentially exert an influence on the developing fetus. These diseases include the following: viral diseases (rubella, HIV), parasitic diseases (toxoplasmosis), hematologic diseases (Rh incompatibility), and endocrine diseases (diabetes mellitus). In this section we examine several of the most influential maternal diseases that can affect the outcome of pregnancy.

Rubella and Congenital Rubella Syndrome

Rubella, sometimes referred to as the German measles, is a highly contagious virus characterized by swollen lymph nodes, mild fever, headache, aching joints, and a pink rash on the face, torso, arms, and legs. In fact, the symptoms can be so mild that 20–50 percent of infected individuals may fail to notice any symptoms at all. Rubella reached epidemic proportions in the United States in 1964 and 1965, when 15.5 million cases of the infection were reported. Additionally, according to the CDC (2017), approximately 20,000 newborns were affected and exhibited symptoms referred to as **congenital rubella syndrome** (CRS). In contrast to the mild symptoms usually experienced by the adult, great damage can be incurred in the developing fetus. The extent of this damage depends in part on when the pregnant woman becomes infected with the virus. The most prevalent defect of CRS, occurring in 80 percent of infected children, is deafness (Alger, 2000). Other potential fetal defects include growth retardation, cataracts, bony lesions, pneumonia, hepatitis, congenital glaucoma, mental retardation, and cardiac anomalies resulting in early heart failure. Fortunately, since the introduction of vaccines, the incidence of rubella and CRS has steadily declined to a median of only 11 cases per year (CDC, 2015b). See Figure 4.4.

Human Immunodeficiency Virus (HIV)

Women who carry the **human immunodeficiency virus** (HIV) risk passing this deadly virus on to their offspring. Perinatal transmission is generally accomplished in one of three ways: (1) in utero from the mother to the fetus; (2) during delivery when the fetus comes in contact with infected blood or infected vaginal secretions; and (3) through breast milk.

Since 1994, oral administration of zidovudine during pregnancy, intravenously during labor, and orally for 6 weeks to the newborn has significantly decreased HIV infection in susceptible children to as low as

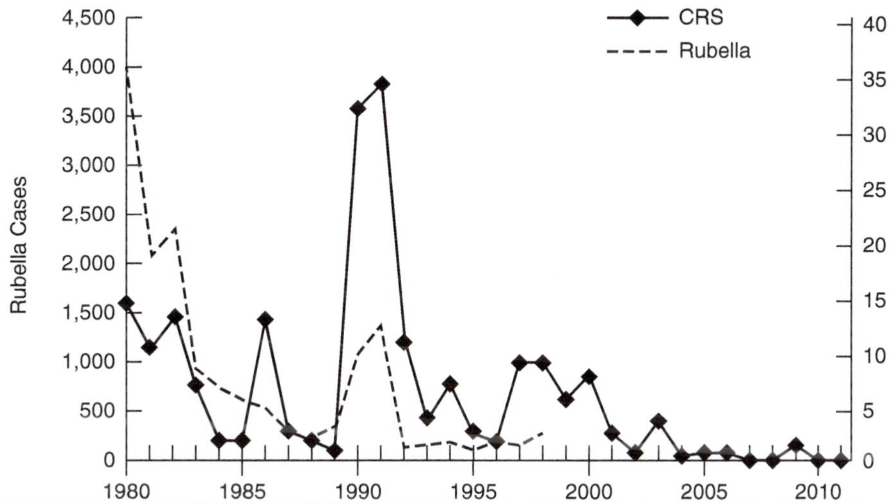

Figure 4.4 Incidence of rubella and congenital rubella syndrome in the United States, 1980 to 2011

Source: CDC (2015b). www.cdc.gov/vaccines/pubs/pinkbook/downloads/rubella.pdf

Table 4.4 Selected neurological findings in HIV-infected children and adolescents

• Encephalopathy
• Mental retardation
• Language delay
• Pyramidal signs (dysfunction of corticospinal spinal cord tracts)
• Hyporeflexia
• Decrease in fine motor coordination
• Positive Babinski

Source: Rocha, Gouvea, Machado, et al. (2005).

2 percent (Marino, 2015). Surviving infants infected with HIV are at greater risk of demonstrating neurodevelopmental delays compared to unexposed infants (LeDoare, Bland, & Newell, 2012). Furthermore, a positive association exists between HIV-positive adults and deficits in motor speed dexterity (Montoya, Campbell, Paolillo, et al., 2019). Table 4.4 lists several of the neurological complications associated with HIV infection in infants and adolescents.

When HIV infection becomes full-blown AIDS, the immune system generally deteriorates rapidly, and death is usually caused by the body's inability to fight off infection.

Toxoplasmosis

The fetus can be infected by protozoan parasites, of which the most common is **Toxoplasma gondii.** Members of the feline (cat) family are the primary hosts for this organism. Pregnant women are introduced to the organism when they are exposed to infectious oocysts present in soil contaminated by cat feces or when they ingest undercooked meats containing the active organism. This virus has frequently been called the "silent infection" because only 10 percent of infected newborns show clinical evidence of the disease at birth (Alford, Pass, & Stagno, 1983).

When toxoplasmosis is acute, 85 percent of live births will experience mental retardation and convulsions; 75 percent will experience effects on motor abilities. Other reported effects include deafness (13 percent) and visual impairments (50 percent), which may be present at birth or take many years to become detectable (Alford et al., 1983). The incidence of primary maternal toxoplasmosis in the United States is only about 11 percent (CDC, 2018b).

Rh Incompatibility and Erythroblastosis Fetalis

In addition to the antigens called A and B, which create the four major blood groups (A, B, AB, and O), red blood cells can contain an additional antigen, the **Rh factor.** Approximately 85 percent of the population have this antigen. These individuals are said to have Rh-positive blood; those people lacking this blood protein possess Rh-negative blood. That all individuals do not possess an Rh factor in their red blood cells is of special concern for a select group of parents. There is a potential problem when an Rh-positive man and an Rh-negative woman conceive an Rh-positive child. If, during the course of gestation, Rh-positive blood cells escape from fetal circulation to enter maternal circulation, the mother's Rh-negative blood will view the Rh-positive cells as foreign bodies. The mother's body will then be stimulated to produce antibodies against the Rh-positive cells. These antibodies may enter the fetal circulation and destroy the fetal red blood cells.

Maternal and fetal circulation do not mix under typical circumstances; however, some experts suggest that fetal blood cells may enter maternal circulation by escaping from broken vessels in the placental villi. Because the placental vessels do not generally rupture until later in pregnancy, the mother typically develops antibodies postnatally, sparing her first offspring. However, in order to protect subsequent children, the mother should receive an injection of **anti-D IgG immunoglobulin** immediately after her first delivery. Treatment within 72 hours after delivery is adequate for protection in 98 percent of cases.

Rh-positive offspring exposed to the antibodies of their Rh-negative mother are born with a condition called **erythroblastosis fetalis,** also called congenital hemolytic disease. Characteristics of this disorder include anemia, an increased number of immature red blood cells in circulation, generalized edema, and jaundice.

The probability of a susceptible couple conceiving an Rh-positive child depends on whether the father carries the Rh antigens on both members of his paired chromosomes (**homozygous**) or on just one of the two chromosomes (**heterozygous**). If the father is a homozygous carrier, all of his children will be Rh-positive; a heterozygous carrier has a 50 percent chance of producing an Rh-positive child. Approximately 12 percent of all marriages involve Rh-positive men and Rh-negative women.

Diabetes Mellitus

Infants born to mothers with **diabetes mellitus** remain a high-risk population in spite of improving management (insulin regulation and diet therapy). Complications during pregnancy are attributed to the fetus's exposure to a constantly altering metabolic environment. This metabolic environment can range from **normoglycemia** (typical blood sugar) to **hypoglycemia** (low blood sugar) to intermittent or constant **hyperglycemia** (high blood sugar). A particular problem is fetal hyperinsulinemia (excessive insulin) induced by maternal hyperglycemia. This condition may result in

1. **macrosomia** (birth weight above the 90th percentile for gestational age or greater than 8.8 lb (4,000 g), making a vaginal delivery difficult;
2. inhibition of maturation of lung surfactant (a material composed of lipids and protein found in the fluids lining the surface of the lung that provides protection from injuries and infections);
3. muscle weakness or cardiac arrhythmias as a result of decreased serum potassium;
4. possible permanent neurological damage brought on by neonatal hypoglycemia.

Of these four outcomes, the most frequently addressed is macrosomia.

Of particular interest to health professionals are findings that suggest that macrosomia in infants of mothers with diabetes may be an important factor in accounting for the development of both diabetes and obesity in later life. For example, Jazayeri (2015) has reported that children born large for gestational age to diabetic mothers had an increased risk of developing metabolic syndrome by 11 years of age. Similarly, Zhao and colleagues (2016) have reported a positive association between gestational diabetes with increased odds of childhood obesity at 9 to 11 years of age. Fortunately, a recent meta-analysis concluded that maternal exercise during pregnancy could significantly reduce the risk of acquiring gestational diabetes mellitus (Yu, Xie, Shen, et al., 2018). Table 4.5 highlights selected effects in infants born to mothers with diabetes.

GENETIC FACTORS

Genetic factors affecting typical prenatal growth and development can take one of two forms. That is, atypical development can be caused by a chromosomal or a gene-based disorder.

Table 4.5 Selected effects in infants born to mothers with diabetes

• Central nervous system deformities
• Spina bifida
• Hydrocephalus
• Congenital anomalies
• Heart defects
• Skeletal and central nervous system defects
• Macrosomia
• Musculoskeletal deformities
• Respiratory distress syndrome
• Traumatic birth injury
• Asphyxia
• Facial nerve injury
• Brachial plexus injury
• Caesarean section due to cephalopelvic disproportion

Chromosomal Disorders

Every typical cell within our bodies contains 46 chromosomes, with the exception of the reproductive cells (sperm and ova), which contain only 23 chromosomes. When the sperm and ovum join during conception, each contributes its 23 chromosomes, to form a new individual whose cells will also contain the usual 23 pairs of genetic material. When the sex chromosomes reproduce through cell division (meiosis), there can be problems if, during the division, a pair of chromosomes does not separate properly. This lack of chromosomal separation is called **meiotic nondisjunction**, the result of which is that one sperm or egg cell contains two members of a particular chromosome while the other sperm or egg cell contains none. If, during conception, the cell containing the extra chromosome unites with a typical sex cell, the new individual will possess 47 chromosomes. This individual is said to be trisomic, meaning that one of the chromosomes has three rather than the usual two members.

The most frequent cytogenetic defect is **Down syndrome** (**DS**). The technical name for this syndrome is trisomy 21, indicating that chromosome number 21 has three chromosomes instead of the usual two. The prevalence of this defect is estimated to be 9 per 10,000 live births (Presson, Partyka, Jensen, et al., 2013). The number of infants born with DS is nearly five times greater among births to women over 35 years of age (38.6 per 10,000) than births to younger women (7.8 per 10,000; Shin, Besser, Kucik, et al., 2009). Apparently, with aging the woman's eggs have a greater chance of improper chromosome division.

The most striking behavioral outcome of this syndrome is cognitive delay, which can be either mild or severe. Individuals with DS generally obtain IQ scores between 20 and 60 and function at a maximum average mental age of 8 years. Table 4.6 lists other prominent characteristics of this genetic defect, although individuals with Down syndrome may exhibit these characteristics to a varying degree or not at all. Pay special attention to the fact that the fundamental motor pattern, walking, is generally delayed until 2 years of age, compared with an onset at 1 year of age in typically developing children.

Gene-Based Disorders

Unlike chromosomal disorders, which affect the entire collection of genes that make up the chromosomal chain, gene-based disorders are caused by a mutation within a selected gene along this chain. In this section we describe the following gene-based disorders: phenylketonuria, cystic fibrosis, sickle-cell trait and sickle-cell disease, and fragile X syndrome.

Table 4.6 Symptoms and signs of trisomy 21 (Down syndrome)

• Walking delayed 1 or more years
• Slow speech development
• Cognitive delays
• Slow development of fine motor control
• Delayed toilet training
• Lower than typical birth weight
• Hypotonia (too little muscle tone)
• Short stature
• Puberty often delayed
• Susceptibility to respiratory infections
• Heart disease common
• Prominent anatomical features
• Close-set eyes
• Short, thick neck
• Small, rather square head

Phenylketonuria

Phenylketonuria (**PKU**) was discovered in 1934 by Asbjorn Folling, a Norwegian doctor. PKU has been the topic of literally thousands of research papers, mainly because the discovery of this disorder led to the prevention of the intellectual disabilities associated with PKU. Mental manifestations are the most commonly reported clinical features of the disorder, but some individuals may exhibit neurological dysfunctions and extraneural symptoms, including motor impairments such as tight muscles and muscle tremors.

PKU is caused by a disturbance in the amino acid metabolism as a result of inheriting a gene that suppresses the activity of the liver enzyme phenylalanine hydroxylase. This enzyme is responsible for converting dietary L-phenylalanine into the amino acid tyrosine. If there is not enough of this conversion, the body tissues accumulate dangerous levels of L-phenylalanine, resulting

IMPROVING THE ONSET OF WALKING IN INFANTS WITH DS

Ulrich, Ulrich, Angulo-Kinzler, and Yun (2001) discovered that infants with DS were capable of exhibiting well-coordinated, alternating stepping patterns at approximately 11 months of age when held in the upright position. Because alternating stepping movements resemble walking, the researchers believed that stepping practice in the form of parent-assisted treadmill walking could influence the onset of independent walking in children with DS. They felt that, in accordance with dynamical systems theory, assisted treadmill walking would emphasize not only neural connections but also the training of multiple subsystems, such as muscular strength, proprioception, joint structure, motivation, and temperament, and that these subsystems are as important as the nervous system in determining specific motor behaviors (Ulrich & Ulrich, 1999).

As a result of this hypothesis, Ulrich and colleagues (2001) developed an infant treadmill-walking intervention program. Subjects with DS were admitted to the study when they were capable of sitting alone for 30 seconds. The treadmill intervention program consisted of parent-assisted walking at a speed of 0.46 mph (0.74 km/h) for 8 minutes/day, 5 days/week, until the infant was capable of independent walking. Analysis indicated that DS subjects assigned to the intervention group, on average, walked independently 101 days sooner than did subjects in a control group who did not participate in the intervention program.

in irreversible changes in the central nervous system.

Unlike the other birth disorders discussed here, PKU cannot be evaluated by visual inspection; blood levels of phenylalanine must be measured in the laboratory. For accurate blood level measures to be obtained, newborns should be evaluated no sooner than 8 days after birth, because the level of phenylalanine in the blood of phenylketonuric children rises after birth until the concentration reaches a dangerous level. Screening too early may result in failing to diagnose 5–10 percent of phenylketonuric children.

As early as the mid-1950s, the medical community demonstrated that many of the symptoms of PKU could be favorably modified and even prevented by placing the child on a low phenylalanine diet. For treatment to be most effective, the disorder should be diagnosed as early as possible. Major differences have been found between early- and late-treated groups of children with PKU. Left untreated, PKU is associated with significant delays in motor milestones including crawling, walking, and even talking (Waisbren, Noel, Fahrbach, et al., 2007).

Cystic Fibrosis (CF)

Individuals with **cystic fibrosis (CF)** have inherited two copies of the defective CF gene, one from each parent. This devastating disease affects approximately 30,000 children and adults in the United States and approximately 70,000 worldwide (ALA, 2018). Characteristically, this disease causes thick, sticky mucus to be secreted within the lungs. This mucus causes reoccurring bouts of pulmonary infection. In addition, the thick mucus frequently will clog the pancreas and interfere with typical digestion. From a movement perspective, individuals with CF often experience shortness of breath, and they fatigue easily. With repeated bouts of lung infection, scar tissue accumulates within the lungs and worsens the condition. To date, there is no cure for CF. However, the drug pulmozyme has proven to be effective in both improving lung function (Mainz, Schien, Schiller, et al., 2014) and reducing lung infections (Stuckey, Clark, Chang, et al., 2015).

Sickle-Cell Trait and Sickle-Cell Disease

Sickle-cell trait (SCT) is a genetic disorder of the red blood cells caused by a mutation in a parental gene for hemoglobin (Hb). An individual is said to possess the SCT if he or she possesses one typical gene (A) and one atypical gene (S). Individuals with the SCT are generally asymptomatic (Martineaud, Samb, Gueel, et al., 2002), and the trait does not appear to pose a significant barrier to athletic performance (NCAA, 2014). However, a far more serious condition, **sickle-cell disease (SCD)**, occurs when the offspring inherits two defective genes (SS). In this situation, the red blood cells will change from the characteristic doughnut shape to the classic "sickle" shape—giving the name to the disease. As illustrated in Figure 4.5, when both parents carry the SCT, the chance of producing an offspring with SCT is 50 percent; of producing an offspring with SCD, 25 percent; and of producing an offspring with neither, 25 percent. Also illustrated in Figure 4.5 are the potential consequences of sickle-cell disease. Briefly, such consequences come about for several reasons: the destruction of red blood cells; the clumping of the sickle-shaped cells, which leads to circulatory problems because of the cells' inability to travel through small blood vessels; and an unusually high concentration of sickle-shaped cells in the spleen. Current treatments involve red blood cell transfusions and use of a new drug, hydroxyurea, which is capable of turning on the production of healthy Hgb. This disease predominately affects individuals of African descent.

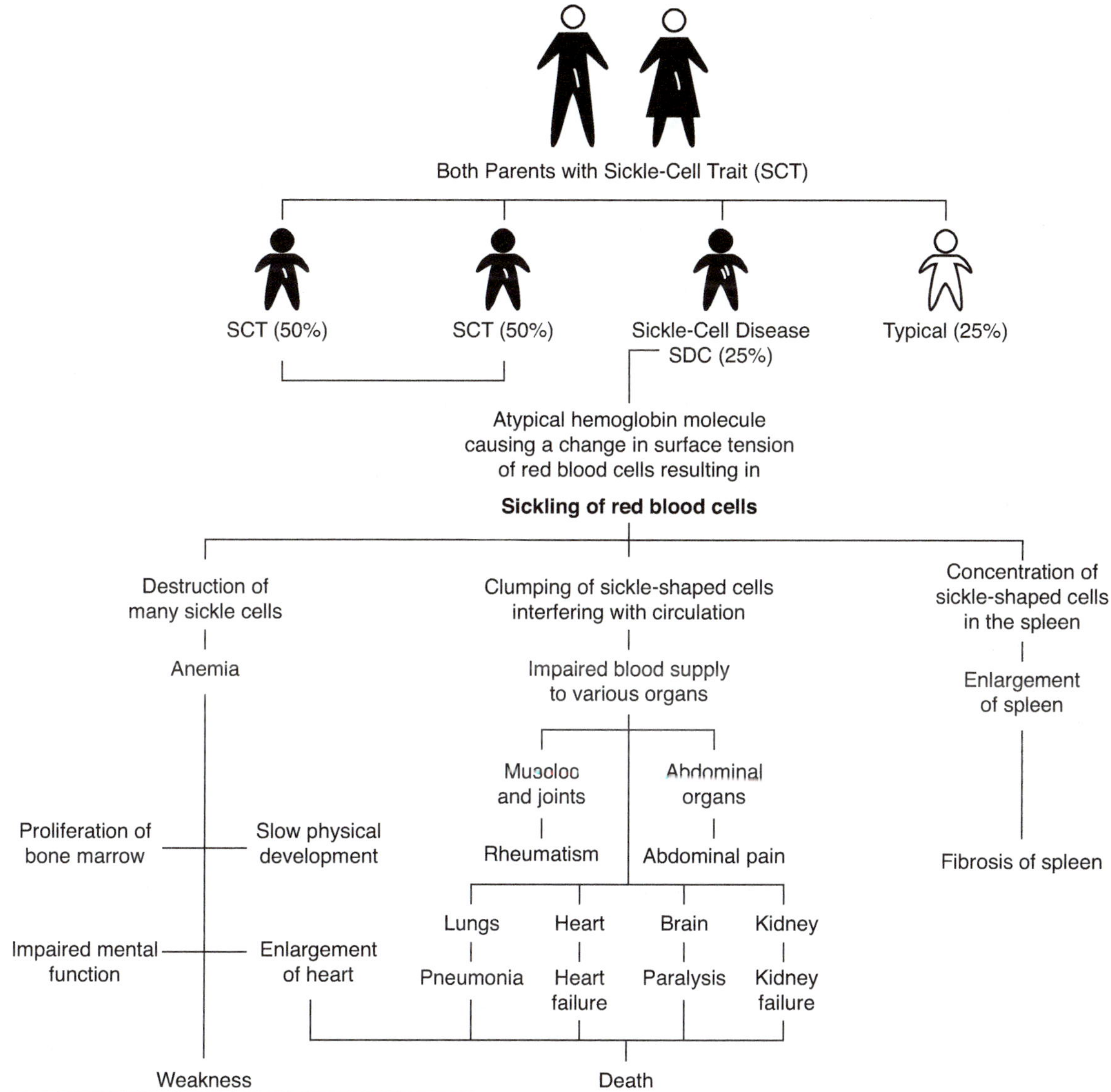

Figure 4.5 Sickle-cell incidence and outcomes

Fragile X Syndrome (FXS)

Fragile X is a family of gene-based conditions that have in common a mutation in the FMR1 gene. This gene mutation can result in **fragile X syndrome** (**FXS**), which is the leading cause of autism. Accompanying this mental impairment is a delay in early motor skill acquisition, including sitting, crawling, and walking. In contrast to the average child, who will be capable of independent walking at an average age of 1 year, most boys with FXS will not walk until 2 years of age (National Fragile X Foundation, 2009). Other potential motor problems related to FXS include low muscle tone; poor balance; poor motor planning, making game playing difficult; and flat feet and hyper-extensibility of joints, which can cause awkwardness in motor movements. Children diagnosed with FXS can benefit from physical therapy and adapted physical education.

PRENATAL DIAGNOSTIC PROCEDURES

Though the list of potential teratogens seems to increase daily, most babies are born healthy. In fact, only about 4 percent will be born with atypical characteristics. Among those, most will experience effects so slight as to have a minimal impact on daily functioning. Aiding in the battle against the small number of atypical characteristics that occur is an array of diagnostic tools. Though these tools are not "cures" for the prenatal characteristics they can detect, they can alert expectant parents and healthcare professionals to the need to take special precautions for the remainder of the pregnancy. In some cases, these tools may provide valuable information to help couples decide whether to continue the pregnancy.

Although medical technology is constantly creating new diagnostic tools, the five most current prenatal diagnostic tools are: ultrasound, amniocentesis, chorionic villus sampling, the alpha-fetoprotein test, and the triple marker screening blood test. These tools are especially important for women who are believed to be at risk for giving birth to a child with atypical characteristics. A woman might be a high-risk candidate if:

- she will be over age 35 at the time of delivery;
- she has already given birth to (or has a partner who has had) a child with a genetic disease or birth defect;
- she has a family history of genetic disease or birth defects;
- she has a medical history of certain genetic traits or chronic diseases (e.g., sickle-cell anemia or diabetes).

Women who are not at high risk may also have these tests administered. However, these tests can be expensive and, in the case of amniocentesis and chorionic villus sampling, can pose a small risk of harming the fetus. With the exception of the alpha-fetoprotein test, where the law mandates offering these tests to all pregnant women, the tests should be administered judiciously.

Ultrasound

Ultrasound, also referred to as a sonogram, is administered by placing a small transmitter on the abdomen of the pregnant woman. Typically, the abdomen is lubricated so the transmitter can be easily maneuvered into the position that provides the best picture of the fetus. The transmitter emits high-frequency sound waves that echo off the fetus, and these sound waves are transformed into computer-enhanced images on a monitor. Though ultrasound does not produce a particularly clear image, it does create a clear enough picture to allow measurement of the baby's head, which can help determine the exact length of gestation (see Figure 4.6). Ultrasound pictures can also show the placement and structure of the placenta, as well as detect the baby's gender, multiple pregnancies, and some atypical anatomical characteristics. The advantages of an ultrasound test are that it causes no pain, requires no injection, and takes only about 30 minutes. According to the American Institute of Ultrasound in Medicine, there are no confirmed adverse biological effects on either patients or operators (Rosen & Hoskins, 2000).

Amniocentesis

Unlike ultrasound, **amniocentesis** requires that a needle be inserted through the abdominal wall. This procedure, which was first used for fetal diagnosis in 1967, employs a thin needle to remove approximately two tablespoons of amniotic fluid drawn from the small amniotic sac around the fetus. This fluid contains fetal cells, which can be examined to determine the presence of some disorders. Because

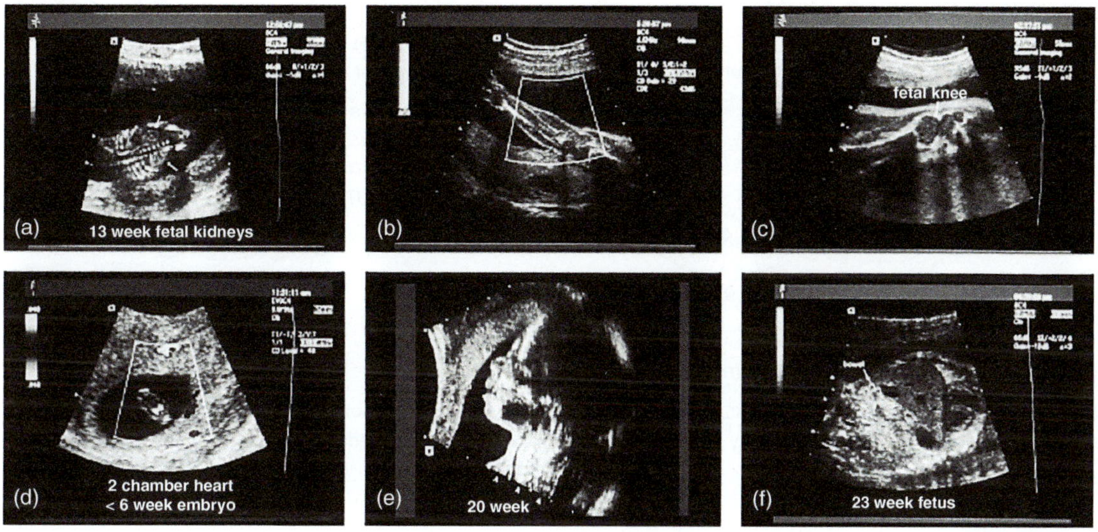

Figure 4.6 The sonogram is a valuable diagnostic tool that enables medical professionals to view the fetus. Fetal kidneys (a), fetal arm (b), fetal knee (c), two-chamber heart of <6-week embryo (d), 20-week fetal head and neck (e), and 23-week fetal bowel (f)

Images courtesy of Acuson Corporation.

amniocentesis is an intrusive test, ultrasound is used to locate the best site for puncture, to locate the placenta, and to guide the needle safely to the best pool of amniotic fluid.

Though amniocentesis is believed to present minimum risk to the mother and fetus, the needle has been known to damage the fetus on occasion. The test is usually performed between 15 and 20 weeks of gestation. Second trimester amniocentesis carries a small risk of miscarriage of about 0.1–0.3 percent. This risk increases when the procedure is performed prior to 15 weeks of pregnancy (Mayo Clinic, 2019). For these reasons, this test is generally employed only when the mother is at high risk for giving birth to a child with atypical characteristics. The process takes about 20 minutes and can detect numerous chromosomal disorders (e.g., Down syndrome), the gender of the baby, and neural-tube defects (e.g., spina bifida, the failure of the bony structure of the spine to close completely around the spinal cord) with a high degree of accuracy.

Chorionic Villus Sampling (CVS)

Chorionic villus sampling (CVS) offers one major advantage over amniocentesis: it can be administered between 11 and 14 weeks of gestation, so that any atypical characteristics are detected earlier. At that time, the amniotic fluid contains too few viable cells per milliliter for amniocentesis to be reliable and safe. Like amniocentesis, CVS is designed to gather cell samples for examination. However, rather than sampling the amniotic fluid, CVS is intended to take samples of the small hair-like projections of the placenta (see Figure 4.7). These projections, known as *villi*, can reveal the same information available through amniocentesis. CVS is administered by inserting a needle through the abdomen or through the cervix of the pregnant woman. Both methods employ ultrasound to guide the needle.

Though CVS offers the advantage of earlier administration and, thus, earlier detection of atypical characteristics, it is also potentially

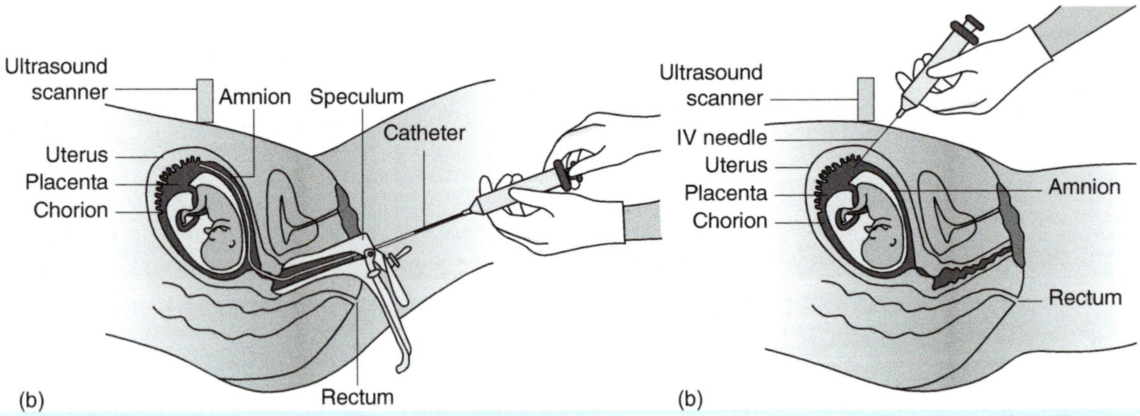

Figure 4.7 Two different methods are employed to gather a tissue sample in chorionic villus testing. (a) A plastic catheter is inserted through the cervix and guided by ultrasound. (b) A biopsy needle is inserted through the abdominal wall and guided by ultrasound

riskier than amniocentesis. Three times as many miscarriages are caused by CVS than by amniocentesis. Nevertheless, that risk is still less than 1 percent (Mayo Clinic, 2019). Therefore, CVS is recommended only for the pregnant women with the highest risk. For such women, any dangers of CVS are generally believed to be outweighed by the benefit of discovering early in the pregnancy that the baby may need special prenatal care.

Alpha-Fetoprotein Test

The **alpha-fetoprotein test** is a simple blood test performed at approximately 15 to 20 weeks into the pregnancy. This blood test measures the amount of alpha-fetoprotein (AFP) in the blood. High AFP levels can indicate the presence of neural-tube defects; low levels may signal a chromosomal disorder such as Down syndrome. The test finds about 90 percent of babies with anencephaly (congenital absence of part of the brain) and about 75 percent with spina bifida (Wayne State University Physician Group, 2019). Because the majority of women who have atypical AFP levels give birth to typical babies, the AFP test is usually employed as a screening device to determine if additional prenatal diagnostic testing should be done. The presence of twins or a small miscalculation in the time of gestation can cause misinterpretation of AFP levels.

Triple Marker Screening

Until recently, no useful tests were available for identifying Down syndrome in pregnant women younger than age 35. However, it is now possible to screen maternal blood serum to test for the amount of human chorionic gonadotropin, unconjugated estriol, and the previously mentioned alpha-fetoprotein. These substances, which vary in amount during the course of the pregnancy, are produced by both the mother's placenta and the fetus and as a screening package are referred to as the **triple marker.** Unlike amniocentesis with its attendant risk, the triple marker screening simply requires a small amount of blood to be drawn from the mother's arm. In most instances, the test is offered to younger mothers during the second trimester. The rate of accuracy is currently between 40 and 60 percent. While this rate of detection is acceptable for women under 35 years of age, it is unacceptable for older pregnant women. For those older than 35, amniocentesis, with its 99 percent rate of detection, is still the preferred screening procedure.

MATERNAL NUTRITION

Adequate prenatal nutrition is essential for the well-being of both the mother-to-be and the growing fetus. The prenatal diet must cover the increased metabolic load that accompanies pregnancy. These additional calories are needed to support the growth of the placenta and the developing fetus. Indeed, total caloric intake appears to be one of the foremost factors affecting infant birth weight. To supply the extra energy needed during pregnancy, sedentary women need to increase their caloric intake by approximately 300 calories/day (ACSM, 2018), for a total of 85,000 additional calories over the course of the pregnancy (Worthington-Roberts, 2000). Women who continue strenuous physical activity during pregnancy must make additional adjustments. How much of an adjustment depends on the caloric cost of the activities performed. In general, an active pregnant woman should ingest additional calories equivalent to the energy expended during physical activity plus the 300 calories/day maintenance load. If weight gain falls below expected levels during the course of pregnancy, it may be necessary to increase caloric intake further.

How much weight should a woman gain over the course of pregnancy? The answer to this question is influenced by the woman's body mass index (BMI) prior to conception (see Appendix B). According to the Institute of Medicine (IOM, 2009), if the pregnant woman is underweight (BMI 18.5), she should gain 28–40 lb (12.7–18.1 kg), but if her BMI is healthy (BMI 18.5–24.9), then the total gestational weight gain should be 25–35 lb (11.3–15.9 kg). In contrast, if the woman is overweight (BMI 25.0–29.9), then total gestational weight gain should be 15–25 lb (6.8–11.3 kg). Obese women (BMI ≥30.0) should gain 11–20 lb (5.0–9.1 kg). However, controversy exists regarding the appropriate weight gain for pregnant women who are overweight or obese. Some experts believe that as long as the fetus is developing typically, gaining less weight than recommended will not adversely affect the maternal outcome (ACOG, 2013).

Table 4.7 shows the recommended distribution of this total gestational weight gain. Ideally, the weight gain should result in an offspring weighing approximately 7.0–7.5 lb (3.2–3.4 kg). Research by Stotland and colleagues (2005) indicated that 24.1 percent of women who were overweight exceeded their target weight gain during pregnancy, compared to only 4.3 percent of women with typical weight. This is unfortunate since research suggests that women who gained weight during pregnancy in excess of the IOM guidelines encountered greater risk of adverse maternal and neonatal outcomes (Truong, Yee, Caughey, et al., 2015). Among women who were underweight, 51.2 percent failed to gain enough weight during pregnancy. Thus, better education is needed to implement the Institute of Medicine's (2009) guidelines for gestational weight gain.

The importance of eating a balanced diet during pregnancy cannot be overemphasized. The developing fetus must receive adequate nutrition in utero, particularly because the developing brain achieves 25 percent of its mature weight prior to birth.

It is important that the mother receives an adequate supply of vitamins and minerals because deficiencies in these nutrients can cause physical and mental damage to the baby and, in some instances, fetal death. Table 4.8 lists the recommended daily allowances of selected nutrients. Pay particular attention to the recommended percentage increase in most of these nutrients for women who are pregnant. These essential nutrients should be acquired by eating a variety of foods, and every attempt must be made to avoid intake of "empty calories." Vitamin and mineral supplements should be taken only under the watchful eye of

Table 4.7 Recommendations for total and rate of weight gain during pregnancy, by prepregnancy BMI

Prepregnancy BMI	BMI* (kg/m^2) (WHO)	Total WEIGHT GAIN RANGE	Rates of weight gain,+ second trimester (mean range)	Rates of weight gain,+ third trimester (mean range)
Underweight	<18.5	28–40 lb (12.7–18.1 kg)	1 lb/week (0.45 kg/week)	1–1.3 lb/week (0.45–0.6 kg/week)
Healthy weight	18.5–24.9	25–35 lb (11.3–15.9 kg)	1 lb/week (0.45 kg/week)	0.8–1 lb/week (0.36–0.45 kg/week)
Overweight	25.0–29.9	15–25 lb (6.8–11.3 kg)	0.6 lb/week (0.27 kg/week)	0.5–0.7 lb/week (0.23–0.32 kg/week)
Obese (includes all classes)	≥30.0	11–20 lb (5.0–9.1 kg)	0.5 lb/week (0.23 kg/week)	0.4–0.6 lb/week (0.18–0.27 kg/week)

*To calculate BMI, go to www.nhlbisupport.com/bmi/.

+Calculations assume a 1.1–4.4 lb (0.5–2.0 kg) weight gain in the first trimester.

Source: Data compiled from Institute of Medicine (2009).

Table 4.8 A comparison of recommended daily allowances for selected nutrients for nonpregnant and pregnant women

Nutrient	Nonpregnant level	Pregnant level	Percent change
Protein	46 g	71 g	+42
Calcium	1,000 mg	1,000 mg	0
Vitamin A	700 mcg	770 mcg	+10
Vitamin D	5 mcg	5 mcg	0
Vitamin E	15 mg	15 mg	0
Vitamin C	75 mg	85 mg	+13
Folic acid	400 mcg	600 mcg	+50

a physician, for an association has been found between selected supplements and neural-tube defects, including spina bifida, anencephaly, and encephalocele (protrusion of the brain through a congenital defect in the skull).

BIRTH WEIGHT

In the past, the medical community considered any newborn weighing less than 5.51 lb (2,500 g) premature. Today, standards classify infants weighing less than 5.51 lb (2,500 g) as low birth weight (LBW) and those weighing less than 3.31 lb (1,500 g) as very low birth weight (VLBW). Extremely low birth weight (ELBW), is used to classify those weighing less than 1.10 lb (500 g) at birth.

Low birth weight is not necessarily associated with premature birth; that is, not all LBW newborns are premature. Further, complications associated with small full-term infants differ significantly from those a premature infant experiences. Because of this distinction, gestational age and weight are no longer used independently to describe or label an infant as premature. Instead, it must be established whether the cause of the LBW is a shortened gestation period or growth retardation resulting from intrauterine impoverishment. This is an important distinction because the clinical outcomes of the two conditions are quite different. More specifically, low birth weight caused by intrauterine impoverishment is associated with mental retardation, whereas spastic diplegia (cerebral palsy) is more closely associated with prematurity.

Figure 4.8 illustrates the three major diagnostic groupings of birth weight. Note that infants with a low birth weight for their gestational age can be born either full term (40 weeks) or preterm (37 weeks or less). These infants exhibit weights two standard deviations below their expected birth weight for their length of gestation and are generally termed **small for gestational age (SGA)**. Excluding other congenital problems, infants who are SGA experienced growth retardation from inadequate nutrition in utero and are at great risk of mental disabilities. The infant's lack of adequate nutrition in utero can have a devastating effect on brain development, particularly because brain cells have completed proliferation by 20 weeks in utero.

Researchers are interested in the long-term effects of LBW on later motor behavior and physiological function. Isaacs and Pohlman (1988) first compared 5- to 9-year-old children who were either low or typical birth weight babies on fundamental motor skills and reaction time. The typical body weight group performed significantly better on locomotor and object control skills, though no statistically significant differences were noted for reaction time. The researchers were careful to indicate that the child-rearing attitudes of the various parents varied greatly. In fact, parents of low birth weight babies often expressed concern that their children avoid involvement in vigorous physical activity. This, as much as the LBW condition, may have accounted for the children's lower abilities on fundamental motor skills (Isaacs & Pohlman, 1988; Pohlman & Isaacs, 1990).

These early findings have now been extensively supported by more recent research involving children ranging in age from 2 to 13 years and representing each of the three levels of birth weight classification: LBW, VLBW, and ELBW (Baraldi, Zanconato, Zorzi, et al., 1991; Bareket, Eliakim, Dotan, et al., 1997; de Kieviet, Piek, Aarnoudse-Moens, &

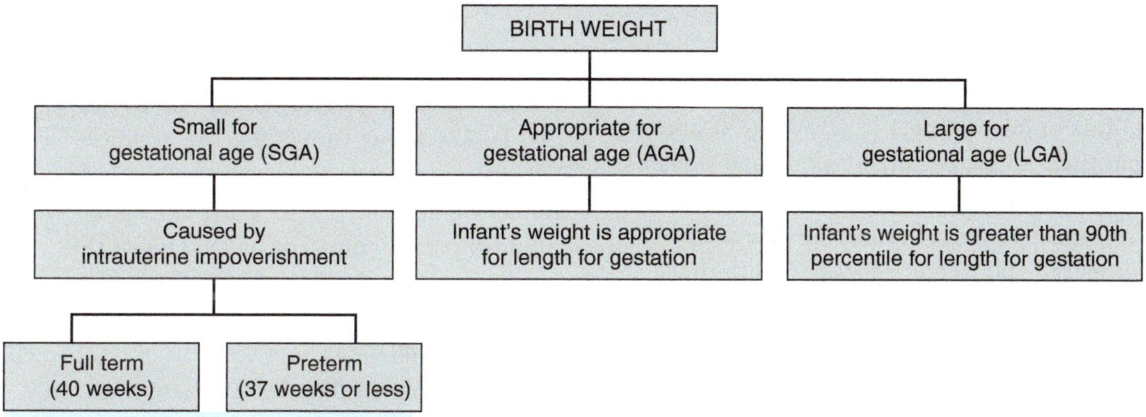

Figure 4.8 Birth weight classifications

Oosteriaan, 2009; Hack, Taylor, Klein, et al., 1994; Johnson, Townsend, Yudkin, et al., 1993; Lie, 1994; Marlow, Roberts, & Cooke, 1989, 1993; Powls, Botting, Cooke, & Marlow, 1995; Stjernqvist & Svenningsen, 1995). For example, de Kieviet and colleagues (2009) sought to examine motor development from birth to adolescence in children who were preterm (≤32 weeks of gestation) or VLBW. In this meta-analysis the researchers examined 41 articles whose subjects were 9,653 children. To be included in the analysis, children in the study must have been assessed by at least one of the following three motor tests: the Bayley Scales of Infant Development II, the Motor Assessment Battery for Children, or the Bruininks-Oseretsky Test of Motor Proficiency. Analysis found that both groups of children (preterm and VLBW) scored significantly lower on all three motor tests than children of typical birth weight. This meta-analysis supports the research mentioned earlier and is one of the first to indicate that this significant motor impairment can persist throughout childhood.

Infants born preterm but of a body weight **appropriate for gestational age (AGA)**, particularly those weighing more than 3.31 lb (1,500 g), tend to be at less risk than infants who were SGA. Children born preterm but AGA show developmental delays in weight, length, and head circumference at 1 year of age, but researchers have found that some catch-up growth occurs during the second year. Regarding the physiological function of infants of less than 3.1 lb (1,500 g), it appears that their ability to catch up in some ways with their peers born AGA is quite complete. For example, Baraldi and colleagues (1991) compared children born VLBW with those born AGA, following them from 7 years to 12 years of age, and found the children born VLBW to be comparable with those born AGA on pulmonary function tests and maximum oxygen consumption. However, the children born SGA exhibited less efficiency in running.

As Figure 4.8 indicates, another birth weight classification is **large for gestational age (LGA)**. The birth weight of infants born LGA is greater than the 90th percentile for their gestational age. Because of the infants' large body size, birth injuries, especially brachial plexus (the network of nerves that transmit signals from the spine to the shoulder, arm, and hand) injuries and fractures of the clavicle (collarbone), are common. Respiratory distress syndrome and developmental delays are also characteristics of this group of infants. Infants of mothers who are diabetic tend to be macrosomic and are, therefore, frequently LGA.

EXERCISE DURING PREGNANCY AND THE POSTPARTUM PERIOD

Exercise during pregnancy and the postpartum period has been associated with beneficial outcomes for both the mother and the baby. In order to ensure these positive outcomes, the U.S. Department of Health and Human Services has published recommendations for women during pregnancy and the postpartum period in the report entitled *Physical Activity Guidelines for Americans* (2018). These recommendations, which address exercise duration and exercise intensity as a function of prepregnancy exercise status, appear in Table 4.9. In addition, the American College of Obstetricians and Gynecologists (ACOG) has published other exercise guidelines (ACOG, 2015). According to ACOG, "An exercise program that leads to an eventual goal of moderate-intensity exercise for at least 20–30 minutes per day on most or all days of the week should be developed with the patient and adjusted as medically indicated" (2015, p, 135). The 2015 guidelines have since been reaffirmed in 2017. Table 4.10 presents selected safe and unsafe physical activities during pregnancy.

Table 4.9 Recommendations for exercise duration and intensity for women during pregnancy and the postpartum period

Healthy women who are not already highly active or doing vigorous-intensity activity should get at least 150 minutes (2 hours and 30 minutes) of moderate-intensity aerobic activity per week during pregnancy and the postpartum period. Preferably, this activity should be spread throughout the week.
Pregnant women who habitually engage in vigorous-intensity aerobic activity or are highly active can continue physical activity during pregnancy and the postpartum period, provided that they remain healthy and discuss with their health-care provider how and when activity should be adjusted during pregnancy and after the baby is born.

Source: U.S. Department of Health and Human Services (2018).

Table 4.10 Selected safe and unsafe physical activities during pregnancy

Safe activities to start or continue during pregnancy
Walking
Swimming
Stationary cycling
Yoga & pilates: Avoid positions which decrease venous return
Jogging or running: if performed regularly prior to becoming pregnant
Racquet sports: only if balance is not affected in order to prevent falls
Activities to avoid during pregnancy
Contact sports
Any activity with a high risk of falling
Scuba diving
Sky diving
Hot yoga or hot Pilates

Source: American College of Obstetricians and Gynecologists (2015).

Maternal Health

The exercise recommendations addressed earlier were based on what is currently known about the effects of exercise during pregnancy and the postpartum period for both the mother and the developing baby. Three extensive literature reviews highlight the state of our current knowledge (ACOG, 2015; Lewis, Avery, Jennings, et al., 2008; Pivarnik & Mudd, 2009). Below are selected conclusions drawn from these literature reviews and other supportive research regarding the effects of exercise during pregnancy on maternal and fetal health (see Figure 4.9).

Preeclampsia

Pregnancy-induced hypertension is referred to as preeclampsia. Practically all research suggests that exercise during pregnancy is associated with a reduced risk of this

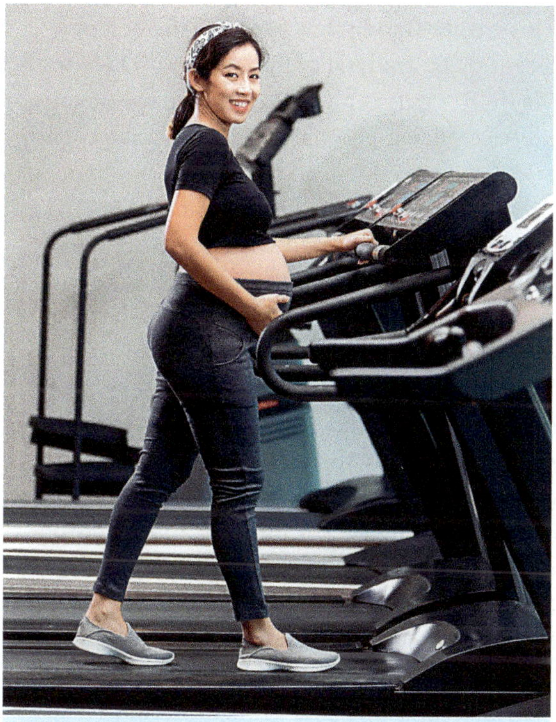

Figure 4.9 Exercise during pregnancy may offer benefits for both mother and child

hypertensive disorder. Only one study, the Danish National Birth Cohort investigation, has reported a particularly contradictory finding (Osterdal, Strom, Klemmensen, et al., 2009). Women who reported exercising more than 420 minutes/week during the first trimester had a significantly increased risk of developing severe preeclampsia, but those women in the study who reported lesser amounts of physical activity were not affected. Therefore, it appears that there may be an upper limit to the amount of exercise that can be performed prior to the potential development of preeclampsia.

Gestational Diabetes

Exercise both prior to and during pregnancy has been associated with a preventive effect against the development of gestational diabetes. Dempsey, Butler, Sorensen, and colleagues (2004) reported a 46 percent risk reduction in gestational diabetes in women who engaged in exercise during the first 20 weeks of pregnancy. This earlier finding has been reaffirmed in a recent meta-analysis of 135 studies (Davenport, Meah, Ruchat, et al., 2018). More specifically, exercise during pregnancy was associated with a 39 percent reduction in the odds of having a baby weighing greater than normal, a complication associated with gestational diabetes.

Weight Gain During Pregnancy

Women who exercise during pregnancy are less likely to exceed the weight gain ranges recommended by the Institute of Medicine (refer back to Table 4.7 on p. 118). Researchers also suggest that it is important to maintain a normal body weight between pregnancies (Sumithran, Houlihan, Shub, et al., 2018). This is because one in five women who were of a normal weight during their first pregnancy will be overweight or obese in their second pregnancy. Thus, maintaining an appropriate body weight before, during, and after pregnancy is important in reducing the associated risk of excess body weight during subsequent pregnancies.

Fetal Distress

Extended periods of a slow heart rate (fetal bradycardia) have been used as an index to measure fetal distress. Of the few studies currently available for review, none have reported any adverse outcomes as a result of maximal aerobic exercise during pregnancy.

Preterm Delivery

Although additional studies are needed, observational studies have found no association between maternal exercise and preterm delivery. In fact, it appears that maternal exercise is associated with a decreased risk of delivering preterm (Juhl et al., 2008).

Birth Weight

According to Pivarnik and Mudd (2009), the majority of evidence suggests that physical activity during pregnancy decreases birth weight modestly within the typical range and may protect against giving birth to a macrosomic or large for gestational age infant, but it does not contribute to an increased risk of low birth weight or a small for gestational age infant.

Maternal Response to Exercise

In pregnant women the maternal blood plasma volume is increased by 50 percent, and, as a result, cardiac output also increases (Hall, 2015). These specific changes can persist for up to 4 weeks postpartum. Other cardiorespiratory changes include the diversion of blood away from the visceral organs to the working muscles during exercise. Though animal research indicates that when 50 percent of the blood flow is diverted from the viscera there is an increased risk of harm to the fetus, no such research has been conducted on humans. In other words, we do not know at what point exercise might begin to jeopardize the fetal oxygen supply. However, research exists which have found that 30 minutes of strenuous exercise is well tolerated by women and their fetuses (Szymanski & Satin, 2012).

Toward the end of the pregnancy the diaphragm is elevated, which is believed to cause discomfort and dyspnea (difficult or painful breathing). This elevation does not impair the respiratory function of the lungs because the rib cage expands to increase the overall tidal volume of the lungs. Breathing appears readily to accommodate low levels of exercise. High levels of exercise, however, tend to increase oxygen levels less than expected, indicating that pregnant women may not be able to maintain high activity levels as readily as nonpregnant women, especially toward the end of the pregnancy.

As in the nonpregnant exerciser, the body temperature rises when a pregnant woman exercises. This is particularly true if insufficient liquid is ingested, causing dehydration. Therefore, during exercise the pregnant woman should stay well hydrated and should avoid exercising in high heat and humid conditions.

SUMMARY

- Both environmental and genetic factors can alter the typical fetal growth and development process.
- Drugs and medications consumed during pregnancy can affect the developing fetus. They are particularly damaging at certain times during pregnancy, especially during the main embryonic period of development.
- Women should not use recreational drugs during pregnancy. Opioids are among the most harmful drugs to the unborn child. The pregnant woman should also be cautious of prescription and nonprescription drugs; when she must take them, she must work closely with her physician to monitor their use, for many can harm the developing fetus.
- There are numerous maternal diseases that can influence the development of the fetus. These diseases take many forms, including viral, parasitic, hematologic, and endocrine diseases.
- Five frequent genetic disorders are Down syndrome, phenylketonuria, cystic fibrosis, sickle-cell disease, and fragile X syndrome. Down syndrome, a chromosome-based disorder, is caused by the presence of an extra chromosome on chromosome number 21. Phenylketonuria, cystic fibrosis, sickle-cell disease, and fragile X syndrome are gene-based disorders.
- Prenatal diagnostic procedures are available to detect the presence of many atypical characteristics in the fetus. Four of the most common prenatal procedures are ultrasound, amniocentesis, chorionic villus sampling, and the alpha-fetoprotein test. These tests are particularly important for women believed to be at risk for fetal atypicalities because of maternal age, a previous child born with a genetic disease or birth defect, a family history of such births, or a medical history of certain genetic traits. The triple marker test may be used for women under age 35; it is used less often than the other four.
- The pregnant woman must receive adequate nutrition. Maternal weight gain can be a partial indication of the nutritional state of the fetus. How much weight should be gained during the pregnancy is a function of the pregnant woman's BMI status prior to conception. With adequate nutrition, maternal weight gain should produce an offspring weighing approximately 7.0–7.5 lb (3.175–3.4 kg). Babies born to women who do not receive adequate nutrition during pregnancy score lower than average on

mental scales and can also suffer physical impairment.

- There are three basic birth weight classifications: small for gestational age (SGA), appropriate for gestational age (AGA), and large for gestational age (LGA). Babies born SGA are particularly at risk for such associated problems as mental retardation. Recent research has also shown that babies born with low birth weight may lag in motor skill development later in life.
- Women who want to exercise during pregnancy and the postpartum period are encouraged to follow the guidelines established by the ACOG (2015) and the *Physical Activity Guidelines for Americans* (USDHHS, 2018).

key concept review

alcohol-related birth defects (ARBD)
alcohol-related neurodevelopmental disorders (ARND)
alpha-fetoprotein test
amniocentesis
anti-D IgG immunoglobulin
appropriate for gestational age (AGA)
carbon monoxide
chorionic villus sampling (CVS)
congenital rubella syndrome (CRS)
cystic fibrosis (CF)
diabetes mellitus
Down syndrome (DS)
ectoderm
endoderm
erythroblastosis fetalis
fetal alcohol spectrum disorders (FASDs)
fetal alcohol syndrome (FAS)
fragile X syndrome (FXS)
heterozygous
homozygous
human immunodeficiency virus (HIV)
hyperglycemia
hypoglycemia
large for gestational age (LGA)
macrosomia
meiotic nondisjunction
mesoderm
neonatal abstinence syndrome (NAS)
nicotine
normoglycemia
phenylketonuria (PKU)
Rh factor
rubella
sickle-cell disease (SCD)
sickle-cell trait (SCT)
small for gestational age (SGA)
sudden infant death syndrome (SIDS)
teratogen
thalidomide
third-hand smoke
Toxoplasma gondii
triple marker
ultrasound

questions for reflection

1. What are three factors that determine the extent of damage caused by a teratogen? When are teratogens most dangerous and why? In your discussion, refer to each of the three prenatal stages of development.
2. Summarize the features of a child born with fetal alcohol syndrome regarding growth, central nervous system characteristics, and craniofacial anomalies.
3. A woman who is 3 months pregnant smokes an average of three cigarettes per day. Following the birth of her child, she continues smoking and breastfeeds her baby. Why might smoking have an effect on her newborn baby? Summarize the short- and long-term risk factors associated with maternal tobacco smoking.
4. What are the fetal defects associated with rubella infections in the mother during pregnancy?
5. What are the events that lead up to the development of erythroblastosis fetalis?

6. What special nutritional concerns do pregnant women have?
7. What are the potential consequences of sickle-cell disease?
8. Why does a concern exist for children who exhibit small for gestational age and large for gestational age birth weights?
9. What are the guidelines concerning exercise during pregnancy and the postpartum period put forth by the American College of Obstetricians and Gynecologists?

online resources

American Academy of Pediatrics, www.aap.org
American Congress of Obstetricians and Gynecologists, www.acog.org
American Pregnancy Association, www.americanpregnancy.org
Center for Motor Behavior & Pediatric Disabilities, www.umich.edu/~cmbds
Cystic Fibrosis Foundation, www.cff.org
March of Dimes, www.modimes.org
Mother to Baby, www.mothertobaby.org
National Down Syndrome Society, www.ndss.org
National Fragile X Foundation, www.fragilex.org
Teratology Society, www.teratology.org
U.S. National Library of Medicine, www.nlm.nih.gov
Visible Embryo, www.visembryo.com

REFERENCES

Alford, C. A., Pass, R. F., & Stagno, S. (1983). Chronic congenital infections and common environmental causes for severe and subtle birth defects. In S. C. Finley, W. H. Finley, & C. E. Flowers, Jr. (Eds.), *Birth defects: Clinical and ethical considerations*, New York: Alan R. Liss.

Alger, L. S. (2000). Common viral infections. In W. R. Cohen (Ed.), *Cherry and Merkatz's complications of pregnancy*, 5th ed. Baltimore, MD: Lippincott Williams & Wilkins.

American Academy of Pediatrics (2000a). Fetal alcohol syndrome and alcohol-related neurodevelopmental disorders (RE9948). *Pediatrics, 106*, 358–361.

American Academy of Pediatrics (2000b). Changing concepts of sudden infant death syndrome: Implications for infant sleeping environment and sleep position. *Pediatrics*, *e*(3), 650–656.

American College of Obstetricians and Gynecologists (ACOG) (2002). *Pregnancy: Illegal drugs and pregnancy*, Washington, DC: American College of Obstetricians and Gynecologists Patient Education, Pamphlet AP104.

American College of Obstetricians and Gynecologists (ACOG) (2013). Weight gain during pregnancy—Reaffirmed. ACOG committee opinion no. 548. *Obstetrics and Gynecology, 121*, 210–212.

American College of Obstetricians and Gynecologists (ACOG) (2015). Physical activity and exercise during pregnancy and the postpartum period. ACOG committee opinion no. 650. *Obstetrics and Gynecology*, *126*, 135–142.

American College of Sports Medicine (2018). *ACSM's guidelines for exercise testing and prescription*, 10th ed. Philadelphia, PA: Lippincott Williams & Wilkins.

American Lung Association (2018). Learn about cystic fibrosis. Retrieved from www.lung.org/lung-health-and-disease/lung-disease-lookup/cystic-fibrosis/learn-about-cystic-fibrosis.html.

American Pregnancy Association (2010). Triple marker. Retrieved from www.americanpregnancyassociation.org.

Arendt, R., Angelopoulos, J., Salvator, A., & Singer, L. (1999). Motor development of cocaine-exposed children at age two years. *Pediatrics, 103*, 86.

Baraldi, E., Zanconato, S., Zorzi, C., Santuz, P., Benini, F., & Zacchello, F. (1991). Exercise performance in very low birth weight children at the age of 7–12 years. *European Journal of Pediatrics, 150*, 713–716.

Bareket, F., Eliakim, A., Dotan, R., Liebermann, D. G., Regev, R., & Bar-Or, O. (1997). Birth weight and physical ability in 5- to 8-year-old healthy children born prematurely. *Medicine and Science in Sports and Exercise, 29*, 1124–1130.

Center for Behavioral Health Statistics and Quality (2017), *2016 National survey on drug use and health: Detailed tables*. Rockville, MD: Substance Abuse and Mental Health Services Administration. Retrieved from www.samhsa.gov/data/sites/default/files/NSDUH-DetTabs-2016/NSDUH-DetTabs-2016.pdf.

Centers for Disease Control and Prevention (CDC) (2009). Notice to readers: New CDC materials regarding fetal alcohol spectrum disorders. *Morbidity and Mortality Weekly Report, 58*, 403.

Centers for Disease Control and Prevention (2015a). Alcohol use and binge drinking among women of childbearing age – United States, 2011–2013. *Morbidity and Mortality Weekly Report*, *64*, 1042–1046.

Centers for Disease Control and Prevention (2015b). Epidemiology and prevention of vaccine-preventable diseases. Retrieved from www.cdc.gov/vaccines/pubs/pinkbook/rubella/downloads/rubella.pdf.

Centers for Disease Control and Prevention (2017). Rubella in the U.S. Retrieved from www.cdc.gov/rubella/about/in-the-us.html.

Centers for Disease Control and Prevention (2018a). Treating for two: Medicine and pregnancy. Retrieved from www.cdc.gov/pregnancy/meds/treatingfortwo/facts.html.

Centers for Disease Control and Prevention (2018b). Toxoplasmosis: Epidemiology & risk factors. Retrieved from www.cdc.gov/parasites/toxoplasmosis/epi.html.

Centers for Disease Control and Prevention (2018c). *2018 Annual surveillance report of drug-related risks and outcomes – United States*. Retrieved from www.cdc.gov/drugoverdose/pdf/pubs/2018-cdc-frug-surveillance-report.pdf.

Centers for Disease Control and Prevention (2018d). U.S. drug overdose deaths continue to rise; increase fueled by synthetic opioids. Retrieved from www.cdc.gov/media/releases/2018/p0329-drug-overdose-deaths.html.

Centers for Disease Control and Prevention (2019). Progress erased: Youth tobacco use increased from 2017–2018. Retrieved from www.cdc.gov/media/releases/2019/p0211-youth-tobacco-use-increased.html.

Dana-Farber Cancer Institute (2018). After 60 years, scientists uncover how thalidomide produced birth defects: Defects linked to disruption of key protein involved in fetal development; finding will help guide development of new drugs. *ScienceDaily*. Retrieved from www.sciencedaily.com/releases/2018/08/180801131524.htm.

Davenport, M. H., Meah, V. L., Ruchat, S., Davies G. A., Skow, R. J., Barrowman, N., et al., (2018). Impact of prenatal exercise on neonatal and childhood outcomes: A systematic review and meta-analysis. *British Journal of Sports Medicine*, *52*, 1386–1396.

de Kieviet, J. F., Piek, J. P., Aarnoudse-Moens, C. S., & Oosteriaan, J. (2009). Motor development in very preterm and very low-birth-weight children from birth to adolescence. *Journal of the American Medical Association, 302*, 2235–2242.

Dempsey, J. G., Butler, C. L., Sorensen, T. K., Lee, I. M., Thompson, M. L., Miller, R. S., et al. (2004). A case-control study of maternal recreational physical activity and risk of gestational diabetes mellitus. *Diabetes Research and Clinical Practice, 66*, 203–215.

Drake, P., Driscoll, A. K., & Mathews, T. J. (2018). *Cigarette smoking during pregnancy: United States, 2016*. HCHS Data Brief, No 305. Hyattsville, MD: National Center for Health Statistics.

Ferreira, J., Sachs, G. S., & Bombard, A. T. (2000). Teratogenic drugs. In W. R. Cohen (Ed.), *Cherry and Merkatz's complications of pregnancy*, 5th ed. Baltimore, MD: Lippincott Williams & Wilkins.

Gentzke, A. S., Creamer, M., Cullen, K. A., Ambrose, B. K., Willis, G., Jamal, A., et al. (2019). Vital signs: Tobacco product use among middle and high school students – United States, 2011–2018. *Morbidity and Mortality Weekly Report*, *68*, 157–164.

Gold, M. S. (1995). *Drugs of abuse: A comprehensive series for clinicians: Tobacco*, New York: Plenum Medical Book Company.

Hack, M., Taylor, H., Klein, N., Eiben, R., Schalschneider, C., & Mercuri-Minich, N. (1994). School-age outcomes in children with birth weights under 750 g. *New England Journal of Medicine, 331*, 753–759.

Hall, J. E. (2015). *Guyton and Hall textbook of medical physiology*, 13th ed. Philadelphia, PA: Saunders.

Harms, R. W. (2012). Is it safe to take aspirin during pregnancy? Mayo Clinic. Retrieved from www.mayoclinic.org/healthy-lifestyle/pregnancy-week-by-week/expert-answers/aspirin-during-pregnancy/faq-20058167.

Institute of Medicine (2009). *Weight gain during pregnancy: Reexamining the guidelines*, Washington, DC: The National Academies Press.

Interrante, J. D., Ailes, E. C., Lind, J. N., Anderka, M., Werier, M. M., Taylor, L. G., et al. (2017). Risk comparison for prenatal use of analgesics and selected birth defects, national birth defects prevention study 1997–2011. *Annals of Epidemiology*, *27*, 645–653.

Isaacs, L. D., & Pohlman, R. (1988, Oct.). Motor development and performance concerns regarding individuals of low birth weight. Paper presented at the meeting of the Motor Development Research Consortium, University of Illinois, Urbana.

Jazayeri, A. (2015). Macrosomia follow-up. *Medscape*. Retrieved from www.emedicine.medscape.com/article/262679-followup-macrosomiafollowup.

Johnson, A. P., Townsend, P., Yudkin, P., Bull, D., & Wilkinson, A. R. (1993). Functional abilities at age 4 years of children born before 29 weeks of gestation. *British Medical Journal, 306*, 1715–1718.

Juhl, M., Anderson, P. K., Olsen, J., Madsen, M., Jorgensen, T., Nohr, E. A., et al. (2008). Physical exercise during pregnancy and the risk of preterm birth: A study within the Danish national birth cohort. *American Journal of Epidemiology, 167*, 859–866, doi: 10.1093/aje/kwm364.

LeDoare, K., Bland, R., & Newell, M. L. (2012). Neurodevelopment in children born to HIV-infected mothers by infection and treatment status. *Pediatrics, 130*, 1326–1344.

Lewis, B., Avery, M., Jennings, E., Sherwood, N., Martinson, B., & Crain, A. L. (2008). The effect of exercise during pregnancy on maternal outcomes: Practical implications for practice. *American Journal of Lifestyle Medicine, 2*, 441–455.

Lie, K. G. (1994). Sensitivity of perceptual motor measures for very low birth weight (VLBW >1500 g) preschoolers. *Child Care Health Development, 20*, 239–249.

Liew, Z., Ritz, R., Rebordosa, C., Lee, P., & Olsen, J. (2014). Acetaminophen use during pregnancy, behavioral problems, and hyperkinetic disorders. *Pediatrics, 168*, 313–320.

Mahabee-Gittens, E. M., Merianos, A. L., & Matt, G. E. (2018). Preliminary evidence that high levels of nicotine on children's hands may contribute to overall tobacco smoking exposure. *BMF Tobacco Control*, *27*, 217–219.

Mainz, J. G., Schien, C. J., Schiller, I., Schadlich, K., Kolschev, A., Koitschev, C., et al. (2014). Sinonasal inhalation of dornase alfa administered by vibrating aerosol to cystic fibrosis patients: A double-blind placebo-controlled cross-over trial. *Journal of Cystic Fibrosis*, *13*(5), 602–603.

Malek, A., & Mattison, D. R. (2011). Drugs and medication in pregnancy: The placental disposition of opioids. *Current Pharmacological Biotechnology, 12*, 797–803.

Marino, T. (2015). HIV in pregnancy. *Medscape*. Retrieved from www.emedicine.medscape.com/article/1385488-overHIVinpregnancy.

Marlow, N., Roberts, B. L., & Cooke, R. W. I. (1989). Motor skills in extremely low birthweight children at the age of 6 years. *Archives of Disease in Children, 64*, 839–847.

Marlow, N., Roberts, B. L., & Cooke, R. W. I. (1993). Outcome at 8 years for children with birth weight of 1250 g or less. *Archives of Disease in Children, 68*, 286–290.

Martineaud, J. P., Samb, A., Gueel, L., Seck, D., Badji, L., & Cisse, F. (2002). Exercise performance in young subjects with sickle cell disease. *Scripta Medica, 75*, 111–117.

Mayo Clinic (2019). Amniocentesis. Retrieved from www.mayoclinic.org/tests-procedures/amniocentesis/about/pac-20392914.

Montoya, J. L., Campbell, L. M., Paolillo, E. W., Ellis, R. J., Letendre, S. L., Jeste, D. V., et al. (2019). Inflammation relates to poorer complex motor performance among adults living with HIV on suppressive antiretroviral therapy.

Journal of Acquired Immune Deficiency Syndromes, *80*, 15–23.

Moore, K. L., Persaud, T. V. N., & Torchia, M. G. (2016). *Before we are born: Essentials of embryology and birth defects*, 9th ed. Philadelphia, PA: Saunders.

National Collegiate Athletic Association (2014). Sickle cell trait. Retrieved from www.ncaa.org/health-and-safety/medical-conditions/sickle-cell-trait.

National Fragile X Foundation (2009). Gross motor skill development. Retrieved from www.nfxf.org/html/motor.htm.

Osterdal, M. L., Strom, M., Klemmensen, A. K., Knudsen, V. K., Jul, M., Halldorsson, T. I., et al. (2009). Does leisure time physical activity in early pregnancy protect against preeclampsia? Prospective cohort in Danish women. *British Journal of Obstetrics and Gynecology, 115*, 98–107.

Pereira, P. P., Da Mata, F. A., Figueiredo, A. C., de Andrade, K. R., & Pereira, M. G. (2017). Maternal active smoking during pregnancy and low birth weight in the Americas: A systematic review. *Nicotine & Tobacco Research*, *19*, 497–505.

Pivarnik, J. M., & Mudd, L. M. (2009). Physical activity during pregnancy and postpartum: What have we learned? *Research Digest, 10*, 1–8.

Pohlman, R. L., & Isaacs, L. D. (1990). The previously low birth weight infant: Fundamental motor skill outcomes in the 5- to 9-year-old. *Pediatric Exercise Science, 2*, 263–271.

Powls, A. N., Botting, R. W., Cooke, R. W., & Marlow, N. (1995). Motor impairment in children 12 and 13 years old with a birthweight of less than 1250 g. *Archives of Disease: Childfetal Neonatal Education, 73*, F62–F66.

Presson, A. P., Partyka, G., Jensen, K. M., Devine, O. J., Rasmussen, S. A., McCabe, L. L., et al. (2013). Current estimates of Down syndrome population prevalence in the United States. *Journal of Pediatrics*, *163*(4), 1163–1168.

Rocha, C., Gouvea, A., Machado, D., Cunegundes, K., Beltrao, S., Bononi, F., et al. (2005). Neurological findings in a group of children and adolescents exposed and infected by HIV-1. *Arquivos de Neuro-Psiquiatria, 63*, 828–831, doi: 10.1590/S0004-282X2005000500020.

Rodu, B., & Plurphanswat, N., (2018). E-cigarette use among adults: Population assessment of tobacco and health (PATH) study. *Nicotine and Tobacco Research*, *20*, 940–948.

Rosen, T., & Hoskins, I. A. (2000). Environmental and occupational hazards. In W. R. Cohen (Ed.), *Cherry and Merkatz's complications from pregnancy*, 5th ed. Baltimore, MD: Lippincott Williams & Wilkins.

Shin, M., Besser, L. M., Kucik, J. E., Lu, C., Siffel, C., & Correa, A. (2009). Prevalence of Down syndrome among children and adolescents in 10 regions of the United States. *Pediatrics, 124*, 1565–1571.

Singer, L. T., Arendt, R., Minnes, S., Farkas, K., Salvator, A., Kirchner, H. L., et al. (2002). Cognitive and motor outcomes of cocaine-exposed infants. *Journal of the American Medical Association, 278*, 1952–1960.

Stjernqvist, K., & Svenningsen, N. W. (1995). Extremely low-birth weight infants less than 901 g: Development and behaviour after 4 years of age. *Acta Paediatrica, 84*, 500–506.

Stotland, N. E., Haas, J. S., Brawarsky, P., Jackson, R. A., Fuentes-Afflick, E., & Escobar, G. J. (2005). Body mass index, provider advice, and target gestational weight gain. *Obstetrics and Gynecology, 105*, 633–638.

Stuckey, L. J., Clark, A. M., Chang, S., Chang, K. M., Bartos, C. E., & Ojo, T. C. (2015). The effects of dornase alfa on recurrent gram negative infections in adult cystic fibrosis lung transplant recipients. *The Journal of Heart and Lung Transplantation*, *34*(4), S240.

Sumithran, P., Houlihan, C., Shub, A., Churilov, L., Pritchard, N., Price, S., et al. (2018). How common is substantial weight gain after pregnancy? *Obesity Research & Clinical Practice*, *12*, 139–145.

Szymanski, L. M., & Satin, A. J. (2012). Exercise during pregnancy: Fetal responses to current public health guidelines. *Obstetrics & Gynecology*, *119*, 603–610.

Truong, Y. N., Yee, L. M., Caughey, A. B., & Cheng, Y. W. (2015). Weight gain in pregnancy: Does the Institute of Medicine have it right? *American Journal of Obstetrics & Gunecology*, *212*, 362.e1–362.e8, doi: 10.1016/j.ajog.2015.01.027.

Ulrich, D. A., & Ulrich, B. D. (1999, March). Treadmill training facilitates the onset of walking in infants with Down syndrome. Paper presented at the 32nd annual Gatlinburg Conference on Research and Theory in Mental Retardation and Developmental Disabilities, Charleston, SC.

Ulrich, D. A., Ulrich, B. D., Angulo-Kinzler, R. M., & Yun, J. (2001). Treadmill training of infants with Down syndrome: Evidence-based developmental outcomes. *Pediatrics, 108*, Article e84. Retrieved from www.pediatrics.org/cgi/content/full/108/5/e84.

U.S. Department of Health and Human Services (2007). *The health consequences of involuntary exposure to tobacco smoke: A report of the Surgeon General, U,S, Department of Health and Human Services*, Retrieved from www.surgeongeneral.gov/library/secondhandsmoke/factsheets/factsheet6.html.

U.S. Department of Health and Human Services (2018). *Physical activity guidelines for Americans*, 2nd ed. Washington, DC: U.S. Department of Health and Human Services.

Waisbren, S. E., Noel, K., Fahrbach, K., Cella, C., Frame, D., Dorenbaum, A., et al. (2007). Phenylalanine blood levels and clinical outcomes in phenylketonuria: A systematic literature review and meta-analysis. *Molecular Genetic Metabolism, 92*, 63–70.

Wayne State University Physician Group (2019). Alpha fetoprotein screening. Retrieved from www.wsupgdocs.org/family-medicine/waynestatecontentpage.aspx?nd=1727.

Whittington, J. R., Simmons, P. M., Phillips, A. M., Gammill, S. K., Cen, R., Magann, E. F., et al. (2018). The use of electronic cigarettes in pregnancy: A review of the literature. *Obstetrical & Gynecological Survey*, *73*, 544–549.

Women's Royal Hospital (2017). Guidelines: Drug and alcohol – neonatal abstinence syndrome (NAS). Retrieved from https://thewomens.r.worldssl.net/images/uploads/downloadable-records/clinical-guidelines/drug-and-alcohol-neonatal-abstinence-syndrome-NAS_160517.pdf.

Worthington-Roberts, B. S. (2000). Nutrition. In W. R. Cohen (Ed.), *Cherry and Merkatz's complications of pregnancy*, 5th ed. Baltimore, MD: Lippincott Williams & Wilkins.

Yazdy, M. M., Desai, R. J., & Brogly, S. B. (2015). Prescription opioids in pregnancy and birth outcomes: A review of the literature. *Journal of Pediatric Genetics*, *4*, 56–70.

Yu, Y., Xie, R., Shen, S., & Shu, L. (2018). Effect of exercise during pregnancy to prevent gestational diabetes mellitus: A systematic review and meta-analysis. *The Journal of Maternal-Fetal & Neonatal Medicine*, *31*, 1632–1637.

Zhao, P., Liu, E., Qiao, Y., Katzarzyk, P. T., Chaput, J. P., Fogelholm, M., et al. (2016). Maternal gestational diabetes and childhood obesity at age 9–11: Results of a multinational study. *Diabetologia*, *59*, 2339–2348.

5 EFFECTS OF EARLY STIMULATION AND DEPRIVATION

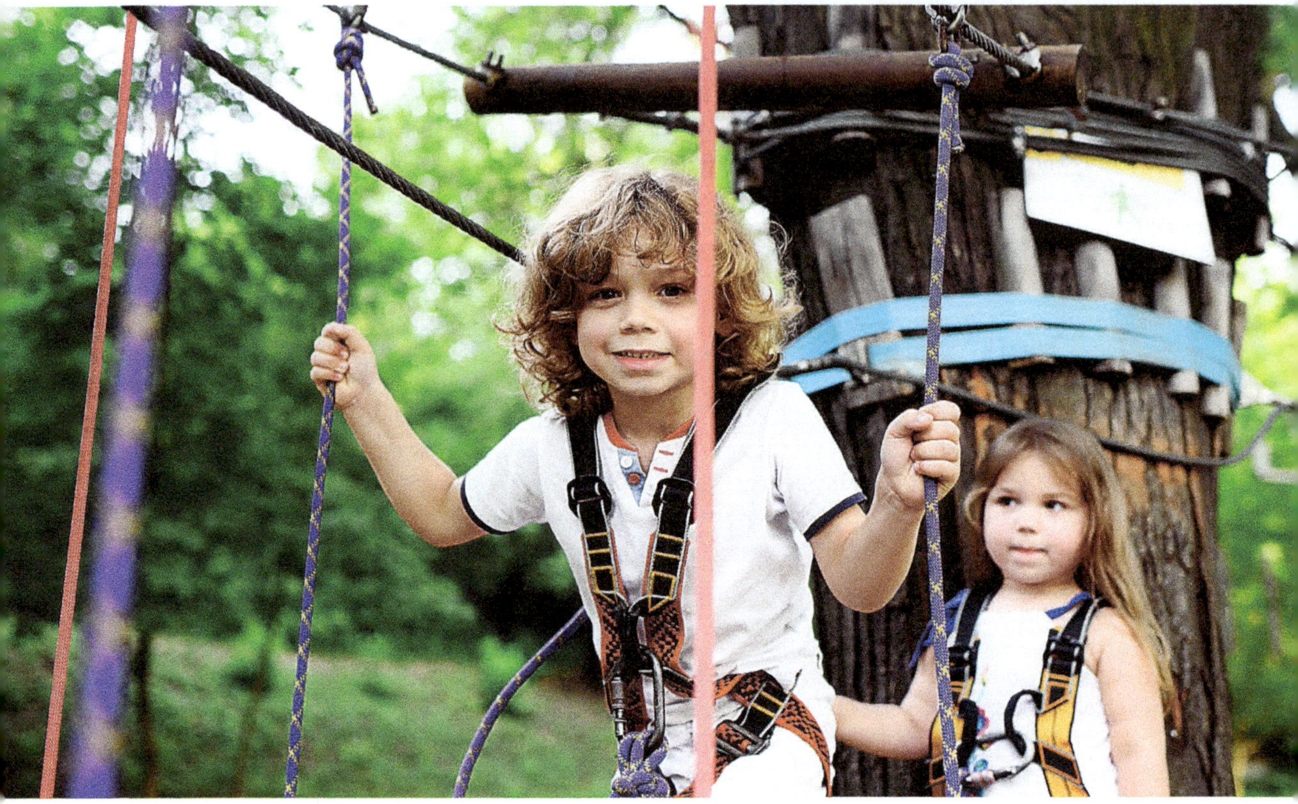

Chapter Objectives

From the information presented in this chapter, you will be able to

- Describe some effects of early stimulation
- Describe some programs to enhance early motor development
- Describe McGraw's famous twin study involving early stimulation and deprivation
- Explain several classic case studies involving deprivation and discuss what they may indicate for human deprivation or stimulation
- Describe some effects of early deprivation
- Explain the concepts of critical periods, readiness, and catch-up as they relate to human development

David Elkind is a professor, psychologist, and prolific author who observes that many parents are convinced that earlier is better in terms of the training and education of their children. The trend toward early education has become ingrained in many sectors of our society, where a common attitude is that it is rarely too early to start children in programs such as reading, math, swimming, violin, or even martial arts. This, according to Elkind, has resulted in a confounding of the perceived need for early education and all children's need for quality child care.

Elkind has written many books, including his most recent, entitled, *Giants in the Nursery* (2015). In a 2007 edition of Elkind's book *The Hurried Child: Growing Up Too Fast Too Soon*, the author proclaims that this unfortunate trend has given rise to "an explosion of interest in stimulating and educating infants" (p. x). He writes, "Infancy and early childhood . . . are now the focus of our hurrying" (p. xi). This focus has even extended to the fetus in the womb. An array of prenatal, infant, and early childhood products on the market are designed to enhance untold aspects of our children's development. DVDs, software programs, toys, and gadgets, as well as exercise, swimming, and sports programs, exist for the youngest of children. Millions of dollars are being spent to ensure that our children have every chance to be all they can, yet few of these products have any research to support their efficacy. According to Elkind, the most important interaction a child can have is with a parent or caregiver, and too many of the cascade of new products may be gradually replacing the parents' and caregivers' role in the interaction (Elkind, 2007).

Interestingly, and perhaps logically, the general belief behind this trend is that **stimulation** is always "good" and **deprivation** is "bad." Although we admire parents who "stimulate" their child, we often scorn parents who "deprive" their child. However, can we overstimulate our children, starting too soon with too much? Is some degree of deprivation ever in the child's best interest? When are the best times for stimulation or the worst times for deprivation? Is stimulation helpful for the acquisition of all human behaviors, or are there some behaviors that cannot be facilitated by early exposure to stimulating experiences? These are all questions that researchers consider as they examine the effects of stimulation and deprivation.

EFFECTS OF EARLY STIMULATION

In recent years, parents have been involving their children more than ever in early educational programs—everything from swimming, gymnastics, and violin lessons to the study of reading and foreign languages. The unusual aspect of these programs designed for early stimulation is that in some cases they start as early as birth, or even earlier, as numerous products have been created to stimulate the baby while still in utero. The rush to enroll children in early programs is not new; it was highlighted nearly four decades ago in "Bringing Up Superbaby" (Langway, Jackson, Zabarsky, et al., 1983). This article described what was happening and what was predicted to come regarding this issue. Many of the points raised in this article are even more timely today than they were when the article was published. For example, many of today's babies are born to parents who are older and more affluent than those of earlier generations and who have been assured that any behavior they desire for their child can be taught. Increased knowledge concerning child development and the idea that the environment influences human behavior have motivated parents to seek all possible advantages for their children. In fact, some may believe that kindergarten is "too late" and waiting until then is a waste of many good learning years.

Contrary to the philosophy of Elkind, Glenn Doman was an advocate of this perspective. Doman was the founder of the Institutes for the Achievement of Human Potential and passed away in 2013 (*New York Times*, 2013). He had written numerous books about teaching reading and math skills to babies, in addition to making babies fitter, smarter, and more physically "superb." He even attempts to describe how to "give your baby encyclopedic knowledge" (see Doman & Doman, 2005, 2006; Doman, Doman, & Aisen, 2005; Doman, Doman, & Hagy, 2006). One of his more recent books is entitled *Fit Baby, Smart Baby, Your Baby!* (Doman, Doman, & Hagy, 2012). Although many reading and math skills are often believed to be essentially intellectual, the fine control of eye movement needed for these activities is just one example of the role of motor development in success in these subjects. For optimal success in these skills, Doman recommends initiating instruction by using flashcards during the *first few days* of neonatal life.

Doman has received harsh criticism from the academic and scientific communities for not scientifically substantiating the effectiveness of the techniques he recommends, and popular opinion as to the value of his programs is mixed. Some children have learned to respond appropriately to flashcards, for example, but others simply play with the cards. Critics of such early programs question the advantage of the simple recognition skills enhanced by the flashcards. They further contend that pressure to learn at an early age may actually frighten the child away from future experiences of a similar nature. Some child developmentalists believe the emphasis on achievement so early may hamper the emotional, physical, or creative aspects of the child's development. A 2007 *Boston Globe* article by Neil Swidey on the push for early education was particularly critical of the extreme approach espoused by Doman. In fact, the approach was characterized as possibly being a waste of time. In that article, Swidey noted that Doman had never produced empirical data to support his contentions and that children following his early education approach rarely performed better than other children with motivated parents. Most significantly, Swidey continued, these early pushes for achievement may slow a child's development, a function of a phenomenon he termed "neurological crowding," or simply too much information too soon (Swidey, 2007).

Regardless of such opinions, parents generally believe early educational stimulation is valuable, as evidenced by the quantity and popularity of the early educational programs available today (see Figure 5.1). These programs may have positive effects, but such factors as the child's age, the type of stimulation, and the parents' and child's attitudes are doubtless critical factors in their success or failure.

Research on Early Stimulation

Clearly, stimulating young children at an early age is often beneficial. Research on young children (6 months to 2 years old) who had been severely malnourished in Bangladesh demonstrates this (Nahar, Hamadani, Ahmed, et al., 2009). At the beginning of this study, the children were provided with "standard"

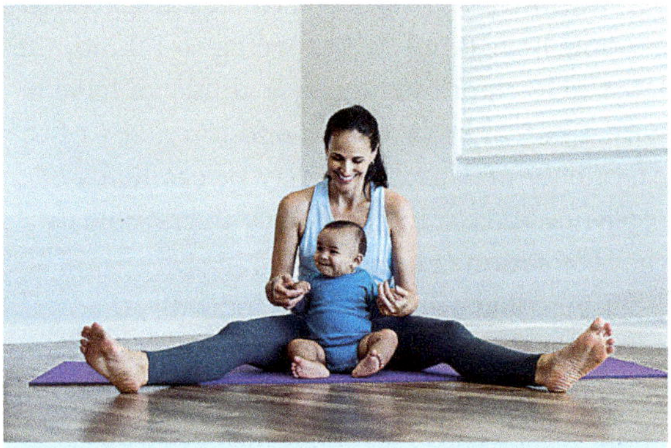

Figure 5.1 Programs of early motor stimulation have become increasingly popular over the past decade

nutritional care and psychosocial stimulation. This stimulation included daily group meetings with the mothers, organized play sessions in a hospital setting, and regular home visits across a 6-month period. Both growth and development were monitored. Though several children tragically died before the culmination of the study, the surviving children were found to have improved significantly beyond a control group of children who did not receive the interventions. The improvements included mental scores, scores on motor ability, and measures of body weight for age. In short, for the severely malnourished children in this research, early stimulation was found to be an effective component of treatment.

As another example of the effects of early stimulation, Lee and Galloway (2012) specifically examined the effects of early daily experiences on the development of head control of 20 healthy babies who were placed in a control or training group. Head control was deemed particularly important as it is one of the first major motor milestones and an important precursor to establishing the visual field, as well as movements involving the trunk and arms, like sitting, reaching, and grasping, and eventually standing. In typical situations in many Western cultures, babies are given considerable external support to maintain head position. The authors indicate that these cultural approaches may affect the rate of acquisition in the development of head control. Starting at 1 month of age, training group babies were provided with postural and movement activities for a third of an hour every day for 1 month. Their movement activities involved increased use of the neck, shoulders, and trunk in addition to reaching activities. They were also carried daily for 20 minutes using a front carrier. The babies in the control group were provided with regular social interaction with a caregiver for 20 minutes daily for 1 month, like the training group. This social activity was designed to compensate for the social interaction that would be experienced by the training group babies. During this time, the control group babies were placed in a supine position and interacted with their caregivers without actually physically contacting them or playing with toys.

All the babies were tested on a standardized developmental test on alternate weeks for 3 months (1–4 months of age). Infants in the training group were found to yield higher test scores, especially on items related to head control. This included keeping their heads vertical and in the midline without external support longer than the control group. The training group also demonstrated more active movement of the head more frequently and across longer distances. This led these researchers to conclude that early postural and movement activities can expedite the development of head control. The likely contributing factors were the positioning of the infant, the way the infant was handled by the caregiver, and the overall interplay between the caregiver and the baby. These findings may be especially important for a baby's demonstrating developmental delays early in life (Lee & Galloway, 2012).

In similar research, Lobo and Galloway (2012) enrolled 2-month-old babies in a 3-week-long program designed to provide enhanced "handling and positioning" (p. 1290) of the babies by their caregivers. The researchers indicated that "enhanced" meant that these were activities well beyond what would be experienced by the babies in a typical day in typical Western culture. Activities specifically encouraged sitting and standing with support, unassisted head control and support, and an emphasis on placing the baby in a prone position. These experiences were provided to the baby by the caregiver for 15 minutes per day for the first 3 weeks of the more than year-long study. A second group of babies (control group) was provided with social interaction for the same period of time that the control babies received their movement experiences—15 minutes per day for 3 weeks. The control group caregivers were also asked to place the baby in a supine, rather than prone, position when possible.

All the babies were tested using a standardized measure of infant motor performance. Results indicated that the babies in the training group, who had received enhanced handling and positioning, were developmentally advanced in a number of ways. The training appeared to enhance motor ability immediately, and the skills were maintained through the first year of life, well after training had ceased. Specific advantages noted in the training group included more mature head control as well as reaching and sitting abilities. The training group also showed better skill in their general play when on the floor, their object manipulation, and even in early forms of locomotion. The researchers believed all of these advances were a result of improved postural control resulting from the training. Postural control is fundamental in the acquisition of many subsequent movement skills during infancy. In addition, the babies in the training group may have benefitted physiologically; their muscle systems were "primed" and their "neurological systems better prepared for action" (p. 1298). Lastly, the authors posited that the training group infants may have benefitted perceptually. As a result of their early experiences, their visual and vestibular systems may have been positively impacted. These findings are particularly important as they may have medical implications for professionals dealing with babies who have special needs. Early interventions of the kind employed in this study may advance the abilities of those who have the greatest need (Lobo & Galloway, 2012).

Though more research is needed on programs of early stimulation, including motor stimulation, many programs do conduct self-evaluations intended to determine how children's development has been enhanced. These evaluations, however, are seldom devised to detect any detrimental effects. Furthermore, developmental gains that are noted are often those that would have occurred anyway with typical exposure to a stimulating home environment. This is not to suggest, however, that such programs should never be considered or employed. We must be careful consumers by seeking programs with qualified professionals, clean and appropriate facilities, reasonable fees, and objectives that seem appropriate for the baby or child to be enrolled. Programs that make indiscriminate claims should be avoided.

Programs Designed to Enhance Early Motor Development

Whole-Child Early Stimulation Programs

In recent years many new programs of early stimulation have evolved, and few have gained the attention and popularity of Gymboree Play & Music (www.gymboreeclasses.com). In fact, according to their website, Gymboree Play & Music is the "global leader" in early childhood programs. The first Gymboree program was designed for children from infancy to 5 years. It was opened in 1976 and by 2017 had grown to 730 locations in 40 countries (Gymboree Play & Music, 2017). The organization is based on the belief that the preschool years may be the most critical time for education and when parents have the least amount of outside help in educating their children. Furthermore, the Gymboree Play & Music philosophy assumes preschoolers need to be provided with certain types of play activities that are believed to be essential to their development but are not readily available at home, on the playground, or in the nursery. The developer describes its environment as being safe and noncompetitive while challenging the psychomotor needs of preschoolers, with a focus on the "whole" child—motor skills, social skills, and self-esteem. Programs are devised to emphasize areas like physical activity, art, music, and school skills, with the goal of enhancing confidence, creativity, curiosity, balance, coordination, school skill, and becoming a competent problem solver (Gymboree Play & Music, 2017).

Most Gymboree Play & Music sessions offer a variety of colorful, scaled-down equipment like ramps, slides and climbers for children to explore with varying degrees of guidance from their parent(s) or Gymboree personnel. Balance beams, balls, scooters, tunnels, rollers, hoops, and ladders are a few of the many pieces of equipment that may be available for exploration during the "free time" segment of each Gymboree session. Gymboree proponents claim that parents benefit from participation by learning their child's needs and increasing their understanding of the child's growth and development. This, proponents say, will help parents meet their child's needs and encourage development in an efficient yet fun way.

Gymboree Play & Music programs emphasize motor activities oriented toward balancing, performing fundamental movements (running, jumping, throwing, catching, and so forth), switching among different modes of locomotion, assuming a variety of body positions, changing direction and speed, socializing (sharing and taking turns), and expressing the imagination freely. According to the current Gymboree website, these classes are beneficial to social, physical, and cognitive development. Thus, they provide an early start to long term developmental success (Gymboree Play & Music, 2017). However, as mentioned earlier, little research exists to substantiate the claims made by this or similar programs. Self-appraisals must be viewed cautiously, as there is an obvious bias. Gymboree makes some significant, though tempered, claims and is careful to point out that fun is paramount. Until controlled research is conducted, however, we will not know whether Gymboree attains its goals or if participants are simply developing skills that are typically part of the developmental process.

Swim Programs for Infants and Preschoolers

For years, one of the most common forms of early motor stimulation has been swim programs for infants and preschoolers (see Figure 5.2). According to Costa and associates, infant water programs have seen a substantial increase in recent years with various goals like decreasing drownings, improving movement ability and socialization (Costa, Barbosa, Ramos, & Marinho, 2016). For infants (birth to 1 year), in particular, there may be little justification for programs designed to teach swimming. Nevertheless, the popularity of swim programs for infants and preschoolers has grown, and many programs have long waiting lists. This popularity is often fueled by a belief on the part of parents or other caregivers that they have to start their children swimming as early as possible even though hard evidence as to the success of these programs in facilitating children's later swimming is disputed. Clearly, some children who have graduated from these swim programs have achieved considerable success in their later swimming endeavors while

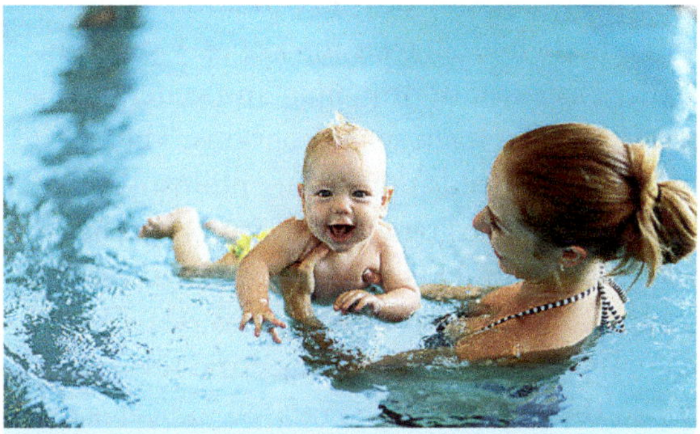

Figure 5.2 Surprisingly to many, infant swim programs are controversial, and professional organizations dispute their sometimes lofty claims

others have left such early programs with no apparent improvement. In fact, in some cases, parents claimed that their children became more fearful of the water!

Often, parents involve infants in "swimming" programs from a desire to improve the child's safety around water, and some early aquatic programs do not profess to teach swimming but rather "drownproofing," "waterproofing," or simply making an infant water-safe. Most experts agree that these terms are inappropriate. In one of their most recent statements on swim programs for infants and toddlers, the American Academy of Pediatrics states, "swimming lessons for infants and toddlers do not protect children from drowning." They further state that children are not prepared to engage in formal swim lessons until after the age of 4 years (AAP, 2019).

Table 5.1 Selected recommendations on infant and toddler swim programs

1.	Children are generally not ready for formal swimming lessons until after their fourth birthday.
2.	Aquatic programs for infants and toddlers should not be promoted as a way to decrease the risk of drowning.
3.	Parents should not feel secure that their child is safe in the water or safe from drowning after participation in infant swim programs.
4.	Whenever infants and toddlers are in or around water, an adult should be within an arm's length for safety purposes.
5.	Aquatics programs should provide information on cognitive and motor limitations of infants and toddlers, the inherent risks of the water, strategies for prevention of drowning, and the role of adults in supervising and monitoring the safety of children in and around water.
6.	Hypothermia, water intoxication, and communicable diseases can be prevented by following existing medical guidelines and do not preclude infants and toddlers from participating in otherwise appropriate aquatic experiences.

Source: American Academy of Pediatrics (2010).

Program recommendations. Selected American Academy of Pediatrics' recommendations regarding infant and toddler swim programs are listed in Table 5.1, including warnings about health considerations with early swimming. These are discussed below.

Despite concerns raised by the American Academy of Pediatrics, a recent Revised Scientific Review (Langendorfer, 2019) revealed another perspective to the considerable controversy surrounding the issue regarding when to start children in aquatics programs. In contrast to the statement generated by the American Academy of Pediatrics, this review stated that children over the age of 1 year can reduce their risk of drowning and generally derive benefits from such programs. This statement contends that strong philosophical differences regarding infant swim programs have long existed between professional medical groups, aquatic professionals, and related agencies. As evidence, this scientific review claims that considerable research indicates that infants and very young children can acquire various basic acquatic skills like breath control, entering and exiting pools, and very preliminary versions of swimming (e.g., dog paddling), with these skills being foundational to more advanced abilities that would ensue with additional instruction at a later age. Despite disagreements regarding infant swim philosophies, most agree that all children should be taught to swim and decisions regarding the age to begin this instruction should involve the child's interest in the water, their maturity for their age, and their initial ability and receptivity to swimming fundamentals (e.g., breath control) as well as their overall health and ability to control their own posture (Langendorfer, 2019).

Health issues. Several health concerns have been attributed to infant swim programs, including hyponatremia (water intoxication), giardia (an intestinal parasite that can be transmitted in pool water), an increased risk of asthma or bronchitis later in childhood, and hypothermia.

Hyponatremia occurs when an individual ingests so much water that the body's electrolytes are reduced and the kidneys cannot filter the excess fluid. Parental education is imperative concerning this dangerous and life-threatening condition because it is avoidable and treatable. Symptoms include reduced core temperature, reduced sodium serum levels, possible seizure, and possible loss of consciousness. Young children are particularly at risk because they have a larger brain relative to their skull size, increasing the chance for edema (accumulation of excess fluids) in the brain. Though water intoxication is relatively rare, occurring less than 100 times per 100,000 children, it is dangerous. It is most common among children younger than 2 years of age. Awareness of the condition, prevention, early detection, and proper medical care can save lives (Hsu, Wang, Chen, et al., 2014). Obviously, hyponatremia is a concern in infant swim programs, especially those that practice forced or frequent submersions or are particularly long. For this reason, parents and caregivers should be advised to monitor the quantity of water that their children consume before, during, and after participation in a water program.

A more common problem with infant swim programs is **giardia**. This parasite resides in the intestines of animals and is passed via animal feces. Found in contaminated soil, food, or water, it can maintain life outside a body for weeks or months. When ingested, giardia can develop into cysts in the intestinal tract and can cause low-grade fever, chills, distended abdomen, and severe diarrhea. It can also be a precursor to more severe maladies, especially among children. Giardia is easily transmitted to others when circulated through the pool water.

A number of precautions can prevent giardia infections among infants and toddlers. These include taking children on frequent trips to the bathroom, changing their diapers often, changing the diapers away from the pool, and teaching children not to swallow pool water. Other helpful strategies include showering before and after being in the pool to wash off infectious bacteria that can be spread through the pool water, and requiring that tight-legged diapers or pants be worn in the water. Infants and toddlers who currently have diarrhea or who have had diarrhea within the past week should be discouraged from using pools (Elkins, 2010).

In addition to hyponatremia and giardia, the gases and aerosols commonly used in indoor swimming environments can be a concern when infants swim in these pools. A group of Belgian researchers studied the effects of these chemicals on infants, being particularly concerned that these irritants may increase the infants' potential for allergic reactions and decrease their general respiratory health later in childhood. The subjects of this study were more than 300 children aged 10–13 years, 43 of whom had been involved in infant swim experiences. Results indicated that the children who had been involved in infant swim experiences showed significantly lower levels of key pulmonary proteins, suggesting pulmonary cell damage, as well as modifications to the permeability of the epithelial barrier of the lungs. According to the researchers, these differences placed the children at an increased risk of asthma and a recurring form of bronchitis later in childhood. The researchers concluded that infant swimming experiences in chlorinated indoor pools can induce airway changes that lead to chronic respiratory conditions (Bernard, Carbonnelle, Dumont, & Nickmilder, 2007). Similar findings resulted from a more recent study on the effect of a pool's chlorine on kindergarten children's respiration. These researchers determined that participation in early aquatic activities increased the liklihood of having inflamed airways and greater sensitivity to dust (Voisin, Sardella, & Bernard, 2014).

Hypothermia, which occurs when the body temperature falls significantly below normal, can also be a concern for very young children in an aquatic program. Young children are particularly susceptible to this condition because they have more surface area per body mass than older children or adults. Thus, heat loss occurs more rapidly. Special caution should be taken to ensure that children stay sufficiently warm when involved in infant water programs. When hypothermia is suspected, children should be re-warmed slowly with blankets and clothing. Warm liquids should also be given to ensure proper hydration. In extreme cases, the child may need emergency treatment. Symptoms of hypothermia include numbness in the extremities (fingers and toes), fingers or lips turning blue, and, in more extreme cases, confusion or disorientation. In a most extreme case, the child may not be able to stand or move typically and may not even know who he or she is (Zablocki, 2001).

Program effectiveness. Despite the shortcomings of some early aquatic programs, exposure to the water at an early age offers many potential benefits to participants. Though supportive data are lacking, early aquatic programs may be valuable in helping a child develop affection for the water at a young age. They may provide an excellent, unique environment for quality parent-child interactions, and being in the water may be comforting to some very young children. Unfortunately, very little research has been conducted to ascertain the effectiveness of infant swim programs with regard to measures of interest (e.g., parental attitudes about their children and water experiences, comfort in the water, later aquatic ability, physical fitness, motor skill development, self-esteem, and so forth). One of the few investigations exploring babies and their water experiences was conducted in Iceland. Specifically, noting an "upsurge in interest among parents" (Sigmundsson & Hopkins, 2010, p. 428), the researchers sought to compare the motor ability of 4-year-old children who had experienced an infant swim program during the first few months of life versus the motor ability of those who had not (the control group). The researchers used a standardized assessment to test all of the children for motor ability. Overall, the researchers found no statistical difference, though the children who had experienced an infant aquatic program demonstrated significantly better prehension as determined by a ball skills test and better balance as demonstrated by a one-leg balance. The researchers acknowledged the limitations of their small sample size but believed their results indicated possible benefits of early water experiences for later motor development. They also advised that much more research is needed to explore the full level of relevance of these kinds of programs in early infancy.

Since so little scientific evidence exists to assist us in understanding these programs, we need much more research on the early development of swimming skills, the effects of early exposure to the water, and hyponatremia. We also need more substantial information concerning the effects of such factors as water condition, facility design, and aquatic teaching methodologies to aid in the establishment of new aquatic teaching curricula. Clearly, we still have much to learn concerning infant and preschool aquatic programs.

Suzuki Method of Learning the Violin

Another of the most popular and enduring early-stimulation programs is the Suzuki method of learning to play the violin. This program, which depends greatly on the early fine motor and intellectual capabilities of its young students, was developed by Shinichi Suzuki in Japan more than 50 years ago.

Suzuki's father owned a violin factory, so as a child Suzuki actually saw the instruments being constructed as he and his siblings played nearby. Suzuki eventually began to ponder how easily we learn language and wondered if the basic principles behind learning language could be applied to learning to play the violin. The process, he believed, should start when we are born by listening to music frequently, even daily, much like we listen to language. Within a few years, formal and actual violin training could begin with constant repetition being integral to the process, again, like we learn to verbally communicate.

Suzuki also believed that parental involvement is integral to getting children to "want to play." Suzuki encouraged parents to first learn to play individual violin pieces, so they can be intimately involved in the instruction as well as serving as a model for the importance and desirability of learning to play the instrument. In the strict Suzuki method, the child would not begin to play the instrument until the parent has mastered, at least, one piece. An emphasis is placed on enjoyment and loving encouragement during the process with the home environment serving as an important cog in instruction. In addition, while Suzuki believed actual instruction with the instrument could begin at around 3 or 4 years of age, a person of any age could benefit from this process (Figure 5.3) (Suzuki Association of the Americas, 2019).

According to Suzuki, the ability to play could be taught to nearly anyone and was not necessarily an innate talent. He also taught that music was critical to being a "good person" who could be a valuable societal contributor with greater appreciation for their fellow person. Because many Suzuki method violin students begin so early and are so small, instruments are adapted to their size enabling them to feel more comfortable with the violin. Thus, they could more capably practice for longer periods of time (Richards, 2017).

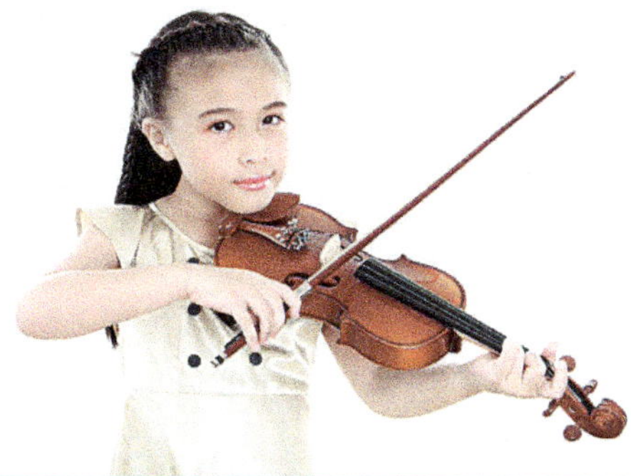

Figure 5.3 The Suzuki method of learning to play the violin emphasizes listening and playing

As is the case with most programs involving the early stimulation of children, much is unknown about the residual effects of the Suzuki method. Although some outstanding violinists began with the program, other Suzuki students lose interest in the instrument. Critics of such programs contend that many children have actually been discouraged from further involvement in music by being inundated with too much violin too young.

Case Study on the Effects of Early Stimulation: Johnny and Jimmy

In 1935, Myrtle McGraw conducted what is now considered a classic investigation directly concerning motor development and the effects of early stimulation. In her research, McGraw closely monitored the twin brothers known as Johnny and Jimmy. She was particularly interested in determining if a child's typical progress in motor development could be altered by certain conditions. Therefore, for the first 22 months of the twins' lives, McGraw gave Johnny toys and considerable stimulation, practice, and experience in a variety of movement activities. Jimmy, however, had few toys and minimal motor stimulation (McGraw, 1935).

McGraw periodically examined the effects of the varying levels of stimulation by exposing the twins to selected movement activities. For example, Johnny was given a tricycle when he was 11 months old. He was also given considerable practice and some instruction at that time. However, McGraw noted that 8 months elapsed before Johnny showed any signs of learning on the tricycle; he then proceeded to master tricycling quickly, within 2 months.

Jimmy was deprived of tricycling until he was 22 months old. However, despite the relatively low levels of stimulation he received, he learned tricycling much faster than Johnny. This led McGraw to conclude that a certain level of readiness is necessary for the acquisition of a motor skill. Jimmy was ready to tricycle at 22 months, but Johnny was not at 11 months (McGraw, 1935). (We discuss the term *readiness* later in this chapter.)

Using the twins as her subjects, McGraw examined many other movement activities, as well. For example, Johnny was taught to roller-skate at less than 1 year of age, and he became skillful at the task. McGraw believed that this achievement was facilitated by his low center of gravity, which enhanced his balance. Jimmy began skating at 22 months but never became a good skater. When their skating experiences ended, both twins' ability declined rapidly. In fact, when they were 3 years old, both twins suffered balance difficulties. Surprisingly, Johnny, the stimulated twin, was described as having more problems skating than Jimmy after their regular skating ended. McGraw credited this to attitudinal differences that were emerging: Johnny had become somewhat reckless, whereas Jimmy maintained a much more cautious approach to movement.

McGraw also observed Johnny and Jimmy ascending and descending slopes of varying grades. Johnny exhibited better skills at ascending the slopes than did Jimmy and also retained his ability better. Furthermore, Johnny appeared to be cleverer at developing climbing strategies and was more graceful in the process. McGraw attributed this superior climbing ability to Johnny's early experience in a diversity of tasks, including slope climbing. When descending the slopes, Jimmy was particularly timid or cautious and occasionally uncooperative. Johnny rarely hesitated to descend and consistently maintained a higher level of ability.

Attitude similarly affected the boys' performance in jumping. For the jumping task, McGraw instructed the twins to jump down from a low pedestal. Frequently, Jimmy, who had far less early experience than his brother, could not be coaxed to jump. Johnny, however, jumped freely and with considerable skill.

McGraw also observed the twins while they were in the water. Both twins were given very early aquatic experiences, which were abruptly halted when they were 17 months old, to be tested periodically in the future. Upon retesting when at 6 years of age, Johnny was found to be much more comfortable and skillful in the water than Jimmy. Whereas Johnny demonstrated a typical horizontal stroking position in a well-coordinated fashion, Jimmy stayed vertical and exhibited jerky swimming actions. Johnny's advanced skill was considered rather unusual because he had never been instructed to perform the relatively sophisticated movements that he exhibited.

The contrast in levels of early stimulation for Johnny and Jimmy may have affected more than their motor development. Although both Johnny and Jimmy were happy and well adjusted, Johnny was frequently favored socially. Perhaps as a result of his jealousy, Jimmy often struck Johnny and would take his toys. At other times, however, Jimmy would exhibit tremendous affection for his brother. In addition, Jimmy was more dependent on his mother and more prone to temper tantrums than was his brother.

A Rorschach (inkblot) test divulged additional information concerning the twins' personalities. Jimmy was more immature emotionally, self-centered, and dependent; Johnny more impersonal, self-confident, too brave at times, and relatively unaggressive.

McGraw's (1935) longitudinal investigation of Johnny and Jimmy was in many respects somewhat unscientific. With only two main subjects in this investigation, we cannot assume that the experiences of Johnny and Jimmy are indicative of what would happen with other subjects of a similar age. Nevertheless, McGraw is frequently credited with an astute and insightful ability to suggest possible explanations for the differences in movement behavior between Johnny and Jimmy. For example, she believed that the degree to which an ability maintains its state depends on its level of fixity. According to McGraw, the **level of fixity** is how well established a skill is when it is discontinued. This phenomenon may have accounted for the twins' maintenance of tricycling ability following a period of inactivity on the tricycle. The high level of skill that they developed upon initial exposure to tricycling facilitated their efforts when they were exposed to the same task later.

McGraw also believed that practice and attitude were important factors affecting skill ability. Johnny's early practice in ascending and descending slopes and his willing attitude appeared to underlie his superior ability in this task. Jimmy had no previous experience to rely on and, perhaps as a result, was hampered by an uncooperative attitude toward this task. Interestingly, though, this attitudinal difference may have had the reverse effect on roller-skating. Johnny was so willing to roller-skate that he became reckless and sloppy as a roller skater compared with his more conservative brother, who was extremely cautious (McGraw, 1935).

Observing Johnny and Jimmy roller-skating led McGraw to conclude that growth affected the facility with which the twins acquired movement ability. As discussed earlier, Johnny became relatively successful at roller-skating as early as 1 year of age. Jimmy was not introduced to the activity until he was 22 months old and never excelled at it. McGraw believed this difference occurred because the two boys had different body sizes when they were introduced to the activity: Jimmy was much taller and, therefore, had a higher center of gravity, making it harder for him to maintain the balance necessary for roller-skating. Johnny, who was younger when he first attempted roller-skating, was shorter, which McGraw believed was an advantage for this particular movement.

EFFECTS OF EARLY DEPRIVATION

The effects of early forms of deprivation, or maltreatment, are important to developmentalists studying all aspects of human behavior. Examples of maltreatment include physical, emotional, or sexual abuse, and neglect and negligent treatment. It can affect physical health as well as such factors as dignity, trust, and sense of power. In fact, early maltreatment can "initiate a negative developmental cascade that continues through life. (Cicchetti, 2016, p. 188). It can disrupt brain function as it can impact neural circuitry, especially in the corpus callosum and cerebellum where actual brain volume can be reduced (Cicchetti, 2016). Thus, emotional and intellectual development can be impaired while poorer self-esteem and impaired long-term social relationships can emerge. Some deprived or maltreated toddlers have exhibited excessive levels of anger, fear, and aggression. They can also tend to be more easily distracted and hyperactive while demonstrating poorer levels of concentration, which may lead to academic concerns upon entering school. Slightly later in life, these same children are more apt to bully others while also being at greater risk of being victims themselves. Interestingly, early maltreatment has also been associated with physical issues (e.g., asthma, heart problems, infectious disease, and generally poorer immune response) and even higher body mass index (Cicchetti & Toth, 2015). These factors can extend into adulthood and, clearly, directly or indirectly impact motor development throughout life.

The type, length, time, and severity of deprivation and maltreatment, and their subsequent effects, are all variables developmentalists strive to understand. Potentially, such information may have beneficial applications for many practical situations, including education and child rearing. However, investigating the effects of deprivation is difficult. Intentionally placing a baby in a poor environment for scientific purposes is unethical and inhumane, so researchers have had to rely on animal research or the study of the unusual and sometimes tragic human cases that have occurred in society. Therefore, only sparse information is available concerning the effects of deprivation on the human being. However, some research, including a number of classic cases involving both animals and humans, has yielded important findings about the effects of various forms of deprivation early in life.

One study focused on the effects of deprivation on motor development, specifically balance and bilateral coordination. Roeber, Gunnar, and Pollak (2013) studied children from institutions with varying conditions and in various parts of the world. The authors indicated that these institutions often do not provide the support necessary for the child's typical development. Thus, children may be affected in any number of domains and have been shown to suffer physical (i.e., growth), intellectual, and even emotional deficits. Children who have been institutionalized for long periods can exhibit more, and more serious, developmental delays. These researchers chose to study effects on motor development, because this topic had not been studied specifically as it relates to deprivation. Children with delayed motor capabilities often face social stigmas, are excluded socially, and eventually experience a lifelong cycle leading to poor social interactions and low self-esteem. Of course, physical fitness and health are also negatively affected. Study participants were 8- and 9-year-olds who had been either (1) internationally adopted and integrated into a family at a median age of just over 18 months after spending at least three-quarters of their lives in an institution; (2) placed with a family early in their young lives, having spent less than a year in an institution; or (3) raised from birth with a family (the control group).

The perceived deprivation of institutionalization was found to have a significant impact on motor development. After seven years with a family, children who had been institutionalized had not achieved the level of bilateral coordination found in the non-institutionalized children. Even the children who had been placed with a family early in their lives continued to lag behind the non-institutionalized children on measures of balance. The researchers found this especially noteworthy as some of the children had been placed with families as early as 2 months of age (Roeber et al., 2013).

For all of these reasons, child maltreatment has become an important worldwide issue as a result of the major impact it can have on one's life. A promising approach to reduce the incidence of maltreatment has been the creation of parenting programs. A meta-analysis of 37 studies examining this phenomenon in the United States, Canada, Australia, New Zealand, England, and Thailand found these programs to be effective in reducing the incidence of maltreatment as well as neglect, overall parental aggression, and particularly stern forms of discipline and punishment (Chen & Chan, 2016).

HOPI CRADLEBOARDS AND INFANT DEVELOPMENT

In the 1930s, Wayne Dennis extensively studied the Hopi tribe. This work culminated with the publication of his book *The Hopi Child* (1940). Of particular interest for motor development was Dennis's description of the Hopis' use of infant cradleboards. As young as 1 month, and often until after the first birthday, babies were swaddled and tied to a board. The baby's arms were usually extended at the sides with only enough room to bend slightly. The legs were also placed in an extended position. Generally, according to Dennis, while on the board the Hopi infants were prevented from performing many movements that would be typical of babies who were not "cradled." For example, while in the cradleboard, babies could not touch their hands to the mouth, watch their hands, or kick their feet.

Initially, the baby was placed in the cradleboard for as long as 23 hours/day. However, progressively more freedom was allowed, starting at about 3 months of age. From 6 months, the baby would not be placed on its abdomen when out of the cradleboard until it was capable of voluntarily turning from a supine to a prone position. Thus, the baby was unable to practice such skills as raising the head or raising the chest off the floor when in a prone position.

Dennis also claimed that Hopi infants were seldom taken from their homes until about 4 months of age. When taken outside the home, babies were usually carried in their mother's arms or on her back, and the cradleboard was left at home. By this time, babies were often so accustomed to the board that they would cry or become restless until returned to it.

As Dennis noted in his book, questions arose concerning the effect of the cradleboard on babies' development. Dennis observed that during the first few months of life Hopi babies maintained a flexed position when temporarily freed from the board. They also exhibited several other activities expected of babies that are not cradleboarded, such as playing with their feet and hands. In fact, the sequence of acquisition of many voluntary movement skills seemed to follow the sequence that would typically occur without the "deprivation" of the cradleboard. According to Dennis, Hopi infants developed such skills as sitting, creeping, and walking in the usual sequence and at the same times as non-cradleboarded children (Dennis, 1940).

Deprivation Dwarfism

The effects of early emotional or social deprivation are much more pervasive than were once expected. For example, infants hospitalized for a long period frequently become listless, apathetic, and depressed. Even more surprising is that infants under extended hospital care in unstimulating environments often fail to gain weight and may develop respiratory infections and fever. A result can be a condition known as **deprivation dwarfism**, *psychosocial dwarfism*, or *psychosocial short stature*. It is a rare condition, induced by emotional stress, that can lead to long-term short stature (Wattchow, Lee, & Brock, 2014) and can have a permanent impact on the individual.

This condition results in reduced, failed or significantly reduced growth during infancy, childhood, or adolescence. It is associated with emotional deprivation or a severe psychosocial rearing environment where an unsatisfactory relationship exists between the child and the caregiver. Experts believe the environmental effects can lead to endocrine dysfunction that, in turn, impacts growth (Kumaran & Kershaw, 2014). Sirotnak (2008) indicates that the physiology of this malady is complicated, often involving reduced nutrition and a malfunction of the endocrine system that ultimately diminishes growth and development. Endocrine disturbances include disturbances of the growth hormone and thyroid function that directly affect growth, with specific reductions in growth of the long bones of the body. The most common physical implication is reduced height to less than the third percentile for the child's age. In some cases the cranial sutures (bands of tissue that connect the bones of the skull) have been observed to widen, along with unusual symptoms such as sleep disruption and reduced sensitivity to pain. Symptoms of the condition can also include psychological and cognitive disruptions and a fixation on food and water consumption even when adequate amounts of both have been consumed. Delays in speech, cognition, and motor development are common, along with withdrawal, apathy, self-injury, irritability, and a tendency toward temper tantrums (Sirotnak, 2008).

The existence of this condition can be confirmed by removing the child from the environment. Catch-up growth (discussed later) is typically demonstrated, with accompanying improvements in behavior and normalization of hormonal disruptions. Catch-up occurs to varying degrees, depending on the age of the child, the severity of the condition, and the time of removal from the severe situation (Sirotnak, 2008).

As one example, a 2014 case study described a 16-year-old girl, Anna, who presented with psychosocial short stature. In fact, her height growth was in the first percentile and her weight was in the third percentile; other family members were more typically sized (Wattchow, Lee, & Brock, 2014). Anna had experienced some degree of isolation starting at birth, when her mother became physically ill and the baby was taken in by her grandparents. The mother described her relationship with her daughter as "superficial" (p. 63). Anna appeared to be fairly healthy through most of her childhood, until her family moved to another country, where she experienced marginalization and social isolation, even bullying. She was further traumatized when her family home was invaded and Anna witnessed the sexual assault of her older sister. Anna was later sexually assaulted herself, resulting in emotional instability and further withdrawal from family relationships. Her mother and father's relationship was strained, and her mother was regularly absent from the family.

In addition to having a small stature, Anna spoke primitively, was prone to trancelike states, and demonstrated "disturbed behavior" (p. 64). The case study's authors speculated that Anna's short stature resulted from the long-standing mother-daughter detachment and the severe trauma she had experienced in her life. Anna was ultimately placed under medical care with emphasis on strengthening the family bond—just the opposite of removal from the family environment, which ordinarily occurs in these situations. However, according to the authors, the family had become more stable and was fully supportive of working toward their daughter's health and well-being. Her prognosis is uncertain (Wattchow et al., 2014).

Deprivation dwarfism was also well documented in a classic article by Gardner (1972). Gardner described two orphanages directed by individuals of different temperament—one cheerful and loving, the other stern and uncaring. During one 6-month period, the relative weight gains of the children in the two orphanages were noted. The children under the care of the cheerful director (first orphanage) were larger overall relative to their respective ages. Soon after these measurements were taken, the stern director from the other orphanage took the place of her more cheerful counterpart at the first orphanage. Ironically, this change of directors coincided with an increase of food at the first orphanage. Despite this increase in food, the emotional effect of the harsh new matron seemed to influence the children's growth negatively: they showed reduced relative weight gain when compared with the children from the second orphanage. However, this decrease in growth did not occur for all of the children in the first orphanage: eight children from the second orphanage, who were the stern matron's favorites, accompanied her to the first orphanage. These children gained weight equivalently to the children in the first orphanage when it had been directed by the more caring individual. This dramatic situation illustrates the effects of adverse conditions on human growth. Although the exact operative mechanism is unclear, apparently harsh early circumstances during infancy or early childhood can lead to reduced growth.

Gardner described another unusual case of deprivation dwarfism. This situation involved twins, a brother and sister, who showed typical growth during their first 4 months, at which point their mother became pregnant with another child, who was unexpected and unwanted. To complicate this situation, the father lost his job and left home, leaving the mother to care for the twins. The mother became frustrated and began to focus her hostility on her son. By the time he was 13 months old, he was approximately the size of a 7-month-old, whereas his twin sister had attained typical growth. The boy was removed from the hostile environment and medically treated, which enabled him to regain his typical size by the age of 3.5 years (Gardner, 1972).

Case Studies on the Effects of Deprivation

Anna: A Case of Extreme Isolation

Kingsley Davis (1946) described one of the most tragic of all reported cases of early deprivation. The study involved another young girl named Anna. Anna was isolated in an attic-like room of her home with minimal stimulation of any kind for almost 6 years. She was an illegitimate child who resided with her mother and grandfather. Anna was the unwitting victim of a family dispute. Her grandfather opposed having an illegitimate child in his home, while Anna's mother argued in favor of her staying. Unfortunately, under the mother and grandfather's compromise, Anna stayed in the house but lived in the attic from the age of 5.5 months to approximately 6 years. In the attic, Anna received minimal care, barely enough to maintain her existence. When Anna was eventually discovered, she was in terrible condition. She showed minimal signs of intelligence, could not walk or talk, and was extremely malnourished. Davis described her legs as being "skeletonlike" and her abdomen "bloated."

Upon her discovery, Anna was taken to a county home. During her stay at that institution, she showed minimal signs of improvement. She had developed motorically somewhat, as she could eat by herself and was able to walk. Her speech and intellectual abilities were still severely impaired (Davis, 1946).

Approximately two years after being discovered in the attic, Anna was taken to a private home for children with intellectual disabilities. There she continued to progress, although slowly. Her prognosis was described as unfavorable because she still showed no signs of speech other than random guttural sounds. Davis further described Anna as having an extremely poor attention span, periodically making nonpurposeful rhythmical movements, and watching her hands "as if she had seen them for the first time" (Davis, 1946).

When Anna was about 8 years old, she was examined by a clinical psychologist, who found that her vision and hearing were typical and she showed progressing motor ability; she had begun to climb stairs. Her speech was in the babbling stage, and her mental age was determined at approximately 19 months. Her social maturity was judged roughly equivalent to a typical 23-month-old child. The examining psychologist predicted that Anna would eventually achieve the mental ability of a 6- or 7-year-old. However, he also noted that these tests were perhaps of questionable value in Anna's extreme case (Davis, 1946).

By the age of 9 years, Anna had progressed motorically. She could bounce balls and socialize somewhat. She could eat with considerable control, although her eating was confined to the use of a spoon, an eating technique typical of a much younger child. Most surprisingly, Anna had begun to speak in occasional full sentences, but she was still described as possessing the language abilities of a 2-year-old (Davis, 1946).

When she was 10, a final report on Anna revealed that she could string beads and build with blocks, showing evidence of progressing fine motor control. In addition, Anna walked and ran but was said to be rather clumsy. Her speech had evolved into frequent attempts at communication, although she rarely spoke in complete sentences (Davis, 1946).

Anna died at the age of 11. Although the case study describing Anna's condition answered only a few questions concerning the effects of extreme deprivation, it did stimulate many new thoughts and avenues of exploration concerning the effects of deprivation on the human condition. For example, what was the effect of Anna's isolation? How did Anna's actual state differ from what she would have been like in more typical circumstances? What would have happened to Anna had she been discovered earlier or later? Davis (1946) postulated that Anna's relatively early discovery may have enabled her to develop some skills that otherwise would have been impossible. Had Anna been discovered even earlier, however, she might have developed more capable communication and increased her general intellectual abilities. Anna's early death was unfortunate for both humane and scientific reasons. Had she lived longer, we may have obtained partial answers to some of these questions.

Victor: A Case of Living in the Wild

Throughout history, stories have been told of children being raised in the wild. According to certain versions, some of these children were even raised by wild animals, but because they are not documented, most of these stories are now considered myth or folklore. However, one account that has been well documented is the case of Victor, a young boy who was found in the woods of France sometime around 1799. Victor, at what was believed to be 11 to 12 years of age, was found by three "sportsmen." He was immediately taken to a nearby village, where he was left in the care of a widow. He remained there for only a week, as he soon escaped back into the nearby mountains. However, occasionally he would wander near villages, and he was eventually captured and sent to a hospital and then to Paris for study. In Paris, Victor was placed under the care of a young physician named Itard. Dr. Itard believed Victor's condition to be a result of "lack of experience" from his isolation starting as early as 4 to 5 years of age. Itard immediately attempted to provide remedial experiences to help Victor catch up.

According to reports, Victor initially appeared to have intellectual disabilities. He was described as "wild and shy," and he constantly sought opportunities to escape. He was further described as "disgustingly dirty," very inattentive and impatient, indifferent, and possessing very little affection for those around him. In fact, he was often known to bite and scratch. He moved "spasmodically" and frequently swayed back and forth. His eyes were unsteady and expressionless, and he rarely appeared to notice even loud sounds or music. Except for occasional guttural noises, he did not speak. He appeared to have very little memory and was unable to imitate. According to Itard, "His whole life was a completely animal existence" (1972, p. 35). He demonstrated an aversion to common foods and disliked wearing clothes and sleeping in a bed.

Victor's mode of locomotion was particularly interesting; he did not walk but tended to "trot or gallop," making walking with him very difficult. Itard also said Victor would smell anything handed to him and described Victor's chewing as being rodent-like. The rapid action of the "incisors" led Itard to the conclusion that Victor's diet had been predominantly vegetarian. Victor's body was quite scarred. Many scars appeared to be the result of animal bites, while others were apparently the result of scratches acquired from years of living outdoors (Itard, 1972).

To determine Victor's level of intellectual ability, Itard placed food out of Victor's reach. Victor seemed to be intellectually incapable of using nearby chairs or other implements to assist him in reaching the food. Itard also placed bits of food beneath inverted cups to test Victor's memory of the location of the food. Again, Victor showed only a "feeble" capacity intellectually, though he finally began to track the cups with his eyes. Itard also attempted to show Victor how to use toys, but, according to Itard, Victor was impatient and often simply hid or broke the toys. Finally, Itard attempted to teach him to talk, though Victor appeared to achieve little verbally beyond using certain words to express pleasure. Though Victor showed moderate overall improvement over the course of his life, he never completely caught up. Victor died at about age 40 (Itard, 1972).

KEY CONCEPTS IN STIMULATION AND DEPRIVATION THEORIES

As discussed earlier, researchers have studied some classic, fascinating, and at times tragic situations to increase our understanding of the effects of stimulation and deprivation on human development. However, because such cases involved different forms of stimulation or deprivation, few solid conclusions can be drawn. Nevertheless, many theories concerning early stimulation and deprivation have been proposed. Much of the theory to date concerns the concepts of critical periods, readiness, and catch-up (see Table 5.2).

Critical Periods

For years, experts have recognized that human development includes certain critical periods. A **critical period**, often called a sensitive period, is a time when specific conditions or stimuli are required for optimal, or even typical, development to ensue, or a developmental period where specific experience has a greater effect on certain human abilities than at other times (Britto & Perez-Escamilla, 2013). If a child is exposed to the appropriate stimuli during this time of optimal sensitivity, a particular human

Table 5.2 Three important concepts in the study of early stimulation and deprivation

• Critical period: A time of particular or maximum sensitivity to environmental stimuli
• Readiness: The establishment of the minimum characteristics necessary for a particular human behavior to be acquired
• Catch-up: The human power "to stabilize and return" to a predetermined behavior or growth pattern "after being pushed off trajectory" (Tanner, 1978, p. 154)

behavior is likely to emerge or at least be facilitated (Newman & Newman, 2018).

Unfortunately, there are few known specifics concerning critical periods. In fact, the idea of the existence of such periods is extremely theoretical, although considerable evidence suggests their presence. Evidence is scarce, however, as to exactly how long critical periods last and which human behaviors they influence.

Note that critical periods are tied to rather specific times in a person's life. During these times, the appropriate stimuli must be present or the potential for optimal development is lost. This concept does not indicate that total capacity for any kind of development will be squelched if the critical period is left unstimulated. Therefore, even if the appropriate stimulation is not present during the critical period, mastery of a given skill may still be possible, although accomplishment may be less than the person's genetic potential would otherwise have allowed.

The development of smiling in humans, a fine movement, is considered evidence of critical periods. A smile often occurs initially and spontaneously at approximately 5–14 weeks of age. At that time it can be evoked by any number of stimuli from familiar or unfamiliar individuals. For example, the sight of a human face, a touch, or a high-pitched voice frequently evokes a smile during this 9- to 10-week period early in infancy. At about 20 weeks, however, a different smiling pattern begins to emerge, in which only familiar faces elicit the smile. Children seem to lose sensitivity to the events that were once capable of causing their smiles to appear (Newman & Newman, 2018). The heightened sensitivity that existed for several weeks seems to diminish.

Classic animal research has been conducted to help fill the information void concerning critical periods. In one classic study, Nottebohm (1970) examined the motor task of vocalization in birds to determine if and when there was a critical period for the wild chaffinch to learn birdsong. Under typical circumstances, this bird learns vocalization from adult birds and establishes a form of birdsong that is basically stable after the age of 1 year. However, Nottebohm noted that when the bird was deprived of hearing typical birdsong, its song became modified or atypical. In fact, the more limited the bird's exposure to the necessary stimulus of hearing birdsong, the more likely the bird was to modify the vocalization to a more rudimentary form. However, if the bird was deprived of hearing birdsong after one full season of typical behavior, the deprivation seemed to have no further effect in altering the vocalization patterns. Apparently, for the wild chaffinch the first 10 months to 1 year is a critical period for the development of birdsong. If the bird acquires the appropriate ability during that time, the behavior becomes fairly stable; if the behavior is not acquired, it may never optimally develop.

These examples illustrate four of the essential elements of the idea of critical periods:

1. For the environmental stimulation to be effective, the organism must have achieved a state of readiness.
2. There is a specific time limit. Multiple critical periods may exist for a given behavior, but each behavior has a particular period when the stimulation is of optimal value. If the appropriate stimulation does not occur during this critical period, the opportunity for optimal development may be lost forever.
3. The effects of the stimulation during the critical period create a permanent and durable imprint. Therefore, even though an individual may temporarily discontinue a particular behavior, optimal reestablishment may be possible as a result of the presence of appropriate stimuli during the critical period. Similarly, if appropriate stimuli were not present during the critical period, a

permanent negative residue may remain. The individual would then be permanently incapable of optimally developing that behavior.

4. Apparently, critical periods may exist for many aspects of human behavior. Although the idea of critical periods has been popularized in relation to cognitive skills, it also appears to be extremely important in the development of social and motor skills, as well as physical growth.

Many theories have been proposed to explain the phenomenon of critical periods. For example, Levin, Zeanah, Fox, and Nelson (2014) proposed that critical periods are reflected in human behavior, though they are physiologically embedded in the circuitry of the nervous system. At certain points in human development, these circuits are more plastic, or malleable, than at others. Thus, at these points, circuits are more likely to be influenced by life experiences than at other times. Missed opportunities for establishing these neural circuits can have lifelong effects on one or more domains of human development. The actual structure of the neural circuits is fundamentally altered when a person experiences a profound environmental experience. This change in neural structure causes the related behavior to become more stable and preferred. Thus, our understanding of critical periods should focus on, and result from, an understanding of both human neural physiology and the resultant human behavior. Studying both of these will help us understand the important role of experience and environment in shaping human behavior.

Readiness

The term **readiness** is often used in conjunction with the term *critical period*. Recall that the latter term is sometimes defined as a period of optimal preparation or readiness for the development of a new behavior. As this definition implies, an ultimate state of readiness can be considered a critical period. However, readiness more commonly implies that the individual has become prepared, or ready, to acquire a particular behavior. In other words, the person has reached a certain point in an ongoing process that has enabled the establishment of the minimum characteristics necessary for the acquisition of a particular movement skill or other human behavior. Sufficient information and ability have been accumulated and the necessary physical characteristics have been acquired so that the new movement can be performed. Acquisition of the necessary physical characteristics implies that the person has attained a certain level of growth and that requisite neurological patterns have been created so that the new motor skill can be employed effectively. For readiness to be complete, however, the person must also be motivated to perform the behavior, implying both internal and external forms of motivation. That is, the person must want to perform the movement skill while also receiving appropriate encouragement from such external sources as the family.

As an example, Patel and colleagues (2017) discuss what is required to be ready for sport participation in young children. Given that sport activities are an excellent forum for social interaction and learning prosocial behaviors, development of unique cognitive skills, enhancing intellectual processing speed, the expected motor skills (e.g., learning new skills like running, throwing, etc.) and physical benefits (e.g., getting stronger, faster, enhancing coordination), sport involvement can be integral to a child's development. However, how do we know when a child is ready to join in? According to Patel, Soares, and Wells (2017), factors like the attained level of physical growth, relative motor ability for their age, their physical maturity, cognitive ability and pre-existing knowledge of the game are critical. To effectively assure that the child is sufficiently ready to participate, however, requires the parent to be aware, realistic, and somewhat knowledgeable of these characteristics in their own child. If this information is appropriately applied, the child is more likely to have a more positive experience at all levels (Patel et al., 2017).

As another example, remember McGraw's examination of the tricycling abilities of the twins Johnny and Jimmy. Johnny, who had received much stimulation and many experiences early in life, was introduced to tricycling when he was 11 months old. He was incapable of performing the skill at that time and showed no signs of learning it for the next 9 months. However, Jimmy, who had received minimal stimulation as an infant, tricycled almost immediately when presented with a tricycle at 22 months. The hypothesis McGraw proposed was that Johnny, regardless of his early stimulation, was not ready to tricycle at 11 months of age. Jimmy, at 22 months, despite his relatively deprived infancy, had acquired the physiological characteristics necessary to tricycle. Despite the varying levels of stimulation the two twins had experienced, Jimmy was ready to tricycle at 22 months, whereas 11 months was too early for Johnny.

As this example suggests, a strict interpretation of the concept of readiness implies that early experience of or instruction in a particular movement activity prior to the achievement of readiness may not be particularly valuable. Before instruction can be worthwhile, the prerequisite skills must be within the child's repertoire. This being true, current trendy early educational programs may, in many cases, be fruitless.

However, not everyone accepts a strict readiness theory. Some believe that the real burden is on the teacher or caregiver and that the child is always ready to acquire a new behavior, with the key to eliciting the desired behavior being the provision of the appropriate stimuli. Unfortunately, the perfect, or even appropriate, stimuli for the development of most behaviors are unknown and will continue to be for years to come.

The outlook is equally unsettling for those who do subscribe to the theory of readiness, particularly regarding motor development. Currently, we may not know all the signs that indicate readiness, or if we do, we may not be able to recognize when they are present. In fact, we really have no assurance that such signs even exist because the concept of readiness is theoretical. Therefore, we can only estimate the most appropriate time for exposing a child to movement experiences and instruction. Knowledge and recognition of signs that indicate a state of readiness would greatly facilitate our ability to efficiently provide instruction in movement skills.

Catch-Up

Both stimulation and deprivation can have various effects on many aspects of human development. Depending on any number of variables, many of which are unknown, the effects vary from one situation to the next. For example, in cases of severe deprivation, one person may exhibit permanent behavioral damage while another person exhibits only temporary effects. This may be attributable to the phenomenon known as catch-up. **Catch-up** refers to the return to an inherent developmental trajectory after a deviation from that path (Berk, 2018). Sometimes referred to as resilience, catch-up refers to the positive adaptation following and despite serious early developmental adversity. This phenomenon occurs in response to severe deprivation or maltreatment, such as the deprivation dwarfism discussed earlier. Catch-up is evidence that the human being is capable of acquiring new behavior or increasing physical growth much more rapidly than usual during a period of recovery. Figure 5.4 illustrates catch-up growth, though catch-up can occur in any domain of human development. Nevertheless, catch-up is most noticeable in the area of growth where it can be clearly quantified or seen. Catch-up growth was first noted nearly 70 years ago in children who had impaired growth from kidney disease and grew faster than normal during recovery. It is also frequently observed in babies who are born particularly small for their age because of insufficient prenatal nutrition (Singhal, 2017). According to Cicchetti (2016), these "self-righting tendencies may be strong" in humans (p. 203) as certain sectors of the brain attempt to overcome negative influences on other parts.

Interestingly, the result of catch-up growth may not always be positive. In a meta-analysis on its health impact, researchers reviewed nine studies that examined accelerated post-natal growth. These authors indicated that catch-up is common and generally positive during the first two years of life among babies who are born small for date. However, if the catch-up occurs after that time, these children can have longer-term health consequences such as obesity, related metabolic issues, and an increase in certain diseases. They also stipulate that this phenomenon is still in its initial stages of research and much remains to be learned about how and why this seems to occur (Martin, Connelly, Bland, & Reilly, 2016).

In other research examining catch-up growth among Filipino children from 2–12 years of age, just over 60 percent of the 2,000 children involved in the study were "stunted" based on World Health Organization standards (Adair, 1999). Thirty percent of the 2-year-olds who were stunted were no longer considered so at 8.5 years, with the percentage increasing slightly by age 12. Interestingly, low birth weight was found to be a factor that reduced the likelihood of catch-up later in childhood. Factors found to increase the likelihood of catch-up included having a taller mother, being a first child, being longer at birth, having less severe growth impairment early in life, and having fewer siblings. In conclusion, this study found that some degree of catch-up growth is likely for many children during childhood. This finding contrasts with early research suggesting that catch-up growth after age 2 was limited (Adair, 1999).

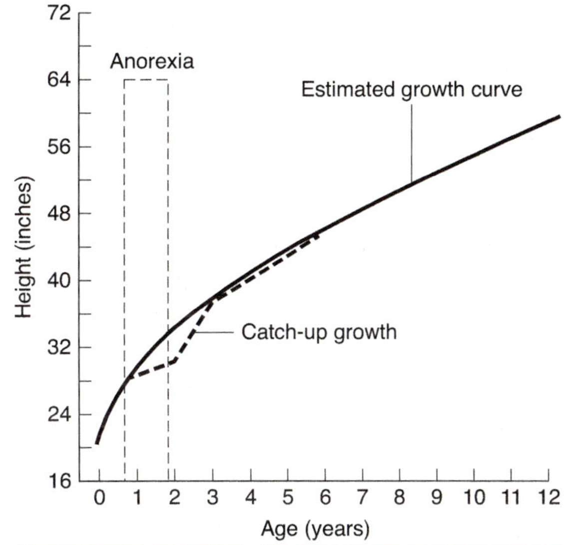

Figure 5.4 A hypothetical example of a child's catch-up growth following a period of anorexia (severe nutritional deprivation)

Source: Adapted and reprinted from Prader et al. (1963). Copyright 1963, with permission from Elsevier.

As evidenced by Adair's study, the term *catch-up* is most frequently used in conjunction with physical growth. The term *catch-up growth* is common in the literature concerning human development. However, catch-up can also occur intellectually, socially, and motorically. When any domain of human development is directly affected by deprivation, motor development is also modified to some degree; as discussed in Chapter 1, all domains of human development are reciprocally related. For all domains, the degree of recovery, or catch-up, appears to depend on the severity, the length, and the timing of deprivation. Despite the remarkable recoveries that some experience, individuals who catch up may never fully realize their genetic potential because of the time they lost during the period of deprivation and recovery.

Anna, the victim of severe isolation, that we discussed earlier, is an excellent example of catch-up and its variability. Recall that after nearly 6 years in isolation in the attic-like room of her home, Anna was incapable of most behaviors expected of the typical 6-year-old. However, with improved care and proper treatment following her discovery, Anna caught up in many ways, particularly physical size. Although she was extremely small and frail when discovered, Anna was actually described as "large for her age" in the years to follow (Davis, 1946). Similar catch-up occurred for certain gross motor skills. Anna could not walk when she was approximately 6 years old, but she was described as being capable at running, ball bouncing, and climbing in the years that followed. No doubt Anna had caught up physically and motorically. Unfortunately, her language and intellectual skills showed much less progress.

One of the most interesting examples of a form of catch-up involves Harlow's classic studies of the rhesus monkey (Suomi & Harlow, 1978). Harlow either totally or partially isolated the monkeys from any kind of social contact for 3, 6, and 12 months. Although the total or partial isolation led to similar behavioral patterns, the longer periods of isolation created much more devastating effects. The 3-month isolates appeared to be in a state of emotional shock when allowed to interact socially. They were fearful of other monkeys and avoided contact with them. This group of monkeys also exhibited the idiosyncrasies of self-clutching, self-biting, rocking, and pulling their own hair. Despite these rather unusual behaviors, the monkeys eventually recovered when allowed to play daily with a group of typical same-age monkeys.

The 6-month isolates yielded a poorer prognosis. They exhibited the same behavioral traits as the 3-month isolates, but this second group showed poorer ability to recover. They avoided their age-mates during playtime, showing social interest only in the other isolates.

As expected, the 12-month isolates exhibited even more behavioral differences. Along with exhibiting the same characteristics as the other isolates, the 12-month group showed greater apathy and were more severely withdrawn. They were extremely passive and defenseless to attacks from their age-mates who had not been isolated.

Follow-up investigations revealed that the monkeys that were isolated 6 months or longer continued to exhibit unusual behavior. Their social behavior during their adolescence and adulthood was considered bizarre, as exemplified by their difficulties in sexual relationships and performance. The severity of the problems among the monkeys isolated for 6 months or longer initially led Harlow to conclude that the first 6 months of social interaction may be a critical period. In other words, if social interaction were prohibited during that time of life, complete or optimal development of social behavior may never be possible (Suomi & Harlow, 1978).

However, in another study, Suomi and Harlow (1972) found that the socially isolated monkeys could be rehabilitated. This was accomplished by exposing their subjects to 26 weeks of "therapy" with 3-month-old monkeys. Because the younger monkeys were less offensive and generally less active than older ones, they tended to approach the isolates more cautiously. After an initial period of acquaintance, the young monkeys would even cling to the isolates. Such affection from the young "therapy monkeys" seemed to normalize the isolates' behavior to the point that they were considered recovered by the end of the 26 weeks. This study provides an example of a simian form of catch-up in the social domain.

SUMMARY

- Programs involving early education for children have become particularly popular in recent years, as part of a trend to provide early and positive forms of stimulation for children. Though nearly all parents would ordinarily seek to avoid depriving their children, some degree of deprivation may, on occasion, be in a child's best interest, while the value of many "stimulating" programs remains unsubstantiated by the little research that exists on early stimulation and deprivation.
- Gymboree has been one of the most popular whole-child programs designed to enhance early motor development, though no research exists to support the provider's claims. Infant and preschool aquatics programs are also extremely popular, though controversial, as they have been linked to water intoxication, giardia infections, hypothermia, and asthma and bronchitis in later childhood. Current interest in and issues associated with infant and preschool aquatic programs have led the American Academy of Pediatrics to create guidelines for these programs. The Suzuki method of teaching the violin is another popular early education program. Research concerning the effectiveness of these early stimulation programs is lacking.
- Myrtle McGraw's research involving the twins Johnny and Jimmy yielded many valuable conclusions concerning the effects of early stimulation. McGraw concluded that level of fixity, readiness, practice, attitude, and physical growth are all particularly important factors that influence human movement at an early age.
- Early deprivation also has a dramatic impact on early development in all domains of human behavior. Deprivation dwarfism is the retardation of physical growth following a period of severe deprivation or adverse treatment despite sufficient levels of nutrition.
- Anna, the victim of severe deprivation during isolation, was seriously impaired as a result of her mistreatment. With improved care and special treatment, she was capable of catching up motorically, although her language and intellectual skills were extremely delayed.
- One of the most interesting cases of deprivation concerned Victor, a boy who was found at an early age after having lived in the wild for years. He could not talk, trotted or galloped rather than walked, chewed "like a rodent," and was delayed intellectually. Despite repeated attempts at remediation, he showed little improvement in his intellectual skills, and he died at the young age of around 40 years.
- A critical period is a time of special sensitivity to environmental stimuli. If a child is appropriately stimulated during this period, the associated behavior is most likely to emerge or be facilitated.
- The term readiness implies that a person, having achieved a certain point in an ongoing process, now possesses the minimum characteristics necessary for acquisition of a certain behavior. Readiness depends on an adequate level of physical growth, the requisite neurological patterns, and sufficient internal and external motivation.
- Catch-up is a human being's ability to return to a predetermined pattern of behavior or growth following a severe period of deprivation or mistreatment. Although typically associated with physical growth, catch-up also appears to occur with motor development, as well as social and intellectual development.

key concept review

catch-up
critical periods
deprivation
deprivation dwarfism
giardia
hyponatremia
hypothermia
level of fixity
readiness
stimulation

questions for reflection

1. Describe the controversy over early-intervention motor development programs. Cite any research you can to provide detail in your explanation.
2. Describe Gymboree programs. Would you involve one of your children in a Gymboree program? Why or why not? What advice would you give to other parents regarding these programs?
3. What is giardia? If you were a parent with a child in an infant aquatics program, what would you do about the risk of giardia infection?
4. If you were in charge of an infant swim program, what would be your goals and what guidelines would you implement? On what basis would you make these decisions?
5. What did McGraw find in her research on Johnny and Jimmy? Give specific findings for the concepts of attitude, practice, readiness, growth, and level of fixity.
6. Over 200 years ago, a young boy named Victor was found in the woods in France. He was believed to be about 12 years old and had grown up in the wild. Describe Victor's state when he was found. Provide specific reference to his verbal skills, his locomotor skills, and his intellectual ability.
7. What is meant by the term *catch-up?* Give at least two examples of this concept from this chapter and one from your real-life experiences. Is it always positive?

online resources

American Academy of Pediatrics, www.aap.org
American Academy of Pediatrics Policy Statements, www.aappublications.org/search/policy/%20toc_section%3AFrom%20the%20American%20Academy%20of%20Pediatrics%20sort%3Apublication-date?see_more_page=1&see_more_page_title=AAP%20Policy&facet%5Bseries-name%5D%5B0%5D=Policy%20Statement
Division for Early Childhood of the Council for Exceptional Children, www.dec-sped.org
Gymboree, www.gymboreeclasses.com
Suzuki Association of the Americas, www.suzukiassociation.org

REFERENCES

Adair, L. S. (1999). Filipino children exhibit catch-up growth from 2 to 12 years. *Journal of Nutrition*, *129*(6), 1140–1148.

American Academy of Pediatrics (2010). Swimming programs for infants and toddlers. *Pediatrics*, *126*, 178–185.

American Academy of Pediatrics (2019). Swimming programs for infants and toddlers. Retrieved from www.aap.org/en-us/about-the-aap/aap-press-room/aap-press-room-media-center/Pages/Swimming-Programs-for-Infants-and-Toddlers.aspx (accessed February 26, 2019).

Berk, L. E. (2018). *Development through the lifespan*. 7th ed. Boston: Pearson.

Bernard, A., Carbonnelle, S., Dumont, X., & Nickmilder, M. (2007). Infant swimming practice, pulmonary epithelium integrity, and the risk of allergic and respiratory diseases later in childhood. *Pediatrics*, *119*, 1095–1103.

Britto, P. R., & Perez-Escamilla, R. (2013). No second chances? Early critical periods in human development. *Social Science & Medicine*, doi.org/10.1016/j.socscimed.2013.09.001.

Chen, M., & Chan, K. L. (2016). Effects of parenting programs on child maltreatment prevention: A meta-analysis. *Trauma, Violence and Abuse*, doi-org.libaccess.sjlibrary.org/10.1177/1524838014566718.

Cicchetti, D. (2016). Socioemotional, perosonality, and biological development: Illustrations from a multilevel developmental psychopathology perspective on child maltreatment. *Annual Review of Psychology*, *67*, 187–211.

Cicchetti, D., & Toth, S. (2015). Child maltreatment. In R. M. Lerner (Ed.), *Handbook of child psychology and developmental science*, 7th ed. New York: John Wiley and Sons, Inc.

Costa, M. J., Barbosa, T. M., Ramos, A., & Marinho, D. A. (2016). Effects of a swimming program on infants' heart rate response. *The Journal of Sports Medicine*, *56*, 1–7.

Davis, K. (1946). A final note on a case of extreme isolation. *American Journal of Sociology*, *52*, 432–437.

Dennis, W. (1940). *The Hopi child*. New York: Appleton-Century.

Doman, G., & Doman, J. (2005). *How to multiply your baby's intelligence*. Garden City Park, NY: Square One.

Doman, G., & Doman, J. (2006). *How to teach your baby to read*. Garden City Park, NY: Square One.

Doman, G., Doman, J., & Aisen, S. (2005). *How to give your baby encyclopedic knowledge*. Garden City Park, NY: Square One.

Doman, G., Doman, D., & Hagy, B. (2006). *How to teach your baby to be physically superb: Birth to age six*. Garden City Park, NY: Square One.

Doman, G., Doman, J., & Hagy, B. (2012). *Fit baby, smart baby, your baby!* Garden City Park, NY: Square One.

Elkind, D. (2007). *The hurried child: Growing up too fast too soon*. Cambridge, MA: De Capo Press.

Elkind, D. (2015). *Giants in the nursery*. St. Paul: Redleaf Press.

Elkins, M. (2010). Get a grip on giardiasis. *Nursing*, *40*, 66.

Gardner, L. I. (1972, July). Deprivation dwarfism. *Scientific American*, *227*(1), 76–82.

Gymboree Play & Music (2017). Discover the Power of Play. Retrieved from www.gymboreeclasses.com (accessed February 26, 2019).

Hsu, W., Wang, C., Chen, S., Lu, Y., Hu, C., et al. (2014). Water intoxication and induced status epilepticus in two children. *Journal of Medical Sciences*, *34*, 77–80.

Itard, J. M. G. (1972). First development of the young savage of Abeyron. In W. Dennis (Ed.), *Historical readings in developmental psychology*. New York: Appleton-Century-Crofts.

Kumaran, A., & Kershaw, M. (2014). Hyperphagic psychosocial short stature: A clinical review. *Paediatrics and Child Health*, *24*(12), 567–571.

Langendorfer, S. J. (2019). Revised scientific review: Minimum age for swimming lessons. *International Journal of Aquatic Research and Education*, doi: 10.25035/ijare.11.03.xx.

Langway, L., Jackson, T., Zabarsky, M., Shirely, D., & Whitmore, J. (1983, March 28). Bringing up superbaby. *Newsweek*, 60–66.

Lee, H., & Galloway, J. C. (2012). Early intensive postural and movement training advances head control in very young infants. *Physical Therapy*, *92*, 935–947.

Levin, A. R., Zeanah, C. H., Fox, N. A., & Nelson, C. A. (2014). Motor outcomes in children exposed to early psychosocial deprivation. *The Journal of Pediatrics*, *164*, 123–129.

Lobo, M. A., & Galloway, J. C. (2012). Enhanced handling and positioning in early infancy advances development throughout the first year. *Child Development*, *83*, 1290–1302.

Martin, A., Connelly, A., Bland, R. M., & Reilly, J. J. (2016). Health impact of catch-up growth in low-birth weight infants: Systematic review, evidence appraisal, and meta-analysis. *Maternal & Child Nutrition*, doi.org/10.1111/mcn.12297.

McGraw, M. (1935). *Growth: A study of Johnny and Jimmy*. New York: Appleton-Century-Crofts. (Reprinted in 1975 by Arno Press.)

Nahar, B., Hamadani, J. D., Ahmed, T., Rahman, A., Huda, S. N., & Grantham-McGregor, S. M. (2009). Effects of psychosocial stimulation on growth and development of severely malnourished children in a nutrition unit in Bangladesh. *European Journal of Clinical Nutrition*, *63*, 725–731.

Newman, B. M., & Newman, P. R. (2018). *Development through life: A psychosocial approach*. 13th ed. Boston: Cengage.

New York Times (2013). Glenn Doman obituary, doi:legacy.com/obituaries/nytimes/obituary.aspx?pid=165110411.

Nottebohm, F. (1970). Ontogeny of bird song. *Science*, *167*, 950–956.

Patel, D. R., Soares, N., & Wells, K. (2017). Neurodevelopmental readiness of children for participation in sports. *Translational Pediatrics*, doi: 10.21037/tp.2017.05.03.

Prader, A., Tanner, J. M., & Von Harnack, G. A. (1963). Catch-up growth following illness or starvation. *Journal of Pediatrics*, *62*, 654–659.

Richards, M. (2017). Influences of Shinichi Suzuki on Japanese music education. Thesis. Liberty University. Retrieved from https://digitalcommons.liberty.edu/honors/655/.

Roeber, B. J., Gunnar, M. R., & Pollak, S. D. (2013). Early deprivation impairs the development of balance and bilateral coordination. *Developmental Psychobiology*, *56*, 1110–1118.

Sigmundsson, H., & Hopkins, B. (2010). Baby swimming: Exploring the effects of early intervention on subsequent motor abilities. *Child: Care, Health, and Development*, *36*, 428–430.

Singhal, A. (2017). Long-term adverse effects of early growth acceleration or catch-up growth. *Annals of Nutrition and Metabolism*, doi.org/10.1159/000464302.

Sirotnak, A. P. (2008). Child abuse and neglect: Psychosocial dwarfism. *Emedicine Journal*. Retrieved from www.medscape.com/article/913843-overview.

Suomi, S. J., & Harlow, H. F. (1972). Social rehabilitation of isolate-reared monkeys. *Developmental Psychology*, *6*, 487–496.

Suomi, S. J., & Harlow, H. F. (1978). Early experience and social development in rhesus monkeys. In M. E. Lamb (Ed.), *Social and personality development*. New York: Holt, Rinehart & Winston.

Suzuki Association of the Americas (2019). About the Suzuki method. Retrieved from https://suzukiassociation.org/about/suzuki-method/shinichi-suzuki/ (accessed February 24, 2019).

Swidey, N. (2007, October 28). Rush, little baby: How the push for infant academies may actually be a waste of time—or worse. *Boston Globe Magazine*. Retrieved from www.boston.com/news/globe/magazine/articles/2007/10/28/rush_little_baby/?page=full.

Tanner, J. M. (1978). *Fetus into man: Physical growth from conception to maturity*. Cambridge, MA: Harvard University Press.

Voisin, C., Sardella, A., & Bernard, A. (2014). Risks of new-onset allergic sensitization and airway inflammation after early age swimming in chlorinated pools. *International Journal of Hygiene and Environmental Health*, *217*, 38–45.

Wattchow, N., Lee, H., & Brock, P. (2014). Psychosocial short stature with psychosis: A case report. *Australasian Psychiatry*, *23*, 63–65.

Zablocki, E. (2001). Come on in, the water's . . . freezing. WebMD, *Fitness & Exercise*. Retrieved from www.webmd.com/fitness-exercise/2001 0412/young-swimmers-hypothermia-risk.

PART III

Physical Changes across the Lifespan

6 GROWTH AND MATURATION

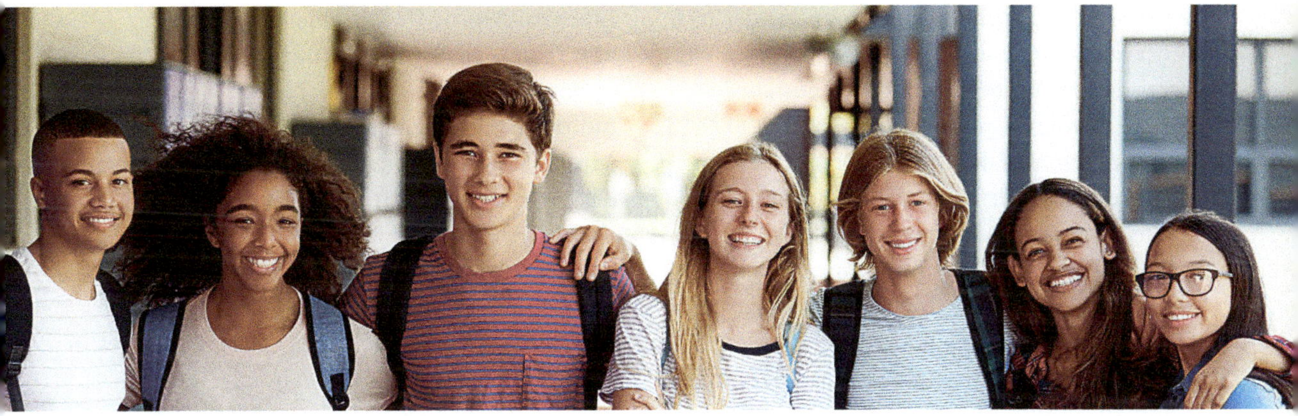

Chapter Objectives

From the information presented in this chapter, you will be able to

- Explain why it is important to study human growth and maturation
- Describe techniques for measuring body length and stature
- Describe anticipated changes in body length and stature across the human lifespan
- Describe techniques for measuring body weight in ambulatory and nonambulatory individuals
- Describe anticipated changes in body weight across the human lifespan
- Calculate body mass index (BMI) and describe changes in BMI across the human lifespan
- Describe gender differences associated with "adolescent awkwardness"
- Describe techniques for measuring changes in body proportions
- Describe anticipated changes in proportional body growth for the ratio of head length to total body length, head circumference, sitting height, shoulder and hip width, and physique classifications
- Describe the relationship between somatic body proportions and motor performance
- Describe instrumentation used to assess skeletal health
- Describe the typical course of skeletal development and the two mechanisms that operate in the development of bone postnatally
- Explain the role of exercise in development of bone and maintenance of skeletal health
- Describe the difference between chronological age and developmental age and explain four methods for determining developmental age
- Explain the relationship between maturation (developmental age) and motor performance

What is the average height of a 5-year-old? How much taller will this child be in one year's time? What is this youngster's expected body weight? What are the expected growth trends regarding height and weight during both middle and late adulthood? Which gender has longer legs, longer arms? What effect does exercise have on the dynamics of human growth? Is there a positive relationship between these physical characteristics and the acquisition and performance of motor skills?

This chapter sheds light on these and other questions and explains how to measure the human body. However, before answering these types of questions, let's first explore why it is important to study and understand the patterns of human growth presented in this chapter.

WHY STUDY HUMAN GROWTH?

As a student of motor development across the human lifespan, you may be wondering why it is important to study human growth and maturation. Let's examine a few reasons. For most individuals, physical growth is a predictable and orderly process. Therefore, understanding these predictable paths will help to determine whether or not a particular individual is growing typically. Throughout this chapter we present a number of growth charts published by the Centers for Disease Control and Prevention (CDC). Scientists, educators, therapists, and other healthcare professionals refer to these growth charts to help answer that question: "Is this individual growing typically?" A departure from the predicted path of growth is often the first sign of an atypical condition. Such atypical conditions can include malnutrition, endocrine system malfunction, heart and other diseases, and physical and psychological abuse, to name just a few. Once alerted to a potential problem, the professional can then search further for potential causes and perhaps institute a corrective intervention.

You might ask, but how can information on the structural development of the human body further our understanding of human lifespan motor development? To see the answer to this question, revisit the section "Models of Lifespan Motor Development" in Chapter 1 and review the information related to dynamical systems theory, Newell's model of motor development, and the Mountain of Motor Development. These models of motor development were designed to help explain changes that occur in our movement behavior across the human lifespan. Furthermore, and perhaps most important, each of these three models subscribes to the notion that changes in movement behavior can be, in part, explained by "constraints." Remember, constraints are factors that limit, contain, or help shape the development of movement. This chapter looks at some of the most important human structural constraints (stature, body weight, physique, and changes in body proportions) known to influence both motor development and motor performance.

LENGTH AND STATURE

Measuring Growth in Length and Stature

From birth to about 2 years, or until the child can stand without assistance, we measure total body length (**recumbent length**) while the child is supine (see Figure 6.1). A special slide ruler is used to measure the distance between the **vertex** (highest point on the skull) and the soles of the feet. The measurement should be recorded to the nearest 1/8 in or 1 mm.

When the child is capable of standing without assistance, the preferred measurement of total body length is standing height (**stature**), the distance between the vertex and the floor (see Figure 6.2). The child should be barefoot when the measurement is taken, and this measure should be recorded to the nearest

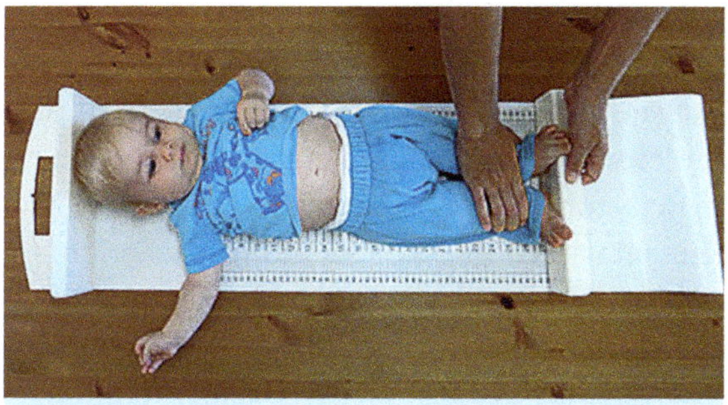

Figure 6.1 Measuring recumbent length
Source: Courtesy of TopEnd Sports and Robert Wood.

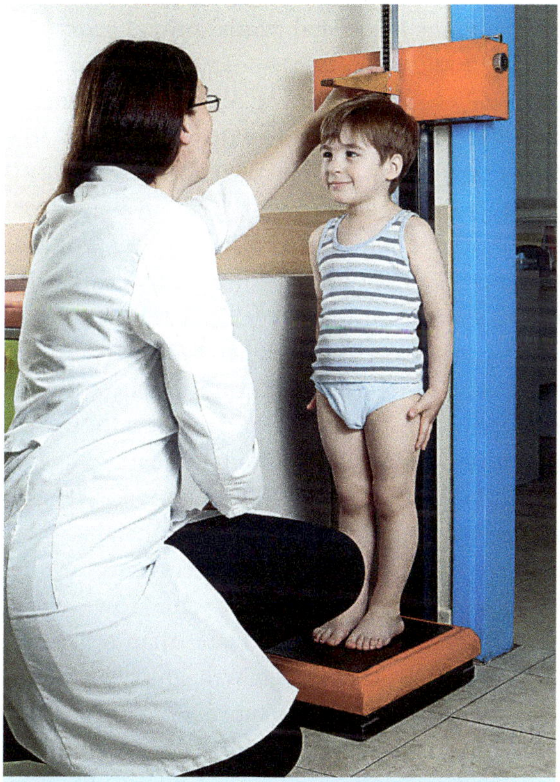

Figure 6.2 Measuring stature with the use of a triangular headboard

1/8 in or 1 mm. Note that a triangular headboard, which forms a right angle between the vertex and the measurement scale, is used to increase accuracy.

Standard techniques for determining stature will not be accurate if the individual is not capable of standing erect or has severe spinal curvature. This is frequently the case for older adults or individuals with disabilities. However, stature can be estimated from the recumbent measure known as **knee height**. Figure 6.3 illustrates the technique for measuring knee height. Note that the individual bends the left knee to a 90-degree angle. The blades of the sliding caliper are then placed under the heel and over the anterior portion of the thigh. Pressure is then applied to compress the soft tissue (skin, fat, and muscle) before a reading is taken. To ensure reliability and accuracy, two consecutive measurements should be taken, and the two measurements should agree within 0.5 cm. Once we have obtained the knee-height value, we can use one of the following gender-specific equations to estimate stature:

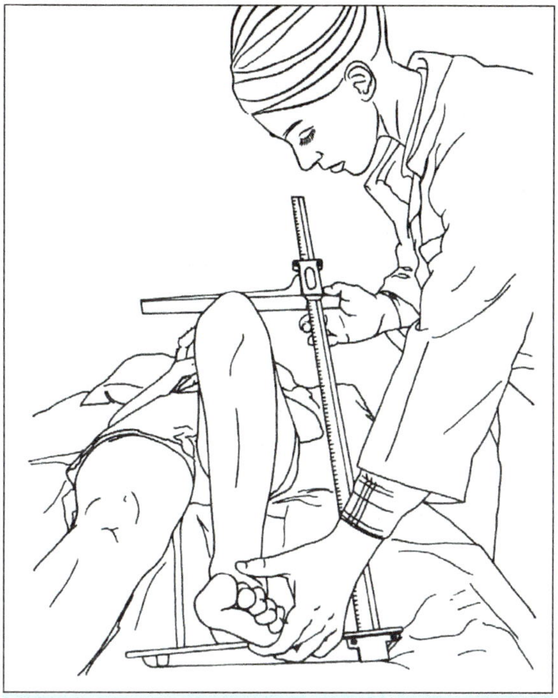

Figure 6.3 Measuring knee height

Stature (men) = 64.19 – (0.04 × age) + (2.02 × knee height)

Stature (women) = 84.88 – (0.24 × age) + (1.83 × knee height)

To solve the equation, round the age to the nearest whole year and record the knee height in centimeters. To convert inches to centimeters, simply multiply inches by 2.54. Conversely, if you desire to estimate stature in inches, simply divide the number derived from the equation by 2.54. For example, if the knee height of a 75-year-old man is 50.5 cm, then we would calculate his stature as follows:

$$64.19 - (0.04 \times 75) + (2.02 \times 50.5)$$
$$= (64.19 - 3) + 102.01$$
$$= 61.19 + 102.01$$
$$= 163.2 \text{ cm}$$
$$163.2 \text{ cm} / 2.54 = 64.25 \text{ in}$$

Milestones in the Growth of Length and Stature

Human prenatal life begins when a male sperm merges with a female egg, forming a zygote, which measures only 0.006 in (0.14 mm) in diameter. During the next 38–40 weeks of intrauterine life, the fetus grows almost 5,000 times longer. In fact, at no time during the human life cycle is growth in body length greater than that which occurs during the fourth prenatal month. However, growth rapidly decelerates during the remaining prenatal period. Mean body length increases approximately 90 percent between the 10th and 14th weeks of gestation but only slightly more than 10 percent during the last 4 weeks of gestation.

Following 280 days of gestation, there is little gender difference in median birth lengths. Boys generally measure about 20 in (50.8 cm) long; girls generally measure about 19.75 in (50.2 cm) long. By the end of the first year of infancy, boys will be approximately 30 in (76.2 cm) long, girls approximately 29.25 in (74.3 cm) long. Thus, during the first year of postnatal life, body length can be expected to increase approximately 50 percent.

During the second year, gains in body length average 4.75 in (12 cm). After age 2, stature increases at a slower rate, until the onset of the adolescent growth spurt. This deceleration in growth continues during most of the elementary school years, with one exception: some children experience a **mid-growth spurt** in height between 6.5 and 8.5 years. This mid-growth spurt occurs more frequently in girls than in boys (Malina, Bouchard, & Bar-Or, 2004). This unexplained deviation in growth rate is less dramatic than the adolescent spurt, and little is known about it.

The many hormonal changes that occur during adolescence cause boys and girls to grow taller rapidly. In fact, about 20 percent of the adult stature is attained during this 2.5- to 3-year growth spurt. The onset of this growth spurt usually occurs in girls at about 9 years of age and in young boys at about 11 years of age (Roche & Sun, 2003). For boys, the mean age of obtaining peak height velocity (PHV: period during the growth spurt when height is increasing at its maximum rate) has been found to occur at about 13.7 (standard deviation, SD 1.4) years and for girls about 12 years of age (SD 1.4; Roche & Sun, 2003; Granados, Gebremariam, & Lee, 2015). Peak height velocity for girls is 9.8 centimeters per year and for boys 11.3 centimeters per year. However, some children will mature faster than others; the time of onset of the growth spurt can vary by as much as 3 years or more. Because girls generally enter adolescence before boys, it is not at all uncommon for young girls to be slightly taller than young boys (average is 1 in taller) between 10 and 13 years of age (Roche & Sun, 2003). During this adolescent phase of development, boys' height increases about 4 in (11.3 cm)/year. The female spurt is somewhat slower: girls grow about 3 in (9.8 cm)/year. Most of the height gained during the adolescent spurt results from a lengthening of the trunk, not a lengthening of the legs. Peak leg-length growth usually occurs 6–9 months earlier. "Thus a boy stops growing out of his trousers (at least in length) a year before he stops growing out of his jackets" (Tanner, 1990, p. 67).

By the time the young woman is about 18 years old and the young man about 21 years, most of their adult height has been attained. After age 30, stature remains relatively stable for about the next 10 years. After about 40 years of age, there is an apparent decrease in height. This decrease in height is caused by age-related changes in the body's bones, muscles, and joints. Most influential is intervertebral disk degeneration and decreased thickness of joint cartilage in the lower extremities. The rate of loss is about one-half inch per decade after the age of 40 and this rate accelerates even more after 70 years of age. Additionally, continued vertebral column degeneration will sometime lead to spinal curvature. Thus, over the lifespan, one could lose between 1–3 inches in height (National Institutes of Health, 2018).

Table 6.1 highlights important milestones in growth for various ages. Appendix B presents mean stature across the human lifespan.

Table 6.1 Important milestones in body length and stature

Age	Selected growth information
Conception	0.006 in (0.14 mm) in diameter
Birth (median length)	Boys: 20 in (50.8 cm) Girls: 19.75 in (50.2 cm)
6 months (median length)	Boys: 26.75 in (67.8 cm) Girls: 26 in (65.9 cm)
Year 1 (median length)	Boys: 30 in (76.2 cm) Girls: 29.25 in (74.3 cm) Length increases approximately 50% during the first year.
Year 2	Length increases about 4.75 in (12.1 cm).
Years 3–5	Growth rate decelerates to about 2.75 in (7.0 cm)/year.
Year 6-adolescence	Growth rate decelerates to about 2.25 in (5.7 cm)/year.
Adolescence	20 percent of adult stature is attained during this 2.5- to 3-year period. Growth spurt onset: Boys, 11 years; Girls, 9 years (mean age) PHV onset: Boys, 13.7 years; Girls, 12 years Approximately 4 in (11.3 cm)/year growth for boys and 3 in (9.8 cm)/year for girls
18 years	Women: growth in stature ceases (mean age).
21 years	Men: growth in stature ceases (mean age). Average adult stature of 69.4 in (176.3 cm) is roughly 3.5 times that of the newborn.
20–30 years	Growth of vertebral column may add another 1/8 in (0.45 cm) to stature.
30–40 years	Stature is relatively stable.
Above 40 years	Stature may decrease about ½ in. per decade.

Illustrating Growth in Stature

Growth in stature can be graphically illustrated. Figure 6.4 is a typical individual's **distance curve** for stature. The distance curve plots accumulative growth obtained over time. In contrast, Figure 6.5 illustrates percentile velocity curves for both boys and girls on the variable stature. The **velocity curve** plots increments of change per unit of time, making the curve useful for identifying periods of fast and slow growth. (See the box entitled "Constructing a Velocity Curve," p. 166.) A close examination of the velocity curves will reveal the possibility of obtaining negative values. It is incorrect to interpret these negative values as representing decreases in stature. Instead, negative values result from measurement error. For a more detailed

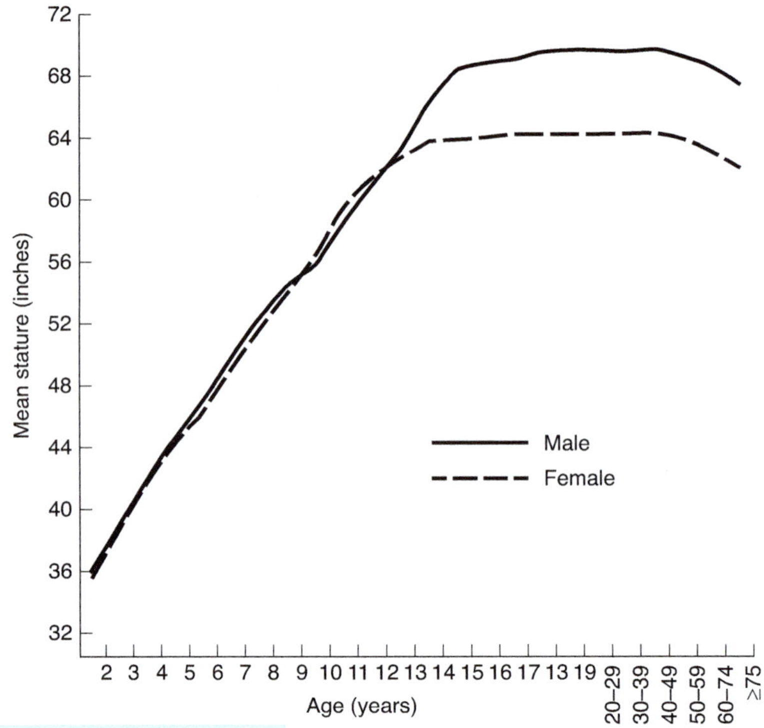

Figure 6.4 Typical distance curve for stature
Source: Based on NCHS data (2004).

discussion of this phenomenon, see Roche and Himes (1980).

Determining Typical Growth

To determine if an individual is growing typically, we compare individual data to norm-referenced data. The National Center for Health Statistics (NCHS) has prepared percentile charts for this purpose. Figure 6.6 gives NCHS percentile charts for stature for both boys and girls between 2 and 20 years of age (Kuczmarski, Ogden, Grummer-Strawn, et al., 2000; Kuczmarski, Ogden, Guo, et al., 2002; see Figure 6.5 for NCHS velocity curves). Visual comparison of charted data to the percentile rankings can quickly alert a care provider to growth abnormalities. Growth retardation may indicate disease, malnutrition (Roche & Sun, 2003), child abuse (Wales & Taitz, 1992), or delayed maturation, among other conditions. If growth retardation is suspected, the youngster should be referred to a physician for further screening. Appendix A presents a complete set of growth charts released as part of the National Health and Nutrition Examination Surveys (NHANES) III national data set. As stated earlier, the NCHS growth charts have been prepared for children between 2 and 20 years of age. When comparisons are needed for children under 2 years of age, the CDC now endorses the use of the World Health Organization growth charts for this younger age group, available at www.who.int/childgrowth/standards/en/.

Predicting Adult Stature

Aside from parental curiosity, there are several important reasons for predicting adult stature. These include the medical management of erratic growth due to disease. For example,

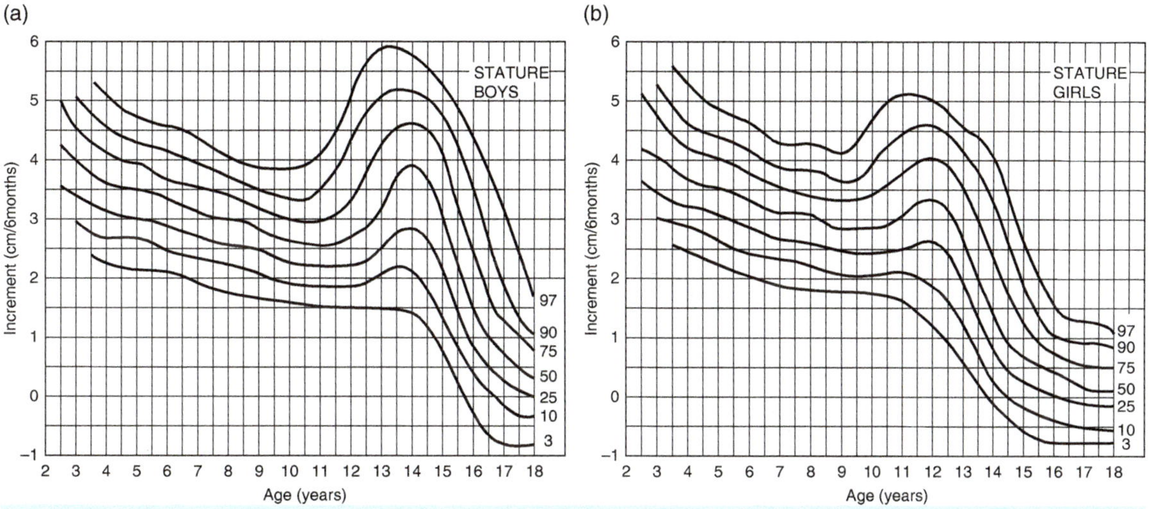

Figure 6.5 National Center for Health Statistics growth velocity charts for boys (a) and girls (b) on the variable stature.
Source: Used with permission of Ross Products Division, Abbott Laboratories Inc., Columbus.

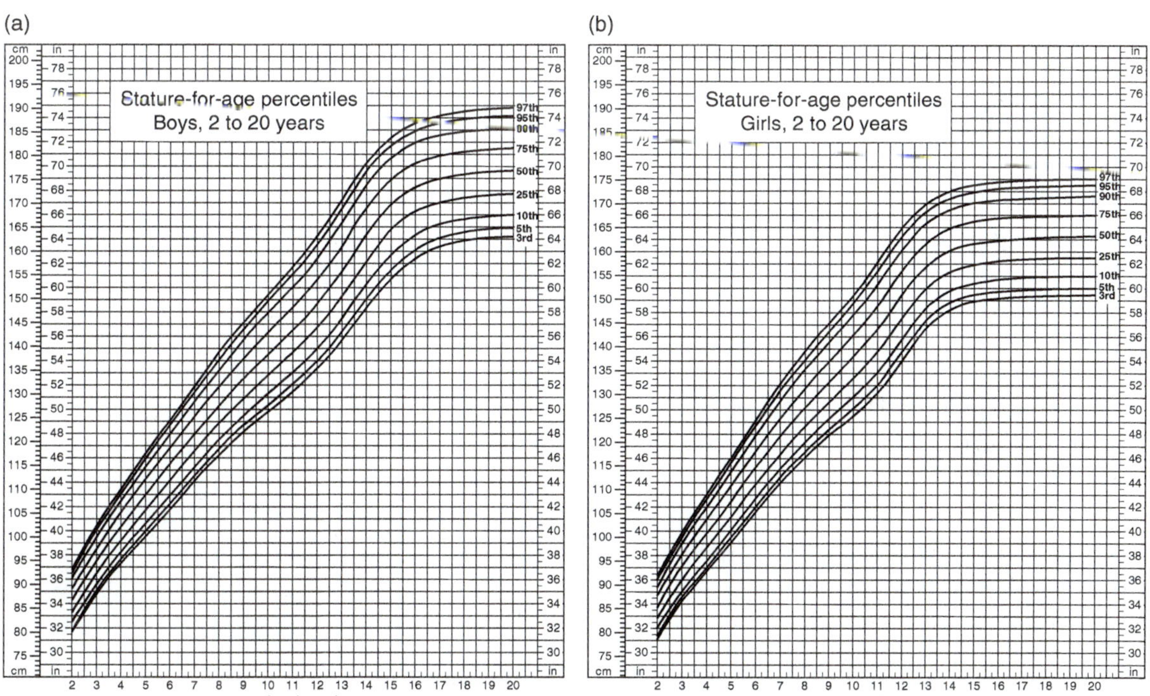

Figure 6.6 Growth charts (U.S.): Stature-for-age percentiles, boys (a) and girls (b), 2 to 20 years.
Source: Developed by the National Center for Health Statistics (2000) in collaboration with the National Center for Chronic Disease Prevention and Health Promotion. Kuczmarski et al. (2000; 2002).

CONSTRUCTING A VELOCITY CURVE

The velocity curve plots increments of change per unit of time—that is, how much growth occurred since the last identified assessment—and illustrates periods of fast and slow growth. For example, using the data in Appendix B, if 6-year-old children are on average 46.9 in (119.1 cm) tall and 7-year-old children are on average 49.1 in (124.7 cm) tall, these children have grown, on average, 2.2 in (5.6 cm) over the course of the year. To construct the velocity curve, we continue to calculate increments of change for each age unit of interest (7 to 8 years, 8 to 9 years, 9 to 10 years, and so forth), then plot the units of change on a graph where the *x* and *y* axes are labeled as in Figure 6.5. For each time increment (year, in this case), we plot the midpoint (6.5 years, 7.5 years, and so on). Once the data points are plotted, we connect them by drawing a line. The result is a velocity curve.

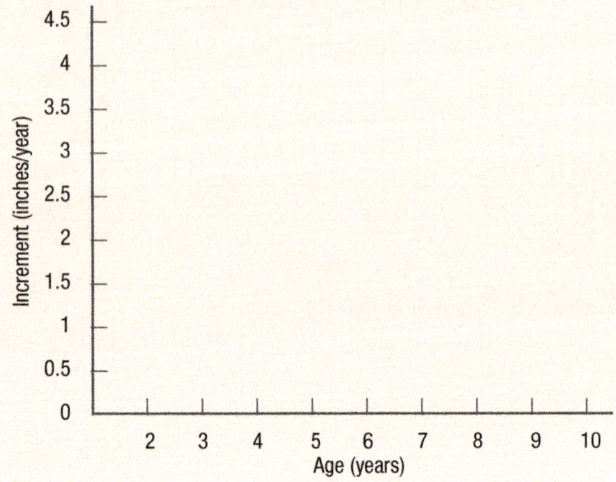

endocrinologists who treat patients diagnosed with idiopathic short stature frequently depend on algorithms to predict adult stature prior to administrating human growth hormones (Topor, Feldman, Bauchner, et al., 2010). Additionally, although this is not an issue in the United States, some sporting agencies in foreign countries attempt to predict adult stature when channeling youth into government-run sport training institutes.

A number of techniques for predicting adult stature have been proposed, but most are extremely variable (Topor, Feldman, Bauchner, et al., 2010). Take, for example, the following:

Adult Stature = 2 × (child's height in inches at 2 years of age)

This is perhaps the simplest and most widely employed formula used by curious parents, but it is the least reliable. Researchers from the Fels Longitudinal Study have determined that the best predictors of adult stature are the child's current stature, the child's current weight, midparent stature (the average stature of the two parents), and skeletal age (Roche, Wainer, & Thissen, 1975). Unfortunately, this technique is not practical because an X-ray is required to determine skeletal age. This shortcoming was alleviated with the development of the Khamis-Roche method (Khamis & Roche, 1994). This technique for predicting adult stature omits the skeletal age requirement, depending only on the child's gender, height, and weight and midparent stature. This technique has been validated for White Americans between 4 and 17 years of age. The Khamis-Roche estimated adult height calculator is available at www. webmd.com/children/healthtool-kids-height-predictor.

BODY WEIGHT

Measuring Body Weight

The instrument of choice for obtaining body weight is an electronic digital scale. The child stands in the middle of the scale with shoes and as much clothing as possible removed. If the child is fully clothed, an adjustment of approximately 1 lb (0.45 kg) is made. A platform scale should be used to measure the body weight of infants who are not capable of standing without assistance (see Figure 6.7). If the infant is crying or moving excessively, an accurate measure may be difficult to obtain. In such a case, another technique would be to weigh the parent on an adult electronic scale, weigh the parent again while she or he holds the infant, and then subtract the parent's weight from the parent-child weight to obtain the child's weight. Most infants will be more relaxed when held by a parent in the upright position, resulting in a more accurate measurement. In addition, other types of scales are available for individuals who are bedridden or adults who cannot stand without assistance (see Figure 6.8).

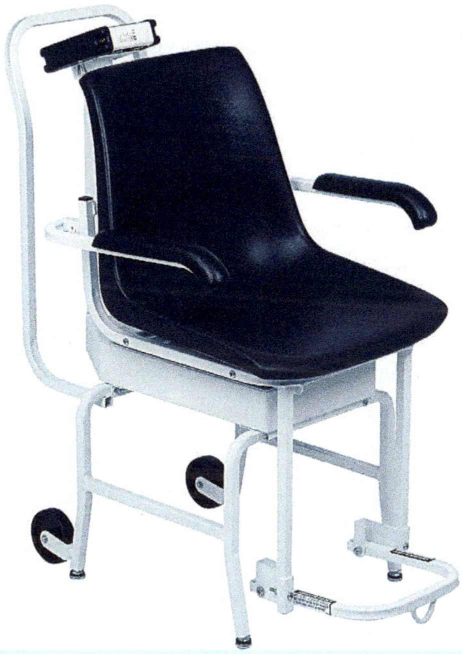

Figure 6.8 Chair scale

Source: Courtesy of Medgeneral Medical Supplies.

Milestones in Body Weight

At conception, the ovum weighs approximately 0.005 mg; it would take more than 5 million of these cells to equal just 1 oz (28.3 g). By the midpoint of the prenatal period (19 weeks), the mean body weight of a typically developing fetus is about 8.5 oz (241 g). At the end of the 38th week of gestation, the fetus is nearly 13 times heavier (6.8 lb / 3.1 kg) than it was at 19 weeks.

Median birth weights of girls and boys are 7 lb (3.23 kg) and 7.5 lb (3.27 kg), respectively. Only rarely does a newborn weigh more than 11 lb (5 kg). Weight at birth, however, tends to be more variable than length at birth. Apparently length, more than weight, is influenced by genetic makeup. Many extraneous factors have been shown to influence birth weight. For instance, lighter mothers tend to have lighter babies, irrespective of the father's weight; later-born children tend to be heavier than firstborns; mothers from low socioeconomic groups tend to give birth to babies who are lighter than babies born to mothers from higher socioeconomic groups; and twins are typically roughly 1.5 lb (0.7 kg) lighter than singletons. Thus, birth weight reflects intrauterine life to a greater degree than does birth length (Roche & Sun, 2003).

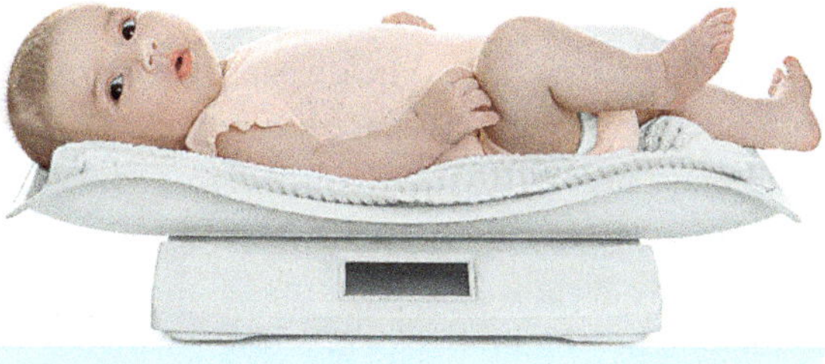

Figure 6.7 Platform scale

During the first week of postnatal life, the infant may lose as much as 5–10 percent of its body weight. This weight loss is attributed to a loss of body water, not fat mass (Toro-Ramos, Paley, Pi-Sunyer, & Gallagher, 2015). During the remaining first 6 months of postnatal life, the infant gains about 2/3 oz (20 g)/day. At this rate of gain, the infant will double its birth weight at 6 months. This rate of weight gain slows toward the middle and latter part of the first year. At the end of the first year, boys, on average, weigh about 25 lb (11.33 kg) and girls about 24 lb (10.93 kg) (Fryar, Gu, Ogden, et al., 2016). Thus, birth weight can be expected to triple during the first year.

Rate of weight gain continues to decelerate during the second year of life. The average child can be expected to gain about 5.5 lb (2.5 kg) during this year. This rate of gain remains steady for the next three preschool years, with the typically developing child averaging about 4.5 lb (2 kg) in weight gain per year. For the next four to six years or until the onset of adolescence, annual weight gain increases slightly to 6.5 lb (3 kg)/year. However, there is a great deal of variability in these rates.

Adolescence can bring about sharp increases in body weight. In fact, during the first three years of this period, boys add about 45 lb (20 kg) to their body weight, on average, and girls add about 35 lb (16 kg). Much of this added body weight is attributable to height increases and changes in body composition. (See Chapter 7 for a discussion of the growth of adipose and muscle tissue.) Age of **peak weight velocity** (**PWV**; maximum rate of growth in body weight) generally occurs after **peak height velocity** (**PHV**; Malina, 2014). Mature body weight is approximately 24–26 times that of birth weight and appears to be trending upward. This is verified from data collected in the most recent National Health and Nutrition Examination Survey (NHANES) that reports a significant linear increase in the body weight of both men and women between 1999 and 2016 (Fryar, Kruszon-Moran, Gu, et al., 2018).

After maturity, adults have some control over whether they add, lose, or maintain their body weight. One exception is adult weight gain following pregnancy: some of the weight gained during pregnancy appears to be permanent, and the amount may increase with each successive child (Gunderson, 2009). However, research has found that women who gain more weight than recommended during pregnancy are at greater risk of being obese one decade later, compared to their counterparts (Rooney & Schauberger, 2002). After a person reaches adult weight, it is difficult to interpret changes in body weight because so much depends on the person's nutritional and exercise status. For instance, muscle and system atrophy can cause weight loss, but some sedentary but well-fed older adults may actually gain weight. Nonetheless, the body composition of older people (fat weight versus muscle weight) is markedly different from that of young adults. Table 6.2 highlights important milestones in weight changes from conception up to adulthood.

Additionally, reference data for mean body weight across the human lifespan are presented in Appendix B.

Illustrating Changes in Body Weight

As with stature, changes in body weight can be graphically illustrated. Figure 6.9 is a typical distance curve showing differences in body weight between male and female humans. In contrast, Figure 6.10 illustrates percentile velocity curves for both boys and girls on the variable weight. Figure 6.11 presents the NCHS percentile charts for the variable body weight.

COMBINING BODY WEIGHT AND HEIGHT: BODY MASS INDEX

Measures of weight and height are frequently combined to yield a measure known as the **body mass index** (**BMI**), a concept introduced in Chapter 4. To calculate the BMI, simply divide body weight in kilograms by the square of the height in meters (see the box entitled "Calculating body mass index", p. 172). This

Table 6.2 Important growth changes in body weight

Age	Selected growth information
Conception	Ovum weighs roughly 0.005 mg
19th week of gestation	8.5 oz (241 g)
38th week of gestation	Fetus is 20 times heavier than at 19 weeks (6.8 lb/3.1 kg)
Birth	Mean weight of boys: 7.5 lb (3.27 kg) Mean weight of girls: 7 lb (3.23 kg) Small mothers tend to have small babies. Later-borns are heavier than firstborns (average difference of 6.8 oz). Twins are approximately 1.5 lb (0.7 kg) lighter on average than singletons.
1–3 days	Weight loss is upwards of 10 percent of birth weight.
10 days	Weight is equal to birth weight or slightly heavier.
First 6 months	Gains about 0.66 oz (20 g)/day Birth weight generally doubles at 6 months.
Second 6 months	Gains decelerate to about 0.5 oz (15 g)/day.
Year 1	Mean weight of boys: 25 lb (11.33 kg) Mean weight of girls: 24.1lb (10.93 kg) Birth weight triples during first year.
Year 2	Boys gain about 5.9lb (2.68 kg) Girls gain about 4.4 lb (2 kg)
Years 3–5	Gains about 4.5 lb (2 kg)/year
Year 6-adolescence	Slight increase in rate of weight gain to 6.5 lb (3 kg)/year
Adolescence	Boys add about 45 lb (20.4 kg) of body weight and girls about 35 lb (15.9 kg) of body weight during the first 3 years of adolescence.
Year 20 & over	Mean weight of men: 197.8lb (89.7 kg) Mean weight of women: 170.5 lb (77.3 kg) Mature body weight is approximately 24 to 26 times birth weight. In adulthood weight becomes more a matter of nutritional and exercise status. Some weight gains during pregnancy appear permanent.

simple measure is valuable because when it exceeds 30 kg/m, it is associated with the prediction of future health risks, including increased incidence of cardiovascular disease, diabetes, hypertension, hypercholesterolemia, and certain cancers (ACSM, 2018). The only exception is found among congestive heart failure patients whose survival tends to improve when BMI > 30 kg/m. This has become known as the **obesity paradox** (Antonopoulos & Tousoulis, 2017). However, BMI cannot be used to determine percentage of body fat. This is because body fatness and BMI are not directly related. Both are influenced by both age and gender. For example, for any given BMI value, women will possess more

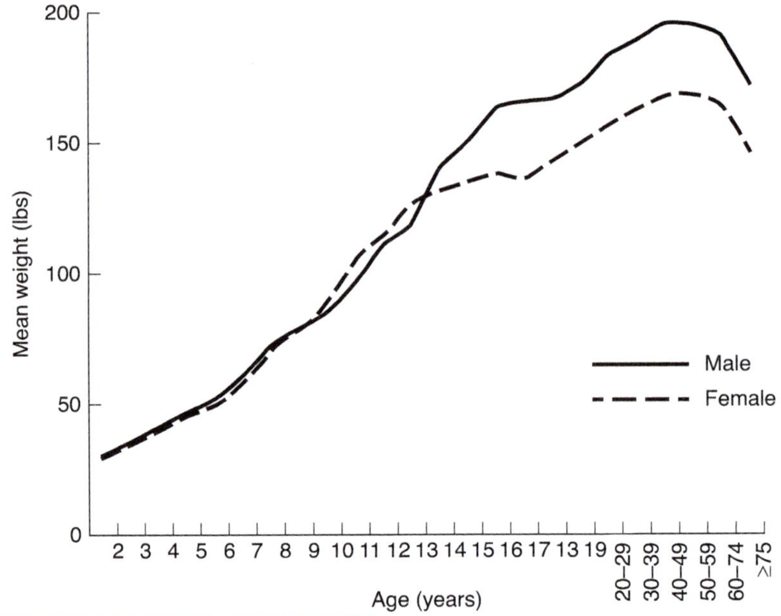

Figure 6.9 Typical distance curve for body weight.

Source: Based on NCHS data (2004).

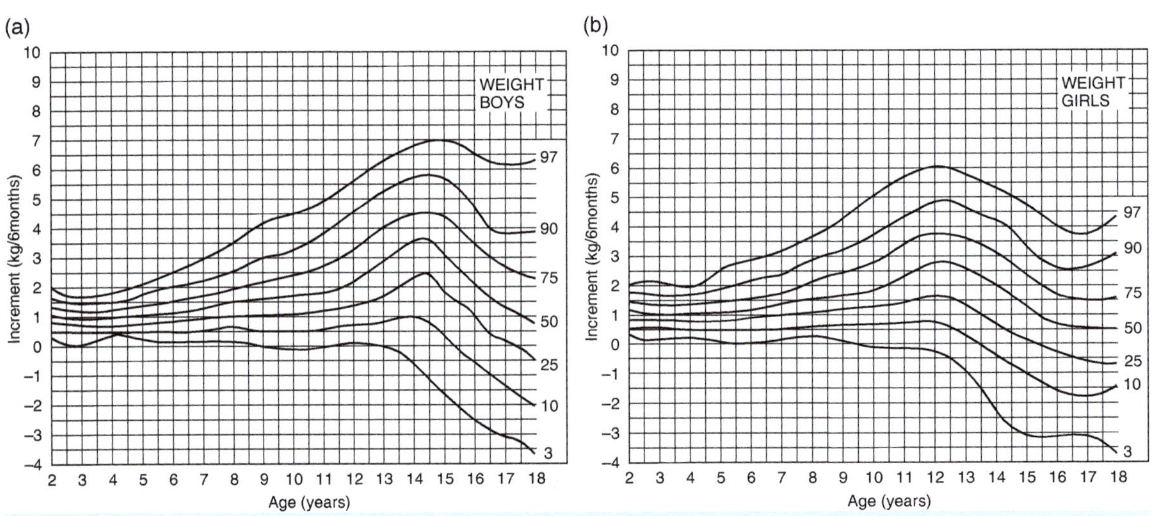

Figure 6.10 National Center for Health Statistics growth velocity charts for boys (a) and girls (b) on the variable of body weight.

Source: Used with permission of Ross Products Division, Abbott Laboratories Inc., Columbus, OH 43215. From data used in the 1981 charts from the Ross Growth and Development Program: Incremental Growth Charts—Girls and Incremental Growth—Boys, © 1981 Ross Products Division, Abbott Laboratories Inc.

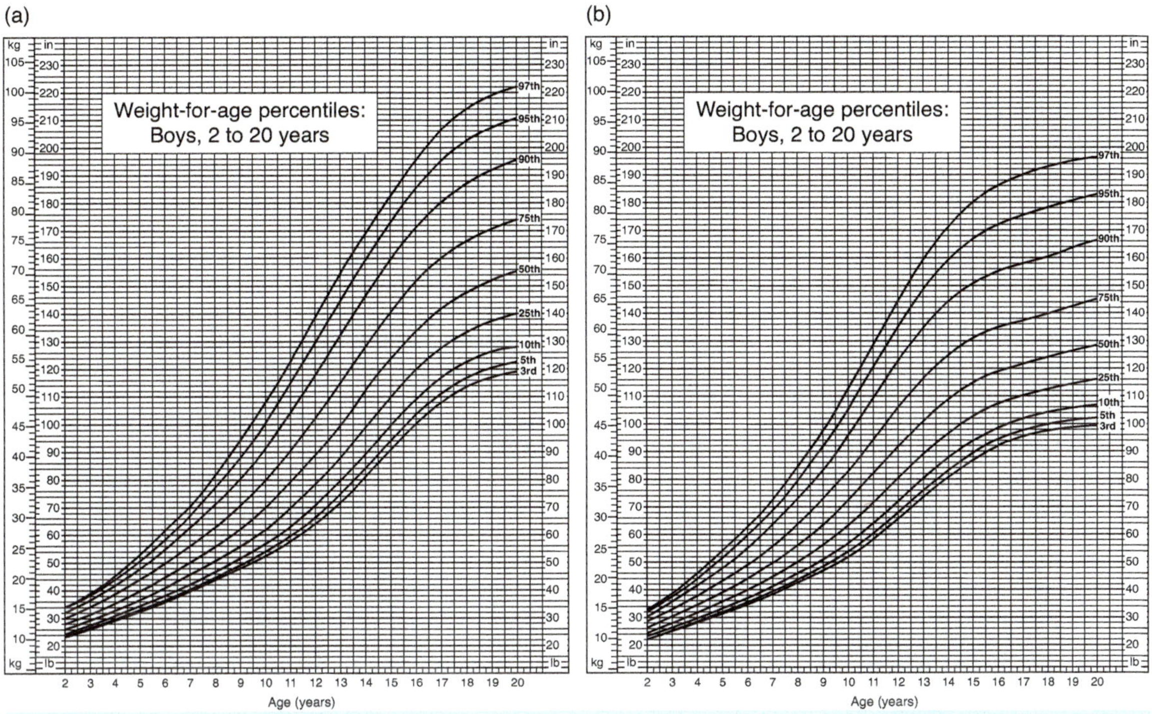

Figure 6.11 Growth charts (U.S.): Weight-for-age percentiles, boys (a) and girls (b), 2 to 20 years.

Sources: Developed by the National Center for Health Statistics (2000) in collaboration with the National Center for Chronic Disease Prevention and Health Promotion. Kuczmarski et al. (2000, 2002).

body fat than men, and an older individual will have more body fat than a younger individual. Thus, although BMI values serve as a means to monitor a population's risk of health and/or nutritional disorders, an individual's BMI alone is not diagnostic (Malina, 2012).

As illustrated in Figure 6.12, which presents BMI percentiles for boys and girls, BMI decreases during the preschool years and reaches a minimum around 5 or 6 years of age. Thereafter, BMI increases throughout most of adulthood, reaching a maximum velocity at about 13 years in girls and about 14 years in boys (Guo, Huang, Maynard, et al., 2000). During this period of rapid growth, increases in BMI are mainly the result of increases in total body fat in girls and in fat-free mass in boys (Maynard, Wisemandle, Roche, et al., 2001). However, BMI values may regress in older adulthood (see Appendix B).

The upward trend that occurs after the low point on the BMI percentile curve is commonly referred to as the **adiposity rebound.** Researchers have discovered that the younger the child is when the adiposity rebound is encountered, the greater is the likelihood that the child will have an increased relative weight gain and BMI as an adult (Edward, Marshall, Saldana, et al., 2017).

In children and adolescents, BMI-for-age is best used as a guide to determine individual nutritional status (underweight, overweight). According to the CDC (2018) and the work of Kuczmarski and colleagues (2000), concerns regarding underweight begin when BMI-for-age is found to be at a percentile rank of less than 5. When the BMI-for-age is greater than the 95th percentile, obesity is of concern. Those children exhibiting a BMI-for-age percentile greater than 85 but less than 95 are considered

CALCULATING BODY MASS INDEX (BMI)

Case: Mary is a 46-year-old woman who weighs 132 lb and is 65 in tall. Calculate Mary's BMI.

1. Convert pounds to kilograms by dividing pounds by 2.2:

$$\frac{132 \text{ lb}}{2.2} = 60 \text{ kg}$$

2. Convert height in inches to height in meters by multiplying inches by 0.0254:

$$65 \text{ in} \times 0.0254 = 1.65 \text{ m}$$

3. Solve the BMI equation by algebraic substitution:

$$\text{BMI} = \frac{\text{weight}}{(\text{height})^2}$$

$$\text{BMI} = \frac{60}{1.65^2}$$

$$\text{BMI} = \frac{60}{2.72}$$

$$\text{BMI} = 22.1 \text{ kg/m}^2 \text{ (rounded to nearest tenth)}$$

Mary's BMI of 22.1 kg/m^2 is within the recommended healthy range (19.5–24.9 kg/m^2).

overweight. In adults, we interpret BMI values by referring to fixed ranges that do not depend on age or gender. The CDC (2017) guidelines for adults are as follows:

- underweight: BMI less than 18.5
- normal weight: BMI 18.5–24.9
- overweight: BMI 25.0–29.9
- obesity: BMI 30.0
- extreme obesity: BMI 40 or more.

Additionally, obesity is frequently subdivided into the following classes:

- Class 1: BMI of 30–34.9
- Class 2: BMI of 35–39.9
- Class 3: BMI of 40 or higher.

Comparisons of national estimates of BMI from the National Health Examination and the NHANES indicate that both American children and adults are getting fatter (Fryar, Gu, Ogden, et al., 2016; Fryar, Kruszon-Moran, Gu, et al., 2018).

CONSTRAINTS ON MOTOR DEVELOPMENT RELATED TO STATURE AND WEIGHT

In the 1930s, Shirley's classic study of 25 babies sparked interest in the relationship between length and weight at birth and the attainment of independent walking. In her study, Shirley concluded, "In general it may be stated that thin, muscular babies and small-boned babies walk earlier than short rotund babies and exceedingly heavy babies" (1931, p. 126).

Growth in overall stature is the sum of growth of the head, neck, trunk, and legs. Since

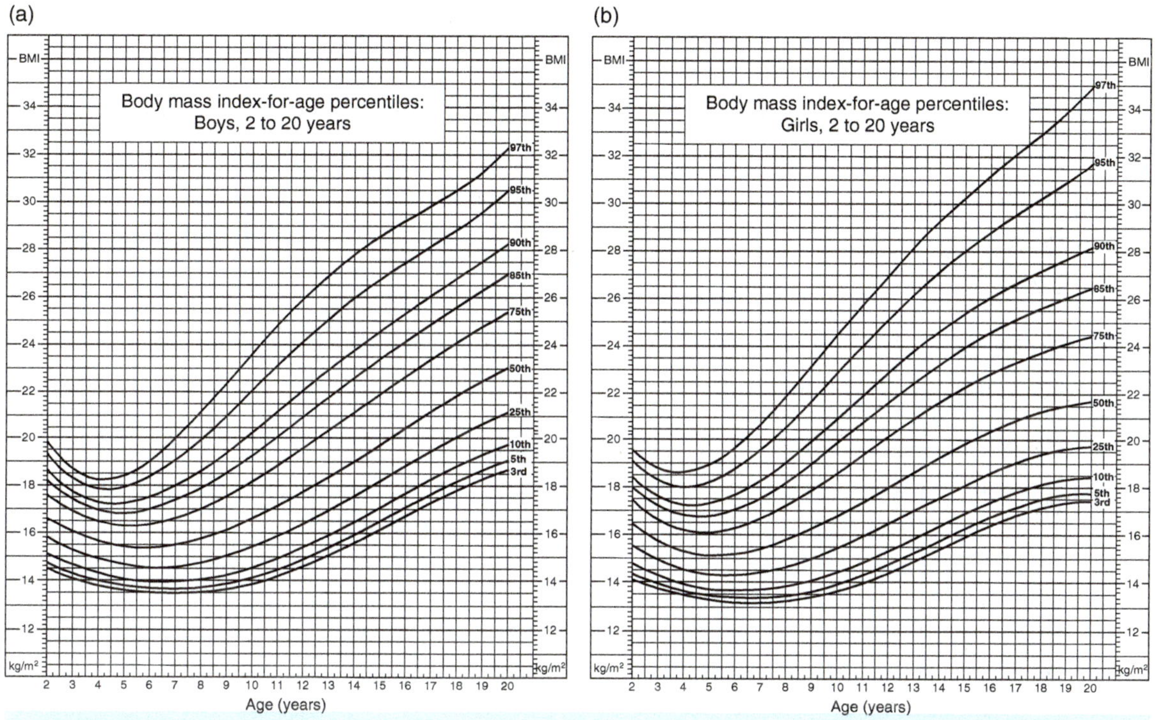

Figure 6.12 Growth charts (U.S.): Body mass index-for-age percentiles, boys (a) and girls (b) 2 to 20 years.

Sources: Developed by the National Center for Health Statistics (2000) in collaboration with the National Center for Chronic Disease Prevention and Health Promotion; Kuczmarski et al. (2000, 2002).

the legs experience maximum growth first, longer legs relative to total stature, has been found to influence both walking (Elbaz, Artaud, Dugravot, et al., 2018) and running speed (Dintiman & Ward, 2011; Malina, 2012). Additionally, with the onset of the adolescent growth spurt, there is a disproportionate rate of growth between the bones of the leg and the surrounding muscles. More specifically, bone growth in length is exceeding the growth of muscle lengthening. This disproportionate growth results in muscle tightening and a reduction in flexibility (Kerssemakers, Fotiadou, de Jonge, et al., 2009). There is also a disproportionate rate of growth in stature compared to gains in muscle weight. More specifically, for boys, there is a delay of about 14 months between PHV and the most rapid period of gains in muscle mass. Thus, adolescent boys are generally weaker than their appearance would suggest (Manna, 2014).

In general, increased body weight is an asset when a person is propelling an external object, such as in the shot put. It can also be beneficial in some sports such as football. In contrast, lighter body weight is more advantageous when the individual's body is the object propelled as in jumping events, many gymnastic maneuvers, and running distances (Silva, 2019). Furthermore, excess body weight and body fatness generally exert a negative influence on performance when the task requires the body to be supported.

Another issue frequently addressed in the professional literature regarding performance changes during adolescence is the concept of **adolescent awkwardness.** This term has been used with regard to PHV. This period is accompanied by a temporary disruption in motor performance. Peak height velocity occurs in girls at a mean estimated age of about 12 years and in boys at 13.7 years (Roche & Sun,

2003; Granados, Gebremariam, & Lee, 2015). Tanner (1990) has noted a period during the growth spurt when balancing abilities may be disrupted for up to 6 months. Beunen, Malina, Van't Hof, and associates (1988), as well as Ostyn, Simons, Beunen, and associates (1980), also found a significant number of boys who declined in performance on four of seven motor tasks during peak height velocity.

This temporary disruption is likely the result of structural constraints being imposed on some individuals. For example, increases in body weight make it more difficult to propel the body through space (jumping). Additionally, muscular strength does not increase at the same pace as the increase in body size (height & weight). In other words, the skeletal muscles can no longer efficiently handle this larger body. Therefore, activities such as the bent-arm hang and other muscular strength/endurance events are more difficult. Also, the rapid growth in leg length may alter the individual's center of gravity, making balancing tasks more difficult. Flexibility may also be compromised as, at PHV, long bone length may increase more rapidly than muscle and tendon length. As a result, the muscles are tighter and joint flexibility is decreased.

Following an extensive review of the literature, Beunen and Malina (1988) concluded that the phenomenon of adolescent awkwardness does exist, but primarily among boys. However, the phenomenon is not universal among boys. That is, not all young males experience a disruption in motor performance during peak height velocity. These researchers report that the percentage of boys exhibiting declines in performance during this growth spurt ranges from 1.4–33.5 percent, depending on the motor task. Table 6.3 illustrates their findings in more detail. Of particular interest is their finding that those boys who exhibited a decline in performance at the time of peak height velocity were generally the best performers at the beginning of peak height velocity. Moreover, follow-up testing during young adulthood revealed that this decline was only temporary (Beunen & Malina, 1988). A more recent systematic literature review (Quatman-Yates, Quatman, Meszaros, et al., 2012) continues to support this finding. For this reason, individuals responsible for motor assessments should be cautious in interpreting motor performance data that have been obtained during this critical growth period.

Once again it must be emphasized that this phenomenon is not universal. In fact, one study involving youth soccer players found that balance, speed of limb movement, trunk strength, upper body muscular endurance, explosive power, running speed, cardiorespiratory endurance, and anaerobic capacity actually peaked at the time of PHV (Philippaerts, Vaeyeng, Janssens, et al., 2006). Thus, each case must be judged independently.

Table 6.3 Percentage of boys exhibiting declines in motor performance during peak height velocity

Task	Number of subjects	Percentage of decliners
Arm pull (static strength)	444	1.4
Plate tapping (speed of limb movement)	441	7.0
Vertical jump (explosive strength)	446	9.5
Sit and reach (flexibility)	444	18.7
Leg lift (trunk strength)	444	26.1
Bent-arm hang (strength)	446	30.5
Shuttle run (agility/speed)	445	33.5

Sources: Based on data reported by Beunen and colleagues (1988) and Ostyn and colleagues (1980). Adapted from Beunen and Malina (1988).

BODY PROPORTIONS

Measuring Changes in Body Proportions

Relevant body proportion measures that involve the head include the head circumference and the relationship of head length to overall body length. As illustrated in Figure 6.13, **head circumference** is obtained by placing the measuring tape anteriorly superior to the eyebrows and posteriorly at the position of the maximum circumference. The tape should be pulled tight to compress the hair.

A second measure of proportional growth is the ratio of **sitting height** to stature (sitting height/stature × 100), which describes the contribution of the legs and trunk to total height. The person being measured should sit on a high bench so that the feet do not touch the floor; she should keep the spine erect and eyes focused straight ahead. The distance between the vertex and the sitting surface is measured.

A third measure of proportional growth is the **biacromial/bicristal ratio** (biacromial breadth/bicristal breadth × 100). Biacromial breadth, a measure of shoulder width, is the distance between the right and left acromial processes; bicristal breadth, a measure of hip width, is the distance between the right and left iliocristales (hipbones). These distances are measured with an anthropometer, a sliding caliper, or a length caliper. The person should stand erect with arms hanging naturally by the sides while being measured.

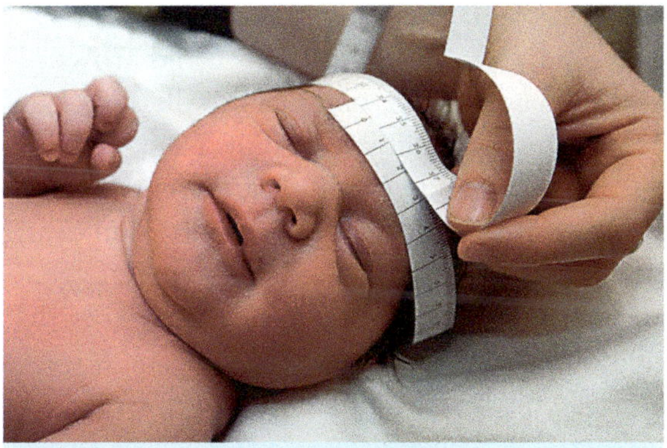

Figure 6.13 Measuring head circumference

Changes in Body Proportions

Here we describe (1) changes in the relationship between head length and total body length; (2) changes in the center of gravity; (3) changes in head circumference; (4) changes in sitting height as it compares with stature; and (5) changes in shoulder width as contrasted with growth in hip width. Lastly, we describe general body shape by examining physique.

Changes in the Ratio of Head Length to Total Body Length

Figure 6.14 illustrates changes in the relationship of head length to total body length. One of the most noticeable characteristics of the newborn is the size of the head in relation to total body length. More specifically, at birth, the head contributes about 25 percent to total body length, while the lower limbs contribute only 15 percent. Because the legs and trunk lengthen in relation to the head, the relative position of the body's midpoint descends with age. In other words, the center of gravity slowly descends through the growing years.

Changes in the Center of Gravity

As mentioned, the head, trunk, and legs do not grow proportionately; therefore, a person's center of gravity varies markedly during childhood. Although the anatomical location of the center of gravity changes with age, it remains a relatively constant proportion of total height. Most kinesiologists agree that this ratio of the center of gravity to total height is 53–59 percent in the adult, a range of only 6 percent. However, in children, the ratio of the center of gravity to total height is higher because children carry a larger proportion of

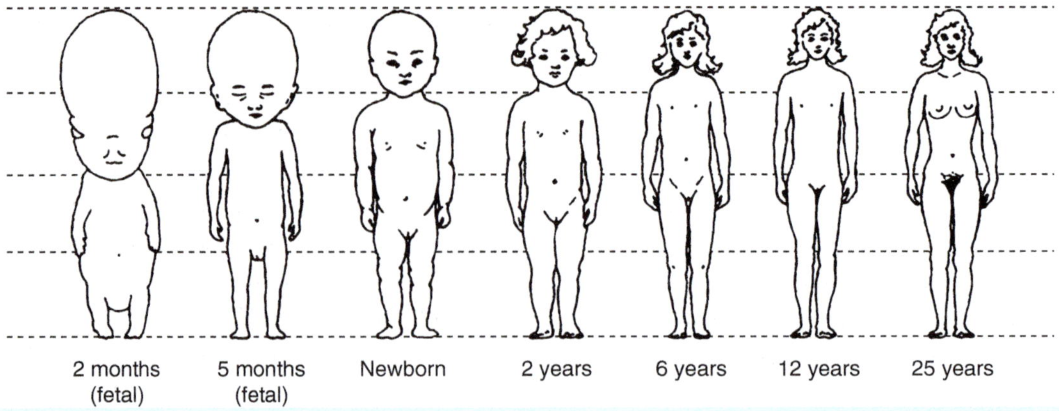

Figure 6.14 Changes in body proportions with age. Notice the great changes in the relative size of the head and the lower limbs

their weight in their upper bodies. As a general rule, the center of gravity in the male is slightly higher than that in the female human.

At birth, the center of gravity is located approximately 8 in (20 cm) above the greater trochanters (large bony projection lateral to the head of the femur). It slowly descends until it rests approximately 4 in (10 cm) above the trochanters at maturity. Although this shift of only 4 in (10 cm) seems relatively small, there is a marked change in the center of gravity's anatomical location. In the newborn, 8 in (20 cm) above the trochanters is an area in the lower level of the thoracic cavity at the xiphoid process (the cartilaginous extension of the lower part of the sternum). By the time children enter elementary school (6 years old), their center of gravity has dropped through the abdominal cavity and is located near the umbilicus. The center of gravity then proceeds to descend at a uniform rate toward the proximal end of the lower extremities. This uniform rate of descent is roughly proportional to the increase in stature. In the adult, 4 in (10 cm) above the trochanters brings the center of gravity to the level of the iliac crest at the second or third sacral vertebra at the base of the spine.

The differences in the center of gravity between the genders and at different ages have a marked effect on motor performance, as discussed later in the chapter.

Changes in Head Circumference

The head circumference is considered a valuable measurement because it can reflect brain development. At birth, the head is approximately one-quarter of total body length. Additionally, the head circumference is greater than the chest circumference. This comparison reflects the advanced development of the brain at this time as compared with other body segments.

Head circumference measured between birth and 2 months is approximately 15.35 in (39 cm), and little difference exists between boys and girls (NCHS, 2012; Fryar, Gu, Ogden, & Flegal, 2016). During the course of the first postnatal year, the head circumference will increase by about 4.7 in (12 cm), and growth in this measurement will then rapidly decelerate to an increase of only 2 in (5 cm) during the second year. In fact, there is only about an increase of 2–2.4 in (5–6 cm) in head circumference between 3 and 20 years of age. Head circumference-for-age percentile growth charts from the CDC for both girls and boys between birth and 36 months of age are presented in Appendix A.

Changes in Sitting Height

At birth, sitting height accounts for 85 percent of total body length. By 6 years of age, sitting height's contribution to total body length has decreased to 55 percent. Typically, the sitting height's contribution to total body length in adulthood is 50 percent. However, there are several exceptions; for example, African American children have slightly shorter sitting heights and longer lower extremities than do White children at all ages (Lowrey, 1986).

Until 10 years of age for girls and 12 years for boys, both sexes exhibit almost the same increases in sitting height (trunk length). Given the overall stature gains during this period, it appears that 55–60 percent of stature gains can be attributed to leg growth in both sexes. Usually, however, boys have longer trunks than do girls until they are about 12 years old. Because boys are generally taller, this means that prior to adolescence, boys have shorter legs than girls relative to total body length (Haubenstricker & Sapp, 1980). During adolescence and adulthood, however, women on average have shorter legs than do men of equal stature (see Figure 6.15).

Changes in Shoulder and Hip Width

Even though there are sex differences in body proportions prior to adolescence, the differences are minimal. During adolescence, however, characteristic sexual dimorphisms become apparent. Perhaps the most noticeable is the relation of shoulder-width growth to hip-width growth. In fact, one of the obvious characteristics of male maturity is a widening of the shoulders. In contrast, girls grow wider through the hips compared to their shoulder development (see Figure 6.16). The bicristal (shoulder width)/biacromial (hip width) ratio is relatively constant in both boys and girls between 6 and 11 years of age. Thereafter, the ratio declines in boys but continues to be relatively stable in girls (Malina, Bouchard, & Bar-Or, 2004; Figure 6.17).

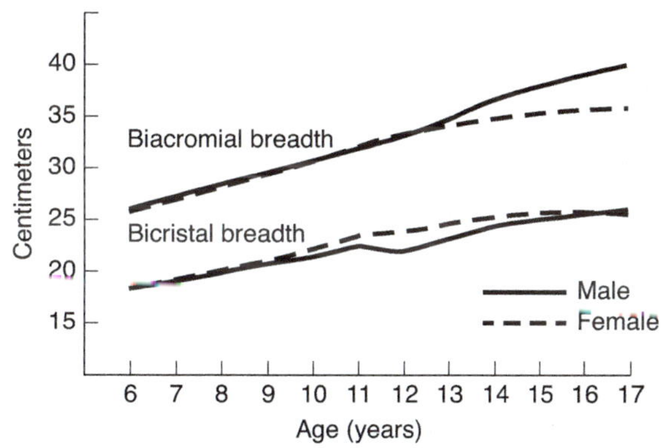

Figure 6.16 Mean biacromial and bicristal breadth

Source: Based on NCHS data reported in Roche and Malina (1983).

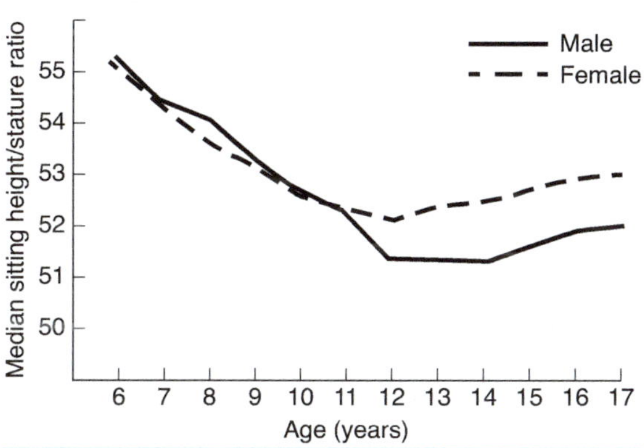

Figure 6.15 Sitting height/stature ratio

Source: Based on NCHS data (1974).

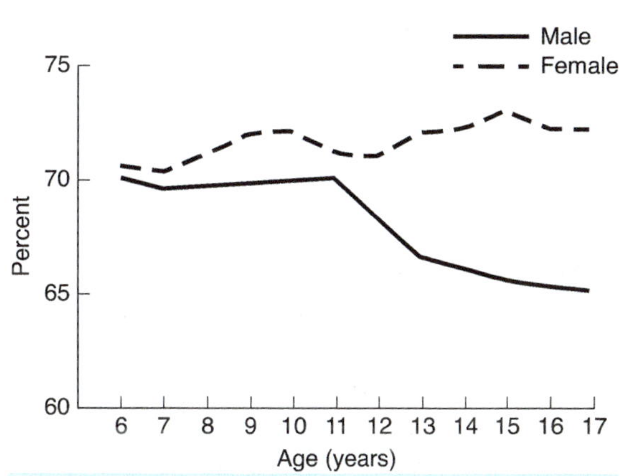

Figure 6.17 Bicristal/biacromial breadth × 100

Source: Based on U.S. Health Examination data reported in Roche and Malina (1983).

Physique

Thus far, our assessment of growth in body proportions across the lifespan has focused on specific body parts. However, it is important to understand overall body form (physique). The classification of the human form dates back to Hippocrates. Sheldon (1940) popularized his method of rating physique, which was based on the premise that three components contribute to the conformation of the entire body. Sheldon described the three components as (1) **endomorphic**—round and soft; (2) **mesomorphic**—muscular; and (3) **ectomorphic**—tall and thin (see Figure 6.18). Each component is assessed from three standardized photographs. Each photograph is rated on a 7-point scale, with 1 representing the least expression and 7 the highest expression of the selected component of physique. For instance, a person with a 7–1–1 physique rating is high in endomorphic qualities and low in both mesomorphic and ectomorphic qualities—in other words, a very obese person.

Heath and Carter (1967) modified Sheldon's approach to include not only photographic but also anthropometric procedures. Practically speaking, this method is most frequently employed in its anthropometric form since it eliminates the moral and ethical problems associated with obtaining nude photographs. **Somatotyping** (classifying physique) calculations are rather complicated; however, this detailed information can be found in the Heath-Carter instructional manual (Carter, 2002) at www.somatotype.org.

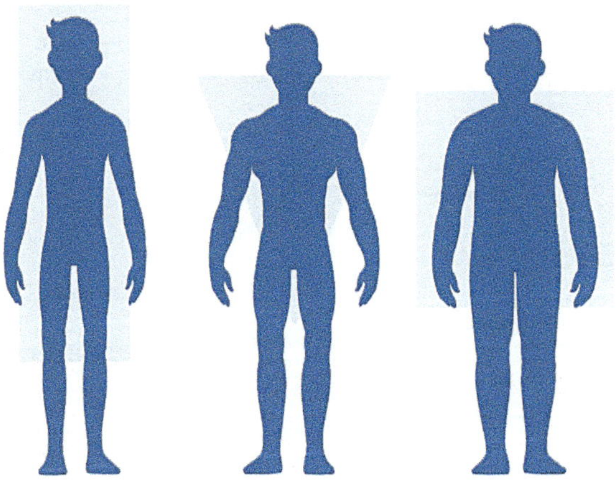

Figure 6.18 Physique: (left) ectomorph; (middle) mesomorph; (right) endomorph

Using data from the Harpenden Growth Study, Malina and colleagues (2004) concluded that changes in physique tend to appear between 3 or 4 and 8 years of age. The physique changes that occur at these times result from a redistribution of subcutaneous fat, the development of lean muscle, and the lengthening of the legs relative to stature. Changes in physique are once again noticed during adolescence as sexual dimorphisms become apparent. Nevertheless, most modifications in somatotype are minor in nature.

Constraints on Motor Performance Related to Body Proportion

Because young children are top-heavy, their high center of gravity and small base of support can limit their early motor performance. Lack of balance is a major obstacle that children must overcome before they can walk. In fact, balance is an important quality necessary for performing all fundamental motor tasks. For instance, during most physical education classes, children are required to manipulate objects, most often some type of playground ball. Whenever a child holds an object such as a playground ball, the weight of the object becomes part of the child's body weight, so the youngster's center of gravity is then displaced in the direction of the added weight. This shift in the center of gravity can influence the child's performance. Consider a kindergarten student who is told to catch a 13-in playground ball. This young child, who already has a relatively high center of gravity, must now maintain control of the thrown projectile while maintaining balance. As a result of the added weight, the child is apt to lose balance in a forward direction, which is most likely why some children drop objects after only momentary control. They catch the object but then must release it to regain their balance.

Generally, Isaacs (1976) believed that a child's high center of gravity sometimes makes it difficult for the child to come to a fast, complete stop when an activity involves a fast forward or backward movement. Furthermore, this high center of gravity may also explain why some young children have difficulty learning to perform such skills as skating and bicycling with instruction alone. Additionally, a child's relatively large head can make it difficult to perform such tumbling skills as a backward roll.

The ratio of trunk length to leg length can also potentially influence motor performance. One longitudinal investigation that examined the influences of physical growth on motor performance suggests that leg length in terms of total body height could have some impact on balance tasks and certain types of power events (Haubenstricker & Sapp, 1980). The superior balancing ability of girls may be partly attributable to a combination of these factors: that is, their shorter legs and broader pelvis establish a lower center of gravity, hence enable better balancing ability. Although these somatic characteristics can enhance balance, they are somewhat disadvantageous in other tasks. For instance, during adolescence, the general structure of the female pelvis places a girl at a disadvantage in both running and jumping events. In addition, Dintiman and Ward (2011) point out that leg length is one of three factors that can account for individual differences in sprinting speed. As mentioned earlier, male leg length in most cases is longer than female leg length following adolescence.

Arm length also appears to influence motor performance. Haubenstricker and Sapp (1980) note that the male's greater shoulder width and arm length could be an advantage to boys in throwing tasks. Thus, it appears that in some activities, such as throwing and striking with force, greater limb length may provide a mechanical advantage for those individuals with this attribute.

Associations between physique and performance can be summarized as follows: a mesomorphic physique is positively associated with motor performance in general and muscular strength. In contrast, a negative association tends to exist between the endomorphic physique and performance in events requiring running, jumping, and agility (Marta, Marinho, & Marques, 2012). The ectomorphic physique tends to be associated with successful athletic performance in endurance events such as long distance running (Tawa & Louw, 2018).

SKELETAL DENSITY

In recent years, skeletal density has become an area of inquiry for many scientists. This increased interest results in part from the aging of our society and the prevalence of bone diseases, especially **osteoporosis**. This disease is characterized by a loss of bone mineral to the point that it renders a bone susceptible to fracture (see Figure 6.19). Therefore, researchers interested in studying this disease

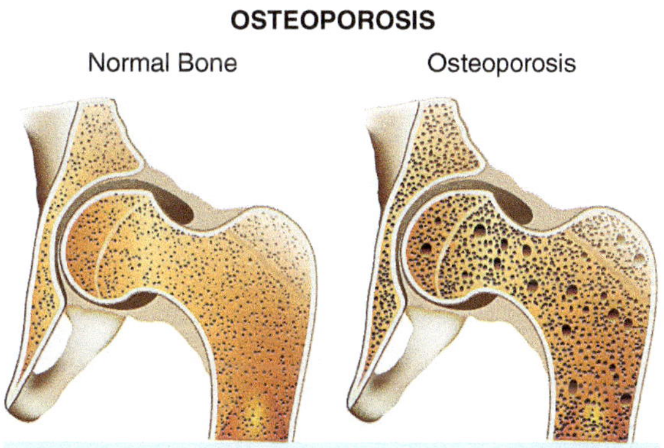

Figure 6.19 (left) Typical bone and (right) osteoporotic bone

are frequently concerned with accurately measuring bone mineral density (BMD), not only within the entire skeletal system but also at susceptible sites, such as the lumbar spine and the neck region of the proximal femur.

Measuring Skeletal Density

The most frequently used instrument to measure bone mineral density (BMD) is the Lunar Prodigy (see Figure 6.20). This instrument uses a technique called **dual-energy X-ray absorptiometry (DEXA)**. DEXA is a noninvasive radiologic technique capable of differentiating body weight into three components: lean soft tissue, fat soft tissue, and bone. In short, it can directly measure and differentiate tissue densities. Figure 6.21 shows a sample DEXA output. The printout includes the scan image, with markers defining the L1 through L4 vertebrae, the numeric BMD values, and comparison with young adult values (T-scores) and with age-matched typical values (Z-scores).

Skeletal Development Milestones

The skeleton makes up 15 percent of a newborn infant's body weight. Prior to birth, the skeleton is made up mostly of cartilage. Through a process called intramembranous bone formation, the embryonic membranes begin to ossify. As early as 2 months in utero, **osteoblastic** (bone-building cell) activity can be observed in the upper arm and thigh at the primary ossification centers. Bone deposition occurs from these centers toward the ends so that at birth, the shaft or **diaphysis** of the long bone has begun to ossify. In fact, all the long bones (radius, ulna, humerus, femur, tibia), as well as the short bones (phalanges, metacarpals, metatarsals), begin to ossify prior to birth. Secondary ossification centers develop in many of the long bones near the end of the prenatal period. More than 400 ossification centers appear before birth, and more than 400 additional centers appear after birth. Chronologically, these sites emerge in girls earlier than in boys. Similarly, **epiphyseal plate** (growth plate) ossification occurs earlier in girls. For example, the median age for ossification in the head of the femur is 167 months for girls and 191 months for boys.

Two mechanisms operate in the development of bone postnatally. First, through a process called **endochondral bone formation**, the bones lengthen at the epiphyseal cartilage discs or

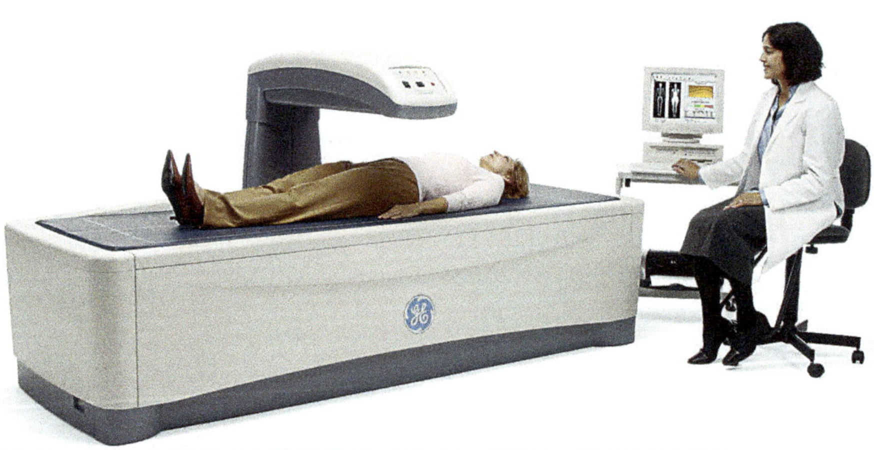

Figure 6.20 The GE Lunar Prodigy, an advanced bone densitometer

Source: Courtesy of Lunar division of GE Healthcare. Copyright © General Electric.

LUNAR DPX-IQ
AP SPINE RESULTS
HP LASERJET PRINTER

Patient, AP Spine — AP SPINE BONE DENSITY

Facility: — Acquired: 12/28/1995 (4.00)
43 years 12/01/1952 — Analyzed: 03/20/1996 (4.1a)
64.8in 125.01bs White Female — Printed: 07/01/1997 (4.3a)
Physician: — paties25.s01

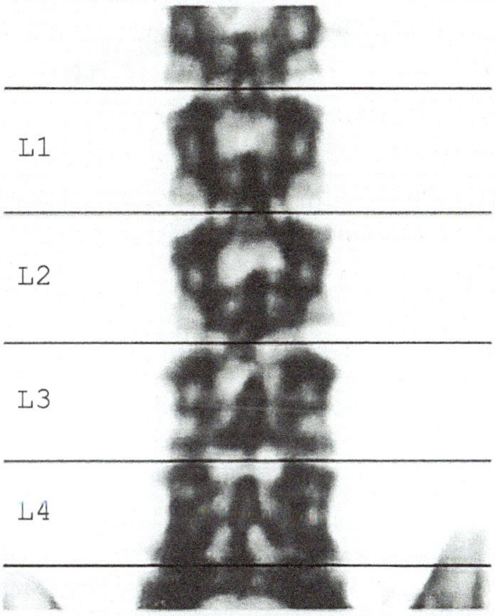

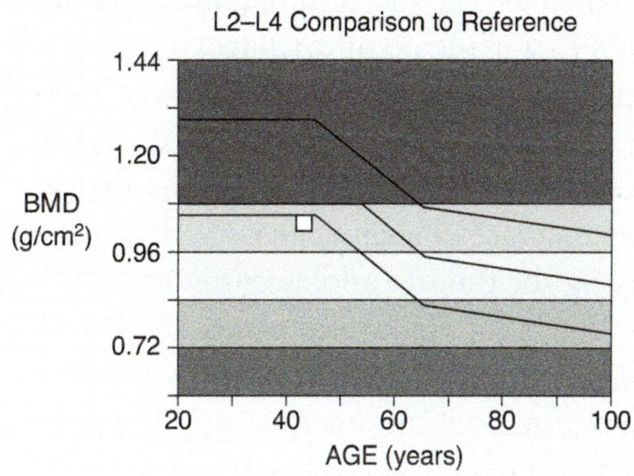

Region	BMD[1,7] g/cm²	Young-Adult[2] %	Young-Adult[2] T	Age-Matched[3] %	Age-Matched[3] Z
L1	0.980	87	-1.2	89	-1.0
L2	1.009	84	-1.6	86	-1.3
L3	0.979	82	-1.8	84	-1.6
L4	1.100	92	-0.8	94	-0.6
L2-L4	1.030	86	-1.4	88	-1.1

Image not for diagnosis.
3.00ma: Hi-Res Medium DPXIQ 0.6 x 1.2mm 1.68mm
784419:435677 265.17:197.67:140.57
%Fat = 14.0(1.364)

1 –See appendix on precision and accuracy.
Statistically 68% of repeat scans will fall within 1 SD. (±0.01 g/cm2)

2 –USA AP Spine Reference Population, Ages 20–45. See Appendices.

3 –Matched for Age, Weight (25–100kg), Ethnic.

4 –Standard BMD for L2–4 is 980 mg/cm2. See J Bone Miner Res 1994:1503–1514.

Comments:

Figure 6.21 Measuring bone mineral density: dual-energy X-ray absorptiometry output

Note: The graph shows the patient's measurement plotted on the normal aging curve, with standard deviation limits. Interday reliability of 13 bone density parameters as measured by DEXA resulted in correlation coefficients ranging from $r = .90$ to $r = .99$ (Tucci, Carpenter, Graves, et al., 1991).

Source: Courtesy of GE Lunar. Copyright © General Electric.

secondary ossification centers. In the long bones, these discs are located at both ends of the bone, while in the short bones (hands and feet), these centers can be found at one end only. The primary ossification centers for the irregularly shaped bones (carpals) develop after birth. These are central ossification centers, which grow outwardly. The epiphysis is a site of osteoblastic activity resulting in new bone growth. It is made up of cartilage, which is eventually replaced by bone in later adolescence. The ossification of the diaphysis reaches the epiphysis and they fuse so that no further increase in length can occur. For most bones, by the time an adolescent is 18 or 19 years of age, the epiphyseal plates are closed. The clavicle and mandible are atypical in that they develop both intramembranously and endochondrally.

A second mechanism, **appositional bone formation,** allows the long bone to increase in diameter. Osteoblasts in the periosteum of the bone will lay down new bone on older bone, while **osteoclasts** (bone-removing cells) reabsorb old bone at the same time. When the rate of deposition is greater than the rate of reabsorption, the bone will increase in diameter.

Throughout the lifespan, **bone remodeling** occurs as a function of both osteoblastic and osteoclastic activity. These two mechanisms of bone remodeling are a response to forces acting on bone, resulting in changes in the bones' size, shape, and density. To remember the difference between the two mechanisms, think of the "b" in *osteoblast* as standing for bone "building" and the "c" in *osteoclast* as standing for bone "chewing."

In general, bone tends to be deposited faster than it is broken down up to about 35 years of age for both men and women. However, the density increases more slowly in women than in men so that, at its peak, the bone density of men exceeds that of women. After age 35, bone mineral is lost at a faster rate than it is deposited, particularly in inactive older adults and at the time of menopause in women; therefore, an osteoporosis prevention program should be started before old age. Recommendations for achieving peak bone mass are presented in Table 6.4.

Table 6.4 Recommendations for achieving peak bone mass

Make a lifelong commitment to physical activity and exercise.
Weight-bearing activities are better than weight-supported activities, such as swimming and cycling.
Activities that increase muscle strength should be promoted, as these will enhance bone density.
Immobilization and periods of immobility should be avoided; where this is not possible (as in bed rest during sickness), even brief daily weight-bearing movements can help reduce bone loss.
In girls, abnormal delay of menarche and chronic irregular menstruation should be avoided, and natural means to restore an energy balance (reduced endurance activity and greater caloric intake) should be advocated to normalize menarche and regulate menstruation where possible. Athletes and coaches should be instructed on the potential skeletal hazards of menstrual dysfunction.
Eating a well-balanced diet that meets the recommended dietary allowance for calcium is also important. The substitution of diet soft drinks for milk should be avoided. Soft drinks are highly acidic with a high phosphorus content that can lead to increased calcium excretion.
Teenagers should avoid smoking cigarettes, as these are antiestrogenic and may interfere with the attainment of normal peak bone mass.
Disordered eating patterns (e.g., anorexia, bulimia) are destructive to the skeleton. These disorders often begin in adolescence and are frequently found in young female athletes, as well as in other adolescent females regardless of activity levels. Parents, coaches, and teachers should be alert to the dangers of extreme eating behavior.

Sources: American College of Obstetricians and Gynecologists (ACOG, 2017); Bailey and Martin (1994, p. 343).

Physical Activity and Skeletal Health

It has been estimated that 54 million men and women over the age of 50 are affected by osteoporosis (Wright, Looker, Saag, et al., 2014). In this section we will examine the role that physical activity plays in helping fight against this public health risk.

The effectiveness of physical activity in maximizing bone mass has typically been judged by examining changes in both bone mineral density and bone geometry following periods of physical activity. Although osteoporosis and low BMD are most often associated with old age, the research suggests that the key to alleviating or reducing their incidence in older adults actually begins during the infancy (Ireland, Muthuri, Rittweger, et al., 2017), childhood, and adolescent years (Hind & Burrows, 2007; Jackowski, Baxter-Jones, Gruodyte-Raciene, et al., 2015; Mitchell, Chesi, Elci, et al., 2016). In fact, it appears that as much as 26 percent of adult BMD is accrued within a two-year window of time around puberty (Tanner stages II, III, and IV; Bailey, Martin, McKay, et al., 2000). In general, physically active children, especially those involved in high-impact weight-bearing activities, possess higher BMD than their less active peers (Burt, Greene, & Naughton, 2017; Gomez-Bruton, Matute-Llorente, Gonzalez-Aguero, et al., 2017).

After the age of 40, bone mass decreases by about 0.5 percent or more per year. Additionally, the withdrawal of estrogen at menopause is responsible for acceleration in the loss of bone mass beyond that which is expected in typical aging. Hormonal replacement therapy may reduce the relative risk of bone fracture by as much as 70 percent, and it appears that physical activity can have the same effect at nearly an equivalent level: women who perform the greatest amount of weekly physical activity (>24 MET [metabolic equivalent—a measure of energy expenditure] hours/week) are able to reduce their risk of hip fracture by 67 percent (Feskanich, Willett, & Colditz, 2002). Because women have a higher prevalence of osteoporosis and other risks associated with low BMD at a younger age than men, far less research has been conducted on men. This is understandable because the prevalence of osteoporosis fractures in men does not significantly increase until the eighth or ninth decade of life (Cummings & Melton, 2002). Nevertheless, the research available on men suggests that exercise can help them maintain and improve BMD (Kelly, Kelly, & Tran, 2000). One 5-year prospective study of both middle-aged and older runners (55–77 years) found that running helped attenuate a decrease in BMD and that the men who experienced the greatest decrease in BMD were those who had also decreased their training volume (Michel, Lane, Bjorkengren, et al., 1992). More specifically, those men who continued to run exhibited a 4 percent decrease in BMD, whereas those who stopped running lost 13 percent of their spinal BMD.

Researchers have also studied the long-term effects of physical activity on bone health by examining the effect of athletes' retirement on BMD. When they compared 22 active and 128 formerly active male soccer players to 138 controls, Karlsson, Linden, Karlsson, and colleagues (2000) found that the active athletes possessed a greater BMD than controls during the first two decades after retirement. The soccer players who had been retired for 5 years still possessed a 10 percent higher leg BMD, and those retired 16 years still had a 5 percent higher leg BMD compared to controls. However, no benefit was noted for those retired for 42 years. This study emphasizes the importance of exercise-induced benefits during the growing years as a means of partially offsetting the typical decrease in BMD with age.

However, according to Karlsson (2007), there is more to the picture. This is because bone health is related not only to BMD but also to the bone's geometry, and exercise appears to produce an enlargement in the bone's diameter that is permanent. This increased bone diameter appears to preserve skeletal strength into late adulthood. One study found that 90 currently active soccer players and weight-lifters (50–92 years of age) who had been retired for 3–65 years possessed a greater bone diameter at the femoral neck and lumbar spine when compared to sedentary age- and gender-matched controls (Karlsson, Alborg, Obrant, et al., 2002). Furthermore, it appears that this increased bone diameter is associated with fewer fractures in older adults (Karlsson, 2007). This finding once again emphasizes the importance of physical activity early in life as a means of reducing risks associated with declining skeletal health in older adults.

The Female Athlete Triad and Skeletal Health

The **female athlete triad** is a medical condition composed of three elements: (1) low energy availability with or without an eating disorder; (2) menstrual dysfunction, including both primary and secondary **amenorrhea**; and (3) osteopenia (ACOG, 2017). This low bone mineral density (osteopenia) in turn can lead to **osteoporosis.** These three related disorders are most prevalent in females, and their prevalence is highest among females who participate in sports that emphasize leanness. As many as 25 percent of elite female athletes who participate in these sports (gymnastics, endurance track events, and weight-class sports) have been reported to have an eating disorder, compared to a 9 percent rate in the general population (Sundgot-Borgen & Torstveit, 2004).

Scientists now recognize that this disorder is present not only in those with eating disorders but also in those females who sustain a restrictive caloric imbalance to the point of causing amenorrhea. An additional mechanism that can trigger amenorrhea is a significant increase in exercise training volume without adequate dietary intake. Amenorrhea affects skeletal health directly by suppressing hormones that promote bone growth and indirectly by removing estrogen's influence on bone absorption. Regardless of how the caloric imbalance is created, the end result is referred to as low energy availability. **Energy availability** is defined as dietary energy intake minus exercise energy expended. Energy availability is important because it provides the fuel for other body functions, including growth, cellular maintenance, thermoregulation, and reproduction. The female athlete triad can be initiated by an eating disorder or any other factor (dieting, overtraining) that causes sustained low energy availability. Recommendations for identifying and treating this disorder are available from ACOG (2017).

MATURATION AND DEVELOPMENTAL AGE

The human organism spends approximately one-quarter of the lifespan in a state of physical growth. Certainly, physical, intellectual, and emotional changes are clearly evident as babies grow into toddlers and school-age children. Physical changes are markedly noticeable in the developmental stage known as adolescence. Adolescence is characterized by rapid physical, biochemical, social, and emotional changes and involves six years, or approximately one-third, of a youngster's growing period. The onset of adolescence and the time necessary to advance from a state of immature to mature development vary from person to person both within and between the sexes.

Determining Maturation

Because changes during adolescence are not always discernible, we generally use

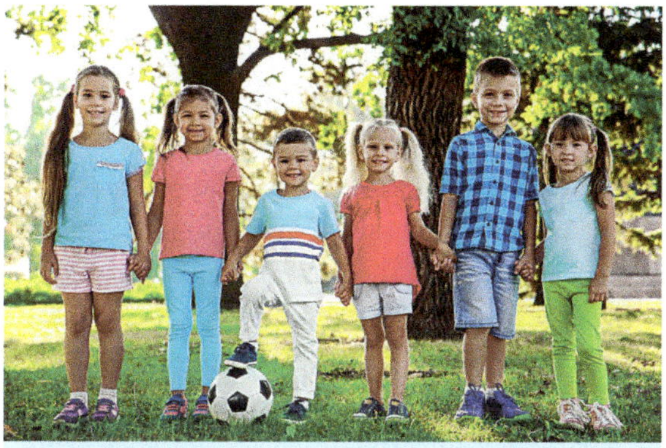

Figure 6.22 Children of the same chronological age can vary in size due to different rates of physical maturation

chronological age to denote a person's level of maturity. **Developmental age**, however, is by far a better indicator of maturity than is chronological age, which simply denotes the length of time from birth but fails to address individual variation in rate of maturation (Figure 6.22). Fortunately, however, landmark parameters tied to physiological events occur in all people. These parameters share a common developmental endpoint and, thus, can serve as indicators as to whether a child is lagging behind peers or springing ahead of them. Height and weight measures are inadequate because people differ in mature stature and weight. A set of predictable physiological parameters includes skeletal maturity, genitalia maturity, and, for girls, age of menarche. Of the three, age of menarche is the most commonly used indicator in girls (Malina, 2014).

Skeletal Maturity

Skeletal age is the most widely accepted measure for determining stage of maturation. During growth, predictable changes in bone structure, observable via radiography, enable professionals to determine skeletal age. As a child matures, primary and secondary centers of bone ossify, rendering them opaque to X-rays. The progressive enlargement of these ossified bone centers can be monitored during the growth years and compared with a set of standard films in which each film in a series represents the bone development of children of a similar age. The area of the body most frequently X-rayed is the left hand and wrist (see Figure 6.23). As you examine the three

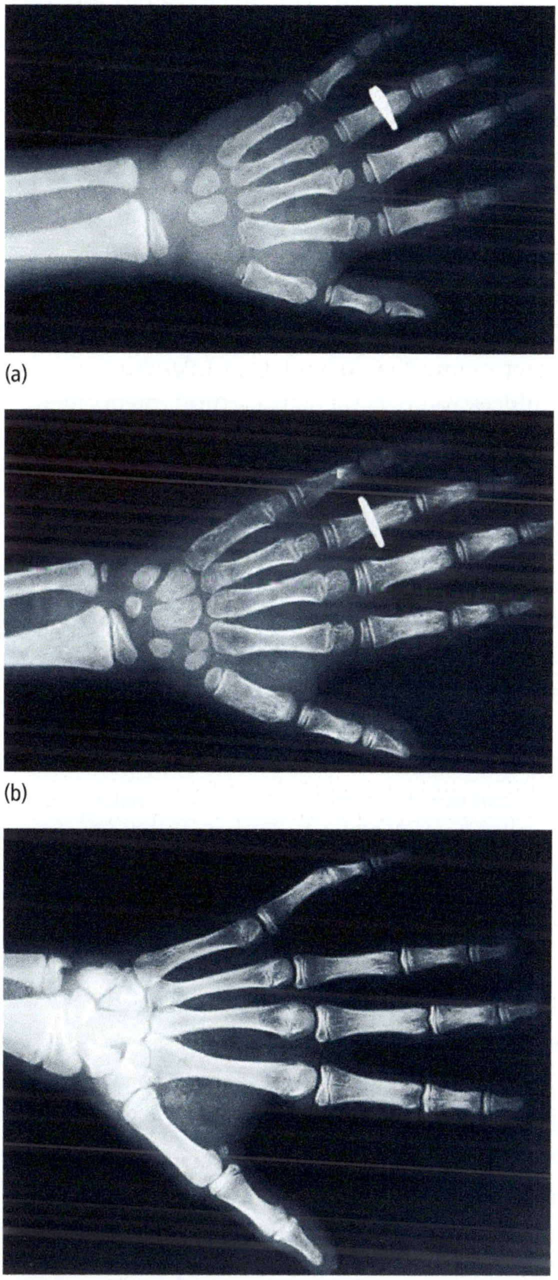

(a)

(b)

(c)

Figure 6.23 Hand-wrist X-rays of (a) a 3-year-old, (b) a 5-year-old, and (c) a 14-year-old.

X-rays, note the increasing number of bones in the lower wrist that become visible as the individual matures.

The first set of standardized radiographs of the hand and wrist were developed in 1937 by T. Todd and published in the same year in the now classic text *Atlas of Skeletal Maturation*. To date, the most carefully prepared atlases have been published by Todd's colleagues at Case Western Reserve University, in particular, the atlas by Greulich and Pyle (1959), which remains in use today. Tanner, Whitehouse, Marshall, and associates (1975) developed a different technique of assessing skeletal maturity (Tanner-Whitehouse Method 2), but the most appropriate method for determining the skeletal age of American children today is the Fels method, mentioned earlier in the chapter (Roche, Chumlea, & Thissen, 1988).

Even though the hand and wrist are the most popular sites for assessing skeletal maturity, some researchers are now recommending other areas of the body be X-rayed, particularly the knee, according to a method known as the Roche-Wainer-Thissen (RWT) technique (Roche, 1992). Roche believed the knee is the most appropriate site if information is sought concerning stature. He also suggested using the knee for individuals up to 4 years of age and toward the end of maturation because during these periods few maturational changes are apparent in the hand and wrist (Roche, 1979).

Age of Menarche

Age of menarche is an important event useful for estimating maturation in girls, even though the event does not generally occur until relatively late in puberty. In fact, the female peak growth spurt in height is complete at this point, so young women are in a period of maximal growth deceleration when this milestone appears. The mean age of this event in developed countries is 13.2 years (standard deviation = 1.0 year), but it occurs slightly earlier in American girls (Roche & Sun, 2003). However, the age span at which menarche occurs tends to be more closely related to skeletal maturity (12–14.5 bone-age years) than chronological age. Even though menarche signifies the attainment of mature uterine development, it does not necessarily denote mature reproductive functioning; early menstrual cycles tend to be irregular, and often an egg is not shed from the ovary.

Researchers rely on one of three methods for determining or estimating the date of the first menstrual flow. The most reliable and accurate technique is longitudinally following a group of girls until the event occurs. Because this technique is so time-consuming, researchers most often estimate date of the event by a second technique, self-reported recall (Lundblad & Jacobsen, 2017). To increase the accuracy of recall, the investigator will oftentimes includes questions that focus on associated events. For example, "What grade were you in?" and "Was the event close to your birthday?" The third method is statistical: calculating normative values for a large female population.

Genitalia Maturity

An ancillary method for rating maturation is evaluating the **genitalia maturity**, or stages of pubertal development, by visual inspection. In girls, this consists of assessing pubic hair and breast development. Menarche commonly occurs when pubic hair and breast development reaches a Tanner stage of 4; however, great variability is possible. In boys, pubic hair and changes in the size of the reproductive organs are evaluated. Tables 6.5 and 6.6 describe each developmental stage. For a complete set of standardized photographs depicting each stage of development, refer to the work of Roche and Sun (2003).

Table 6.5 Development of pubic hair

Female		Male	
Stage 1:	There is no pubic hair.	Stage 1:	There is no pubic hair.
Stage 2:	There is sparse growth of long, lightly pigmented, downy hair, straight or only slightly curled, primarily along the labia.	Stage 2:	There is a sparse growth of long, slightly pigmented, downy hair, straight or only slightly curled, primarily at the base of the penis.
Stage 3:	The hair is considerably darker, coarser, and more curled. The hair spreads sparsely over the junction of the pubes.	Stage 3:	The hair is considerably darker, coarser, and more curled. The hair spreads sparsely over the junction of the pubes.
Stage 4:	The hair, now adult in type, covers a smaller area than in the adult.	Stage 4:	The hair, now adult in type, covers a smaller area than in the adult.
Stage 5:	The hair is adult in quantity and type.	Stage 5:	The hair is adult in quantity and type.

Source: Used with permission of Ross Products Division, Abbott Laboratories Inc., Columbus, OH 43215. From *Children Are Different*, pp. 25–29, © 1978 Ross Products Division, Abbott Laboratories Inc.

Table 6.6 Development of female breast and male genitalia

Female breast		Male genitalia	
Stage 1:	The breasts are preadolescent. There is elevation of the papilla only.	Stage 1:	The penis, testes, and scrotum are of childhood size.
Stage 2:	Breast bud stage. A small mound is formed by the elevation of the breast and papilla. The areolar diameter enlarges.	Stage 2:	There is enlargement of the scrotum and testes, but the penis usually does not enlarge. The scrotal skin reddens.
Stage 3:	There is further enlargement of breasts and areola with no separation of their contours.	Stage 3:	There is further growth of the testes and scrotum and enlargement of the penis, mainly in length.
Stage 4:	There is a projection of the areola and papilla to form a secondary mound above the level of the breast.	Stage 4:	There is still further growth of the testes and scrotum and increased size of the penis, especially in breadth.
Stage 5:	The breasts resemble those of a mature female as the areola has recessed to the general contour of the breast.	Stage 5:	The genitalia are adult in size and shape.

Source: Used with permission of Ross Products Division, Abbott Laboratories Inc., Columbus, OH 43215. From *Children Are Different*, pp. 25–29, © 1978 Ross Products Division, Abbott Laboratories Inc.

Maturation's Interrelationship with Motor Performance

Researchers have recognized that more physically mature individuals will generally perform selected motor tasks more proficiently than their less mature counterparts. For instance, it has been shown that success in youth baseball is related to skeletal maturity. More specifically, data collected during a Little League World Series indicated that 71 percent of the participants had advanced skeletal ages relative to their chronological ages, while only 29 percent of the participants were delayed in skeletal age (Krogman, 1959). Hale (1956) reported somewhat similar findings when he assessed the pubertal development of 112 participants during the 1955 Little League World Series. Not only did he find a majority of the young participants either in puberty (37.5 percent) or postpuberty (45.5 percent), he also found that the most important positions—pitcher, first base, and left field—were played by postpubescent individuals. In addition, the postpubescent youngsters held the all-important fourth position in the batting order. Thus, these postpubescent athletes were bigger and stronger than their prepubescent opponents. Level of maturation as determined by pubertal assessment has been found to correlate positively with strength in adolescent boys (Bastos & Hegg, 1984).

In studying young male elite athletes, Malina concluded that early maturation, with its concomitant size and strength advantages, constitutes an asset positively associated with success in several sports. However, as adolescence approaches its termination, the maturity status of the youths is of less significance, as the catch-up of late-maturing boys reduces the size differences so apparent in early adolescence (1984, p. 56).

This is essentially what Clarke (1971) found in his now classic Medford Growth Study—namely, that the superior elementary school athlete may no longer be outstanding in junior high school and that the superior junior high school athlete may not have been outstanding in elementary school. In fact, once the late-maturing person has reached a state of postpubescent development, he is generally larger and may have more athletic success than his counterparts simply because he has had a longer growth period.

Although early maturation may give boys an early athletic advantage, the opposite generally is true for girls. With the exception of swimming, female athletic participation is associated with delayed biological maturation. Malina, Bouchard, Shoup, and associates (1979) first suggested that delayed biological maturation may give young girls a slight competitive edge in such Olympic events as volleyball. Beunen, Beul, Ostyn, and colleagues (1978) studied the relationship between age of menarche and motor performance in 398 Belgian schoolgirls. They found the motor performances of late-maturing girls superior to the motor performances of early- and average-maturing girls on such tasks as trunk strength, functional strength, running speed, and speed of limb movement. Thus, "in general, motor performance is negatively related to biological maturity status in girls but positively related to biological maturity status in boys" (Beunen & Malina, 1988, p. 522). A more recent review continues to support this finding (Manna, 2014).

Note that the studies reported above are classical, as denoted by their publication dates. In today's society these studies, in which the researchers examined genitalia maturity, are difficult to conduct due to ethical and privacy concerns. Researchers desiring to continue this line of research have attempted to overcome these ethical and privacy concerns, as in the work of Jones, Hitchen, and Stratton (2000). These researchers were interested in studying the relationship of biological maturity to performance on selected tasks (vertical jump, hand grip strength, and cardiorespiratory endurance as measured by a multistage 20-m shuttle run). With sexual maturity as the biological marker of interest, the researchers overcame ethical and privacy concerns by employing a self-assessment. For this self-assessment, the subjects viewed photographs of secondary sex characteristics as described by Tanner. The subjects were required to review these photographs carefully and decide which one most closely reflected their own current status. Statistical analysis revealed that different stages of maturity were positively associated with performance on each of the criterion tasks. However, when height (stature) and body weight (mass) were taken into consideration, these positive relationships held true for the boys but not the girls. This finding suggests that increases in height and body weight are primarily responsible for variations in girls' physical performance. The authors concluded that sexual maturity is positively associated with physical performance, but more so in boys than in girls.

SUMMARY

- Growth in both stature and weight rapidly decelerates after the fourth prenatal month. Stature and weight growth then remain relatively constant during the childhood years, only to accelerate again in the phase of development known as adolescence. This rapid change in body size is sometimes accompanied by a period of adolescent awkwardness, especially in boys. However, this decline in motor performance is only temporary and is not universal among all adolescents.
- During childhood, children are top-heavy; that is, they have a high center of gravity. This high center of gravity can affect children's stability.
- The wider shoulders and longer arms of boys and men give them an advantage in throwing events. On the other hand, women and girls are generally superior in balancing, perhaps because of their shorter legs and broader pelvis.
- Growth data can be visually inspected by plotting the data on a distance curve or velocity curve. A distance curve plots accumulative growth obtained over time; a velocity curve plots the rate of change in growth per unit of time.
- Physical activity affects bone density and bone width but does not influence bone length. Osteoporosis is generally thought of as being associated with old age. However, it appears that physical activity during the growth years, particularly high impact activity, is associated with improved bone mineral density outcomes in the elderly.
- Developmental age is a better indicator of maturity than is chronological age. Level of maturity can be determined by reference to skeletal maturity, age of menarche, and genitalia maturity.
- Level of maturation can influence motor performance. In general, research indicates that postpubescent boys initially outperform prepubescent boys. However, once late-maturing boys reach adolescence, their performance is comparable to that of early-maturing boys. Although early maturation is associated with superior athletic performance for boys, the opposite is generally true for girls, except for female swimmers.

key concept review

adiposity rebound
adolescent awkwardness
age of menarche
amenorrhea
appositional bone formation
biacromial/bicristal ratio
body mass index (BMI)
bone remodeling
chronological age
developmental age
diaphysis
distance curve
dual-energy X-ray absorptiometry (DEXA)
ectomorphic
endochondral bone formation
endomorphic
energy availability
epiphyseal plate
female athlete triad

genitalia maturity
head circumference
knee height
mesomorphic
midgrowth spurt
obesity paradox
osteoblastic
osteoclast
osteopenia
osteoporosis
peak height velocity (PHV)
peak weight velocity (PWV)
recumbent length
sitting height
skeletal age
somatotype
stature
velocity curve
vertex

questions for reflection

1. Can you summarize changes in body length and stature, as well as changes in body weight across the human lifespan? Pay particular attention to changes that occur during the adolescent growth spurt.
2. What is the difference between a distance curve and a velocity curve?
3. Can you calculate a body mass index (BMI) and state the desired BMI range associated with optimal health?
4. What is adolescent awkwardness, and what is peak height velocity? How are they related? How common is adolescent awkwardness, and what types of motor performance seem most affected by this phenomenon?
5. What changes in sitting height occur for male and female persons from birth through adulthood?
6. Can you describe and illustrate the relative change in the body's center of gravity from 2 fetal months through adulthood?
7. What is the Heath-Carter somatotyping process, and how does this process differ from that used by Sheldon?
8. What is the interrelationship between body proportion and motor performance from childhood through adolescence?
9. Can you describe the use of dual-energy X-ray absorptiometry (DEXA) for measuring skeletal health?
10. Can you describe bone development, including discussions of the following terms: *diaphysis, epiphyseal plate, endochondral bone formation*, *osteoblast, osteoclast*, and *appositional bone formation*? Also, at what age is bone broken down faster than it is deposited?
11. What are five recommendations for achieving peak bone mass?
12. Can you describe the condition referred to as female athlete triad?
13. Can you list and explain three methods of determining physical (biological) maturity? What is Tanner's approach for determining biological maturity?
14. What differences exist between male and female persons regarding the relationship between motor performance and biological maturation?

online resources

American College of Obstetricians and Gynecologists, www.acog.org
American Society for Bone and Mineral Research, www.asbmr.org
Body Mass Index Calculator, www.cdc.gov/nccdphp/dnpa/bmi/calc-bmi.htm
CDC Growth Charts, www.cdc.gov/growthcharts
Centers for Disease Control and Prevention, www.cdc.gov
Kid's Height Predictor, www.webmd.com/children/healthtool-kids-height-predictor
National Center for Health Statistics, www.cdc.gov/nchs
National Osteoporosis Foundation, www.nof.org
Osteoporosis Canada, www.osteoporosis.ca
Somatotyping: Heath-Carter, www.somatotype.org

REFERENCES

American College of Obstetricians and Gynecologists (2017). The female athlete triad. Committee Opinion No. 702, *Obstetrics & Gynecology*, *129*, e160–e167.

American College of Sports Medicine (2004). Physical activity and bone health. *Medicine and Science in Sports and Exercise*, *36*, 1985–1996.

American College of Sports Medicine (2018). *ACSM's guidelines for exercise testing and prescription.* 10th ed. Baltimore, MD: Lippincott Williams & Wilkins.

Antonopoulos, A. & Tousoulis, D. (2017). The molecular mechanisms of obesity paradox. *Cardiovascular Research*, *113*, 1074–1086.

Bailey, D. A., & Martin, A. D. (1994). Physical activity and skeletal health in adolescents. *Pediatric Exercise Science*, 6, 330–347.

Bailey, D. A., Martin, A. D., McKay, H. A., Whiting, S., & Mirwald, R. (2000). Calcium accretion in girls and boys during puberty: A longitudinal analysis. *Journal of Bone and Mineral Research*, *15*, 2245–2250.

Bailey, D. A., McKay, H. A., Mirwald, R. L., Crocker, P. R., & Faulkner, R. A. (1999). A six-year longitudinal study of the relationship of physical activity to bone mineral accrual in growing children: The University of Saskatchewan bone mineral accrual study. *Journal of Bone Mineral Research, 14*, 1672–1679.

Bastos, F. C., & Hegg, R. V. (1984). The relationship of chronological age, body build and sexual maturation to hand-grip strength in school boys, ages ten through seventeen years. *Proceedings of the 1984 Olympic Scientific Congress*, Eugene, OR.

Beunen, G., Beul, G., Ostyn, M., Renson, R., Simons, J., & Gerven, D. (1978). Age of menarche and motor performance in girls aged 11 through 18. *Medicine and Sport, 11*, 118–123.

Beunen, G., & Malina, R. M. (1988). Growth and physical performance relative to the timing of the adolescent spurt. In K. B. Pandolf (Ed.), *Exercise and sport sciences reviews*. New York: Macmillan.

Beunen, G., Malina, R. M., Van't Hof, M. A., Simons, J., Ostyn, M., Renson, R., et al. (1988). *Adolescent growth and motor performance: A longitudinal study of Belgian boys*. Champaign, IL: Human Kinetics.

Burt, L. A., Greene, D. A., & Naughton, G. A. (2017). Bone health of young gymnasts: A systematic review. *Pediatric Exercise Science*, *29*, 456–464.

Carter, J. E. L. (2002). *The Heath-Carter anthropometric somatotype: Instructional manual.* Surrey, Canada: Tep & ROSSCRAFT.

Centers for Disease Control and Prevention (2017). *Defining adult overweight and obesity*. Retrieved from www.cdc.gov/obesity/adult/defining.html

Centers for Disease Control and Prevention (2018). *Defining childhood obesity: BMI for children and teens*. Retrieved from www.cdc.gov/obesity/childhood/defining.html.

Clarke, H. H. (1971). *Physical and motor tests in the Medford Boys' Growth Study.* Englewood Cliffs, NJ: Prentice-Hall.

Cummings, S. R., & Melton, L. J. (2002). Epidemiology and outcomes of osteoporotic fractures. *Lancet*, *359*, 1761–1767.

Dintiman, G., & Ward, R. (2011). *Encyclopedia of sport speed*. Kill Devil Hills, NC: The National Association of Speed and Explosion.

Edward, H., Marshall, S. A., Saldana, S., Skelton, J. A., Suerken, C. K., Arcury, T. A., et al. (2017). Determinants of adiposity rebound timing in children. *Journal of Pediatrics*, 184, 151–156.

Elbaz, A., Artaud, F., Dugravot, A., Tzourio, C., & Singh-Manoux, A. (2018). The gait speed advantage of taller stature is lost with age. *Scientific Reports*, doi: 10.1038/s41598-018-19882

Feskanich, D., Willett, W., & Colditz, G. (2002). Walking and leisure-time activity and risk of hip fracture in postmenopausal women. *Journal of the American Medical Association*, *288*, 2300–2306.

Fryar, C. D., Gu, Q., Ogden, C. L., & Flegal, K. M. (2016). Anthropometric reference data for children and adults: United States, 2011–2014. *Vital and Health Statistics*, 3(39), National Center for Health Statistics.

Fryar, C. D., Kruszon-Moran, K., Gu, Q., & Ogden, C. L. (2018). *Mean body weight, height, waist circumference, and body mass index among adults: United States, 1999–2000 through 2015–2016*. No. 122. Hyattsville, MD: National Center for Health Statistics.

Gomez-Bruton, A., Matute-Llorente, A., Gonzalez-Aguero, A., Casajus, J. A., & Vicente-Rodriguez, V. (2017). Plyometric exercise and bone health in children and adolescents: A systematic review. *World Journal of Pediatrics*, *13*, 112–121.

Granados, A., Gebremariam, A., & Lee, J. M. (2015). Relationship between timing of peak height velocity and pubertal staging in boys and girls. *Journal of Clinical Research in Pediatric Endocrinology*, *7*, 235–237.

Greulich, W. W., & Pyle, S. I. (1959). *Radiographic atlas of skeletal development of the hand and wrist*. 2nd ed. Palo Alto, CA: Stanford University Press.

Gunderson, E. P. (2009). Childbearing and obesity in women: Weight before, during, and after pregnancy. *Obstetrics and Gynecology Clinics of North America*, *36*, 317–332.

Guo, S. S., Huang, C., Maynard, L. M., Demerath, E., Towne, B., Chumlea, W. C., & Siervogel, R. M. (2000). Body mass index during childhood, adolescence and young adulthood in relation to adult overweight and adiposity: The Fels Longitudinal Study. *International Journal of Obesity*, *24*, 1628–1635.

Hale, C. J. (1956). Physiologic maturity of Little League baseball players. *Research Quarterly*, *27*, 276–284.

Haubenstricker, J. L., & Sapp, M. M. (1980). A longitudinal look at physical growth and motor performance: Implications for elementary and middle school activity programs. Paper presented at the meeting of the American Alliance for Health, Physical Education, Recreation, and Dance, Detroit, MI.

Heath, B. H., & Carter, J. E. L. (1967). A modified somato-type method. *American Journal of Physical Anthropology*, *27*, 57–74.

Hind, K., & Burrows, M. (2007). Weight-bearing exercise and bone mineral accrual in children and adolescents: A review of controlled trials. *Bone*, *40*, 14–27.

Ireland, A., Muthuri, S., Rittweger, J., Adams, J. E., Ward, K. A., Kuh, D., et al. (2017). Later age at onset of independent walking is associated with lower bone strength at fracture-prone sites in older men. *Journal of Bone and Mineral Research*, *32*, doi.org/10.1002/jbmr.3099.

Isaacs, L. D. (1976). The anatomical changes of the center of gravity during development: Implications to physical education. Unpublished manuscript, University of Maryland.

Jackowski, S. A., Baxter-Jones, A. D., Gruodyte-Raciene, R., Kontulainen, S. A., & Erlandson, M. C. (2015). A longitudinal study of bone area, content, density, and strength development at the radius and tibia in children 4–12 years of age exposed to recreational gymnastics. *Osteoporosis International*, *26*, 1677–1690.

Jones, M. A., Hitchen, P. J., & Stratton, G. (2000). The importance of considering biological maturity when assessing physical fitness measures in girls and boys aged 10 to 16 years. *Annals of Human Biology*, *27*, 57–65.

Karlsson, M. K. (2007). Does exercise during growth prevent fractures in later life? *Medicine and Sport Science*, *51*, 121–136.

Karlsson, M. K., Alborg, H. G., Obrant, K., Nyquist, F., Lindberg, H., & Karlsson, C. (2002). Exercise during growth and young adulthood is associated with reduced fracture risk in old age. *Journal of Bone and Mineral Research*, *17*, S297.

Karlsson, M. K., Linden, C., Karlsson, C., Johnell, O., Obrant, D., & Seeman, E. (2000). Exercise during growth and bone mineral density and fractures in old age. *Lancet*, *355*, 469–470.

Kelly, G. A., Kelly, K. S., & Tran, Z. V. (2000). Exercise and BMD in men: A meta-analysis. *Journal of Applied Physiology*, *88*, 1730–1736.

Kerssemakers, S. P., Fotiadou, A. N., de Jonge, M. C., Karantanas, S. H., & Maas, M. (2009). Sport injuries in the paediatric and adolescent patient: A growing problem. *Pediatric Radiology*, *39*, 471–484.

Khamis, H. J., & Roche, A. F. (1994). Predicting adult stature without using skeletal age: The Khamis-Roche method. *Pediatrics*, *94*, 504–507.

Krogman, W. M. (1959). Maturation age of 55 boys in the Little League world series. *Research Quarterly*, *30*, 54–56.

Kuczmarski, R. J., Ogden, C. L., Grummer-Strawn, L. M., Flegal, K. M., Guo, S. S., Wei, R., et al. (2000). *CDC growth charts: United States advance data from vital and health statistics*. No. 314. Hyattsville, MD: National Center for Health Statistics.

Kuczmarski, R. J., Ogden, C. L., Guo, S. S., Grummer-Strawn, L. M., Flegal, K. M., Mei, Z., et al. (2002). *CDC growth charts: United States, 2000*. Vital and Health Statistics, National Center for Health Statistics. Washington, DC: Department of Health and Nutrition Services.

Lowrey, G. H. (1986). *Growth and development of children*. 8th ed. Chicago: Year Book Medical Publishers.

Lundblad, M. W., & Jacobsen, B. K. (2017). The reproducibility of self-reported age at menarche: The Tromso study. *BMC Women's Health, 17* (62), doi: 10.1186/s12905-017-0420-0.

Malina, R. M. (1984). Maturational considerations in elite young athletes. *Proceedings of the 1984 Olympic Scientific Congress*. Eugene, OR.

Malina, R. M. (2012). Body mass index. In Institute of Medicine (Ed.), *Measuring progress in obesity prevention: Workshop report* (pp. 42–48). Washington, DC: The National Academies Press.

Malina, R. M. (2014). Top 10 research questions related to growth and maturation of relevance to physical activity, performance, and fitness. *Research Quarterly for Exercise and Sport, 85*, 157–173.

Malina, R. M., Bouchard, C., & Bar-Or, O. (2004). *Growth, maturation, and physical activity.* 2nd ed. Champaign, IL: Human Kinetics.

Malina, R. M., Bouchard, C., Shoup, R. F., Demirjian, A., & Lariviere, G. (1979). Age at menarche, family size, and birth order in athletes at the Montreal Olympic Games, 1976. *Medicine and Science in Sport, 11*, 354–358.

Manna, I. (2014). Growth development and maturity in children and adolescent: Relation to sports and physical activity. *American Journal of Sports Science and Medicine*, 2, 48–50.

Marta, C., Marinho, D. A., & Marques, M. C. (2012). Physical fitness in prepubescent children: An update. *Journal of Physical Education and Sport, 12*, 445–457.

Maynard, L. M., Wisemandle, W. A., Roche, A. F., Chumlea, W. C., Guo, S. S., & Siervogel, R. M. (2001). Childhood body composition in relation to body mass index: The Fels Longitudinal Study. *Pediatrics*, *107*, 344–350.

Michel, B. A., Lane, N. E., Bjorkengren, A., Bloch, D. A., & Fries, J. F. (1992). Impact of running on lumbar bone density: A 5-year longitudinal study. *Journal of Rheumatology, 19*, 1759–1763.

Mitchell, J. A., Chesi, A., Elci, O., McCormack, S. S., Roy, S. M., Kalkwarf, H. J., et al. (2016). Physical activity benefits the skeleton of children genetically predisposed to lower bone density in adulthood. *Journal of Bone Mineral Research*, *31*, 1504–1512.

National Center for Health Statistics (1974). Body dimensions and proportions: White and Negro children 6–11 years, United States. *Vital and Health Statistics*, ser. 11, no. 143.

National Center for Health Statistics (2012). Anthropometric reference data for children and adults: United States, 2007–2010. *Vital and Health Statistics*, ser. 11, no. 252.

National Institutes of Health (2018). Aging changes in body shape. *MedlinePlus*. Retrieved from https://medlineplus.gov/ency/article/003998.htm.

Ostyn, M., Simons, J., Beunen, G., Renson, R., & Van Gerven, D. (Eds.). (1980). *Motor development of Belgian secondary schoolboys.* Leuven, Belgium: Leuven University Press.

Philippaerts, R. M., Vaeyeng, R., Janssens, M., Renterghern, B. V., Matthys, D., Craen, R., et al. (2006). The relationship between peak height velocity and physical performance in youth soccer players. *Journal of Sports Sciences, 24*, 221–230.

Quatman-Yates, C. C., Quatman, C. E., Meszaros, A. J., Paterno, M. V., & Hewett, T. E. (2012). A systematic review of sensorimotor function during adolescence: A developmental stage of increase motor awkwardness? *British Journal of Sports Medicine*, *46*, 649–655.

Roche, A. F. (1979). The measurement of skeletal maturation. In F. E. Johnston, A. F. Roche, & C. Susanne (Eds.), *Human physical growth and maturation*. New York: Plenum Press.

Roche, A. F. (1992). *Growth, maturation and body composition: The Fels longitudinal study 1929–1991*. Cambridge: Cambridge University Press.

Roche, A. F., Chumlea, W. C., & Thissen, D. (1988). *Assessing the skeletal maturity of the hand-wrist: Fels method.* Springfield, IL: Thomas.

Roche, A. F., & Himes, J. H. (1980). Incremental growth charts. *American Journal of Clinical Nutrition, 33*, 2041–2052.

Roche, A. F., & Malina, R. M. (Eds.) (1983). *Manual of physical status and performance in childhood.* Vol. 1. New York: Plenum Press.

Roche, A. F., & Sun, S. S. (2003). *Human growth: Assessment and interpretation*. Cambridge: Cambridge University Press.

Roche, A. F., Wainer, H., & Thissen, D. (1975). Predicting adult stature for individuals. *Pediatrics, 3*, 1–115.

Rooney, R. L., & Schauberger, C. W. (2002). Excess pregnancy weight gain and long-term obesity: One decade later. *Obstetrics and Gynecology, 100*, 245–252.

Sheldon, W. H. (1940). *The varieties of human physique*. New York: Harper & Row.

Shirley, M. M. (1931). *The first two years: A study of twenty-five babies*. Minneapolis, MN: University of Minnesota Press.

Silva, A. M. (2019). Structural and functional body components in athletic health and performance phenotypes. *European Journal of Clinical Nutrition, 73*, 215–224.

Sundgot-Borgen, J., & Torstveit, M. K. (2004). Prevalence of eating disorders in elite athletes is higher than in the general population. *Clinical Journal of Sports Medicine, 14*, 25–32.

Tanner, J. M. (1990). *Fetus into man*. Cambridge, MA: Harvard University Press.

Tanner, J. M., Whitehouse, R. H., Marshall, W. A., Healy, M. J., & Goldstein, H. (1975). *Assessment of skeletal maturity and prediction of adult height (TW 2 method)*. New York: Academic Press.

Tawa, N., & Louw, Q. (2018). Biomechanical factors associated with running economy and performance of elite Kenyan distance runners: A systematic review. *Journal of Bodywork and Movement Therapies, 22*, 1–10.

Todd, T. W. (1937). *Atlas of skeletal maturation*. St. Louis, MO: Mosby.

Topor, L. S., Feldman, H. A., Bauchner, H., & Cohen, L. D. (2010). Variation in methods of predicting adult height in children with idiopathic short stature. *Pediatrics, 126*, 938–944.

Toro-Ramos, T., Paley, C., Pi-Sunyer, F., & Gallagher, D. (2015). Body composition during fetal development and infancy through the age of 5 years. *European Journal of Clinical Nutrition, 69*, 1279–1289.

Tucci, J., Carpenter, D., Graves, J., Pollock, M. L., Felheim, R., & Mananquil, R. (1991). Interday reliability of bone mineral density measurements using dual energy X-ray absorptiometry. *Medicine and Science in Sports and Exercise, 23*, S115.

Wales, J., & Taitz, L. (1992). Patterns of growth in abused children. In M. Hernandez & J. Argente (Eds.), *Human growth: Basic and clinical aspects*. Amsterdam: Elsevier Science Publishers.

Wright, N. C., Looker, A. C., Saag, K. G., Randall, S., & Dawson-Hughes, B. (2014). The recent prevalence of osteoporosis and low bone mass in the United States based on bone mineral density at the femoral neck or lumbar spine. *Journal of Bone Mineral Research, 29*, 2520–2526.

7 PHYSIOLOGICAL CHANGES: HEALTH-RELATED PHYSICAL FITNESS

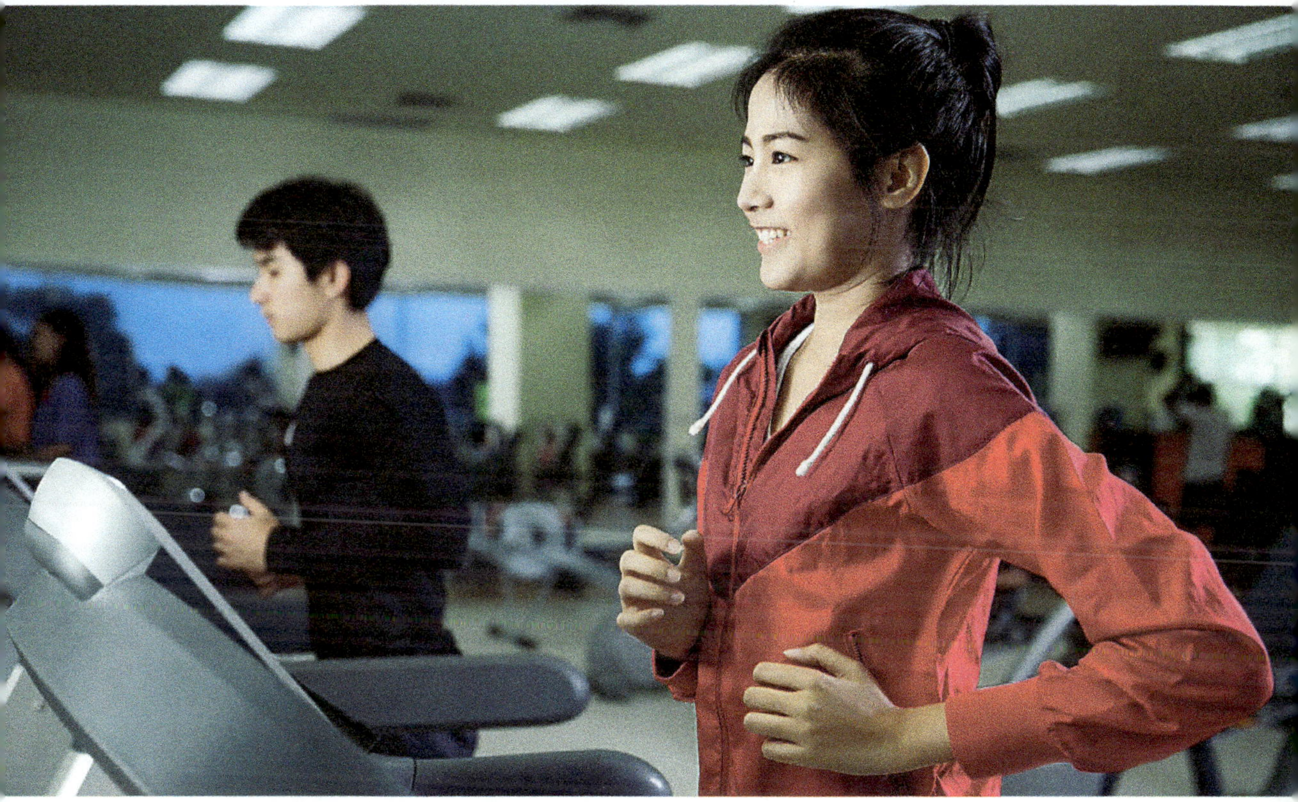

Chapter Objectives

From the information presented in this chapter, you will be able to

- Describe how the components of cardiorespiratory fitness change across the human lifespan and how these changes are influenced by increases in physical activity
- Describe the developmental changes in muscular strength/muscular endurance across the human lifespan and how these changes are influenced by maintaining an active lifestyle
- Describe the developmental changes in flexibility across the human lifespan and how these changes are influenced by participating in a flexibility training program
- Describe the developmental changes in adipose tissue across the human lifespan, explain the prevalence of overweight and obesity, and identify the influence of being overweight or obese on both motor development and motor performance
- Identify gender differences in each component of health-related physical fitness
- Describe the role of interactive technology in promoting physical activity

Within the last three decades, what is commonly referred to as health-related or physiological fitness has become a focus of increasing concern. The primary thrust behind this movement is the widespread notion that U.S. children and youth are less fit today than children of 45 years ago. In addition, results from the most recent National Health and Nutrition Examination Survey (NHANES, 2015–2016) indicate an increase in the prevalence of obesity among children, adolescents, and adults in the United States (Hales, Carroll, Fryar, & Ogden, 2017). This should come as no surprise since only 22.9 percent of U.S. adults between 18 and 64 years were found to have met the U.S. Department of Health and Human Services' 2008 National Guidelines for both aerobic and muscular strength activity (Blackwell, & Clarke, 2018). Similarly, more than 80 percent of adolescents fail to engage in adequate aerobic activity (U.S. Department of Health and Human Services, 2018).

Because of the links established between physical activity and health, prestigious organizations now stress the importance of maintaining an active lifestyle. The *Physical Activity Guidelines for Americans* (U.S. Department of Health and Human Services, 2018) emphasize the importance of engaging in regular physical activity throughout the entire lifespan in order to reduce the risk of many adverse health outcomes. A copy of this milestone publication, which includes the guidelines for children and adolescents, adults, older adults, women who are pregnant, and individuals with disabilities, is available at https://health.gov/paguidelines/second-edition/pdf/Physical_Activity_Guidelines_2nd_edition.pdf. Clearly, maintaining an active lifestyle is linked to good health. In fact, the World Health Organization now recognizes physical inactivity as the fourth leading risk factor for global mortality (World Health Organization, 2010).

The most frequently identified components that make up health-related fitness include cardiorespiratory endurance, muscular strength and endurance, flexibility, and body composition. This chapter examines each of these components and changes to them that occur over the lifespan. We look at the evolution of each, paying particular attention to how an active lifestyle affects them. In addition, we examine both laboratory data and field-test performance data.

CARDIORESPIRATORY FITNESS

Cardiorespiratory fitness is the efficiency of the heart, lungs, and vascular system in delivering oxygen to the working muscle tissues so that prolonged physical work can be maintained. A person's ability to deliver oxygen to the working muscles is affected by many physiological parameters, including heart rate, stroke volume, cardiac output, and maximal oxygen consumption. Here we examine changes that occur in each parameter as a result of maturation, aging, and physical training.

Heart Rate

Heart rate (HR), the number of times the heart beats each minute, is a physiological parameter that undergoes much change during the lifespan. The fetal heart begins to beat about the fourth prenatal week. Characteristically, fetal HR is rapid and frequently irregular.

At rest, children's HRs are consistently higher than adults'. In fact, the newborn infant's HR averages about 130 beats/min, ranging between 120 and 140 beats/min. With time (age), however, this resting heart rate progressively decelerates. For example, by 1 year of age, the average resting HR will have declined by an average of 40 beats/min. This trend is evident until late adolescence, when young men exhibit an average HR of 57–60 beats/min and young women average between 62 and 63 beats/min (Malina, Bouchard, & Bar-Or, 2004). Thus, resting HR can be expected to decline by about 50 percent from birth to maturity. The average HR among 20-year-old men and women averages 75 and 79 beats/min, respectively. Thereafter, there is little change in resting HR until around 60 years of age, when the HR again decreases slightly.

There is a linear relationship between physical work and HR. That is, up to a point, increases in workload increase HR. During labor contractions, fetal HR frequently exceeds 200 beats/min. Furthermore, newborn crying, a form of physical work, induces rates greater than 170 beats/min. In preadolescent children, HR responses to submaximal work decline with age.

Unlike submaximal HR, which declines with age, maximal HR does not decline until after maturity. The maximal HR of both children and adolescents is from 195 to 220 beats/min. For young adult men and women, the maximal HR generally peaks at values just under 200 beats/min. Maximal heart rate declines at approximately 0.87–1.02 beats/min/year of age, and the rate of this decline is independent of gender (Ozemek, Whaley, Finch, & Kaminsky, 2017). However, maintaining a high to moderate level of cardiorespiratory fitness may slow this decline (Ozemek, Whaley, Finch, & Kaminsky, 2016).

The following formula provides a general estimate of maximal HR in young and middle-aged adult populations:

$$\text{Maximal HR} = 220 - \text{age (years)}$$

However, evidence suggests that as individuals age, maximal HR is more accurately predicted by the following equation (Tanaka, Monahan, & Seals, 2001):

$$HR_{max} = 208 - 0.7 \times \text{age (years)}$$

Example: Calculate the predicted HR_{max} of a 70-year-old male.

$$HR_{max} = 208 - (0.7 \times 70)$$

$$HR_{max} = 159 \text{ beats/min}$$

Researchers believe that the decline in HR with age is attributable to a decrease in myocardial (heart) sensitivity to catecholamines, prolonged diastolic filling time, and changes in the contractile properties of the cardiac muscle (Dai, Hummel, Salazar, et al., 2015).

Stroke Volume

With each contraction of the heart, a certain volume of blood, called **stroke volume** (SV), is ejected from the left ventricle into general circulation via the aorta. The size of the stroke volume is limited by many factors, including heart size, contractile force of the myocardial tissue, vascular resistance to blood flow, and venous return (the rate at which blood is returned to the right side of the heart).

At all levels of physical work, SV is substantially lower in children than in adults, most likely because of the child's smaller heart, which partly explains children's need for higher HRs. At birth, SV is only 3–4 ml per ventricular contraction. This value increases 10-fold by adolescence, to about 40 ml, and it remains quite stable until the adolescence growth spurt, when it rapidly accelerates to about 60 ml at rest (Malina et al., 2004). In the typical untrained male adult, the SV is usually between 60 and 100 ml/beat. This range is significantly elevated in highly trained people. Even at rest, the aerobically trained person's SV is 100–120 ml/beat.

Maximal SV is achieved during submaximal work, somewhere between 40 percent and 60 percent (mean = 50%) of aerobic power. A further increase in workload is not likely to increase SV significantly. During exercise, untrained men can expect to attain an SV of 100–120 ml/beat. Conversely, highly trained men are capable of obtaining average values of 150–170 ml/beat. In contrast, maximal SV in untrained and trained women is generally between 80 and 100 ml/beat and between 100 and 120 ml/beat, respectively. Nevertheless, at all levels of work, SV is about 25 percent lower in women, on average (McArdle, Katch, & Katch, 2006).

Like most other physiological parameters, age can affect SV. A person's SV at rest can decline by as much as 30 percent between the ages of 25 and 85. Older individuals who perform aerobic exercise regularly can minimize this decline in SV because regular aerobic training increases blood volume, reduces vascular resistance, and increases heart preload, all of which help maintain a higher SV.

Cardiac Output

Cardiac output is the amount of blood that can be pumped out of the heart in 1 minute. Thus, cardiac output is the product of heart rate and stroke volume. Cardiac output is less in children than in adults, for both resting and exercising states. Although children are capable of obtaining a higher exercise HR than adults, their elevated HR is not enough to compensate for the marked difference in stroke volume.

At rest, adults have a cardiac output of approximately 5 l/min. With the onset of exercise, cardiac output rises in both children and adults until it reaches a new steady state. Two of the most important factors affecting ultimate maximal cardiac output are level of physical condition and age. The untrained adult generally achieves a maximal cardiac output of 20–25 l/min; a trained adult can achieve a maximal cardiac output 10 l/min greater than can the untrained adult.

Because both HR and SV decrease with age, resting cardiac output does, as well. Specifically, there is a 58 percent reduction between the ages of 25 and 85 in the amount of blood the heart can pump in a given unit of time. Thus, resting cardiac output, on average, declines approximately 1 percent per year after age 25. There is a somewhat similar pattern for maximal cardiac output: cardiac function typically declines 20–30 percent by age 65, but like other cardiorespiratory parameters, this decline can be minimized through regular aerobic exercise.

Maximal Oxygen Consumption

An increase in the level of physical work brings a corresponding increased need for oxygen among the active muscles. Thus, the human body's ability to sustain physical work for extended periods is directly related to its ability to transport oxygen to the working muscle tissue. The largest amount of oxygen that a human can consume at the tissue level is the **maximal oxygen consumption (VO_2max)**. This physiological measure is considered the best single measure of **physical working capacity**.

Abundant information is available about VO_2max consumption in adults and older children, but we have little data on children younger than 6 years. It is difficult to study this population because it is hard to motivate young children to an all-out effort. Nevertheless, several researchers have undertaken the challenge of obtaining data on VO_2max consumption in this population. Mrzena and Macek (1978) required two groups of children between 3 and 5 years of age to walk or run on a treadmill. Group 1 performed for 5 minutes at each of the following speeds: 3, 4, and 5 km/hour. In contrast, group 2 performed at 4 km/hour, but instead of increasing treadmill speed, the researchers increased the treadmill's grade by 5 degrees every 5 minutes until the treadmill was at a 15-degree grade. In group 1, the highest oxygen consumption value a child attained was 22.06 ± 4.7 milliliters per kilogram of body weight per minute (ml/kg/min). Oxygen consumption was higher in the second group, where the highest value attained was 28.7 ± 4.84 ml/kg/min.

Results involving children older than 6 years are fairly consistent. The VO_2max for boys is fairly constant during childhood and the adolescent years. Boys generally exhibit a spurt in maximal oxygen consumption at puberty, but it is believed that this increase is more directly related to increases in body size than to a true increase in oxygen extraction. In fact, Rowland's (1996) classic review of the literature found support for the idea that maximal oxygen uptake closely parallels the dimensions of cardiorespiratory organ growth. For example, for boys between 8 and 12 years of age, maximal aerobic capacity rises about 49 percent. During this same period, the average weight of the lungs increases 58 percent, lung vital capacity improves 48 percent, and left ventricular volume increases 52 percent. This phenomenon raises an interesting point: although older children obtain higher VO_2max values than do younger children, the discrepancy in values is no longer as great when we use body weight to standardize the measures.

This point is apparent when we compare the VO_2max of young boys to that of young girls. Young boys evidence much higher values than do young girls when we compare absolute values between the genders without considering body weight. However, when we standardize the scores based on body weight, girls' working capacity is practically the same as young boys', at approximately 50 ml/kg/min (Armstrong, 2006).

Girls' decline in VO_2max early in life is most likely caused by the female's increase in body fat at maturation, lower blood hemoglobin concentrations at puberty, and lesser degree of large-muscle development in the lower extremities. Table 7.1 gives the aerobic capacity of U.S. adolescents.

Table 7.1 Aerobic capacity of U.S. adolescents (ml/kg/min)

Age	Boys		Girls	
	50th %	95th %	50th %	95th %
12	42.3	59.2	39.0	55.1
13	43.4	60.6	38.6	53.9
14	44.5	62.0	38.3	52.8
15	45.7	63.4	38.0	52.1
16	46.3	64.1	37.8	52.0
17	46.4	64.1	37.7	52.9
18	46.5	64.1	37.4	53.8

Source: Data from Eisenmann, Laurson, & Welk (2011).

With age, the body's ability to acquire and deliver oxygen to the working tissues is altered, reducing physical work capacity. The rate of decline in VO_2max is approximately 10 percent per decade between 20 and 79 years of age (Kaminsky, Arena, & Myers, 2015). Thus, a person's physical work capacity at 79 years old is about one-half of what the person attained nearly 60 years earlier. This loss of aerobic power is caused by many factors, including an increase in fat tissue and a concomitant decrease in lean muscle tissue, decreased cardiac output, and a decrease in physical activity. Later in the chapter we discuss how an active lifestyle can alter or delay the decline in VO_2max.

Table 7.2 gives the aerobic capacity (ml/kg/min) of men and women between 20 and 79 years of age. Note that the table contains two sets of data. Data presented in parenthesis were derived from the Fitness Registry and the Importance of Exercise: A National Data Base (FRIEND). FRIEND represents the first cardiorespiratory fitness reference database that was obtained from a directly measured cardiorespiratory exercise test. The other database was obtained from the widely cited Cooper Institute and was derived through the use of an estimated cardiorespiratory fitness value calculated from treadmill speed and grade.

Table 7.2 Aerobic capacity of men and women (ml/kg/min)

Age	Men		Women	
	50th %	95th %	50th %	95th %
20–29	43.9 (48.0)	55.5 (66.3)	37.8 (37.6)	49.6 (56.0)
30–39	42.4 (42.4)	54.1 (59.8)	36.7 (30.2)	47.4 (45.8)
40–49	40.1 (37.8)	52.5 (55.6)	34.5 (26.7)	45.3 (41.7)
50–59	37.1 (32.6)	49.0 (50.7)	31.4 (23.4)	41.0 (35.9)
60–69	33.8 (28.2)	45.7 (43.0)	28.8 (20.0)	37.8 (29.4)
70–79	30.9 (24.4)	43.9 (39.7)	27.6 (18.3)	37.2 (24.1)

Source: Reference values in parenthesis from the Fitness Registry and the Importance of Exercise: A National Data Base (Kaminsky, Arena, & Myers, 2015). Reference values not in parenthesis are from the Cooper Institute (2009).

Physical Activity and Cardiorespiratory Fitness in Childhood

Our understanding of the effects of physical activity on cardiorespiratory fitness in young children is both fragmented and limited. Also, many findings are contradictory, most likely because of the different conditioning protocols among studies and the use of a host of various methodological factors. For instance, when researchers study the effects of long-term training, they must distinguish between training effects and those effects caused primarily by the natural growth and maturation process. Researchers have recognized that many of the reported changes following physical training occur naturally through maturation, whereas others actually do result from the training. For example, lower resting and submaximal HRs are known to be byproducts of physical training. Moreover, many physiological parameters naturally decline with age. Because of the difficulty of interpreting research results, observed effects should be viewed as occurring *with* conditioning and training, not necessarily *as a result of* conditioning or training.

Rowland (1985) critically analyzed the research literature regarding aerobic responses to endurance training in preadolescent children. After reviewing the eight available studies, he reported gains in VO_2max ranging from 7–26 percent, with a mean gain of 14 percent. The data from these studies appear to indicate that adult training protocols are effective in improving aerobic capacity in children. Mandigout, Melin, Lecoq, and colleagues (2002) came to the same conclusion when they found that 13 weeks of aerobic training with two sessions/week for 15–20 minutes at an intensity of 80 percent failed to improve VO_2max in prepubertal children of 10–11 years of age. However, when frequency and duration were increased to align with adult recommendations (3 days/week for 25 to 35 minutes), the children's VO_2max improved by 7 percent on average.

A growing amount of other evidence, however, leads us to question the benefit of endurance training for improving aerobic capacity in preadolescent children. For example, Payne and Morrow (1993) performed a meta-analysis in an attempt to shed light on this important question regarding the effects of exercise on VO_2max in preadolescent children. Their findings were based on the analysis of 28 studies resulting in 70 effect sizes. In a pretest/posttest design, the subjects improved VO_2max by only about 2 ml/kg/min, or a 4 percent improvement. These results indicated that changes in VO_2max in preadolescent children are small to moderate.

Even though evidence does not support the value of endurance training in preadolescent children, some experts argue that training does improve performance. Most believe that training can improve performance by

CARDIORESPIRATORY ENDURANCE FIELD-TEST DATA ON CHILDREN AND ADOLESCENTS

In 2012, the cardiorespiratory fitness of American children and adolescents was assessed through a nationwide sample as part of the long-standing National Health and Nutrition Examination Survey. Unlike previous nationwide samples, the NHANES National Youth Fitness Survey (NYFS) employed a criterion-referenced standard based on the healthy fitness zones associated with the FITNESSGRAM (see Chapter 16). Based on this assessment, we can say the following regarding the current state of cardiorespiratory fitness in American children and adolescents (Gahche, Fakhouri, Carroll, Burt, et al., 2014):

- In 2012, 42.2 percent of American youth aged 12–15 years had an adequate level of cardiorespiratory fitness.
- The number of youth who exhibited an adequate level of cardiorespiratory fitness decreased as body weight status increased.
- The percentage of youth who exhibited an adequate level of cardiorespiratory fitness decreased from 52.4 percent in 1999/2000 to 42.2 percent in 2012.
- The percentage of youth who exhibited an adequate level of cardiorespiratory fitness did not differ by race and Hispanic origin, or by family income-to-poverty ratio.

improving mechanical efficiency. For example, training can improve mechanical aspects of a child's running style without an associated rise in aerobic capacity, with the end result being better run times (Indranil, 2014).

Nevertheless, for health reasons, it is recommended that children between 6 and 17 years of age should be involved in 60 minutes of moderate or vigorous physical activity daily and that at least three of those days should involve vigorous activity (U.S. Department of Health and Human Services, 2018).

Physical Activity and Cardiorespiratory Fitness in Adulthood

The effects of aerobic exercise on the cardiorespiratory system of young and middle-aged adults has been well documented. Authorities agree that to attain substantial health benefits, a person should perform at least 150–300 minutes of moderate-intensity exercise per week, or 75–150 minutes per week of vigorous-intensity exercise (U.S. Department of Health and Human Services, 2018). Such a program will increase physical work capacity. As a result of aerobic exercise, during submaximal work, SV will increase, HR will decrease, cardiac output will increase, and VO_2max will increase; in addition, HR recovery following physical work will be faster (Farrell, Joyner, & Caiozzo, 2011). Not only has aerobic exercise been found to influence the above-mentioned physiological variables, but it has also been found to protect against diseases typically acquired in late adulthood. For example, higher levels of cardiorespiratory fitness in middle-aged adults has been associated with a decreased risk of stroke (Pandey, Patel, Willis, et al., 2016), a 16 percent lower risk of depression, and a 56 percent lower risk of cardiovascular mortality following a diagnosis of depression (Willis, Leonard,

Barlow, et al., 2018), a lower risk of both lung and colorectal cancer (Lakoski, Willis, Barlow, et al., 2015), and a 32–35 percent lower risk of all-cause mortality (Saint-Maurice, Coughlan, Kelly, et al., 2019). Additionally, findings from the Cooper Center longitudinal study suggest that higher levels of cardiorespiratory fitness appear to help mediate body mass index associated risks in middle age adults (Pandey, Cornwell, Willis, et al., 2017).

Frequently asked questions regarding exercise training in late adulthood include, "What effect does a physical exercise training program have on the physical work capacities of these individuals?" and "Can long-term training offset the decline in physical work capacity that comes with aging and sedentary behavior?" We do know that the rate of decline in physical work capacity in the general adult population has been established as about 1 percent/year between 25 and 75 years of age. Obviously, not all individuals age at the same rate. Take, for example, the athletic feats shown in Table 7.3. These performances were accomplished by individuals participating in the U.S. National Senior Games in 2017.

Most authorities believe that what makes the physical performance of these individuals so different from that of the general population is their active lifestyle. It has been suggested that as much as 50 percent of the functional declines that mediate physical performance are attributable to disuse rather than aging. For example, in a longitudinal study, Kasch, Boyer, Van Camp, and associates (1990) found only a 13 percent decline in VO_2max in men 45–68 years old who had maintained an active lifestyle over the previous 18 years. However, a somewhat similar group of men (52–70 years old) who did not exercise showed a 41 percent decline in maximal oxygen consumption during the period under study.

Older individuals often wonder whether it is too late to establish a regimen of aerobic activity. Shephard "has projected that commencement of regular fitness training at the time of retirement may delay the age at which environmental demands exceed physical capabilities (i.e., the age of dependency) by as much as 8 years" (cited in Stones & Kozma, 1985). Furthermore, Shephard (1987) suggested that if an older individual increases her or his VO_2max by approximately 20 percent, it "offers the equivalent of 20 years of rejuvenation—a benefit that can be matched by no other treatment or lifestyle change" (p. 5). Shephard's earlier view regarding the importance of maintaining an active lifestyle has recently been supported by scientific evidence. More specifically, Saint-Maurice and colleagues (2019) studied the association between patterns of leisure-time physical activity (LTPA) during adolescence, early-, middle-, and late-adulthood and all-cause or cause-specific mortality. This cohort study, which involved 315,059 subjects, found that maintaining LTPA from adolescence through late-adulthood was associated with a 36–39 percent lower risk of all-cause mortality. Perhaps most important, the study found that

Table 7.3 Selected winning times for the 1500 m run for men and women at the Summer National Senior Games, 2017 (minutes)

	Age (Years)							
	50–54	55–59	60–64	65–69	70–74	75–79	80–84	85–89
Men	4:31	4:42	4:59	5:21	5:21	6:16	8:14	8:48
Women	6:10	6:00	6:05	6:02	6:38	8:10	8:26	14:01

Source: NSGA (2017).

those individuals who did not become physically active until later in adulthood (ages 40–61 years) witnessed a somewhat similar reduction in all-cause mortality (32–35 percent). In summary, individuals who can maintain an active lifestyle throughout middle and late adulthood may slow down the rate of deterioration, improve their aerobic capacity, and lower their risk of all-cause mortality.

MUSCULAR STRENGTH

Minimal **muscular strength** is important because the contraction of skeletal muscle makes human movement possible. We use the term minimal muscular strength, but researchers to date have not been able to qualify this term. In fact, to do so is impossible because each human movement requires different degrees of strength. For instance, the 14-month-old toddler possesses enough lower-extremity strength to walk but lacks the strength needed to propel the body through space, a requirement of running. People, regardless of age, who lack the necessary strength needed to launch the body from a supporting surface are said to be **earthbound.** This inability to project the body through space limits the number of ways a person can move in the environment, which is why earthbound children's ability to acquire many of the fundamental movement patterns is frequently delayed. Furthermore, older children and adults whose movement is restricted by inadequate levels of muscular strength generally find themselves leading a sedentary life. In brief, muscular strength is needed for the execution of all motor tasks.

Defining and Measuring Muscular Strength

Strength is the ability to exert muscular force. This muscular force can be exerted under various conditions. A muscular force exerted against an immovable object, with no or very little change in the length of the exercised muscle, is called **static** or **isometric.** A muscular force exerted against a movable object, with a change in the length of the exercised muscle, is called **dynamic.** Pushing against a wall is an example of static force; lifting a barbell is a dynamic force.

Age-Related Changes in Muscular Strength

Little data is available regarding strength in preschool children. However, many investigators have examined this component of fitness in populations older than 5 years. Most frequently, the dependent variable in these studies has been grip strength. This measure of static force production is used more frequently than any other test of muscular strength because it is easy to administer and is reliable.

Studies examining changes in grip strength during childhood and the adolescent years are consistent in their findings. A review of the literature by Keogh and Sugden (1985) revealed that grip strength in boys increased 393 percent from 7 to 17 years of age. Grip strength was assessed in the recent NHANES NYFS (Ervin, Wang, Fryar, et al., 2013). See the accompanying box, p. 204.

Gender differences in muscular strength become most apparent after puberty. In boys, puberty is associated with the introduction of the male sex hormones, which influence muscularity. During this time of development, boys become leaner and young girls begin to develop more body fat. Prior to adolescence, muscle weight is about 27 percent of total body weight, but after sexual maturity, muscle development increases to about 40 percent of total body weight (Malina et al., 2004). In adulthood, even when body size is taken into consideration, women are not generally as strong as men. Overall, women's total maximal absolute body strength is about 63.5 percent of

MUSCULAR STRENGTH/ENDURANCE FIELD TEST DATA ON CHILDREN AND ADOLESCENTS

As mentioned previously, muscular strength was assessed as part of the NHANES NYFS (Ervin et al., 2013). In this survey children aged from 6–11 years and 12–15 years were assessed. The assessment included measures of core strength (plank test), two measures of upper-body strength (grip strength, modified pull-ups), and lower-body strength (knee extension test). Table 7.4 presents the data from this nationwide survey. The key findings are as follows:

- There were no significant differences by gender in core, lower-body, or upper-body measures of strength for the 6–11-year-old boys and girls. However, the 12–15-year-old boys had higher values than the adolescent girls on all measures of strength.
- The adolescent boys and girls had higher scores than the younger boys and girls on the core lower-body strength measures and on upper-body strength, as measured by grip strength.
- The adolescent boys completed more modified pull-ups than did the younger boys. There was no significant difference in the number of modified pull-ups completed between the adolescent and younger girls. See Figure 7.1 for the modified pull-up assessment apparatus.

Table 7.4 Muscular strength in U.S. children and adolescents

Test	6–11 Years		12–15 Years	
	Boys	Girls	Boys	Girls
Plank	60 sec	61 sec	91 sec	77 sec
Knee extension	43 lb	44 lb	86 lb	77 lb
Modified pull-up	5	4	10	4
Grip strength	71 lb	68 lb	143 lb	116 lb

Source: Ervin et al. (2013).

men's strength (McArdle et al., 2006). The interested reader is referred to the work of Fleck and Kraemer (2014) for a detailed analysis of gender differences in both absolute and relative strength.

During early and middle adulthood, grip strength remains relatively constant. Men between 25 and 45 years exhibit an average grip strength of about 54 kg. However, during the next 44 years, grip strength declines significantly. This association of aging with loss of muscle mass and, therefore, muscle strength appears to occur in two stages. First, a rather slow regression in muscle mass of about 10 percent occurs between 25 and 50 years of age. The rate of loss accelerates between 50 and 89 years of age, resulting in an additional loss of about 36 percent. Thus, men lose more than one-half of their muscular grip strength by 85–89 years of age. In comparison, women have been found to lose approximately 58 percent of their muscular grip strength between 50 and 89 years of age (Roush, Gombold, & Bay, 2017).

Muscular Strength Training

Any discussion regarding the effect of resistance training on the development of

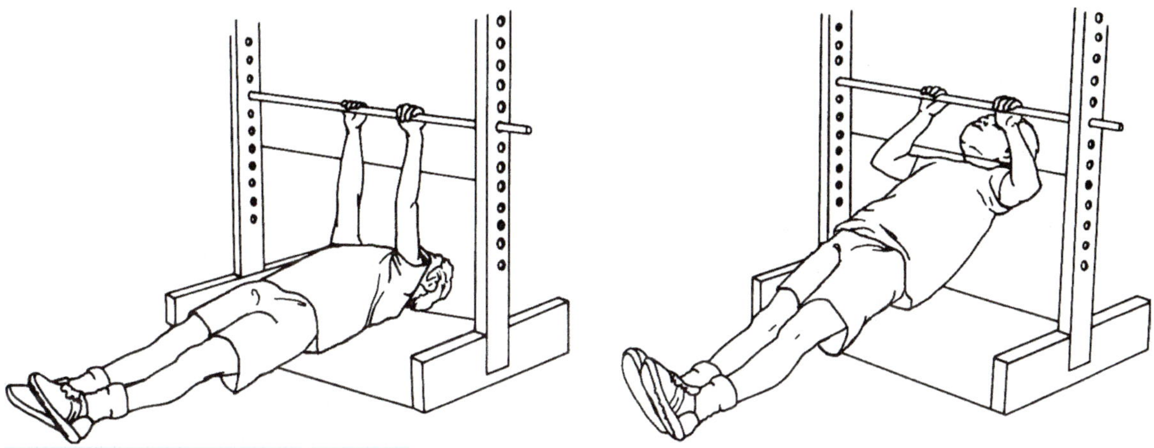

Figure 7.1 Modified pull-up apparatus

muscular strength must account for differences in training outcomes attributable to maturity level. For this reason, we divide our discussion on trainability into three sections: prepubescence, adolescence/early and middle adulthood, and late adulthood.

Prepubescence

Controversy has existed regarding the use of resistance training for the purpose of developing muscular strength in prepubescent populations. This controversy involves three questions. First, can prepubescent children significantly increase their muscular strength through participation in a resistance-training program? Second, if gains in muscular strength are possible, does this increase in strength enhance skilled athletic performance? Finally, does the benefit of increased strength outweigh the potential of sustaining injury (e.g., injury to growth plates) during participation in a resistance-training program?

Gains in muscular strength from training. The first question arises because popular belief suggests that without a sufficient level of circulating **testosterone,** significant gains in muscular strength are not possible. This belief was first reinforced when Vrijens (1978) found no significant strength gains in 16 prepubescent individuals following an 8-week training program. However, other studies have reported significant strength gains in prepubescent subjects following participation in resistance-training programs (Faigenbaum, Milliken, Loud, et al., 2002; Faigenbaum, O'Connell, Glover, et al., 2000; Faigenbaum, Westcott, Loud, & Long, 1999; Faigenbaum, Westcott, Micheli, et al., 1996; Faigenbaum, Zaichkowsky, Westcott, et al., 1993; Isaacs, Pohlman, & Craig, 1994; Ozmun, Mikesky, & Surburg, 1994; Stahle, Roberts, Davis, & Rybicki, 1995).

For example, Falk and Tenenbaum (1996) reviewed the professional literature regarding resistance training in girls and boys under age 12 and 13, respectively. Of the 28 studies identified, only three reported nonsignificant effects following resistance training. A majority of the studies found increases in strength following a resistance training program, in the range of 13.7–29.6 percent. In a meta-analysis regarding resistance training in both children and youth, Payne, Morrow, Johnson, and Dalton (1997) identified 28 studies yielding 252 effect sizes. Like Falk and Tenenbaum, Payne and colleagues concluded that children and youth can acquire a significant increase in both muscular strength and endurance as a result of participating in resistance training.

Gains in strength and improved athletic performance. Because most of the recent professional literature suggests that prepubescent individuals are capable of significantly increasing their strength with resistance training, the next logical question is whether these strength gains are accompanied by improved athletic performance. Findings from a meta-analysis observed that resistance training was effective in enhancing motor skill performance (running, jumping, throwing) and in fact, younger children showed greater gains in performance than adolescents (Behringer, Vom Heede, Matthews, & Mester, 2011). This finding underscores the importance of implementing a progressive program of resistance training in early life when children possess the highest levels of neural plasticity as explained in more detail in the section entitled Mechanisms of Increasing Muscular Strength on p. 209 (Lloyd, Faigenbaum, Stone, et al., 2014).

Safety of strength training. As mentioned previously, there has been much concern regarding the safety of strength training for prepubescent individuals. This concern has prompted such prestigious organizations as the American Academy of Pediatrics (2008), the UK Strength and Conditioning Association (Lloyd, Faigenbaum, Stone, et al., 2014), as well as the NSCA (Faigenbaum, Kraemer, Blimkie, et al., 2009) to publish position statements regarding strength training for prepubescents.

A clear distinction must be made among resistance training, weight lifting or power lifting, and body building. **Resistance training** involves the use of various resistance exercises to enhance physical fitness or to increase muscular strength, muscular endurance, and power for sports participation. In contrast, **weight lifting** and **power lifting** are considered sports that involve performing maximum lifts, including the snatch, clean and jerk, squat, bench press, and dead lift. **Body building** is also considered a competitive sport, in which participants use resistance training to develop muscle size, body symmetry, and muscle definition. All three associations now recognize that resistance training and even weight lifting (Lloyd, Faigenbaum, Stone, et al., 2014) can benefit the prepubescent individual if it is conducted within the framework of other established guidelines (see Table 7.5). In fact, it is now recognized that youth strength training may actually lay the foundation for injury prevention among at-risk youth. Those most at risk include: the physically inactive, early specializers in youth sports, and young girls. One clinical review has found a 68 percent injury risk reduction among youth who participated in resistance training (Zwolski, Quatman-Yates, & Paterno, 2017).

Some frequently ask, "At what age is training with maximal lifting acceptable?" The United States Powerlifting Association and USA Weightlifting recommend maximal lifting at 14 years of age. Yet the answer to this question is not so simple because chronological age is not an acceptable indicator of biological maturity. Rather than using chronological age, it has been suggested that boys and girls not be allowed to perform maximal lifts until they reach a Tanner stage 5 level of development (see Chapter 6). At this level of developmental maturity, peak height velocity (PHV) will have occurred; therefore, the likelihood of injury to the epiphyses (growth plates) will be reduced. In fact, one meta-analysis of maturation-related influences on strength gains in boys concluded that strength gains in boys is greatest during and after PHV (Moran, Sandercock, Ramirez-Campillo, et al., 2016). Nevertheless, research has found that 1 RM (repetition maximum) testing in young boys and girls (6.2–12.3 years of age) is safe when conducted under appropriate adult supervision (Faigenbaum, Milliken, & Westcott, 2003).

Table 7.5 Selected weight-resistance guidelines for children

1.	Before beginning a strength program, the child should have a physical examination if he or she is not already apparently healthy.
2.	The child must be emotionally mature enough to follow directions from a coach.
3.	The program should be supervised by certified instructors knowledgeable in pediatric strength training.
4.	Fifty to 80 percent of the child's training should be in activities other than strength training.
5.	The exercise session should include 10 to 15 minutes of general warm-up exercises, followed by one or more light to moderate specific warm-up sets on the chosen resistance exercises. A 15-minute cool-down should follow each session.
6.	The session should start with one set of several upper- and lower-body exercises that focus on the major muscle groups. Single- and multi-joint exercises should be included in the training program. Beginning with relatively light loads (e.g., 12 to 15 RM*) will allow for appropriate adjustments to be made.
7.	After the child can accomplish 15 repetitions in good form, weight can be increased by 5 percent to 10 percent.
8.	Progression may also be achieved by gradually increasing the number of sets, exercises, and training sessions per week. Depending on the goal of the training program (e.g., strength or local muscular endurance), 1 to 3 sets of 8 to 15 repetitions performed on two or three nonconsecutive days each week is recommended.
9.	The child should receive instruction regarding correct lifting technique, training guidelines, and spotting procedures. Whenever a new exercise is introduced, the child should start with a relatively light weight, or even a broomstick (no load), in order to learn the correct technique.
10.	All exercises should be carried out through the full range of motion.
11.	Emphasis should be on dynamic concentric contractions.
12.	The concept of periodization (variation in training volume and intensity) should be taught.
13.	The child should use only appropriately sized equipment.
14.	No unsupervised or improper 1RM testing should be performed by children or adolescents.
15.	Due to the intense nature of weightlifting movements, fewer than 6 to 8 repetitions per set are usually recommended.
16.	Because emphasis is placed on correct form and technique, it is recommended that training be conducted in a controlled manner at a moderate velocity.

*RM = repetition maximum.

Sources: Position statements of the American Academy of Pediatrics (2008, Reaffirmed June 2011), the National Strength and Conditioning Association (Faigenbaum et al., 2009). and the UK Strength and Conditioning Association (Lloyd, Faigenbaum, Stone, et al., 2014).

Adolescence/Early and Middle Adulthood

Authorities agree that programs of progressive resistance training will result in improved muscular strength and endurance within adolescent and adult populations. Gains in muscular strength and endurance, however, depend on adherence to established principles of training. The American College of Sports Medicine (2009, 2018) recommends that the healthy adult perform approximately 8–10 exercises involving the body's major muscle groups. These resistance-training exercises should be performed a minimum of two times per week. Each exercise should consist of a minimum of 1 set with 8–12 repetitions.

Near maximal and maximal lifts are acceptable for adolescents (beyond Tanner stage 5) and young adults; however, these individuals must receive training in proper lifting technique. It is particularly important that adolescents and young adults understand the importance of proper breathing during the performance of resistance training. In short, holding the breath or straining with a closed glottis (the opening between the vocal cords; called a Valsalva maneuver) can cause a "blackout" and should, therefore, be avoided.

An additional concern is the use of **anabolic steroids**, sometimes referred to as androgens (Joyner, 2000). The primary androgen, testosterone, aids in the development of muscle mass. Because of this, some athletes believe that taking anabolic steroids will lead to better athletic performance. However, the use of synthetic anabolic steroids is not confined to athletes. A growing number of nonathletic youth are taking steroids as a means of improving their physique. One national study revealed that the prevalence rates for steroid use are 1.2 percent, 1.8 percent, and 2.6 percent for 8th-, 10th-, and 12th-grade boys and 0.9 percent, 0.7 percent, and 0.4 percent for 8th-, 10th-, and 12th-grade girls, respectively (Johnson, O'Malley, Bachman, & Schulenberg, 2006).

When women are administered anabolic steroids, they may develop various male characteristics, such as increased upper-body muscularity, facial hair, a deeper voice, and a reduction of body fat, especially in the breasts and hips. In contrast, when administered to young boys, anabolic steroids accelerate puberty and make possible the premature closure of the growth plates of the long bones. Table 7.6 lists the potential adverse effects of anabolic steroid use (President's Council on Physical Fitness and Sports, 2005).

Table 7.6 Potential adverse effects of anabolic steroids

Males	Females	Both males and females
Baldness	Breast shrinkage	Acne
Prostate changes	Clitoral enlargement	Aggression
Gynecomastia	Increased facial/body hair	Brittle connective tissue
Impotence/sterility	Menstrual irregularities	Cardiovascular disease
	Premature hair loss	Cerebrovascular incidents
	Deepened voice (vocal cord thickening)	Dependency
		Headaches
		Hypertension
		Liver disease
		Psyche and behavior changes
		Short stature (premature growth-plate closure)

Source: President's Council on Physical Fitness and Sports (2005).

Late Adulthood

For individuals in late adulthood, the paramount question is whether strength training is capable of altering, delaying, or even allowing a person to avoid some of the physiological deterioration believed to be associated with aging (see Figure 7.2). Lemmer, Hurlbut, Martel, and colleagues (2000) found that when older men and women (65–75 years) trained for 9 weeks, not only did both genders significantly improve in strength, but the women maintained strength above baseline after 12 weeks of detraining. Most impressive was the finding that the older men maintained strength above baseline even after 31 weeks of detraining.

Fatouros, Kambas, Katrabasas, and colleagues (2005) have reported similar

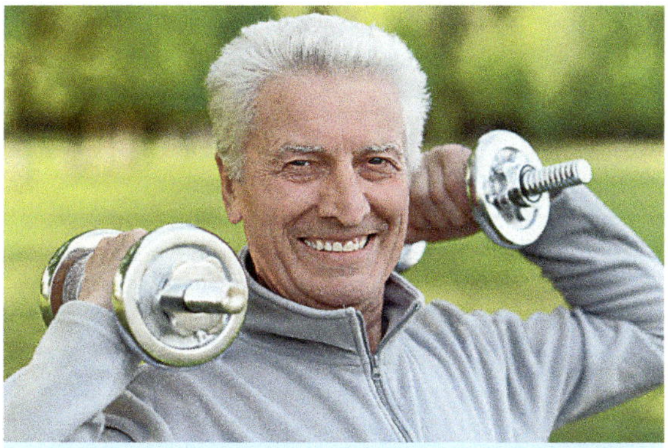

Figure 7.2 Strength training is capable of delaying and even preventing some of the physiological deterioration associated with aging muscle

findings. Specifically, high-intensity strength training in older men (mean age: 71 years) resulted in strength gains of 63–91 percent. Furthermore, strength remained above baseline after 48 weeks of detraining.

Perhaps most important are findings indicating that improvements in muscular strength and endurance following resistance training positively influence the activities of daily living, thus leading to a better quality of life (Fahlman, McNevin, Boardley, et al., 2011). For example, Fiatarone and colleagues (1990) have demonstrated that resistance training can benefit individuals well into the tenth decade of life. The male and female subjects of this study, who were frail and living in an institutional setting, improved quadriceps strength by 31 percent and muscle cross-sectional area by 8 percent following an 8-week resistance-training program. Clinically, these individuals exhibited significant improvement in walking speed, a functional index of mobility.

With physically frail elders, a resistance-training program can be implemented without the use of free weights or commercial weight machines. Instead, the individual's body weight can be used to provide the muscular resistance. One such study employed the use of sit-to-stand exercises. The training protocol required the 75–88-year-old frail subjects to perform 48 sit-to-stand repetitions per session. Following the 12-week training program the subjects increased their knee extensor strength, which in turn facilitated activities of daily living which required the lowering and raising of the body (Fujita, Taaffe, Yoshitake, & Kanehisa, 2019).

Mechanisms of Increasing Muscular Strength

Even though our review thus far indicates that individuals of all ages can improve in strength by following a program of progressive resistance, the mechanisms responsible for change may differ among the various age groups. Voluntary muscular strength can be improved in two main ways: (1) by increasing the size of the muscle (**hypertrophy**) and the specific tensions that can be exerted within the muscle; and (2) by neural adaptations that result in an increased ability of the nervous system to activate muscle tissue. Figure 7.3 illustrates the interplay between neural and muscular adaptations (Sale, 1988). Sale conducted an extensive review of the literature and concluded that children may have more difficulty than older individuals in increasing muscle mass. On the other hand, adaptations within the nervous system of children are similar to or even greater than those in older individuals (Sale, 1989, p. 211).

The reason for prepubescent children's difficulty in increasing muscle mass is not clear at this time. One possible explanation is their low level of circulating **androgens** (sex hormones). Indeed, with the introduction of higher levels of circulating testosterone, which occurs in boys around 13–14 years of age, a corresponding increase in muscle hypertrophy and muscular strength occurs, even in the absence of resistance training. Nevertheless, this theory of circulating androgen level cannot be totally accurate because young adult

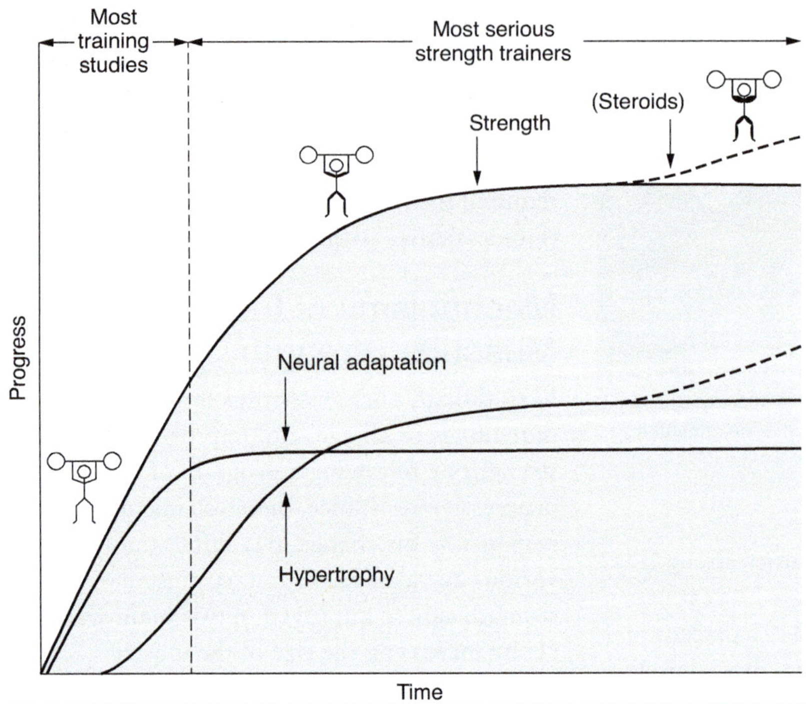

The top curve represents the total changes in strength across time. The other two curves illustrate the contributions of neural adaptation and hypertrophy to the overall change in strength with training. Most training studies examine the early phase of training, in which neural adaptation predominates. In intermediate and advanced training, progress is limited to the extent of muscular adaptation that can be achieved, notably hypertrophy; hence the temptation for some strength trainers to use anabolic steroids when it becomes difficult to induce hypertrophy by training alone.

Figure 7.3 The relative roles of neural and muscular adaptation to strength training

Source: Adapted from Sale (1988). Used with permission of Lippincott, Williams & Wilkins.

women, with their low androgen levels, can increase their muscle mass. Thus, the answer to why prepubescent individuals have difficulty in increasing muscle mass must await further study.

Potential mechanisms of muscle deterioration (**sarcopenia: loss of muscle mass**) in late adulthood are many. For example, age brings a decrease in both the size and the number of muscle fibers, loss of mitochondrial content and function, as well as infiltration of muscle fat (Colon, Molina-Vicenty, Frontera-Rodriguez, et al., 2018). Additionally, muscular deterioration tends to affect the **Type II**, fast-twitch muscle fibers more than the **Type I**, slow-twitch fibers. Because of this reduction in fast-twitch fibers, older adults frequently experience a reduction in the speed of muscular contractions. This may help to explain why these individuals frequently suffer falls. Recognizing a loss of postural balance may be of little value if muscles in the lower extremities are not capable of contracting quickly and with sufficient force to restore postural stability.

FLEXIBILITY

The abilities to ambulate and perform such daily tasks as bending over to pick up an object, tying one's shoes, rising out of a chair, and even eating all have one thing in common: each task requires the bending of various parts of the body. Smooth functioning of the body's joints makes these bending movements possible. **Flexibility**, the range of movement within these joints, is regionally specific. In other words, there is little relationship between the flexibility of one of the body's joints and another. For example, a person with flexible shoulders does not necessarily have a flexible back. Few physical-fitness test batteries include flexibility among the test items because no single flexibility test can estimate total body flexibility. When a flexibility test is included, it

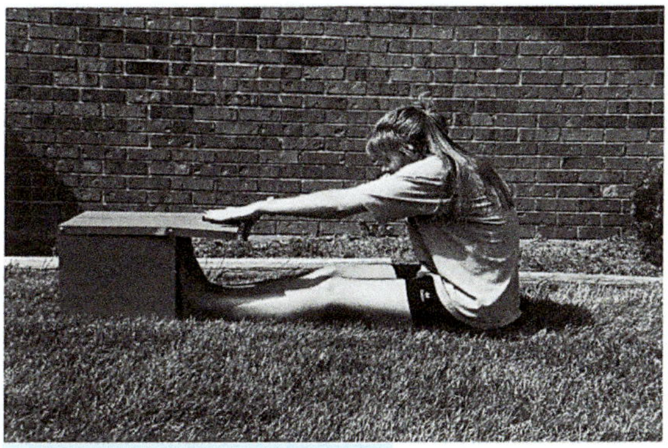

Figure 7.4 Sit-and-reach test

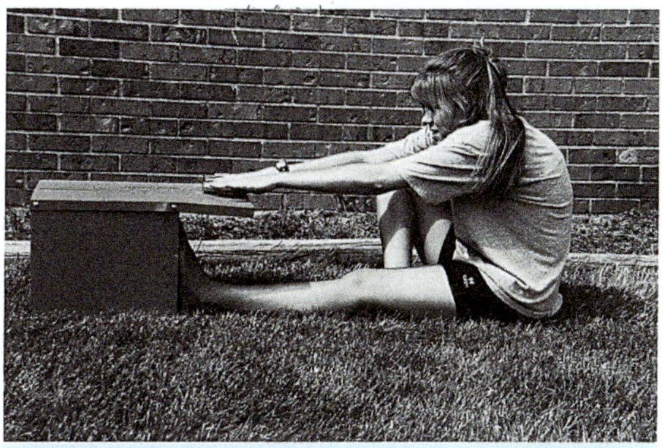

Figure 7.5 The back saver sit-and-reach test evaluates flexibility on one side at a time. This technique places less stress on the lower back.

is generally a test of hamstring, back, and hip flexibility—the **sit-and-reach** test (see Figure 7.4) or the back saver sit-and-reach test (see Figure 7.5). The next section examines the general course of flexibility across the lifespan.

Performance Trends

When the sit-and-reach test is used to measure hamstring, hip, and back flexibility, the data show that peak flexibility is achieved in the late teens or early twenties. Thereafter, the range of motion decreases. This trend is readily apparent in National Children and Youth Fitness Studies (NCYFS) I and II (Ross & Pate, 1987). In these classic studies, norms were established for a nationally representative sample of youngsters 6 through 18 years of age (see Figure 7.6). Generally, the data from these studies show a yearly increase in range of motion during these childhood and adolescent years. Furthermore,

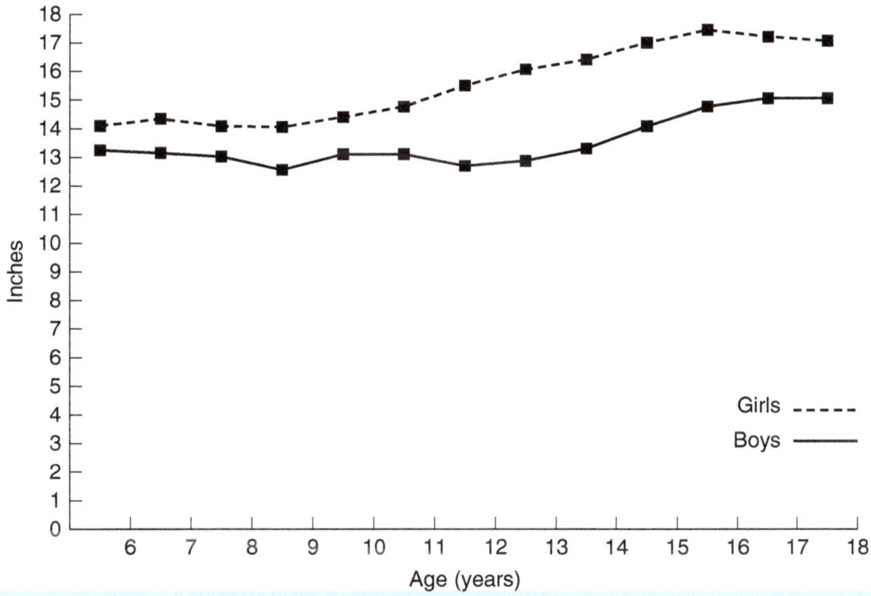

Figure 7.6 Average sit-and-reach scores for boys and girls based on findings of the National Children and Youth Fitness Studies I and II. The zero point was located at 12 in.

Sources: As reported by Ross & Gilbert (1985) and Ross & Pate (1987).

gender differences are apparent: girls attained higher scores than did boys across all ages and across all percentile ranges.

With age, there is an accompanying decrease in the range of motion in many of the body's joints. For example, Stathokostas and colleagues (2013) observed a decrease in shoulder abduction of 5 degrees per decade in men and 6 degrees per decade in women. Rate of decline started to accelerate at about 71 years of age in men (0.80 degrees/yr) and about 63 years of age in women (0.74 degrees/yr). Likewise, a similar trend was observed in hip flexion. Men averaging a decline of about 1.16 degrees per year beginning at 71 years of age, while women averaged a linear decline of about 0.66 degrees per year, across the entire age span studied (55–86 yrs).

Declining Flexibility and Aging: Causes and Therapy

The decrease in joint mobility with age is partly caused by physiological changes to the structures that make up the joints: tendons, ligaments, muscle, synovial fluid, and cartilage. With age, the joints' connective structures become less resilient and crack and fray. Synovial fluid becomes less viscous, and cartilage is frequently damaged from both injury and everyday wear and tear. Degenerative joint disease, such as osteoarthrosis, also contributes to loss of joint functioning. About 80 percent of the population between 55 and 64 years have signs of osteoarthrosis in at least one joint.

Although researchers have not been able to ascertain the extent to which joint changes are caused by age-related processes or by pathological changes, one fact is clear: physical activity is necessary to maintain joint mobility. Moreover, joint flexibility can be improved with flexibility-specific training (Haab & Wydra, 2017; Stathokostas, Little, Vandervoort, & Paterson, 2012). For example, Haab and Wydra (2017) found a significant increase in hamstring flexibility following a 10-week stretch training program. When the elders' (65.1 +/– 7.9 yrs) performance was compared with a younger population (24.0 +/– 4 yrs), they found that the older individuals benefited from the stretch training program just as much as the younger individuals. Improving lower extremity flexibility in the elderly is extremely important since it has been associated with poor balance (Reddy & Alahmari, 2016), and with chronic lower back pain (Hasarangi & Jayawardana, 2018), both of which may contribute to devastating and even life-threatening falls.

BODY COMPOSITION

We live in a technological society—a society that is relying increasingly on special machinery to perform daily tasks. The use of robotics in the workforce has improved productivity, but we seem to be paying a price for this technology: some experts believe this price to be an increasingly sedentary lifestyle. Accompanying this lifestyle we are witnessing a corresponding increase in the prevalence of overweight and overfatness. Adipose (fat) tissue serves many useful and important functions: it insulates the body, it can provide a source of energy reserve, and it serves as a protective cushion for internal organs. Unfortunately, evidence suggests that excess fat in relation to total **body composition** has serious health consequences, including high blood lipid levels, elevated blood pressure, and many other physiological parameters associated with cardiovascular disease (coronary artery disease) and metabolic disease (diabetes mellitus).

Defining Overweight and Obesity

Overweight and *obesity* describe a state of excess body fat greater than what is generally considered healthy for a given height. Thus, this operational definition is based on criteria tied to rates of mortality and morbidity. Use of these two terms is in part based on the calculation of body mass index (BMI) (see Chapter 6). Briefly, BMI is a measure of weight relative to height (BMI = weight in kilograms / (height in meters)^2). In adults, a BMI between 25.0 kg/m^2 and 29.9 kg/m^2 defines **overweight. Obesity** is defined as having a BMI greater than 30 kg/m^2. In adults, waist circumference also indicates obesity. A person is classified as obese when the waist circumference exceeds 102 cm (40 in) in men or 88 cm (35 in) in women (ACSM, 2018).

As with adults, BMI is used to determine overweight or obesity in children (2–19 years of age). However, with children, we refer to the Centers for Disease Control (CDC) growth charts to determine a percentile based on BMI, age, and gender. As discussed in Chapter 6, children who fall between the 85th and 94th percentiles are overweight. Those who score at or above the 95th percentile are considered obese.

It is important to remember that BMI is not a direct measure of body fat but instead is a reasonable indicator of body fatness.

General Growth Trends of Adipose Tissue

Subcutaneous adipose tissue first appears prenatally, toward the end of the second trimester, and rapidly develops during the last 2 months of gestation (Moore & Persaud, 2008). At birth, the amount of fat present is about 11 percent in boys and 14 percent in girls. This fat is stored in about 5 billion adipocytes (fat cells). The number of fat cells increases during childhood. For example, during the 12 months after birth, the percentage of body fat can rise to about 26 percent in boys and 28 percent in girls (Butte, Hopkinson, Wong, et al., 2000). This increase in fat tissue during the first year of life constitutes one of two typical rapid growth spurts of adipose tissue. The second spurt occurs during puberty in boys and during both prepuberty and puberty in girls. The result of this second spurt is a greater fat mass in girls than in boys. On average, the young but mature female adolescent has a body-fat content 50 percent greater than that of her male counterpart of the same age (Rowland, 1996). Authorities believe that the number of adipocytes does not increase following puberty. Instead, changes in fat's contribution to overall body composition depend on the size of each fat cell, rather than the number of fat cells.

There appears to be one period early in the lifespan when body fat declines: at the onset of independent walking. This period of decreasing body fat ends somewhere between 6 and 8 years of age; at this time, body fat is typically about one-half of what it was at 1 year of age (Sinclair, 1998).

A body-fat content 1 or 2 standard deviations above the mean lies outside the range generally recommended for optimal health. Authorities (Jeukendrup & Gleeson, 2019) believed an acceptable level of body-fat content would be 15–20 percent in men and 24–30 percent in women. However, for optimal fitness, body-fat content should be reduced to approximately 11–14 percent in men and 16–23 percent in women. By comparison, most male athletes possess a body-fat content of 5–10 percent, with most female athletes at 8–15 percent. Because fat is an essential body component, it should not drop below 1–5 percent in men and 3–8 percent in women. Slightly higher levels of essential fat are often recommended for women to avoid amenorrhea.

Body weight per se is not an indicator of body composition. Body weight tends to reach its peak at about 45 years of age; during the next 15 years, body weight generally decreases or remains constant. A decrease in body weight may appear to imply a reduction in adipose tissue, but generally this is not the case. For instance, skinfold thicknesses (indicating body composition; see discussion later in the chapter) do not change during this period of weight loss, so the reduction in body weight is attributable to a reduction in lean body mass, not fat mass. The increasingly sedentary lifestyle that generally accompanies aging partly explains this reduction in lean body mass.

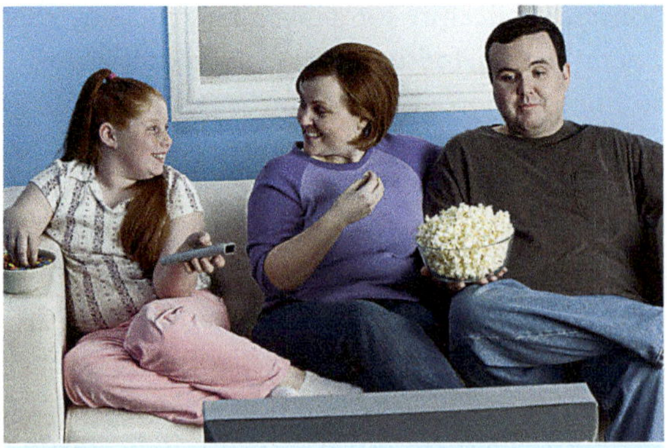

Figure 7.7 The prevalence of obesity is increasing among adults, adolescents, and children

Prevalence of Overweight and Obesity

The prevalence of overweight and obesity in the U.S. population continues to escalate (see Figure 7.7).

Figure 7.8 highlights the prevalence of obesity among American youth aged 2–5, 6–11, and 12–19 over the past four-plus decades. Data for 2015 through 2016 indicate an overall prevalence of obesity of 18.5 percent among American youth (Hales, Carroll, Fryar, & Ogden, 2017). Partially noteworthy is the significant increase in obesity observed in children aged 2–5, particularly young males, compared to the 2011–2012 assessment cycle (8.4 percent vs 13.9 percent). This is disheartening since this represents a 40 percent increase in obesity among these preschool children (Skinner, Ravanbakht, Skelton, et al., 2018). Also alarming is the finding that the percentage of children (aged 6–11) and young adults (aged 12–19) who are obese has more than tripled over the last 40-plus years.

The prevalence of overweight, obesity, and extreme obesity is even greater among adults. The NHANES 2015–2016 data (Hales, Carroll, Fryar, & Ogden, 2017) indicated that 39.8 percent (crude) of American adults were obese (see Figure 7.9). This represents approximately 93.3 million adults in the United States. Most surprising was the finding that obesity in women over 60 years of age

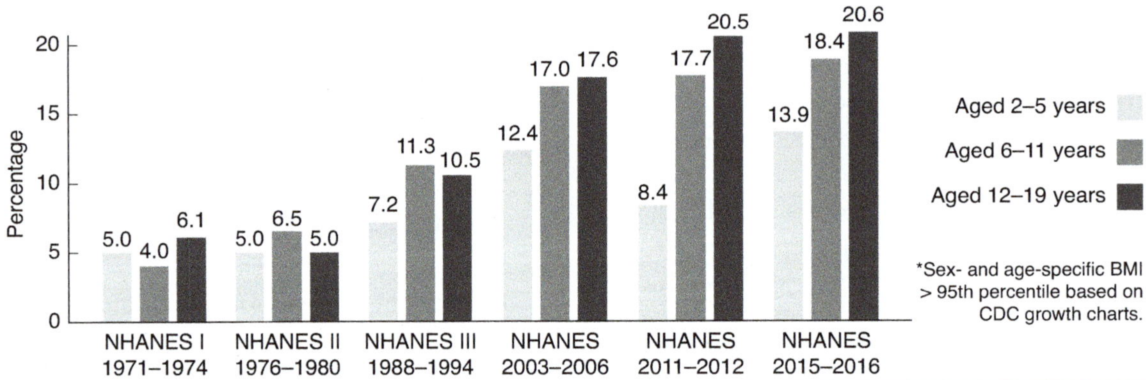

Figure 7.8 Prevalence of obesity* among U.S. children and adolescents (aged 2–19 years): National Health and Nutrition Examination Surveys

Sources: Based on data from Hedley, Ogden, Carroll, et al. (2004); Ogden, Flegal, Carroll, & Johnson (2002); Ogden et al. (2008; 2014); Hales, Carroll, Fryar, & Ogden (2017).

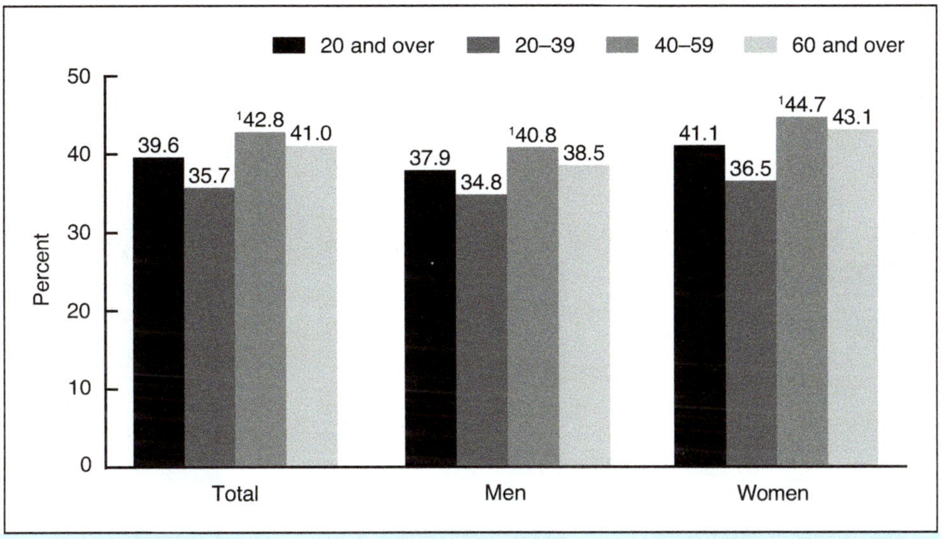

Figure 7.9 Prevalence of obesity among adults aged 20 and over, by sex and age: United States, 2015–2016

[1] Significantly different from those aged 20–39.

Notes: Estimates for adults aged 20 and over were age adjusted by the direct method to the 2000 U.S. census population using the age groups 20–39, 40–59, and 60 and over. Crude estimates are 39.8% for total, 38.0% for men, and 41.5% for women. Access data table for Figure 1 at: https://www.cdc.gov/nchs/data/databriefs/db288_table.pdf#1.

Source: Hales, Carroll, Fryar, & Ogden (2017), using data from CDC-NCHS, National Health and Nutrition Examination Survey, 2015–2016.

increased from 31.5 percent (NHANES, 2011–2012) to 43.1 percent (NHANES, 2015–2016) in a span of only four years.

Figure 7.10 summarizes the prevalence of overweight and obesity among men and women of selected racial and ethnic groups. In general, rates were lowest among non-Hispanic Asian adults (12.7 percent). Among men, the prevalence of obesity was highest among Hispanics (43.1 percent). The highest prevalence of obesity, 54.8 percent, was found among non-Hispanic Black women, followed closely by Hispanic women (50.6 percent).

A major goal of the *Healthy People 2020* initiative is to reduce the proportion of adults and children who are considered obese (Healthy People 2020, 2019). More specifically, the target goal for each age category is as follows: Adults, 30.5 percent; age 2–5 years, 9.4 percent; age 6–11 years, 15.7 percent; and age 12–19 years, 16.1 percent. These targets represent very challenging goals given the history of escalating obesity in the United States.

Association Between Childhood and Adulthood Obesity

Because of the public health concern that obesity is related to increased risk of cardiovascular disease, diabetes, and hypertension, researchers have attempted to examine whether BMI in childhood predicts the likelihood of developing obesity in adulthood.

Defining overweight as BMI >28 for men and BMI >26 for women (note that these figures differ from the 2002 CDC guidelines), Guo, Roche, Chumlea, and colleagues (1994) constructed models to predict the likelihood of being overweight in adulthood based on BMI values measured during childhood (see

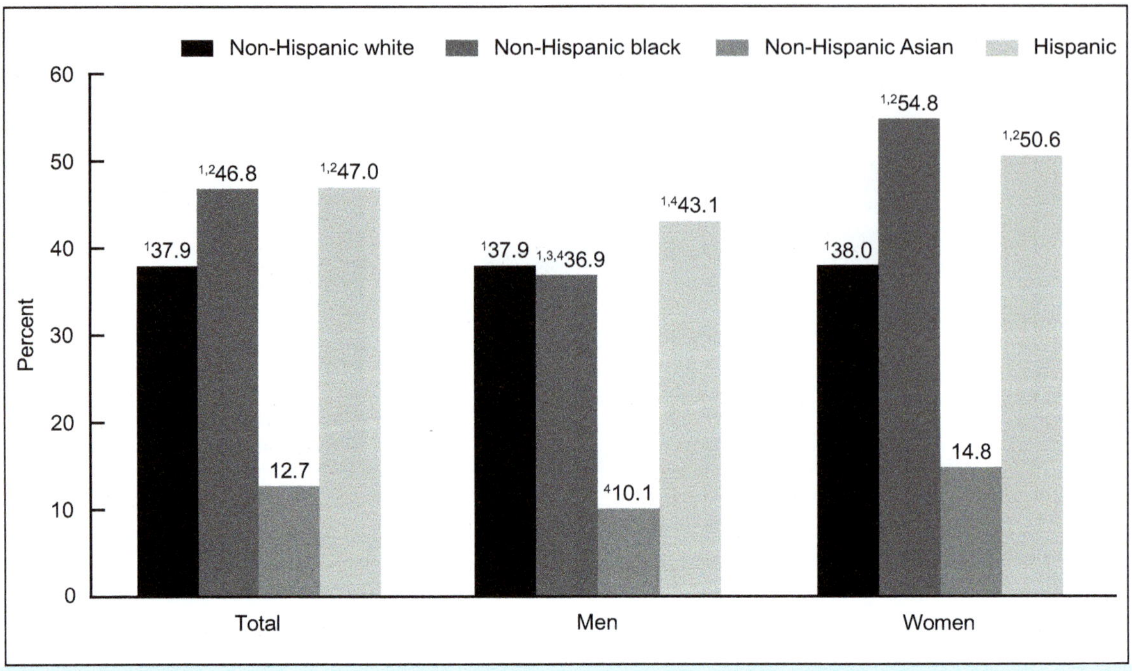

Figure 7.10 Age-adjusted prevalence of obesity, by sex, race, and Hispanic origin, among adults aged 20 and over: United States, 2015–2016

[1] Significantly different from non-Hispanic Asian persons.
[2] Significantly different from non-Hispanic white persons.
[3] Significantly different from Hispanic persons.
[4] Significantly different from women of same race and Hispanic origin.

Notes: All estimates are age adjusted by the direct method to the 2000 U.S. census population using the age groups 20–39, 40–59, and 60 and over. Access data table for Figure 2 at: https://www.cdc.gov/nchs/data/databriefs/db288_table.pdf#2.

Source: Hales, Carroll, Fryar, & Ogden (2017) using data from CDC/NCHS, National Health and Nutrition Examination Survey, 2015–2016.

Figure 7.11). In general, Guo and colleagues found that children with BMI values at the 95th percentile for their age and gender have a higher than 60 percent chance of being obese at age 35. The strength of this association increases with age: these predictions are excellent at age 18, good at 13 years of age, and moderate at ages younger than 13 years. Furthermore, these predictions appear to continue to be valid; that is, "childhood BMI and rate of change in BMI during childhood are a strong predictor of obesity in adulthood" (Zhang, Whelton, Xi, et al., 2019; Magarey, Daniels, Boulton, & Cockington, 2003).

To use Figure 7.11, simply find the child's age on the *X* axis and her or his present BMI on the *Y* axis, and note the point of intersection. You can determine the child's percentile rank based on national data. Pay close attention to the shading of the percentile lines. Use the key to find the risk of the child's being overweight at age 35. For example, a 10-year-old White male child who has a BMI value approaching 24 is at the 95th percentile. According to the shaded scale, this child has a 40–80 percent (mean = 60%) chance of being overweight at 35 years of age. In contrast, a 9-year-old White female child with a BMI value of about 18 has a less than 20 percent risk of being overweight at age 35. This information can assist in the identification of at-risk individuals who might benefit from early intervention.

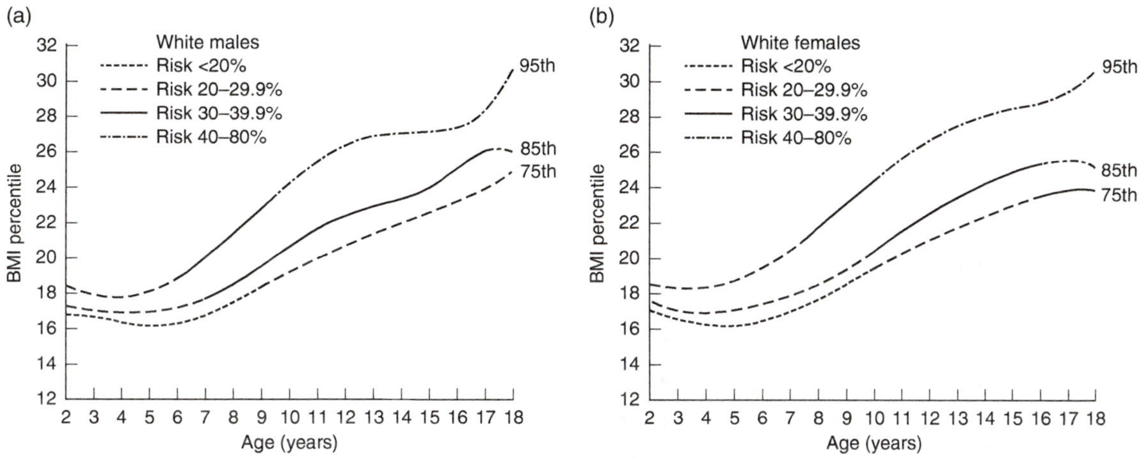

Note: Segments of the 75th, 85th, and 95th percentile lines are differentially shaded to indicate differences in the probability that BMI at 35 years will be >28 for males and >26 for females.

Figure 7.11 Selected percentiles for BMI in boys (a) and girls (b) from the Second National Health and Nutrition Examination Survey

Source: Guo, Roche, Chumlea, et al. (1994). Reproduced with permission of the *American Journal of Clinical Nutrition*. © American Society for Clinical Nutrition.

Laboratory-Test Measures of Body Composition

Hydrostatic weighing (HW) has long been considered the "gold standard" for determining a person's body composition. This technique, which requires total body submersion under water, is based on Archimedes' principle (see Figure 7.12). When an object is submerged in water and its weight is measured, the object will weigh less than it does when out of water. According to Archimedes' principle, this reduction in weight is equal to the weight of the volume of water that the object displaces. After taking a person's weight measurement under water, we can use equations to calculate the person's body density and then to predict the person's percentage of body fat (see ACSM, 2018). The advantage of this method is that the error rate is less than 2 percent; however, the test requires a highly skilled technician to administer it, requires expensive and nonportable equipment, and is not appropriate for individuals who have an aversion to water.

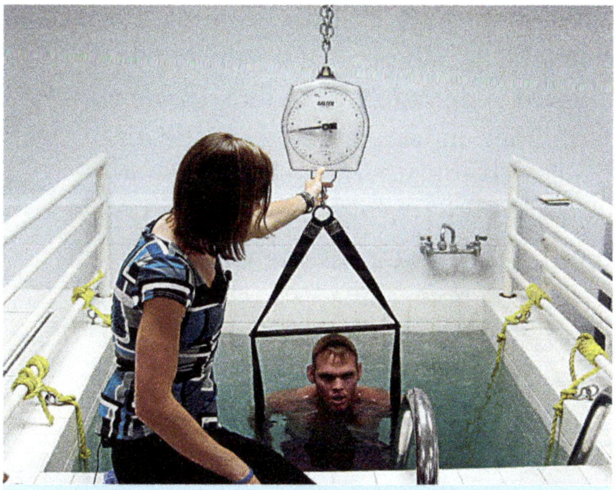

Figure 7.12 Hydrostatic weighing is the preferred method for determining percentage of body fat, but this technique is not practical as a field-test measure

Source: Photo from Housh, Housh, & deVries (2016). Used with permission.

A popular alternative to HW is the use of the **Bod Pod** (see Figure 7.13). Unlike HW, which is based on the displacement of water, the Bod Pod is based on the displacement of air (air-displacement plethysmography). All calculations are computerized, and the test

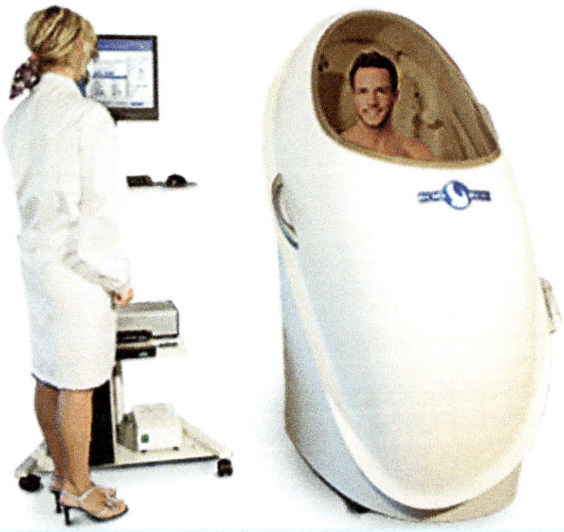

Figure 7.13 The Bod Pod uses air-displacement technology to measure body composition

Source: Courtesy of BodPod.com.

takes only about 5 minutes. Because submersion in water is not required, the test is suitable for all populations including children, older adults, and individuals with disabilities. In fact, one study found air-displacement plethysmography to be more accurate than HW and dual-energy X-ray absorptiometry (DEXA; see Chapter 6) for calculating body composition in children between 9 and 14 years of age (Fields & Goran, 2000).

Field-Test Measures of Body Composition

While HW, the Bod Pod, and DEXA are the preferred methods for estimating percent body fat, these laboratory procedures are not always practical. A more practical alternative is the use of **skinfold calipers** to estimate body composition indirectly. Skinfold calipers are available from numerous manufacturers; avoid cheap plastic calipers, as they are not spring-loaded and their scales are difficult to read. Using calipers that are spring-loaded ensures that a constant calibrated pressure (10 g/mm^2) is applied to the fold of skin and fat tissue.

In both classic National Children and Youth Fitness Studies, the researchers used skinfold calipers to estimate body fat in children between 6 and 18 years of age. Table 7.7 presents the findings of these studies. The values for the 6–9-year-olds were obtained by summing the skinfold thicknesses for the triceps, sub-scapular, and medial calf. In contrast, values for the 10–17-year-olds were obtained by summing only the triceps and subscapular skinfolds. Because of the inclusion of the medial calf measure for the younger group, it is difficult to compare trends between these two age groups. To make comparisons across ages easier, Figure 7.14 shows changes in only the sum of triceps and subscapular skinfolds across both age groups (the medial calf measure has been removed from the younger age group).

Clearly, at all ages, girls possess more body fat than do boys. In general, body fat appears to increase steadily in girls until 15 years of age. In contrast, boys exhibit a steady increase in body fat until about 10 years; thereafter, it remains relatively constant through 18 years of age. Note that the magnitude of difference between the genders widens significantly after 11 years of age, and this widening trend continues until about age 15. At this time, the average sum of triceps and subscapular skinfolds is nearly 10 mm greater in girls than in boys.

Table 7.8 presents data that show a definite decrease in triceps skinfold thickness in men and women 50 years of age and older. Since obesity and malnutrition often occur in late adulthood, it is recommended that body fat changes be closely monitored in older adults. Among these individuals, obesity tends to be the most common reason for approaching the 90th percentile in measures of body fat, whereas malnutrition and serious illness can cause a significant drop in body fat.

Table 7.7 Average sum of skinfolds (mm) for boys and girls based on findings of the NCYFS I and II

Age (years)	6	7	8	9	10	11	12	13	14	15	16	17	18
Sum of triceps, subscapular, and medial calf skinfolds													
Boys	24.56	26.36	28.91	32.07									
Girls	30.55	32.25	36.11	39.16									
Sum of triceps and subscapular skinfolds													
Boys					20.90	21.20	21.60	20.10	20.10	20.10	19.40	20.10	20.20
Girls					22.60	24.80	25.30	26.80	27.90	30.00	28.70	30.20	28.90

Sources: As reported by Ross & Gilbert (1985) and Ross & Pate (1987). Reprinted with permission of Taylor & Francis via CCC.

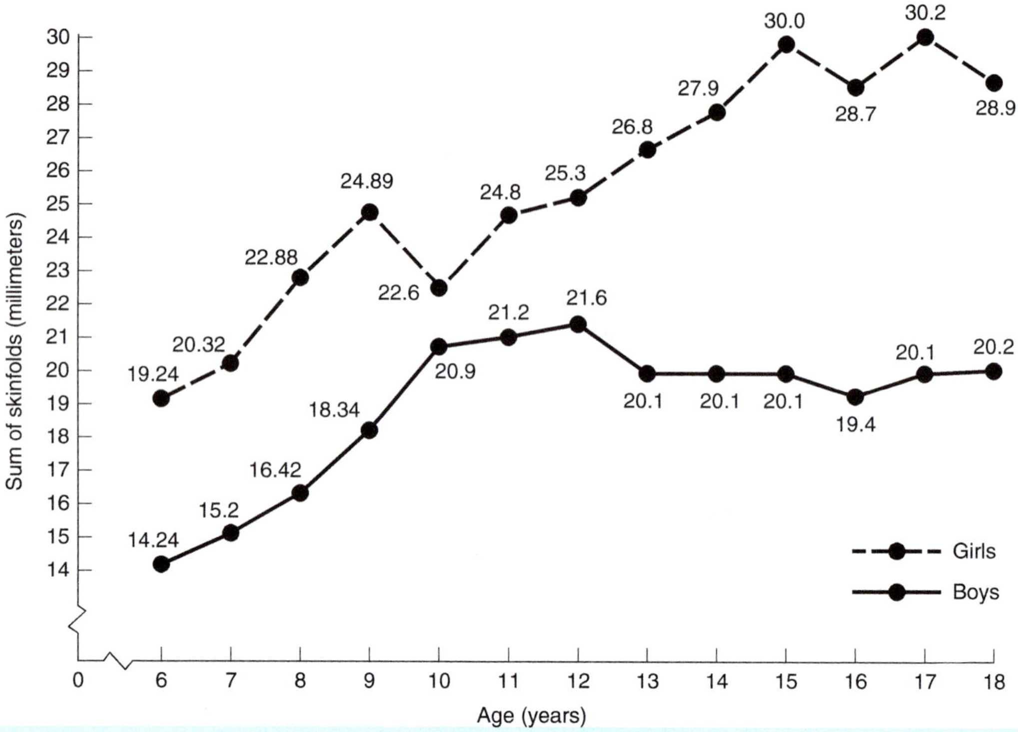

Figure 7.14 Average sum of triceps and subscapular skinfold thicknesses in boys and girls based on findings of the NCYFS I and II

Sources: As reported by Ross & Gilbert (1985) and Ross & Pate (1987). Reprinted with permission of Taylor & Francis via CCC.

Table 7.8 Percentiles for triceps skinfold thickness in men and women 50 years of age and older examined in NHANES (2007–2010)

Age (years)	Men				Women			
	Mean ± SE	90TH	50TH	10TH	Mean ± SE	90TH	50TH	10TH
50–59	15.1 ± 0.37	24.2	13.3	8.2	24.6 ± 0.30	34.0	24.5	15.6
60–69	15.9 ± 0.31	24.9	14.9	8.4	24.7 ± 0.34	33.8	24.9	15.0
70–79	15.7 ± 0.41	24.9	14.6	8.6	23.4 ± 0.33	32.8	22.9	14.3
80+	14.4 ± 0.25	22.0	13.2	8.5	19.4 ± 0.34	27.8	19.0	11.2

Source: Fryar, Gu, & Ogden (2012).

Relationship of Obesity to Motor Development and Performance and Health-Related Fitness

As early as 1931, Shirley noted that of the 25 babies in her study, the heavy ones evidenced more delays in walking than did the lighter ones. Over 80 years later, Slining, Adair, Goldman, and colleagues (2010) reported similar motor delays in infants 3–18 months of age. In fact, high subcutaneous fat and overweight were associated with delayed infant motor development as assessed by the Bayley

Scales of Infant Development-II. Additionally, children between 4 and 5 years of age who are overweight have been found to exhibit poorer performance on both locomotor and object-control skills than their counterparts of typical weight (Morano, Colella, & Caroli, 2011). Isaacs and Pohlman (2000) found that for every 2.2 lb (1 kg) increase in body fat there was a corresponding decrease in vertical jump performance of 0.25 in (0.65 cm) among a group of children between 7 and 11 years of age.

Health-related fitness has also been found to be affected by excess body fat. For example, Chatrath, Shenoy, Serratto, and Thoele (2002) required children between 4 and 18 years of age to take part in an endurance exercise test (the Bruce treadmill protocol). Results revealed that 61 percent of the boys and 81 percent of the girls performed below the 25th percentile, with a strong negative correlation found between BMI and endurance performance, suggesting that obesity contributed greatly to the children's low levels of aerobic fitness. Likewise, researchers in Seoul, Korea, have also observed lower levels of cardiorespiratory fitness in overweight and obese elementary school-age children (Kim, Lee, Jeon, et al., 2016).

Treatment of Overweight and Obesity

A logical extension of our discussion on overweight and obesity is to suggest a treatment plan for safely losing weight. The algorithm presented in Figure 7.15 summarizes our discussion regarding the identification and classification of overweight and obesity based on BMI and waist circumference (NHLBI, 2000). Note that once identification and classification have been made, this chart can provide information regarding potential treatments and follow-up maintenance programs.

As Figure 7.15 suggests, for most individuals a reduction in body weight of about 1–2 lb/week is indicated, which is both reasonable and healthy. This amount of weight loss would require a calorie reduction of between 3,500 and 7,000 calories/week (there are 3,500 calories to a pound) or 500–1,000 calories/day. A dual approach should be employed to accomplish this weight-loss goal, namely, the use of both diet and moderate-intensity exercise (ACSM, 2018)—for example, 30 minutes of moderate-intensity exercise on most days of the week, as shown in Figure 7.15. Although pharmacological (drugs) and surgical approaches are available, they should be considered only as a last resort, e.g., when BMI is in the obese/extremely obese range or multiple health risk factors are involved (see Figure 7.15).

PROMOTING PHYSICAL ACTIVITY: THE ROLE OF INTERACTIVE TECHNOLOGY

Throughout this chapter and in reports in the popular media, the epidemic of overweight and obesity in the United States has been much discussed. In general, children, adolescents, and adults are simply consuming too many calories and expending too little energy. Americans of all ages need to increase their physical activity and reduce their sedentary behaviors. One sedentary behavior that has received much attention is video game playing. For the last 30 years, health professionals have identified sedentary game playing as one major reason so many Americans remain inactive. Research indicates that individuals who are obese and deconditioned are less likely to participate in traditional exercise or sport programs, compared to their counterparts of healthy weight (Dowda, Ainsworth, Addy, et al., 2001).

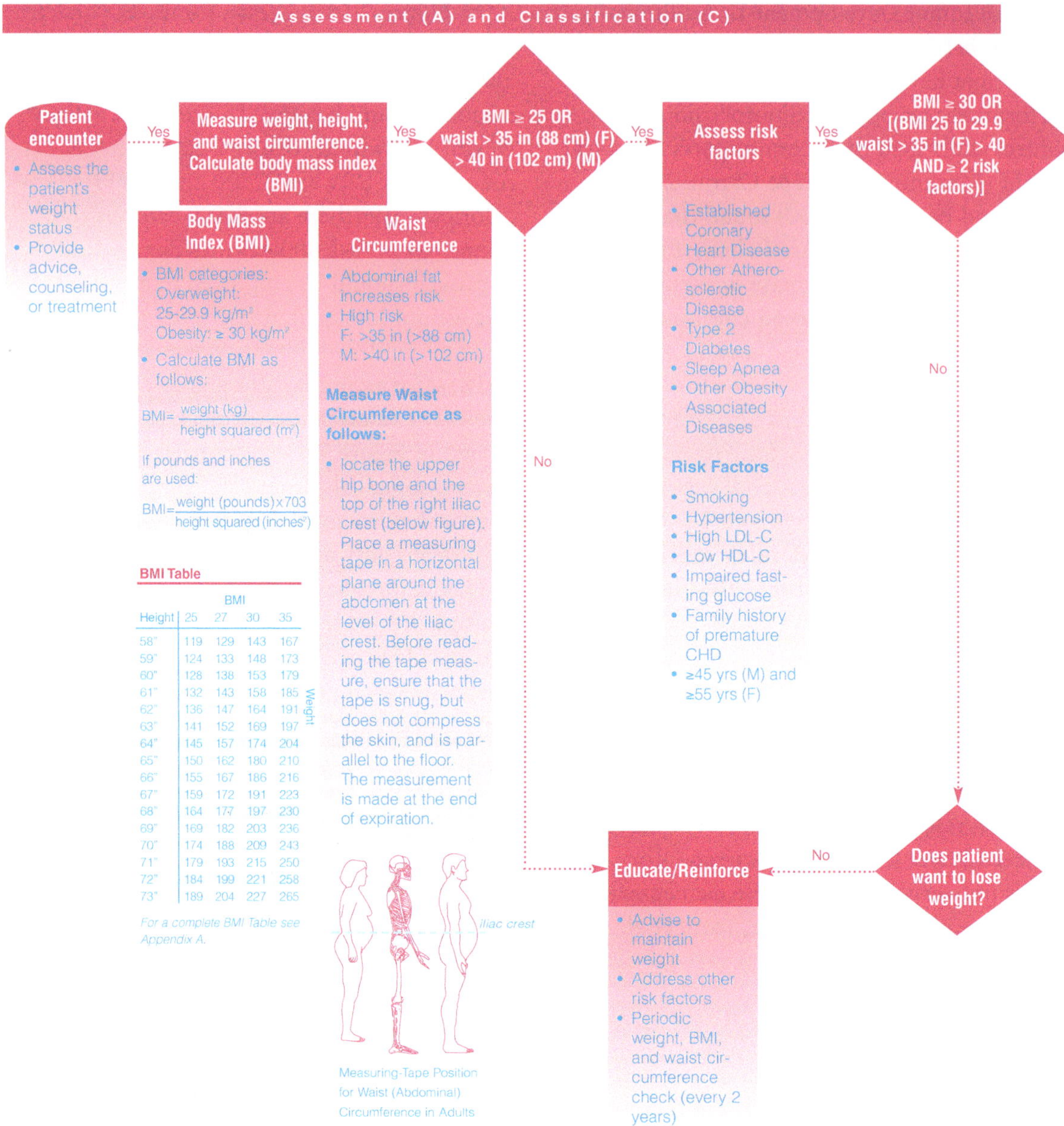

BMI Table

Height	BMI 25	27	30	35
58"	119	129	143	167
59"	124	133	148	173
60"	128	138	153	179
61"	132	143	158	185
62"	136	147	164	191
63"	141	152	169	197
64"	145	157	174	204
65"	150	162	180	210
66"	155	167	186	216
67"	159	172	191	223
68"	164	177	197	230
69"	169	182	203	236
70"	174	188	209	243
71"	179	193	215	250
72"	184	199	221	258
73"	189	204	227	265

Weight

For a complete BMI Table see Appendix A.

Figure 7.15 Identification, evaluation, and treatment of overweight and obesity in adults

Source: National Heart, Lung, and Blood Institute (2000).

Fortunately, some video games now require physically interactive participation. For example, some games simulate dancing; others require interactive sports participation, while still others require one to participate on exercise equipment, most frequently a cycle ergometer. This format of interactive video game playing is referred to as **exergaming.** Exergaming has excited health care professionals as it continues to gain in popularity, not only among children and adolescents but also among adults, including older adults (Sween, Wallington, Sheppard, et al., 2014). Researchers are evaluating the effectiveness of these interactive games as means of encouraging physical activity in

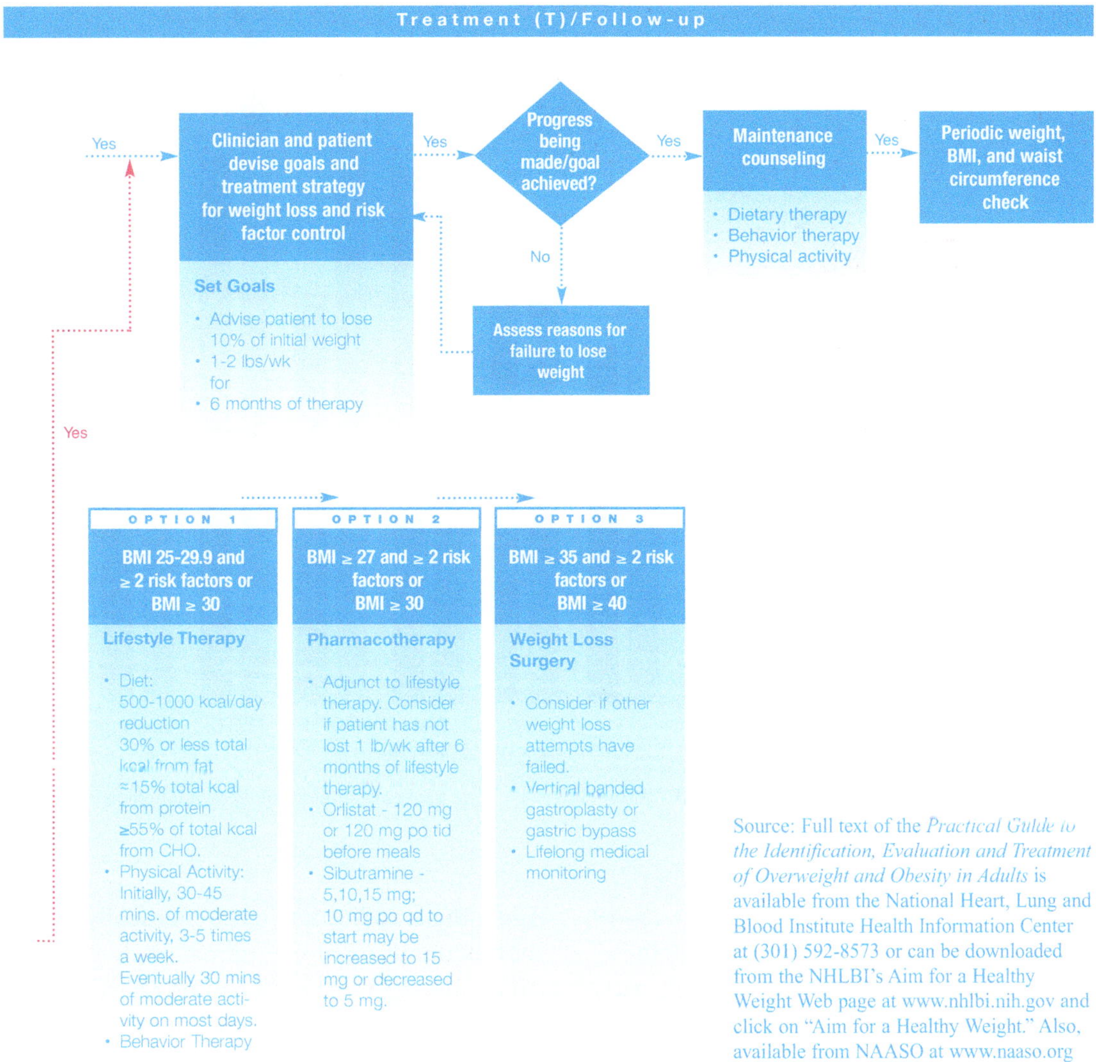

Figure 7.15 Continued

populations of individuals who traditionally have been inactive.

Graf and colleagues (2009) compared differences in energy expenditure in children (aged 10–13 years) as they participated in several physically interactive video games or walked on a treadmill. The interactive video games included Dance Dance Revolution (DDR) and Nintendo Wii Sports, both bowling and boxing. Figure 7.16 illustrates their findings. Note that both DDR (beginning and intermediate levels) and Nintendo Wii Sports boxing elicited energy expenditure similar to and even greater than moderate-intensity treadmill walking. In fact, energy expenditure during these activities was up to three times greater than expenditure at rest. As a result, DDR is becoming a popular addition to many physical activity programs, and it is now estimated that approximately 1,500 schools incorporate the game in their physical education curricula. In Norway, the game has become so popular that it has been registered as an official sport called Machine Dance (Zhu, 2008).

Somewhat similar findings have been reported among adults playing interactive video

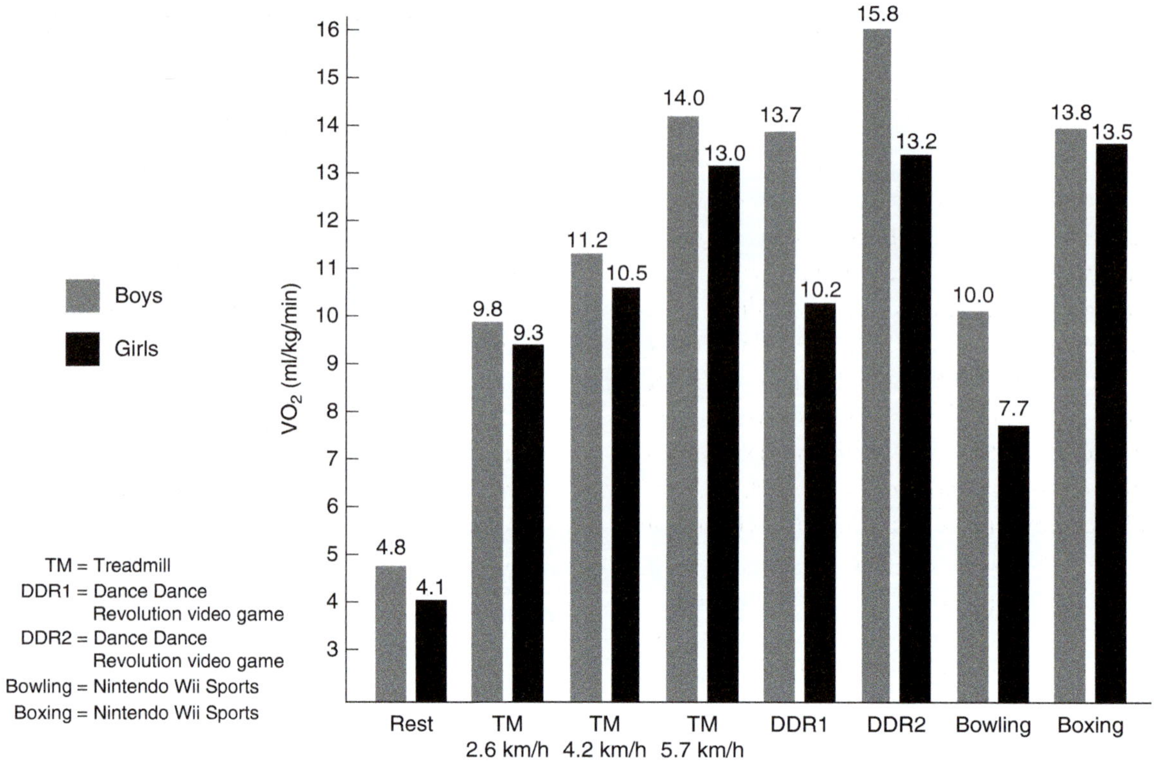

Figure 7.16 Average VO_2 (ml/kg/min) during rest, treadmill walking, and physically interactive video game play

games (Barkley & Penko, 2009). Adults 17–49 years of age were required to participate in three activities: (1) a traditional sedentary video game (Nintendo PunchOut!), which required only hand and finger manipulation of a remote control; (2) a physically interactive video game (Nintendo Wii Sports boxing) requiring total body movement; and (3) treadmill walking at 2.5 mph. An analysis of the data found that energy expenditure (VO_2) and heart rates were highest when the subjects were playing Wii boxing (VO_2: 15.4 ± 4.5 ml/kg/min), followed by treadmill walking (VO_2: 10.4 ± 0.9 ml/kg/min) and sedentary video game play (VO_2: 4.7 ± 0.8 ml/kg/min).

Based on the research currently available, health care professionals are excited about the possibilities offered by these physically interactive video games—particularly their value in motivating extremely sedentary individuals to become more physically active. For example, one longitudinal study reports that video game playing can be effective in promoting self-esteem, which in turn leads to greater real-world sports participation among adolescents (Adachi & Willoughby, 2014). This finding is exciting since it is during the adolescent period that many, particularly young girls, tend to drop out of youth sport participation (see Chapter 14). Likewise, 12-weeks of dance exergaming has been found to significantly improve self-efficacy toward physical activity among overweight and obese adolescent girls (Staiano, Beyl, Hsia, et al., 2017).

In part, because of the success of exergaming among sedentary, overweight, and obese individuals, researchers are now beginning to explore the benefits of **rehabilitation exergaming.** This term is being used to refer to individuals who are sedentary, not because of a lack of motivation, but instead they have been living a sedentary life because some disability has made it impossible to participate in a real-world sport activity. Preliminary results are encouraging because rehabilitation exergaming has been shown to be beneficial for improving energy expenditure in individuals with spinal cord and other neurological disabilities (Mat, Mat, Hasnan, et al., 2017; Mat, Mat, Davis, et al., 2017). Additionally, Nintendo Wii-Fit balance-based video games has proven helpful in improving both the static and performance-related balance parameters in children with mild cerebral palsy (Tarakci, Huseyinsinoglu, Tarakci, & Ozdincler, 2017).

In summary, the greatest strengths of exergaming are that it can increase motivation to engage in physical activity; it can potentially reduce obesity; it can aid in the improvement of aerobic fitness; and it can be adapted to meet the needs of special populations (Benzing & Schmidt, 2018).

SUMMARY

- Cardiorespiratory fitness is the body's ability to deliver oxygen to the working muscle tissues. Increased workloads require a corresponding increase in cardiac output, the amount of blood pumped through the heart in 1 minute. This increased blood flow is made possible by an increase in the heart's rate of contraction and stroke volume, the amount of blood ejected with each beat. Aging affects each of these parameters; HR, SV, and cardiac output all decrease with age.
- The largest amount of oxygen the body can consume at the tissue level is called VO_2max. Generally, VO_2max remains fairly constant during the childhood and adolescent years. Boys may exhibit greater values than girls, but the differences are reduced when variations in body size are considered. The rate of decline with aging is about 1 percent per year after 25 years of age.
- A growing amount of evidence calls into question the benefit of aerobic training for improving aerobic capacity in preadolescent children.
- Strength is the ability to exert force. Static force is produced when there is no change in the length of the exercised muscle; dynamic force is produced when the exercised muscle does change its length. Most studies examining strength changes across the lifespan use grip strength as the dependent variable.
- Most authorities now agree that resistance training can improve muscular strength in prepubescent individuals, especially if approved guidelines are followed. The American Academy of Pediatrics, the UK Strength and Conditioning Association, and the National Strength and Conditioning Association have published position statements and guidelines for prepubescent resistance training. The benefits of muscular fitness are also evident among both young and older adults. Higher levels of muscular fitness are associated with a lower risk of developing functional limitations, fewer cardiorespiratory disease issues, and a lower risk of all-cause mortality.
- Flexibility is the range of motion of a joint. Yearly increases in sit-and-reach flexibility are apparent during childhood and adolescence. Thereafter, decreases in joint mobility become evident. Girls are usually more flexible than boys, and this gender difference widens with age. In older adults, general exercise activity and flexibility exercises may help to slow down the inevitable decrease in joint mobility. Maintaining joint mobility is important to facilitate activities of daily living and may also reduce fall risk.

- Body composition is the ratio of fat tissue to lean muscle mass. Two growth spurts of fat tissue typically occur during childhood, the first during the first year of life and the second during puberty in boys and both prepuberty and puberty in girls. Following this second spurt, females possess more body fat than do males throughout the lifespan.
- The prevalence of obesity in the United States continues to be unacceptable. The NHANES (2015–2016) data set reveals that 39.8 percent (crude) of Americans adults and 18.5 percent of children (aged 2–19 years) are considered obese. Thus, the Healthy People 2020 goal of 30.5 percent for adults and 14.5 percent for children remains a formidable challenge. Researchers have found a positive correlation between childhood obesity and adulthood obesity. In children, excess body fat has been associated with delays in motor development and poor performance on measures of health-related physical fitness.
- The use of interactive technology, commonly referred to as exergaming, has proven to be useful in motivating sedentary individuals to become more active.

key concept review

anabolic steroids
androgens
Bod Pod
body building
body composition
cardiac output
cardiorespiratory fitness
dynamic force
earthbound
exergaming
flexibility
heart rate (HR)
hydrostatic weighing (HW)
hypertrophy
isometric force
maximal oxygen consumption (VO_2max)
muscular strength
obesity
overweight
periodization
physical working capacity
power lifting
rehabilitation exergaming
resistance training
sarcopenia
sit-and-reach test
skinfold calipers
static force
stroke volume (SV)
subcutaneous adipose tissue
testosterone
Type I muscle fibers
Type II muscle fibers
weight lifting

questions for reflection

1. What are the typical VO_2max values for children between 6 and 16 years of age?
2. Can you describe trends in cardiac output after 25 years of age?
3. What is the U.S. Department of Health and Human Services' position regarding the duration, frequency, and intensity of exercise needed to obtain an improvement in cardiorespiratory fitness?
4. Can you describe gender differences in muscle strength in both relative and absolute terms?
5. Can you distinguish between resistance training, weight lifting (power lifting), and bodybuilding?
6. Can you summarize Payne and colleagues' (1997) meta-analysis regarding resistance training in children and youth?
7. Can you summarize the resistance-training guidelines established by AAP, the NSCA, and the UK-SCA?
8. What is the position of the U.S. Powerlifting Association and USA Weightlifting regarding maximum lifting during resistance training for young people?

9. Can you describe potential mechanisms of muscle deterioration, paying particular attention to changes in selective fiber type deterioration? Can you also describe the role of this deterioration in potential falls by older adults?
10. What mechanisms are responsible for increases in muscular strength?
11. What are the causes of declining flexibility with age?
12. Why is obesity so prevalent in the U.S. population?
13. What is the association between childhood obesity and the probability of adult obesity?
14. What is the relationship between body composition and both motor development and motor performance?
15. Describe differences in energy expenditure among the most popular physically interactive video games.

online resources

American College of Sports Medicine, www.acsm.org
American Heart Association, www.heart.org
American Senior Fitness Association, www.seniorfitness.net
Centers for Disease Control and Prevention, www.cdc.gov
Healthy People 2020, www.healthypeople.gov
National Heart, Lung, and Blood Institute, www.nhlbi.nih.gov
National Senior Games Association, www.nsga.com
National Strength and Conditioning Association www.nsca.com
The Obesity Society, www.obesity.org
Physical Activity Guidelines for Americans, www.health.gov/paguidelines/second-edition/pdf/Physical_Activity_Guidelines_2end_edition.pdf
U.S. Department of Health and Human Services, www.hhs.gov

REFERENCES

Adachi, P. J. C., & Willoughby, T. (2014). From the couch to the sports field: The longitudinal associations between sports video game play, self-esteem, and involvement in sports. *Psychology of Popular Media Culture*, doi: 10.1037/ppm0000042.

American Academy of Pediatrics (2008). Policy statement: Strength training by children and adolescents. *Pediatrics*, *121*, 835–840.

American College of Sports Medicine (2009). Progression models in resistance training for healthy adults. *Medicine and Science in Sports and Exercise*, *41*(3), 687–708.

American College of Sports Medicine (2018). *ACSM's guidelines for exercise testing and prescription.* 10th ed. Baltimore, MD: Lippincott Williams & Wilkins.

Armstrong, N. (2006). Aerobic fitness of children and adolescents. *Jornal de Pediatric, 82*, 406–408.

Barkley, J. E., & Penko, A. (2009). Physiologic responses, perceived exertion, and hedonics of playing a physical interactive video game relative to a sedentary alternative and treadmill walking in adults. *Journal of Exercise Physiology online, 12*, 12–22.

Behringer, M., Vom Heede, A., Matthews, M., & Mester, J. (2011). Effects of strength training on motor performance skill in children and adolescents: A meta-analysis. *Pediatric Exercise Science*, *23*, 186–206.

Benzing, V., & Schmidt, M. (2018). Exergaming for children and adolescents: Strengths, weaknesses opportunities and treats. *Journal of Clinical Medicine*, *7*, doi: 10.3390/jcm7110422.

Blackwell, D. L., & Clarke, T. C. (2018). *State variation in meeting the 2008 federal guidelines for both aerobic and muscle-strengthening activities through leisure-time physical activity among adults aged 18–64: United States, 2010–2015*. National Health Statistics Reports, no. 112. Hyattsville, MD: National Center for Health Statistics.

Butte, N. F., Hopkinson, J. M., Wong, W. W., O'Brian-Smith, E., & Ellis, K. J. (2000). Body composition during the first 2 years of life: An updated reference. *Pediatric Research, 47*, 578–584.

Chatrath, R., Shenoy, R., Serratto, M., & Thoele, D. G. (2002). Physical fitness of urban American children. *Pediatric Cardiology, 23*, 608–612.

Colon, C. J. P., Molina-Vicenty, I. L., Frontera-Rodriguez, M., Garcia-Ferre, A., Rivera, B. P., Cintron-Velez, G. C., et al. (2018). Muscle and bone mass loss in the elderly population: Advances in diagnosis and treatment. *Journal of Biomedicine, 3*, 40–49.

Cooper Institute (2009). *Physical fitness assessment and norms for adults and law enforcement.* Dallas: The Cooper Institute.

Dai, S., Hummel, S. L., Salazar, J. B., Taffet, G. E., Zieman, S., & Schwartx, J. B. (2015). Cardiovascular physiology in the older adults. *Journal of Geriatric Cardiology, 12*, 196–201.

Dowda, M., Ainsworth, B. E., Addy, C. L., Saunders, R., & Riner, W. (2001). Environmental influences, physical activity, and weight status in 7- to 16-year-olds. *Archives of Pediatric and Adolescent Medicine, 155*, 711–717.

Eisenmann, J. C., Laurson, K. R., & Welk, G. J. (2011). Aerobic fitness percentiles for U.S. adolescents. *American Journal of Preventive Medicine*, 41, S106–S110.

Ervin, R. B., Wang, C., Fryar, C. C., Miller, M., & Ogden, C. L. (2013). Measures of muscular strength in U.S. children and adolescents, 2012. NCHS data brief, no. 139. Hyattsville, MD: National Center for Health Statistics.

Fahlman, M. M., McNevin, N., Boardley, D., Morgan, A., & Tapp, R. (2011). Effects of resistance training on functional ability in elderly individuals. *American Journal of Health Promotion, 25*, 237–243.

Faigenbaum, A. D., Kraemer, W. J., Blimkie, C. J. R., Jeffreys, I., Micheli, L. F., Nitka, M., et al. (2009). Youth resistance training: Updated position statement paper from the National Strength and Conditioning Association. *Journal of Strength and Conditioning Research, 23*, 1–20.

Faigenbaum, A. D., Milliken, L. A., Loud, R. L., Burak, B. T., Doherty, C. L., & Westcott, W. L. (2002). Comparison of 1 and 2 days per week of strength training in children. *Research Quarterly for Exercise and Sport, 73*, 416–424.

Faigenbaum, A. D., Milliken, L. A., & Westcott, W. L. (2003). Maximal strength testing in healthy children. *Journal of Strength and Conditioning Research, 17*, 162–166.

Faigenbaum, A., O'Connell, J., Glover, S., Loud, R. L., & Westcott, W. (2000). Comparison of different resistance training protocols on upper body strength and endurance development in children. *Medicine and Science in Sports and Exercise, 32* (5 Supplement), S278.

Faigenbaum, A. D., Westcott, W. L., Loud, R. L., & Long, C. (1999). The effects of different resistance training protocols on muscular strength and endurance development in children. *Pediatrics, 104*, e5.

Faigenbaum, A., Westcott, W., Micheli, L., Outerbridge, A., Long, C., LaRosa-Loud, R., et al. (1996). The effects of strength training and detraining on children. *Journal of Strength and Conditioning Research, 10*, 109–114.

Faigenbaum, A. D., Zaichkowsky, L. D., Westcott, W. L., Micheli, L. J., & Fehlandt, A. F. (1993). The effects of a twice-a-week strength training program on children. *Pediatric Exercise Science, 5*, 339–346.

Falk, B., & Mor, G. (1996). The effects of resistance and martial arts training in 6–7-year-old boys. *Pediatric Exercise Science, 8*, 48–56.

Falk, B., & Tenenbaum, G. (1996). The effectiveness of resistance training in children. A meta-analysis. *Sports Medicine, 22*, 176–186.

Farrell, P. A., Joyner, M. J., & Caiozzo, V. J. (2011). *ACSM's advanced exercise physiology.* Baltimore, MD: Lippincott Williams & Wilkins.

Fatouros, I. G., Kambas, A., Katrabasas, I., Mikolaidis, K., Chatzinikolaou, A., Leontsini, D., et al. (2005). Strength training and detraining effects on muscular strength, anaerobic power, and mobility of inactive older men are intensity dependent. *British Journal of Sports Medicine, 39*, 776–780.

Fiatarone, M. A., Marks, E. C., Ryan, N. D., Meredith, C. N., Lipsitz, L. A., & Evans, W. J. (1990). High-intensity strength training in nonagenarians: Effects on skeletal muscle. *Journal of the American Medical Association, 22*, 3029–3034.

Fields, D. A., & Goran, M. I. (2000). Body composition techniques and the four-compartment model in children. *Journal of Applied Physiology, 89*, 613–620.

Fleck, S. J., & Kraemer, W. J. (2014). *Designing resistance training programs.* 4th ed. Champaign, IL: Human Kinetics.

Fryar, C. D., Carroll, M. D., & Ogden, C. L. (2014). Prevalence of overweight, obesity, and extreme obesity among adults: United States, 1960–1962 through 2011–2012. Health E-Stat. Retrieved from www.cdc.gov/nchs/data/hestat/obesity_adult_11_12/obesity_adult_11_12.pdf.

Fryar, C. D., Gu, Q., & Ogden, C. L. (2012). Anthropometric reference data for children and adults: United States, 2007–2010. *Vital Health Statistics*, ser. 11, no, 252. Hyattsville, MD: National Center for Health Statistics.

Fujita, E., Taaffe, D. R., Yoshitake, Y., & Kanehisa, H. (2019). Repeated sit-to-stand exercise enhances muscle strength and reduces lower body muscular demands in physically frail elders. *Experimental Gerontology, 116*, 86–92.

Gahche, J., Fakhouri, T., Carroll, D. D., Burt, V. L., Wang, C., & Fulton, J. E. (2014). Cardiorespiratory fitness levels among U.S. youth aged 12–15 years: United States, 1999–2004 and 2012. Data Brief No. 153. Hyattsville, MD: National Center for Health Statistics.

Graf, D. L., Pratt, L. V., Hester, C. N., & Short, K. R. (2009). Playing active video games increases energy expenditure in children. *Pediatrics, 124*, 534–540.

Guo, S., Roche, A. F., Chumlea, W. C., Gardner, J. D., & Siervogel, R. M. (1994). The predictive value of childhood body mass index values for overweight at age 35y. *American Journal of Clinical Nutrition, 59*, 810–819.

Haab, T., & Wydra, G. (2017). The effect of age on hamstring passive properties after a 10-week stretch training. *The Journal of Physical Therapy Science, 29*, 1048–1053.

Hales, C. M., Carroll, M. D., Fryar, C. D., & Ogden, C. L. (2017). Prevalence of obesity among adults and youth: United States, 2015–2016. NCHS data brief, no. 288. Hyattsville, MD: National Center for Health Statistics.

Hasarangi, L. B. S., & Jayawardana, D. G. S. K. (2018). Comparison of hamstring flexibility between patients with chronic lower back pain and the healthy individuals at the national hospital of Sri Lanka. *Biomedical Journal of Scientific & Technical Research, 5*, doi: 10.26717/BJSTR.2018.05.001171.

Healthy People 2020 (2019). Nutrition and weight status. Retrieved from www.healthypeople.gov/2020/topics-objectives/topic/nutrition-and-weight-status

Hedley, A. A., Ogden, C. L., Carroll, M. D., Curtin, L. R., & Flegal, K. M. (2004). Prevalence of overweight and obesity among US children, adolescents, and adults, 1999–2002. *Journal of the American Medical Association, 291*, 2847–2850.

Housh, T. J., Housh, D. J., & deVries, H. A. (2016). *Applied exercise and sport physiology with labs.* 4th ed. Scottsdale, AZ: Holcomb Hathaway.

Indranil, M. (2014). Growth development and maturity in children and adolescents: Relation to sports and physical activity. *American Journal of Sports Science and Medicine 2*, 48–50.

Isaacs, L. D., & Pohlman, R. L. (2000). Effectiveness of the stretch-shortening cycle in children's vertical jump performance. *Medicine and Science in Sports and Exercise, 32* (5 Supplement), S278.

Isaacs, L. D., Pohlman, R., & Craig, B. (1994). Effects of resistance training on strength development in prepubescent females. *Medicine and Science in Sports and Exercise, 26* (5 Supplement).

Jeukendrup, A., & Gleeson, M. (2019). *Sport nutrition*, 3rd ed. Champaign IL: Human Kinetics.

Johnson, L. D., O'Malley, P. M., Bachman, J. G., & Schulenberg, J. D. (2006). *National results on adolescent drug use.* NIH Publication No. 06–5882. Bethesda, MD: National Institute on Drug Abuse.

Joyner, M. J. (2000). Over-the-counter supplements and strength training. *Exercise and Sport Science Reviews, 28(1)*, 2–3.

Kaminsky, L. A., Arena, R., & Myers, J. (2015). Reference standards for cardiorespiratory fitness measured with cardiopulmonary exercise testing: Data from the fitness registry and the importance of exercise national database. *Mayo Clinic Proceedings, 90*, 1515–1523.

Kasch, F. W., Boyer, J. L., Van Camp, S. P., Verity, L. S., & Wallace, J. P. (1990). The effects of physical activity and inactivity on aerobic power in older men: A longitudinal study. *Physician and Sportsmedicine, 18*, 73–83.

Keogh, J., & Sugden, D. (1985). *Movement skill development*. New York: Macmillan.

Kim, H. J., Lee, K. J., Jeon, Y. J., Ahn, M B., Jung, I. A., Kim, S. H., et al. (2016). Relationships of physical fitness and obesity with metabolic risk factors in children and adolescents: Chungju city cohort study. *Annals of Pediatric Endocrinology & Metabolism*, *21*, 31–38.

Lakoski, S. G., Willis, B., Barlow, C. E., Leonard, D., Gao, A., Radford, N. B., et al. (2015). Midlife cardiorespiratory fitness, incident cancer, and survival after cancer in men: The Cooper Center Longitudinal Study. *JAMA Oncology*, *1*, 231–237.

Lemmer, J. T., Hurlbut, D. E., Martel, G. F., Tracy, B. L., Ivey, F. M., Metter, E. J., et al. (2000). Age and gender responses to strength training and detraining. *Medicine and Science in Sports and Exercise, 32*, 1505–1512.

Lloyd, R. S., Faigenbaum, A. D., Stone, M. H., Oliver, J. L., Jeffreys, I., Moody, J. A., et al. (2014). Position statement on youth resistance training: The 2014 international consensus. *British Journal of Sports Medicine*, *48*, 498–505.

Magarey, A. M., Daniels, L. S., Boulton, T. J., & Cockington, R. A. (2003). Predicting obesity in early adulthood from childhood and parental obesity. *International Journal of Obesity, 27*, 505–513.

Malina, R. M., Bouchard, C., & Bar-Or, O. (2004). *Growth, maturation, and physical activity.* 2nd ed. Champaign, IL: Human Kinetics.

Mandigout, S., Melin, A., Lecoq, A. M., Courteix, D., & Obert, P. (2002). Effect of two aerobic training regimens on the cardiorespiratory response of prepubertal boys and girls. *Acta Paediatrica, 91*, 403–408.

Mat, R. M., Mat, R. H., Davis, G. M., Husain, R., & Hasnan, N. (2017). Exergaming for individuals with neurological disability: A systematic review. *Disability and Rehabilitation*, *39*, 727–735.

Mat, R. M., Mat, R. H., Hasnan, N., Davis, G. M., & Husain, R. (2017). Exergaming boxing versus heavy-bag boxing: Are these equipotent for individuals with spinal cord injury? *European Journal of Physical and Rehabilitation Medicine*, *53*, 527–534.

McArdle, W. D., Katch, F. I., & Katch, V. L. (2014). *Exercise physiology.* 8th ed. Baltimore, MD: Lippincott Williams & Wilkins.

McArdle, W. D., Katch, F. I., & Katch, V. L. (2006). *Essentials of exercise physiology.* 3rd ed. Philadelphia, PA: Lippincott Williams & Wilkins.

Moore, K. L., & Persaud, T. V. N. (2008). *Before we are born: Essentials of embryology and birth defects*. 7th ed. Philadelphia, PA: Saunders.

Moran, J., Sandercock, G. R. H., Ramirez-Campillo, R., Meylan, C., Collison, J., & Parry, D. A. (2016). A meta-analysis of maturation-related variation in adolescent boy athletes' adaptations to short-term training. *Journal of Sports Sciences*, doi: 10.1080/02640414.2016.1209306.

Morano, M., Colella, D., & Caroli, M. (2011). Gross motor skill performance in a sample of overweight and non-overweight preschool children. *International Journal of Pediatric Obesity*, Supplement 2, 42–46.

Mrzena, B., & Macek, M. (1978). Use of treadmill and working capacity assessment of preschool children. In J. Borms & M. Hebbelinck (Eds.), *Pediatric work physiology.* New York: Karger.

National Heart, Lung, and Blood Institute (2000). *The practical guide: Identification, evaluation, and treatment of overweight and obesity in adults.* Bethesda, MD: NIH publication no. 00–4084. Retrieved from www.nhlbi.nih.gov/files/docs/guidelines/prctgd_c.pdf.

National Senior Games Association (2017). 2017 National Senior Games result book. Baton Rouge, LA. Retrieved from www.nsga.com/media/documents/national-results/2017/2017NSGResultsBook.pdf.

Ogden, C. L., Carroll, M. D., & Flegal, K. M. (2008). High body mass index for age among U.S. children and adolescents, 2003–2006. *Journal of the American Medical Association, 299*, 2401–2405.

Ogden, C. L., Carroll, M. D., Kit, B. K., & Flegal, K. M. (2013, October). Prevalence of obesity among adults: United States, 2011–2012. Centers for Disease Control and Prevention. www.cdc.gov/nchs/data/databriefs/db131.pdf.

Ogden, C. L., Carroll, M. D., Kit, B. K., & Flegal, K. M. (2014). Prevalence of childhood and adult obesity in the United States, 2011–2012. *Journal of the American Medical Association, 311*, 806–814.

Ogden, C. L., Flegal, K. M., Carroll, M. D., & Johnson, C. L. (2002). Prevalence and trends in overweight among U.S. children and adolescents, 1999–2000. *Journal of the American Medical Association, 288*, 1728–1732.

Ozemek, C., Whaley, M. H., Finch, W. H., & Kaminsky, L. (2016). High cardiorespiratory fitness levels slow the decline in peak heart rate with age. *Medicine & Science in Sports & Exercise, 18*, 73–81.

Ozemek, C., Whaley, M. H., Finch W. H., & Kaninsky, L. (2017). Maximal heart rate declines linearly with age independent of cardiorespiratory fitness levels. *European Journal of Sport Science, 17*, 563–570.

Ozmun, J. C., Mikesky, A. E., & Surburg, P. R. (1994). Neuromuscular adaptations following prepubescent strength training. *Medicine and Science in Sports and Exercise, 26*, 510–514.

Pandey, A., Cornwell III, W. K., Willis, B., Neeland, I. J., Gao, A., Leonard, D., et al. (2017). Body mass index and cardiorespiratory fitness in mid-life and risk of heart failure hospitalization in older age. *American College of Cardiology: Heart Failure, 5*, doi: 10:1016/j.jchf.2016.12.021.

Pandey, A., Patel, M. R., Willis, B., Gao, A., Leonard, D., Das, S. R., et al. (2016). Association between midlife cardiorespiratory fitness and risk of stroke. *Stroke, 47*, 1720–1726.

Payne, V. G., & Morrow, J. R. (1993). Exercise and VO_2max in children: A meta-analysis. *Research Quarterly for Exercise and Sport, 64*, 305–313.

Payne, V. G., Morrow, J. R., Johnson, L., & Dalton, S. N. (1997). Resistance training in children and youth: A meta-analysis. *Research Quarterly for Exercise and Sport, 88*, 80–88.

President's Council on Physical Fitness and Sports (2005). Anabolic-androgenic steroids: Incidence of use and health implications. *Research Digest, 5*, 1–8.

Reddy, R. S., & Alahmari, K. A. (2016). Effect of lower extremity stretching exercises on balance in geriatric population. *International Journal of Health Sciences, 10*, 389–395.

Ross, J. G., & Gilbert, G. G. (1985). The national children and youth fitness study: A summary of findings. *Journal of Physical Education, Recreation, and Dance, 56*, 45–50.

Ross, J. G., & Pate, R. R. (1987). The national children and youth fitness study II: A summary of findings. *Journal of Physical Education, Recreation, and Dance, 58*, 51–56.

Roush, J. R., Gombold, K. L., & Bay, R. C. (2017). Normative grip strength values in men and women, ages 50 to 89 years' old. *The Internet Journal of Allied Health Sciences and Practice, 16*(1), Article 7. Retrieved from https://nsuworks.nova.edu/ijahsp/vol16/iss1/7.

Rowland, T. W. (1985). Aerobic response to endurance training in prepubescent children: A critical analysis. *Medicine and Science in Sports and Exercise, 17*, 493–497.

Rowland, T. W. (1996). *Developmental exercise physiology.* Champaign, IL: Human Kinetics.

Saint-Maurice, P. F., Coughlan, D., Kelly, S. P., Keadle, S. K., Cook, M. B., Carlson, S. A., et al. (2019). Association of leisure-time physical activity across the adult life course with all-cause and cause-specific mortality. *JAMA Network Open, 2*, doi: 10.1001/jamanetworkopen.2019.0355.

Sale, D. G. (1988). Neural adaptation to resistance training. *Medicine and Science in Sports and Exercise, 20*, S135–S145.

Sale, D. G. (1989). Strength training in children. In C. V. Gisolfi & D. R. Lamb (Eds.), *Perspectives in exercise science and sport medicine: Youth, exercise, and sport.* Indianapolis, IN: Benchmark.

Shephard, R. J. (1987). *Human physiological work capacity.* Cambridge: Cambridge University Press.

Shirley, M. (1931). *The first two years: A study of twenty-five babies.* Minneapolis, MN: University of Minnesota Press.

Sinclair, D. (1998). *Human growth after birth.* 6th ed. Oxford: Oxford University Press.

Skinner, A. C., Ravanbakht, S. N., Skelton, J. A., Perrin, E. M., & Armstrong, S. C. (2018). Prevalence of obesity and severe obesity in US children, 1999–2016. *Pediatrics, 141*, doi: 10.1542/peds.2017-3459.

Slining, M., Adair, L. S., Goldman, B. D., Borja, J. B., & Bentley, M. (2010). Infant overweight is associated with delayed motor development. *Journal of Pediatrics, 157*, 20–25.

Spirduso, W. W. (2005). *Physical dimensions of aging.* Champaign, IL: Human Kinetics.

Stahle, S., Roberts, S., Davis, B., & Rybicki, L. (1995). Effect of 2 versus 3 times per week weight training programs in boys 7 to 16. *Medicine and Science in Sports and Exercise, 27*, S114.

Staiano, A. E., Beyl, R. A., Hsia, D. S., Katzmarzyk, P. T., & Newton Jr, R. L. (2017). Twelve weeks of dance exergaming in overweight and obese adolescent girls: Transfer effects on physical activity, screen time, and self-efficacy. *Journal of Sport Health Science*, 6, 4–10.

Stathokostas, L., Little, R. M. D., Vandervoort, A. A., & Paterson, D. H. (2012). Flexibility training and functional ability in older adults: A systematic review. *Journal of Aging Research*, 2012, Article ID 306818 1–30.

Stathokostas, L., McDonald, M. W., Little, R. M. D., & Paterson, D. H. (2013). Flexibility of older adults aged 55–86 years and the influence of physical activity. *Journal of Aging Research*, doi: 10.1155/2013/743843.

Stones, M. J., & Kozma, A. (1985). Physical performance. In N. Charness (Ed.), *Aging and human performance.* New York: Wiley.

Sween, J., Wallington, S. F., Sheppard, V., Taylor, T., Llanos, A. A., & Adams-Campbell, L. L. (2014). The role of exergaming in improving physical activity: A review. *Journal of Physical Activity & Health*, *11*, 864–870.

Tanaka, H., Monahan, K. D., & Seals, D. R. (2001). Age-predicted maximal heart rate revisited. *Journal of the American College of Cardiology, 37*, 153–156.

Tarakci, D., Huseyinsinoglu, B. E., Tarakci, E., & Ozdincler, R. A. (2017). Effects of Nintendo Wii-Fit video games on balance in children with mild cerebral palsy. *Pediatrics International*, *58*, 1042–1050.

U.S. Department of Health and Human Services (2018). *Physical activity guidelines for Americans*, 2nd ed. Washington, DC: U.S. Department of Human Services.

Vrijens, J. (1978). Muscle strength development in pre- and postpubescent age. In J. Borms & M. Hebbelinck (Eds.), *Pediatric work physiology.* New York: Karger.

Willis, B., Leonard, D., Barlow, C. E., Martin, S. B., DeFina, L. F., & Trivedi, M. H. (2018). Association of midlife cardiorespiratory fitness with incident depression and cardiovascular death after depression in later life. *JAMA Psychiatry*, *75*, 911–917.

World Health Organization (2010). *Global recommendations on physical activity for health.* Geneva: WHO.

Zhang, T., Whelton, P. K., Xi, B., Krousel-Wood, M., Bazzano, L., He, J., et al. (2019). Rate of change in body mass index at different ages during childhood and adult obesity risk. *Pediatric Obesity*, doi: 10.1111/ijpo.12513.

Zhu, W. (2008). Promoting physical activity using technology. *Research Digest, 9*, 1–8.

Zwolski, C., Quatman-Yates, C., & Paterno, M. V. (2017). Resistance training in youth: Laying the foundation for injury prevention and physical literacy. *Sport Health: A Multidisciplinary Approach*, doi: 10.1177/1941738117704153.

8 MOVEMENT AND THE CHANGING SENSES

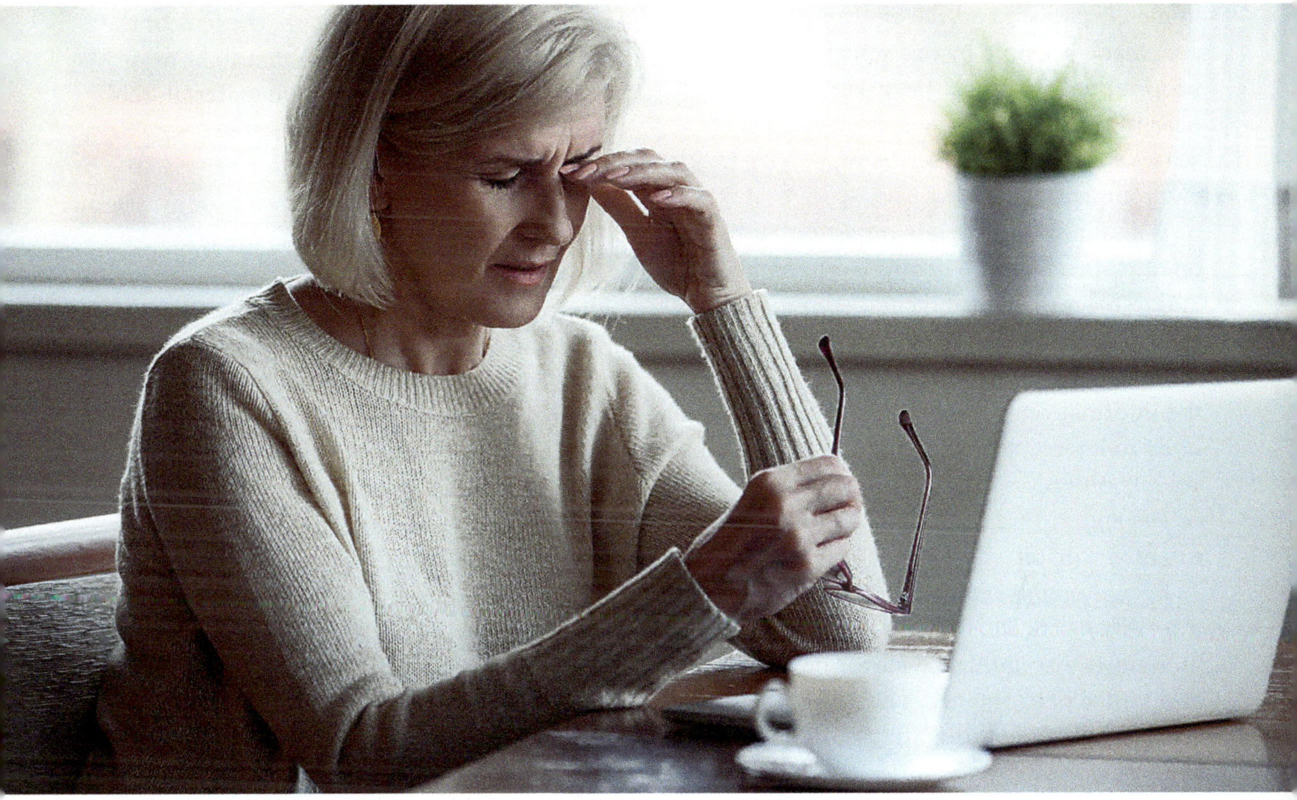

Chapter Objectives

From the information presented in this chapter, you will be able to

- Describe the mechanics of human vision
- Describe the physical development of the eye
- Describe age-related changes in visual acuity, depth perception, field of vision, eye dominance, and tracking and object interception ability and their relationship to skilled motor performance
- Describe the course of motor development and motor performance in children with visual impairments
- Describe the development of the nonvisual senses (proprioceptive, auditory, and cutaneous systems) and identify how these senses influence motor development and motor performance

The human body contains many complicated communication channels that allow us to respond to the multitude of stimuli we encounter, primarily during our waking hours. This communicative link between the human organism and the environment is in part made possible by our senses: vision, proprioception, touch, taste, smell, and hearing. Information we receive from these senses enables us to describe our environment.

Without doubt, we rely on vision more than on any other sense to describe our environment and to react to environmental stimuli. In fact, most movement tasks are initiated as a result of receiving visual information. Vision provides the information we need in order to adjust our body to intercept moving objects. Furthermore, we rely on vision to emulate the movements of others and to find our way around our visually oriented world.

Even though vision is the sensory modality of choice, nonvisual sensory modalities also influence motor development and motor performance. Therefore, this chapter will end with a discussion of the nonvisual sensory modalities and the role they play in both directly and indirectly influencing motor development and motor performance.

UNDERSTANDING THE MECHANICS OF VISION

The photographic camera and the human eye share many common structural features. To produce a sharp photograph, the lens of the camera must be focused so that light rays converge on its light-sensitive material, the digital sensor or photographic film. Similarly, for the human eye to obtain a clear visual image, light entering the eye must converge on the eye's light-sensitive tissue, the **retina**.

Within the retina are two types of photoreceptors: **rods**, which make colorless night vision possible, and **cones**, which make color vision and acuity possible. Cones are predominantly concentrated in a region of the retina known as the **macula**; rods are located in the retina's periphery and, thus, make peripheral vision possible.

Exactly how does light enter the eye and get focused on the retina? The eye adjusts its ocular refractory ability by changing the shape of the lens. The lens of the human eye changes shape whenever the **ciliary muscle** is contracted. This process that maintains a clear retinal image in the presence of varying light conditions is called **accommodation**. Sharpness of vision results when light properly converges on the macula. Figure 8.1 illustrates the major structures of the human eye.

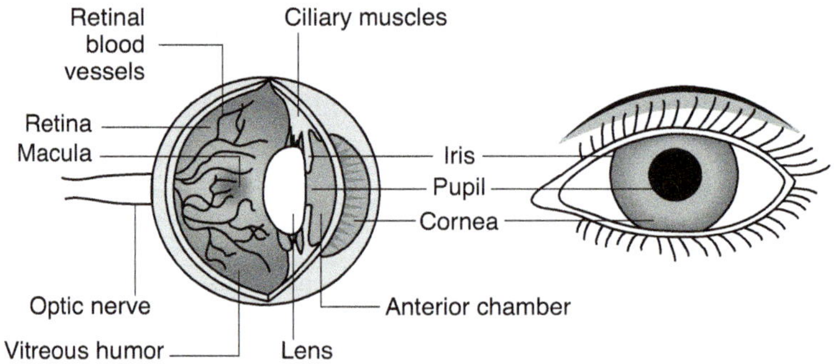

Figure 8.1 Diagram of the human eye

PHYSICAL DEVELOPMENT OF THE EYE

The eye develops as an outgrowth of the forebrain and is an inseparable component of the central nervous system. Of the 12 cranial nerves, 6 play a role in vision. The eye, like the brain, achieves most but not all of its growth prior to birth. Because the eye is shorter at birth than it will be at maturity, the infant's eye is **hyperopic**; that is, light entering the eye focuses behind the retina. Nevertheless, the infant can achieve sharp vision through accommodation.

The eye's cornea increases its diameter until adulthood is reached. Thereafter, the cornea does not grow but does change its curvature to become less spherical.

The retina is fairly well developed at birth but is thicker than an adult's retina and contains mostly rod cells. During the first postnatal month, as the retina thins and cone cells begin to squeeze between the rod cells, the macula becomes more differentiated. By 8 months of age, the macula is histologically mature.

The muscles that control eye movements and the dilator muscles of the pupil are perhaps the slowest structures to develop. Ciliary muscle cells first appear in the eye at about the fifth prenatal month. Thus, except for the macular and dilator muscles of the pupil, by the end of the sixth prenatal month, all eye parts are present and presumably able to function.

DEVELOPMENT OF SELECTED VISUAL TRAITS AND SKILLED MOTOR PERFORMANCE

Despite the relatively advanced size of the eye in utero, the eye is still immature at birth because optimal vision requires good central and peripheral function of the retina, the ability to gauge depth, and the ability to track moving objects. Here, we describe postnatal changes in these selected visual attributes, paying special attention to the influence of these changes on skilled motor performance.

Visual Acuity

Visual acuity is the ability to see detail in an object. The fine details of objects are blurred for a person with poor visual acuity.

To appreciate changes in visual acuity across the lifespan, we must first describe how visual acuity is measured. With the most common technique, a person reads the smallest letters possible on the **Snellen eye chart** (see Figure 8.2). Visual acuity determined by the Snellen eye chart is called **static visual acuity** because both the target and the performer are stationary. Distance visual acuity is expressed in fractional notation that compares the measured individual's visual acuity with the acuity of a typical person. A person with 20/20 vision can see an object 20 feet away with the same level of detail that other people with typical vision can see at 20 feet. A person with 20/100 vision has less than typical static visual acuity: this person can see an object 20 feet away with the level of detail that people with typical vision can see at 100 feet. Use of the Snellen eye chart is not recommended for children under 3 years of age. Software applications are now available for mobile devices for the purpose of assessing static visual acuity in both clinical and community-based field settings (Rono, Bastawrous, Macleod, et al., 2018; Bastawrous, Rono, Livingstone, et al., 2017; Brady, Eghrari, & Labrique, 2015). See the accompanying box, p. 237.

Developmentally, improvement in static visual acuity occurs during the first 4 to 5 years of life (AOA, 2017). However, much variability exists in reported acuity measures both within and across different ages. For instance, visual acuity at birth has been estimated at between 20/200 and 20/400. By 6 months, visual acuity has improved to between 20/50 and 20/200;

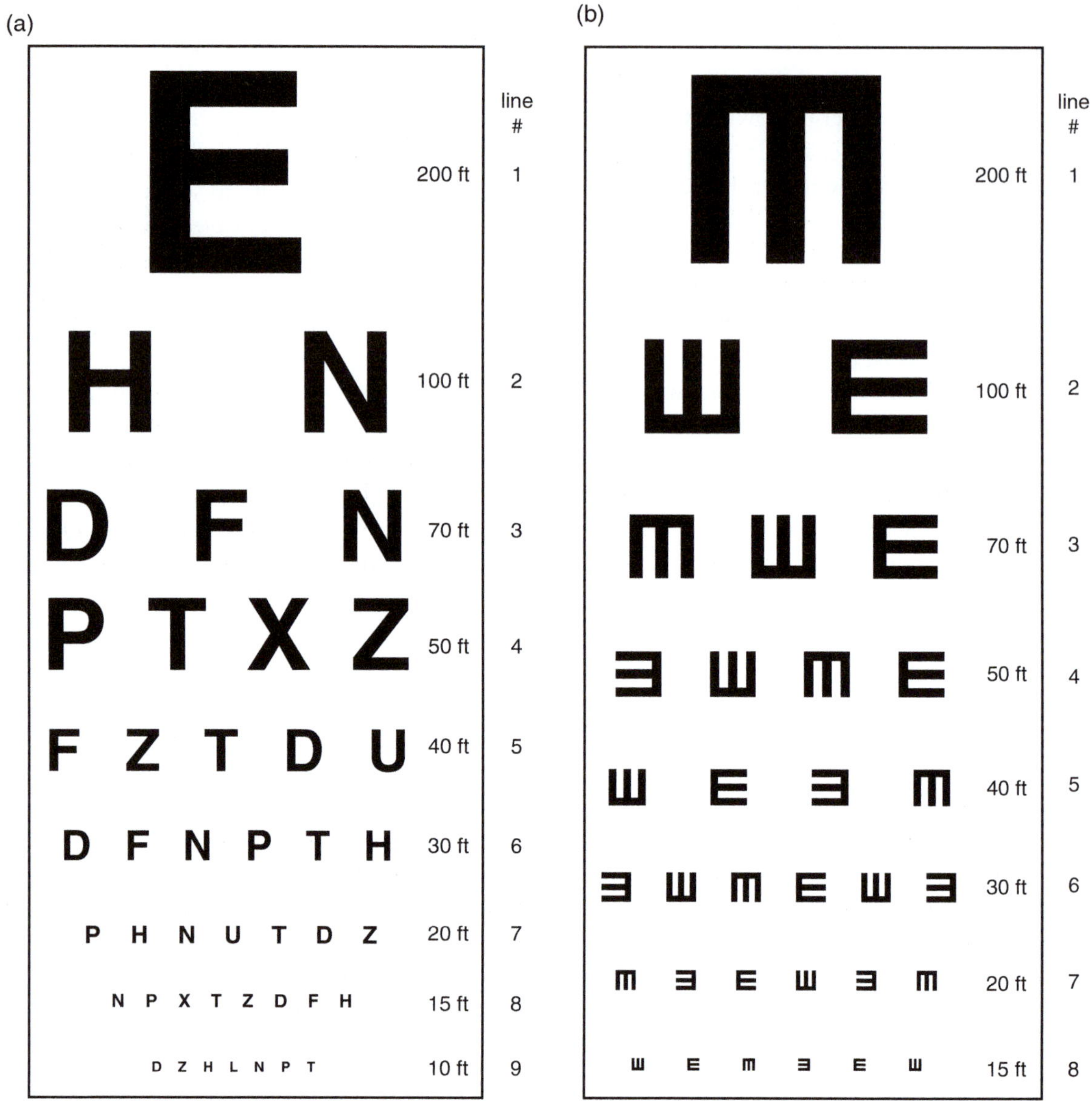

(a) is used to determine static visual acuity for individuals who are able to recognize letters. (b) is used with children in grades K-1 who may not be capable of letter recognition. The child must point in the direction that the "E" symbol faces or state that the symbol faces up, down, right, or left.

Figure 8.2 Snellen eye charts

by 18 months, to 20/40 to 20/100. Typical static distance acuity (20/20) is usually attained some time around 3 years of age. At first glance, it may appear that the infant has very low quality functional vision. In reality, however, infants' visual acuity is sufficient for most of the static visual tasks they confront. For example, a 1-month-old infant has adequate acuity for resolving facial expressions when the baby is held close to a person. Similarly, the acuity of a 6-month-old infant is adequate for stimulating the visual curiosity that causes the child to reach for small objects as grasping skills begin to develop.

PEEK ACUITY PRO: A SMARTPHONE-BASED VISUAL ACUITY TEST

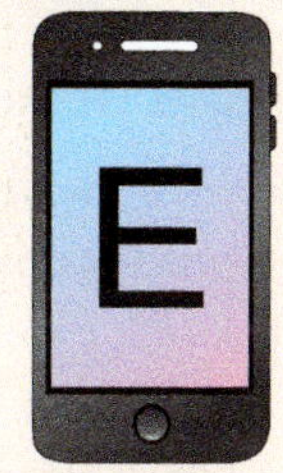

Advances in technology have made it now possible to assess visual acuity using a smartphone. The validity of this has been established through research (Bastawrous, Rono, Livingstone, et al., 2015). To conduct the assessment, the patient is seated approximately 2 to 3 meters from the examiner. The smartphone will display the letter "E" similar to that which appears on the Snellen eye chart. The patient is instructed to simply point in the direction the "E" is facing. To record the response, the examiner will swipe the phone's screen in the direction indicated by the patient, even if the patient's response is incorrect. Therefore, there is no need for the examiner to view the phone's screen. If the patient indicates an inability to recognize the direction of the "E," the examiner will shake the smartphone to record its response. The smartphone will vibrate to signal to the examiner when the assessment is complete. A short video demonstrating an actual assessment can be found at: www.youtube.com/watch?v=Xw3qMLjdpfM

A second type of visual acuity is dynamic visual acuity, the ability to see detail in moving objects. **Dynamic visual acuity** depends on the ability of the central nervous system to estimate an object's direction and velocity and the ability of the ocular-motor system to "catch" and "hold" an object's image on the eye's fovea (center posterior part of the retina) long enough to permit resolution of the object's detail.

Dynamic visual acuity improves rapidly between 5 and 15 years of age, at which point it reaches its peak (Bhootra & Sumitra, 2008). Like many human qualities, dynamic visual acuity declines with age (Li, Beaumont, Rine, et al., 2014), and this decline generally begins at about 20 years of age.

Visual Acuity and Motor Performance

Both static and dynamic visual acuity correlate with the successful performance of specific motor tasks. Thus, this attribute of vision may play a key role in motor task performance. For example, correlations as high as 0.76 have been found between measures of dynamic visual acuity and basketball field-goal shooting percentage during a competitive season (Beals, Mayyasi, Templeton, & Johnson, 1971). Studies by Sanderson and Whiting (1974, 1978) also suggest a possible relationship between dynamic visual acuity and task performance. These researchers found a significant relationship between dynamic visual acuity and performance on a ball-catching task. The ball's velocity was found to place a constraint on performance. For instance, a fleece ball or a whiffle ball travels through space more slowly than a baseball, giving participants more time to process visual information and succeed in catching the ball. This explains why people with low levels of dynamic visual acuity may benefit from the use of special equipment when playing ball-skill activities.

Laby, Rosenbaum, Kirschen, and colleagues (1996) evaluated visual acuity among professional baseball players. Their findings were based on the evaluation of 387 players from the Los Angeles Dodgers over a 4-year period. Eighty percent of the players demonstrated a static visual acuity of 20/15 or higher. Some players even exhibited a static visual acuity of 20/9, which according to the authors approaches the limits of human performance. Only 1.3 percent of the players exhibited static visual acuity of 20/30 or less. These results continue to be supported in a more recent study (Laby & Kirschen, 2017).

Effects of Aging on Visual Acuity

Age-related eye diseases (AREDs) are a leading cause of loss of visual acuity and, if left untreated, can sometimes lead to blindness. In fact, approximately 47,000 Americans become blind each year. The four major AREDs are age-related macular degeneration, glaucoma, cataracts, and diabetic retinopathy. Figure 8.3 shows, through simulated photos, how individuals with age-related eye diseases may see the same subject. We will discuss each ARED, as well as presbyopia, an age-related disorder that also affects vision.

Age-related macular degeneration (AMD). One of the most prevalent causes of loss of visual acuity in older adults is **age-related macular degeneration (AMD)**. According to the National Eye Institute (2019), an estimated 2.07 million people are affected by this visual impairment and by 2030 that number is expected to increase to more than 3 million. AMD can take one of two forms: dry AMD or wet AMD (National Eye Institute, 2008). Dry AMD is the more prevalent, responsible for approximately 90 percent of all AMD cases. This form of AMD results from the breakdown of the light-sensitive cells in the macula. Because the breakdown occurs in the macula, this disease affects central vision. Therefore, although individuals with dry AMD are not capable of driving and may find reading difficult, they are still capable of general mobility. The disease progresses so slowly that most affected people will not lose total central vision. Dry AMD cannot be medically treated. The more devastating form of AMD is wet AMD. With wet AMD, new blood vessels grow behind the retina (neovascularization), and these new vessels tend to be very fragile and oftentimes will leak. This leakage causes a rapid

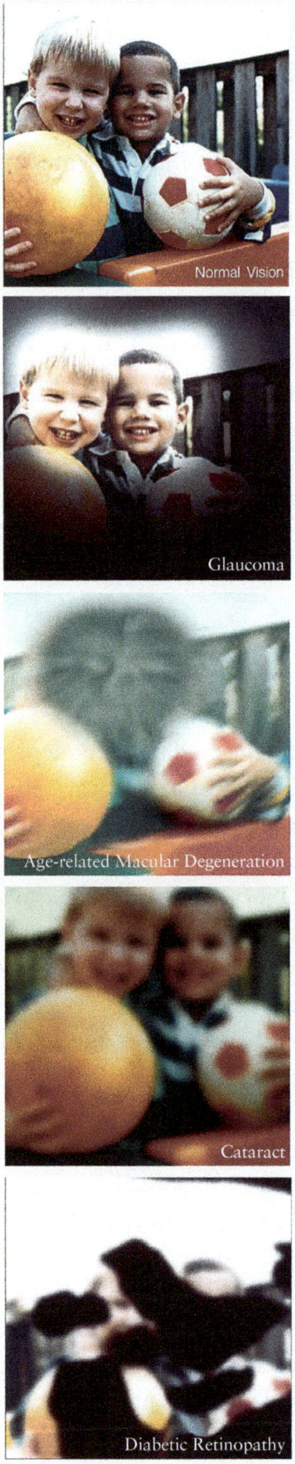

Figure 8.3 Simulated photos of a subject as it might be seen by people with various age-related eye diseases
Source: Courtesy of the National Eye Institute.

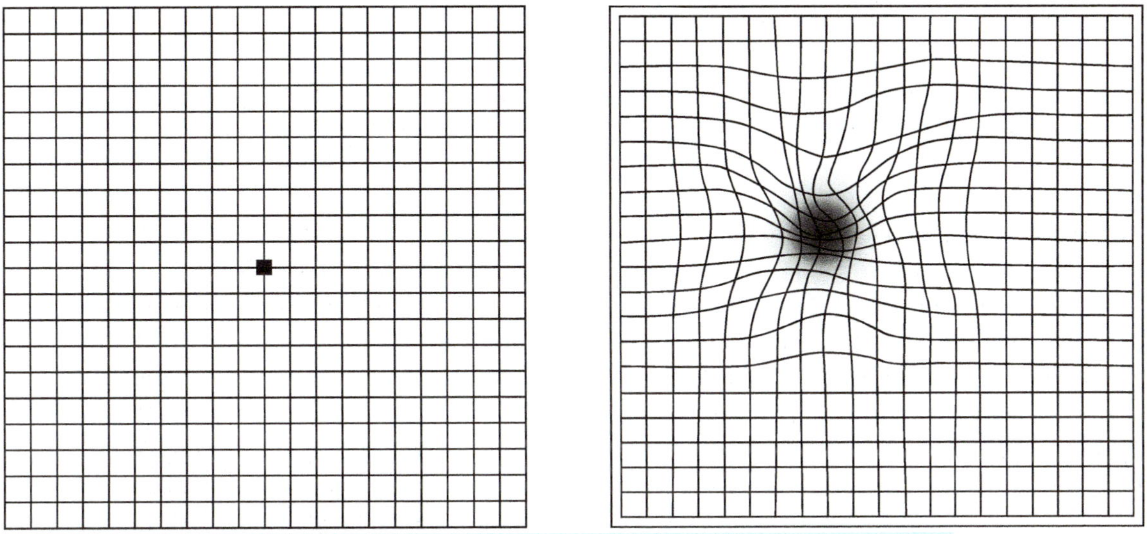

Figure 8.4 On the left is an Amsler grid; on the right is how it might look to someone with AMD
Source: National Eye Institute (2008).

deterioration of the macula. Although only 10 percent of AMD cases are of this form, it is responsible for 90 percent of all AMD blindness (Gorusupudi, Nelson, & Bernstein, 2017).

Visual acuity in people affected with AMD ranges anywhere from 20/50 to total central vision blindness. Several tests are available to detect AMD. One test is visual inspection of the retina for the presence of **drusen**, small yellow deposits in the retina that are an early sign of AMD. To facilitate this visual inspection of the retina, the eye-care professional will chemically dilate the pupils of the eyes. The patient may also be asked to take an **Amsler grid** examination (see Figure 8.4), a test associated with wet AMD. If wet AMD is suspected, a fluorescein angiography will likely be performed. A special dye is injected into an arm vein, and pictures of the inner eye are taken, which will show any retinal blood vessel leakage. If leakage is found, laser surgery is frequently performed in an attempt to stop or reduce it. Additionally, an injection into the eye's vitreous of an antivascular endothelial growth factor can be used to stop abnormal blood vessel growth which can help stabilize and sometimes improve vision.

Risk factors for AMD include: advancing age, heredity, cigarette smoking, long-term sun exposure, and nutritional factors. In fact, results from the Age Related Eye Disease 2 Study have led to a new formulation for eye vitamins. This new formulation includes the carotenioids, lutein and zeaxanthin, which along with other compounds are designed to reduce oxidative stress within the retina and therefore reduce the formation of drusen (Gorusupudi, Nelson, & Bernstein, 2017). Researchers are just beginning to study the link between genes to AMD (Ratnapriya, Sosina, Starostik, et al., 2019).

Glaucoma. A leading cause of loss in visual acuity and blindness, in 2010, **glaucoma** affected approximately 2.7 million Americans and with the aging of the U.S. population, this number is expected to increase to about 7.32 million by 2050 (National Eye Institute, 2019). Blacks are three times more likely than Whites to be affected (National Eye Institute, 2004). In the healthy eye, fluid constantly circulates in and out of the eye's anterior chamber. This chamber sometimes becomes plugged, so that the fluid can no longer freely circulate, and pressure rises within the eye. This eye disease is first manifested by a loss in peripheral vision; if left untreated, it can rapidly progress to affect central visual acuity and damage the optic nerve.

Cataracts. The most common cause of loss in visual acuity, **cataracts** result in the clouding of the eye's lens. Like glaucoma, cataracts generally cause no pain or initial symptoms. However, as the condition progresses, frequent complaints include sensitivity to glare, the fading of colors, and an increased need for additional light when reading. Alcohol use, smoking, and long-term exposure to the sun's ultraviolet rays are believed to increase the risk for developing cataracts (National Eye Institute, 2008). Accordingly, the American Academy of Ophthalmology (2018) recommends the use of sunglasses that block 99–100 percent of both UVA and UVB radiation. Cataracts are not to be confused with senile miosis, which also limits the amount of light that enters the eye. With senile miosis, the restriction of light is caused by a decrease in the pupil's resting diameter. Typically, between 30 and 60 years of age, the amount of light that reaches the retina declines in a linear fashion. In fact, the amount of light that reaches the retina at age 60 is only one-third the amount that reached the retina at age 20 (Bottomley, 2010).

Diabetic retinopathy. Diabetic retinopathy is a complication of diabetes. Diabetes is known to cause changes in all of the body's blood vessels, including those in the retina. As with AMD, **diabetic retinopathy** can cause the vessels of the retina to hemorrhage. This hemorrhage in turn discolors the eye's interior gel (vitreous humor), which is clear when healthy. To complicate matters further, the blood vessels that hemorrhage tend to contract as they heal and oftentimes will detach the retina (National Eye Institute, 2008). For these reasons, it is critical that individuals with diabetes control their blood sugar in order to slow the onset and progression of diabetic retinopathy.

Presbyopia. By approximately 40 years of age, we begin to lose the ability to accommodate near objects. For instance, print can be brought into focus at 4 in (10 cm) at age 30, but by the mid-forties a person generally cannot read print unless it is held beyond arm's length (Boron & Boulpaep, 2009). Not specially classified as an ARED, this inability to focus clearly on near objects is clinically known as **presbyopia**. Presbyopia does not affect distance vision. Some of its symptoms can be overcome with bifocal, trifocal, or progressive lenses. Bifocals correct for distance and near vision; trifocals correct for distance, intermediate, and near vision; and progressive lenses provide a smooth transition between distance, intermediate, and near vision, as well as all in-between vision zones.

Because with age less light reaches the retina, it is important that older adults perform their physical tasks in well-illuminated activity areas. In addition, activity supervisors should be aware that bifocal wearers frequently experience difficulty in both tracking and judging the speed of moving objects.

Binocular Vision and Depth Perception

As mentioned earlier, the ocular muscles that control eye movements are not fully developed at birth. As a result, the newborn frequently moves each eye at random; the newborn has **strabismus**, misaligned eyes. Strabismus is common at birth but should not persist beyond the first year. Usually, the degree of strabismus greatly diminishes during the first week of life, and by the end of the third month most typically developing infants move both eyes in a coordinated manner. However, in some cases, strabismus may require surgical correction. Fortunately, this correction has been shown to improve motor performance in tasks requiring visual motor control, even when performed after the fourth year of life (Caputo, Tinelli,

Bancale, et al., 2008). Approximately 2–5 percent of preschool children exhibit strabismus (Garvey, Dodson, Messer, et al., 2010).

Coordinated eye movements are important because they are the basis of **binocular vision,** which occurs when both eyes move in unison so that each eye focuses the desired image on its macula. Because each eye views the object from a different angle, there is a slight disparity between the two macular images and this disparity can significantly exert a negative influence on motor coordination (Suttle, Melmoth, Finlay, et al., 2011).

Gibson and Walk's (1960) classic **visual cliff** study (see Figure 8.5) was one of the first to demonstrate that infants are capable of organizing depth clues during the first year of life. The researchers constructed a platform with a surface of clear plastic that was raised several feet off the ground. On one side, a checkerboard pattern was placed directly under the clear surface, and on the other side the checkerboard pattern was placed on the floor below the surface, creating the appearance of a drop-off or cliff. Infants aged 6–14 months old were placed in the middle of the platform. When the mothers called their infants from the side with the visual cliff, nearly all the babies backed off and cried, refusing to cross the apparent cliff. However, when the mothers coaxed their infants from the other side, where the pattern was directly under the clear surface, all of the babies ventured across. This finding implied that infants could detect the differences in depth between the two sides.

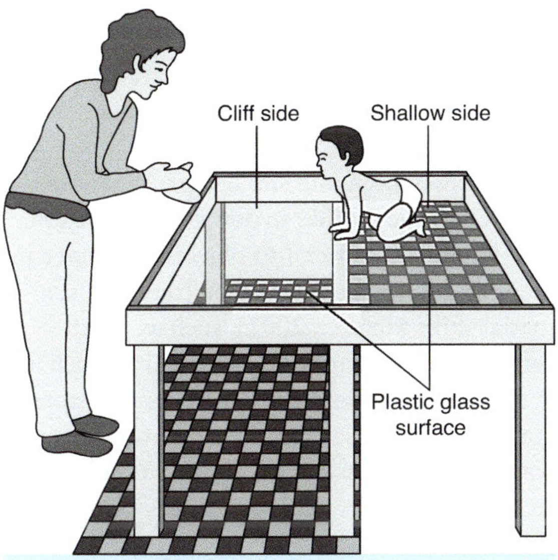

Figure 8.5 Gibson and Walk's visual cliff. Note the mother attempting to coax the infant into crossing the apparent deep (cliff) side.

One question that has interested researchers for many years is whether depth perception is innate or develops with time. There are arguments for both positions, but mounting evidence indicates that some form of depth recognition is possible early in life, as the visual cliff experiment illustrates. Nevertheless, even though depth perception begins to develop early in life, it is slow to mature, as evidenced by the fact that toddlers frequently bump into objects. In any case, depth perception is usually mature by 6 years of age.

There has also been considerable discussion about the importance of active movement for optimal development of depth perception. Held and Hein addressed this question in 1963 in a classic study.

In their research, Held and Hein raised kittens in a completely dark environment for 8 to 12 weeks. The kittens were then separated into two groups: active and passive. A kitten from each group was attached to a cart-like device that rotated around a central axis in a lighted carousel. The active kitten propelled its cart around the axis with its own legs; the passive kitten was simply a passenger, with its legs held immobile. The two carts were connected, so that the passive kitten's cart was propelled by the active kitten's leg movements (see Figure 8.6). Kittens from both groups spent up to 3 hours/day in this situation and were otherwise kept in darkness. In posttests, the active kittens showed signs of having acquired typical depth perception, whereas the passive kittens exhibited impaired depth

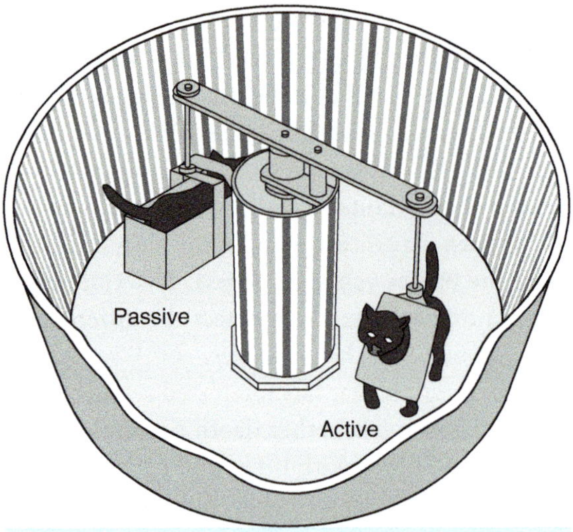

Figure 8.6 Held and Hein involved kittens in active and passive movement. The researchers concluded that active movement benefited the kittens' development of depth perception, whereas passive movement did not.

perception, which eventually improved markedly when they were exposed to light outside of the carousel activity. Held and Hein concluded that active movement plays a vital role in the development of visual-spatial skills such as depth perception. This research has also been used to justify perceptual-motor programs. These programs involve children in movement activities designed to improve skills such as depth perception, often with the aim of enhancing an academic ability such as reading, which typically depends on visual proficiency.

Critics of Held and Hein's research point out that those kittens actively involved in producing movement most likely were also required to maintain greater visual attentiveness (Shaffer, 2001). Therefore, the active kittens may have achieved better depth perception than the passive kittens because they had more visual experience and practice rather than higher levels of actively produced movement, as the original researchers suspected.

Related research by Walk (1981) supports this critical view of Held and Hein's research. On the basis of other research, Walk suggested that active movement may be an essential element in development, but the movement does not need to be self-produced, only viewed. As Held and Hein did, Walk researched kittens to reach these conclusions. The kittens in Walk's research were kept in total darkness for a time following their birth. Then one group of kittens was removed from the darkness and allowed to move actively around the environment and examine the available visual stimuli. A second group of kittens was inhibited from actively moving but allowed to examine passive (stationary) stimuli. A final group of kittens, also inhibited from movement, viewed a stimulus that was in motion. Following exposure to these varying situations, all kittens were tested for depth perception. The kittens that could not actively interact with the environment and that watched the passive stimuli had the poorest level of depth perception. According to Walk, this was most likely attributable to the tendency of these kittens to become bored and fall asleep. However, the kittens that watched the active stimuli remained attentive despite their inability to move actively through their environment. As a result, these kittens developed depth perception comparable to that of the kittens that were allowed to move actively through the environment.

Walk's research and similar investigations have led to the **motion hypothesis**, the idea that individuals must attend to objects that move in order to develop a typical repertoire of visual-spatial skills (Shaffer, 2001), such as depth perception. Contrary to early research, such as in the Held and Hein study, and considerable popular opinion, self-produced movement may not be as critical as once believed in the development of such important abilities as depth perception.

Another question regarding depth perception is its role in skilled motor performance. Unfortunately, the research literature presents conflicting viewpoints regarding the relationship between depth perception and sporting success. One might speculate that the importance of accurate depth perception is task-specific. For example, depth perception may significantly influence basketball shooting performance but may have no significant influence on many other basketball skills. In addition, most likely the central nervous system uses secondary cues (shadows, ball texture, projectile size) to perceive depth, which explains how some athletes with a sight-related disability (i.e., sight in one eye only) maintain a high level of performance without the aid of stereo vision (sight with both eyes).

Field of Vision

Field of vision refers to the entire extent of the environment that an individual can see while looking straight ahead and without changing the fixation of the eye. Two frequently studied aspects of field of vision are lateral and vertical **peripheral vision**. Typical adult lateral peripheral vision is just over 90 degrees from straight ahead, resulting in a visual field that covers slightly over 180 degrees. In contrast, typical adult vertical peripheral vision is approximately 60 degrees above the visual midlines and approximately 75 degrees below the visual midline (Ang, 2015). Consequently, young adults are capable of detecting movements that significantly deviate from central vision.

In comparison, the infant's field of vision is extremely limited. For example, when fixating on a light located in their central field of vision, infants younger than 2 months will not refixate on a second light until it is within 15 degrees laterally. When the second light is allowed to blink, the neonate's lateral peripheral vision enlarges to 25 degrees, and at 7 weeks of age it has expanded to 35 degrees (Macfarlane, Harris, & Barnes, 1976).

Davids (1987) has expressed concern that reported functional peripheral vision values have predominantly been collected in laboratory situations and, as a result, lack ecological validity. *Ecological validity* refers to the likelihood that research findings obtained in a laboratory will carry over to a real-world setting. He believes it is important to measure the development of peripheral vision in more ecologically valid settings because such measurements may influence our expectations of children's performance in ball games in which peripheral vision is used. According to Davids, the problem with laboratory assessments is their failure to include an appropriate central task during the peripheral vision assessment. Indeed, earlier work has noted that the presence of a central task can significantly affect peripheral vision performance (Ikeda & Takevchi, 1975).

Davids (1987) examined peripheral vision processing capabilities in both children and adults (age groups: 9-, 12-, 15-year-olds, and adults). His study was unique in that peripheral vision processing was assessed not only by itself (as a single task, similar to most laboratory tasks) but also in ecologically valid settings where subjects were presented peripheral information during the performance of a ball-catching task (dual task performance; see Figure 8.7). An analysis of the data revealed that 9-year-old subjects made significantly more catching errors during the dual task than did subjects in the other three age groups. However, during the single-task performance there was no difference in peripheral visual sensitivity between the 9-year-olds and the adults.

Davids' findings suggest that earlier laboratory estimates regarding the size of children's functional visual field have been overestimated. Only the adult subjects (over 18 years) were capable of effectively coping with the dual processing demands presented in this study. It appears that the size of the functional peripheral visual field is reduced when the child performer is confronted with a real-world

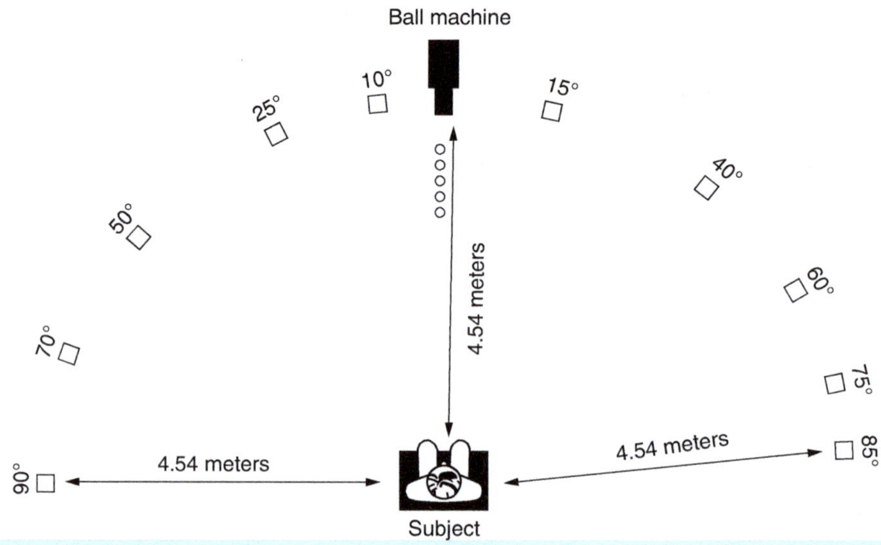

Figure 8.7 Davids' (1987) experiment examining peripheral vision processing during the performance of a catching task

central task, such as catching a ball. According to Davids (1987):

> The implications for teachers and coaches of ball games are that due consideration must be given to the central task when instructing young athletes to respond to peripheral visual cues such as gaps in the field, positioning of players, and location of boundaries and targets.
>
> (p. 283)

Many of the changes associated with age-related eye diseases (AMD, glaucoma, cataracts, etc.) affect the size of a person's field of vision. Retinal cells are lost not only in the area of the macula but also in the retina's periphery. In adulthood, there is about a one to three degree reduction in the visual field per decade. Thus, by approximately 70–80 years of age, one may have a visual field that has been reduced by 20–30 percent (Heiting, 2019). Anatomical and physiological changes within the visual system itself are not the only causes of decreased field of vision. Changes in facial structure can also reduce the size of the visual field. For instance, with age the upper eyelid may droop, a clinical condition known as **senile ptosis.** This condition can significantly limit vertical peripheral vision. In addition, loss of fat tissue around the orbital sockets can make the eyeball sink, restricting vision in all directions.

Eye Dominance

It is well known that humans show dominance for handedness, and within the last decade much has been written about right versus left hemispherical brain dominance. A lesser-known fact regarding human makeup is **eye dominance,** the tendency of one eye to lead the other in tasks involving visual tracking and visual fixation.

Eye dominance is believed to be established early in life. About 75 percent of children will develop a dominant eye by 3 years of age, and by 5 years the percentage of children who have developed a dominant eye increases to about 95 percent (cited in Whiting, 1971). Approximately two-thirds of the population is right-eye dominant (Eser, Durrie, Schwendeman, & Stahl, 2008).

The most frequently used test to determine eye dominance is the "hole-in-card" test. To administer this test, one simply cuts a .25-in (0.6 cm, diameter) hole in the middle of a sheet of cardboard measuring 11 in (28 cm) square. Standing 7 ft (2.14 m) from a blackboard, the individual holds the cardboard at arm's length and, while keeping both eyes open, looks through the hole and locates a .5-in (1.3 cm)-diameter dot that is drawn on the blackboard. The individual then closes one eye. If the dot remains in view, then the open eye is the dominant eye. If the dot disappears, then the eye that was closed is the dominant eye.

Most studies examining the association between eye dominance and motor performance have included handedness as an additional variable. Individuals who are right-eyed and right-handed or left-eyed and left-handed are said to possess **unilateral dominance**, which means their dominant eye is on the same side of the body as their dominant hand. In contrast, a person who is either right-eyed and left-handed or left-eyed and right-handed has **crossed-lateral dominance**.

A majority of the studies investigating this topic have found unilateralism to correlate to higher scores than cross-lateralism in a variety of tasks (Laborde, Dosseville, Pascale, & Margas, 2009; Payne, 1988). Nevertheless, a great deal of speculation exists among baseball coaches, suggesting that the performer with cross-lateral dominance may have a distinct advantage in such tasks as batting. It is believed among baseball coaches that this purported advantage results because the dominant eye of the hitter with cross-lateral dominance is closer to the pitcher. Moreover, this leading eye is not restricted by having to look across the bridge of the nose. However, this pattern of cross-lateral dominance has not been found to be associated with a positive effect on baseball batting averages (Laby, Kirschen, Rosenbaum, & Mellman, 1998).

Although an overwhelming majority of the research has reported superior performance among individuals with unilateral dominance, Razeghi, Nia, Bushehri, and Maleki (2012) caution that those with cross-lateral dominance also perform well in a variety of activities. This suggests that the interaction between eye and hand dominance and its effect on sport performance may be functions of the particular visual demands of specific sports. Therefore, no attempts should be made to change an individual's dominance from cross-lateral to unilateral.

Tracking and Object Interception

To gain control over a projectile, the performer must visually track the object to be intercepted. The primary purpose of **tracking** the object is to gain important information regarding the object's flight. A properly functioning ocular-motor system is needed to track the object, and a properly functioning motor system is needed to act on the object.

The ocular-motor system is composed of two eye-movement systems. First, the **smooth ocular-motor pursuit system** is capable of matching eye-movement speed to the speed of the projectile, to maintain a stable retinal image. Second, the **saccadic eye-movement system,** in which the eye makes jerky movements, detects and corrects differences between the projectile's location and the eye's fixation. When objects are traveling very fast (79 to 108 ft/sec or 24 to 33 m/sec), the saccadic system is primarily used.

Developmentally, the infant is not capable of freely moving the eyes across an arc of 180 degrees until some time between 40 and 52 weeks of age (Corbin, 1980), which explains why tracking is first accomplished primarily with head movements and then through a series of eye-head movements. By 5 or 6 years of age, children can efficiently track objects moving in the horizontal plane. When children are between 8 and 9 years of age, they can track balls that travel in an arc (Morris, 1980).

As dynamic visual acuity improves, so does the ability to track fast-moving objects, because whenever an object is moving at an angular velocity at which smooth eye movements are no longer possible, the pursuit task becomes a function of dynamic visual acuity.

The coordinated interception of a moving object is a task frequently studied in research laboratories. This process behind object interception is commonly referred to as **coincidence-anticipation**. Most frequently, the instrument of choice to measure coincidence-anticipation is the Bassin anticipation timer (Crocetta, Guarnieri, Antunes, et al., 2018; see Figure 8.8). The apparatus consists of one yellow warning light and two "runways" attached end to end. Each runway consists of 16 red LEDs that are .25 in (0.6 cm) in diameter and spaced 1.75 in (4.5 cm) apart, which are lit sequentially to give the appearance of a moving stimulus. Most often, the objective of the task is to depress a button placed at the end of the runway so that the response coincides with the lighting of the last runway lamp. To succeed at this task, the subject must initiate the response one reaction time and one movement time before the lighting of the target lamp. In addition, Isaacs (1987, 1990) described a procedure whereby two independent Bassin anticipation timers are interfaced, making the equipment capable of measuring a type of coincidence-anticipation that involves the intersection of two converging targets.

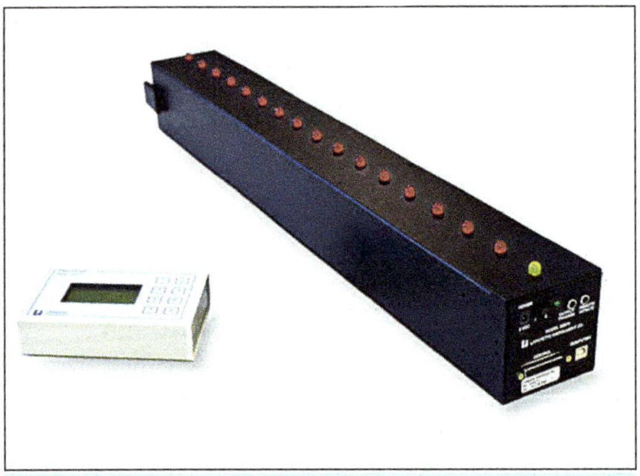

Figure 8.8 The Bassin anticipation timer
Source: Courtesy of Lafayette Instrument Company.

Many factors can influence how well a person can make a motor response coincide with the arrival of an external object, including object speed, object predictability, viewing time, gender, and age (Magill & Anderson, 2013; Shea, Shebilske, & Worchel, 1993). Briefly, coincidence-anticipation improves with age and is greatly influenced by practice. Interestingly, Kuhlman and Beitel (1997) found that practice, as reflected by sport participation and video game experience, may be a better predictor of coincidence-anticipation than is age. This finding has been confirmed by Uchida, Kudoh, Higuchi, and colleagues (2013). It also appears that boys tend to perform more accurately than girls (Isaacs, 1983; Sanders, 2011) and that both very slow- and very fast-moving objects cause increases in performance errors. Thus, one could speculate that both children and adults may respond most accurately to object speeds that they confront in their everyday experience.

Based on these findings, it appears that a slowly projected ball may not necessarily always be the easiest to catch. Furthermore, when a child is first learning to catch, the teacher should consistently toss the ball directly toward the child instead of using an arched delivery. This may explain why Isaacs (1984) found that young T-ball players missed 85 percent of all fly balls.

Teachers of motor skills should also be aware that each visual trait described in this chapter may be improved with visual training (Wilson & Falkel, 2004).

Motor Development of Children with Visual Impairments

Chapters 9 through 13 discuss at length the acquisition of selected reflexes and motor skills. This section describes the development of selected motor acts in children who have a visual impairment. Indeed, the effects of blindness on the motor development and motor performance of children are far more devastating than those of other sensory disabilities, such as hearing impairments.

The general public tends to associate **blindness** with a total loss of vision, but this is a misconception. The official definition of blindness is based on distance vision as measured by the Snellen eye chart and does not take into consideration near vision. Thus, a person who is legally blind may be capable of considerable vision when objects are placed close to the eyes. In general, residual vision in people who are legally blind can range from total blindness, where light is not perceived, to a Snellen distance vision of 20/200, which is the equivalent of an 80 percent loss of vision. Therefore, whenever we speak of blindness, we should specify the degree of residual vision remaining, if any. The effects of blindness on a child's motor development depend on the type and degree of residual vision.

The effects of blindness on motor development also depend on the age of onset. Individuals who are congenitally blind or who become blind before they are 5 years old do not retain a workable visual imagery. Thus, people who are congenitally blind must learn to function in the world without the advantage of the information provided through sight. Conversely, those individuals who lose their sight later in life have experienced vision and are capable of remembering it, giving them advantages in dealing with life's demands. Obviously, blindness exerts its greatest effects on motor development and motor performance when a newborn experiences total blindness (that is, 0 percent residual vision). The following sections discuss the specific influence of congenital blindness on early motor development and the development of both fundamental and object control skills.

Head and Trunk Control

Several weeks after birth, infants with sight attempt to raise their head off the crib mattress; soon thereafter the child begins to arch the back and elevate the chest. Because of visual curiosity, infants elevate the trunk for increasingly longer periods. Thus, for these infants, visual curiosity elicits the movements that aid in the development of head, neck, and trunk control. Infants without sight, however, tend to cry and fuss in the prone position. Parents often place them on their back in an attempt to pacify them, but this position does not help the development of head and upper-body control because this position does not encourage head, neck, and trunk movement. Even when these infants stay in the prone position, they arch the head and neck less frequently than do infants with sight because there is little or no vision to initiate purposeful movement at this young age.

Independent Sitting

Somewhere between 4 and 8 months of age, most infants with sight are capable of sitting alone. Infants without sight are also capable of sitting alone at this time if their parents have adequately prepared them for this milestone. However, if these infants have spent prolonged periods of time supine, they will not have had the opportunity to develop the necessary head, neck, and trunk control to sit alone.

Creeping

By approximately 10 months of age, infants with sight are capable of supporting themselves on their hands and knees, making creeping possible. Visual curiosity entices these infants to creep toward objects that are within sight but out of reach. Obviously, such visual curiosity is absent in the infant without sight. If this infant is to develop typically, a sensory modality other than vision must be used to instigate the infant's creeping and exploration of the unseen environment. Parents of an infant without sight should stimulate the child's curiosity by enticing the child to move toward noise-making toys.

Independent Walking

Both children with and without sight are capable of standing and walking with support at approximately the same time. Nevertheless, the achievement of independent walking is usually significantly delayed in those without sight (Adelson & Fraiberg, 1976). In fact, children with partial vision tend to walk sooner than children who are totally blind or those who possess only light perception. When independent walking is achieved, children both with and without sight characteristically exhibit an insecure gait with a wide base of support, flat-footed contact with the supporting surface, and toeing out. These characteristics are part of the expected sequence of events in learning to walk, but some individuals without sight exhibit these immature characteristics throughout the lifespan.

Prehension

Prehension, the ability to grasp and seize objects with the hands, is an important aspect of a child's motor development. Prehensile abilities enable a child to gather information about the environment in new ways. Increased and varied exploration is possible because of the child's ability to seize and manipulate objects with the hands. This new mode of exploration lets the child discover properties of objects and allows the child to use objects as implements to achieve goals.

Vision is important for the development of prehension for three reasons. First, the initial phase of self-directed reaching is visually evoked; that is, the child reaches upon viewing some object in the environment. This form of reaching is an improvement over the random grasping that occurs earlier in the child's life. Second, vision is used to facilitate hand closure around an object once the child has manual contact with the desired object. Third, during the act of reaching, vision enables the child to correct errors throughout the reach.

Thus, for the child without sight the primary modality for stimulating prehensile skills is absent (Troster & Brambring, 1993). Because reaching for sound-producing objects generally will not occur until the last quarter of the first year of life, it is important that parents encourage their child without sight to manipulate objects that have been placed in her or his hand. In addition, manual guidance by the parents is important; it is imperative that finger dexterity and sensitivity be acquired early in development because they establish a readiness for Braille instruction at school age.

A classic investigation by Adelson and Fraiberg (1976) compared the gross motor achievements of 10 infants who were congenitally blind with those of peers with sight. The children were observed for 2 years, and comparisons were made in reference to selected items from the Bayley Scales of Infant Development. Table 8.1 presents the median age comparisons for children with and without sight on selected Bayley Scale items. Note that nearly all the infants without sight were found to be on schedule when compared with their counterparts with sight on items requiring postural control. These items include sitting alone momentarily, making stepping movements when the hands are held, and standing alone. Attaining these items on schedule suggests typical development of trunk control and the ability to bear weight and perform stepping movements with support. Note, however, that the greatest motor delays in mobility included tasks involving independent walking, a finding confirmed by Celeste (2002).

Table 8.1 Comparison of children with and without sight on selected Bayley Scale items

Item	Median age (months)	
	With sight	Without sight
Elevates self by arms, prone	2.1	8.75
Sits alone momentarily	5.3	6.75
Rolls from back to stomach	6.4	7.25
Sits alone steadily	6.6	8.00
Raises self to sitting position	8.3	11.00
Stands up using furniture (pulls up to stand)	8.6	13.00
Makes stepping movements (walks with hands held)	8.8	10.75
Stands alone	11.0	13.00
Walks alone, three steps	11.7	15.25
Walks alone across room	12.1	19.25*

*One child had not achieved this task by age 2 years.
Source: Adapted from Adelson and Fraiberg (1976).

However, there were five items in which the subjects without sight showed significant delays: elevating self by arms when prone, raising self to sitting position, standing up using furniture (pulls up to stand), walking alone (three steps), and walking alone across room. With the exception of elevating self by arms when prone, all involve self-initiated mobility. Thus, the authors concluded that if children without sight are to develop within the typical limits of their peers with sight in self-initiated mobility, they need sound as an adaptive substitute for sight; this substitution should occur toward the end of the first year of life.

Fundamental and Object Control Skills

Researchers have found that children who are blind perform significantly worse than their sighted peers on both fundamental motor skills and object control skills. More specifically, Wagner, Haibach and Lieberman (2013) utilized the Test of Gross Motor Development to assess fundamental and object control skill performance in both sighted and blind children between 6 and 12 years of age. Findings revealed that blind children performed significantly worse than the sighted children in the following fundamental motor skills: running, galloping, hopping, leaping, jumping, and sliding. Similarly, the blind children performed significantly worse than the sighted children in the following object control skills: striking, dribbling, catching, kicking, throwing, and rolling. Among all of these gross motor skills, running, leaping, kicking, and catching were the most affected.

In a follow-up study, these researchers, in part, studied the influence of severity of visual impairment on the performance of the fundamental and object control skills (Haibach, Wagner, & Lieberman, 2014). The findings revealed that children with some residual vision performed better than those children classified as being totally blind. However, the researchers did note that unlike sighted children, those with significant visual impairments failed to improve performance with age. They attributed this finding to a lack of opportunity to regularly participate in activities involving the use of these gross motor skills. The authors offered the following suggestions for teaching these skills to children with significant visual impairments: Use a whole-part-whole method of teaching in order to reduce task complexity, allow the children extra instruction and practice time, and use modified equipment such as balls, targets, and boundaries that employ auditory input as opposed to visual input.

Additionally, employ the use of tactile modeling and physical guidance (Alex, Petersen, Lieberman, et al., 2019; Lieberman, Ponchillia, & Ponchillia, 2013).

Play Behavior of Children with Visual Impairments

For the child with sight, play is a spontaneous and creative act carried out for its own sake, usually consisting of self-imposed games where new movement skills are learned and current movement skills are refined. Children pick up new movement ideas by imitating the movements of other children. Thus, play is an important learning medium. In contrast, children without sight tend to be inactive and show little drive to explore their environment. If left on their own, many engage in physical activity involving little more than rocking the body, pressing the eyes, and tapping the fingers. Because blindness is known to cause motor delays, providing an adequately stimulating environment can help shorten these delays in motor development (Levtzion-Korach, Tennenbaum, Schnitzer, & Ornoy, 2000).

As noted earlier, the degree of blindness can influence a child's rate of development across all domains (motor, cognitive, affective). For example, Hatton (1995) reported that children whose visual function was 20/800 experienced reduced performance in both motor and adaptive skills compared to children exhibiting a visual deficit as great as 20/500. Therefore, it is important—within reason—not to overprotect the child without sight. These children should be given the opportunity to engage in numerous movement experiences and should be encouraged to explore their unseen world.

THE NONVISUAL SENSES

While the visual system is typically the predominant system in motor development and motor performance, it is by no means the only sensory modality that can exert an influence. Unfortunately, less information is available on the other sensory modalities that are known to influence motor development and motor performance. Nevertheless, in this section we describe the proprioceptive system and its accompanying vestibular apparatus, as well as the auditory and cutaneous systems.

The Proprioceptive System

The **proprioceptive system** makes it possible for us to be aware of our own movements and to perceive the location of our body parts in space without visual reference to them. These feats are made possible by a group of sensory receptors located in the joints, muscles, tendons, and labyrinth of the inner ear. These specialized receptors include the muscle spindles, the Golgi tendon organs, and the vestibular apparatus. These sensory receptors respond to changes in joint angles, changes in the lengths and tension relationships of muscles, and movements of the head. Because these receptor cells are activated by mechanical deformation, they are frequently referred to as mechanoreceptors. Let us briefly examine the function of each.

Muscle Spindles

The **muscle spindles** are cigar-shaped structures that are attached in parallel with the muscles' largest fibers, known as the *extrafusal muscle fibers*. Contained within the spindle itself is a smaller muscle fiber known as an *intrafusal muscle fiber*. Because the fibers lie parallel to one another and are attached to the sheath of the extrafusal fibers, it is possible for the muscle spindle to gauge the amount of tension within the muscle itself. That is, when the larger extrafusal muscle fibers are stretched, they in turn stretch the smaller intrafusal fibers of the muscle spindle. This stretch will cause activation of the spindle, resulting in afferent

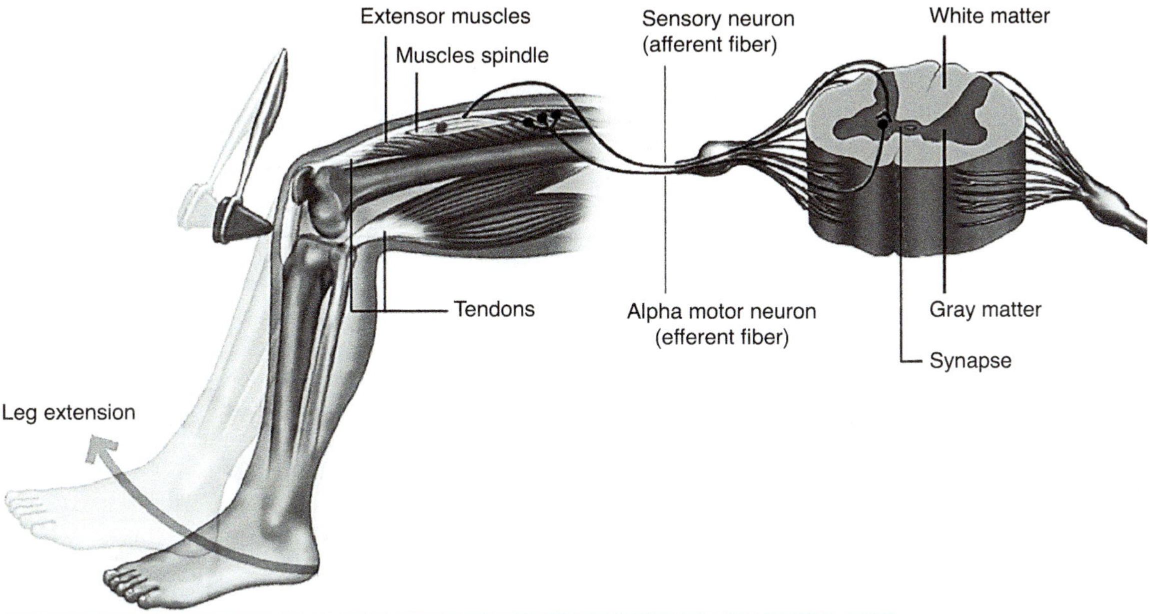

Figure 8.9 The classic knee jerk is a stretch reflex initiated by muscle spindle stimulation

discharge. The effect of an afferent discharge is to stimulate the skeletomotor neurons, which in turn will cause a contraction of the muscle's larger extrafusal fibers, thus reducing the stretch on the intrafusal muscle fibers. The classic knee jerk is an example of this phenomenon (see Figure 8.9).

Individuals who have suffered a stroke or spinal cord injury will frequently experience an overly sensitive muscle spindle. This can cause the flexor muscles of the arms and legs to possess too much muscle tension (hypertonus). This increased muscle tone results in stiffness and atypical posture, both of which can diminish motor development and motor performance. For these individuals, it is important to keep the affected muscles as flexible as possible by performing stretching activities.

Golgi Tendon Organs

The **Golgi tendon organs** are small stretch receptors located near the junction of the muscle and the muscle's tendon (the musculo-tendinous junction). Their primary roles are to detect tension in the tendon and to provide the central nervous system with continuous information regarding force development in both static and dynamic conditions. When excessive tension stimulates the Golgi receptors, signals are rapidly sent to the spinal cord to elicit a reflexive inhibition of the involved muscles. This muscle inhibition protects against an excessive overload of the muscle and connective tissue.

Vestibular Apparatus

The **vestibular apparatus**, which is located in the inner ear, is responsible for registering head motion and accompanying body motion. Any time the head is turned or moved through space, the vestibular receptors will be stimulated. As Figure 8.10 illustrates, the vestibular system is composed of two subsystems, the **semicircular canals** and the **otolith organs** (utricle and saccule). The semicircular canals are fluid-filled ducts that lie at right angles to one another. Because they are capable of registering changes in head motion, they are sometimes referred to as angular

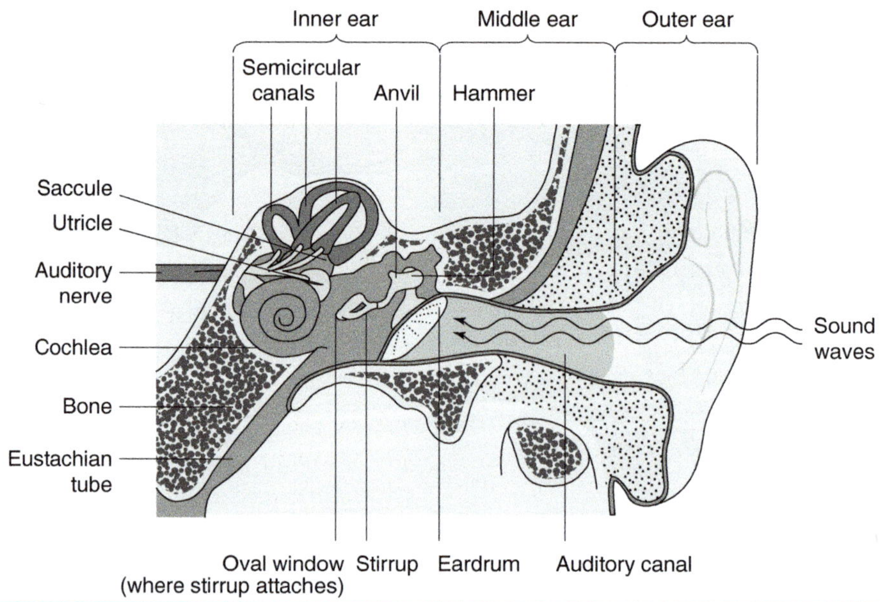

Figure 8.10 The vestibular system is composed of two subsystems: the semicircular canals and the otolith organs (saccule, utricle). The auditory system includes the other organs of the outer, middle, and inner ear.

accelerometers. Unlike the semicircular canals, which primarily detect rotational motion, the otolith organs are primarily responsible for detecting linear acceleration, as they provide information concerning the body's position in relation to the force of gravity. This system is also important in the righting reflex and the coordination of visual fixation.

The proprioceptive system plays an important role in motor development and skilled motor performance. Briefly, proprioception contributes to the development of body awareness, spatial awareness, and directional awareness. In addition, the vestibular apparatus is critical in the development of both static and dynamic balance, a topic that is discussed at some length in Chapter 15.

The Auditory System

Auditory perception is the process whereby auditory stimuli are received, selected, organized, and interpreted. It can affect sport performance, such as the ability to hear an opponent coming from behind, and health-related activities, such as the ability to hear traffic when walking or running. Furthermore, as discussed in the previous section, a portion of the auditory system—the inner ear—is also part of the vestibular apparatus, and it plays a role in balance, which also affects movement performance.

The sensory organ that makes auditory perception possible is the ear (see Figure 8.10). Note that the human ear is composed of three main parts: the outer, middle, and inner ear. Any source of sound sends vibrations through the air (sound waves), which are collected through the ear opening and then travel down the ear canal and onto the eardrum. The eardrum's vibrations are transmitted to the inner ear's cochlea, which in turn stimulates the auditory nerve, which sends the nerve impulses to the brain for interpretation (sensation of hearing).

Prenatally, babies are capable of hearing during the last few months of pregnancy. Therefore, at birth, the newborn is structurally equipped for hearing; however, hearing is generally compromised for several days as the inner canal is usually filled with fluid. Additionally, the sensory threshold is believed to be higher in newborns than in mature adults. That is, a louder auditory stimulus is needed to stimulate a newborn's auditory perception.

Auditory development during the first 3 months of postnatal life is characterized by the child's enjoyment of hearing the parents' voices. At this age, babies generally respond more strongly to the mother's voice than the father's, as it is associated with food and comfort. This may help explain why most people will use an exaggeratedly high-pitched voice when speaking to babies.

From 4 to 7 months of age, babies begin to recognize some components of speech instead of simply recognizing tone of voice. This milestone is critical for speech development. During the seventh month, babies should become able to recognize and respond to their own name. Babbling, the baby's first attempt at speech should be encouraged.

From 8 to 12 months, babies start to produce recognizable sounds and exhibit a more sophisticated babbling that resembles attempts at real conversation. Also during this time, babies should become capable of responding to simple verbal requests, such as looking toward "Dad" when asked "Where's Daddy?" and waving "bye" upon command. Attempts to reproduce sounds made by parents should be encouraged.

From 1 to 2 years of age, infants and toddlers continue to improve their ability to recognize and respond to commands. Children of this age can be expected to respond to the names of family members and familiar objects. When children do not exhibit the developmental milestones mentioned in this section, some hearing impairment may exist. Of the more than 3 million American children with hearing impairments, approximately 1.3 million are under the age of 3. It is imperative that hearing impairments be recognized early so that corrective action can be taken; early intervention limits the impairments' effect on language and speech development.

The Cutaneous System

The **cutaneous system**, which provides tactile sensitivity, receives its information from sensory receptors located at the body's surface, the skin (see Figure 8.11). Once thought of as just the sense of touch, the cutaneous system is now known to consist of at least four skin senses: pressure, coldness, warmth, and pain. Because of its sensitivity to temperature and pain, this sensory system is what alerts us to potentially adverse environmental conditions.

Researchers studying the development of the cutaneous system typically look for one of three possible responses to tactile stimulation: reflex, withdrawal, or approach. For example, the *reflex behaviors* known as the sucking reflex, the searching reflex, the Babkin reflex, and the Babinski reflex, as well as the palmar grasp and plantar grasp reflexes, are all typically elicited by tactile stimulation (see Chapter 9). *Withdrawal responses* generally manifest themselves when the infant or child attempts to turn the head or move a limb away

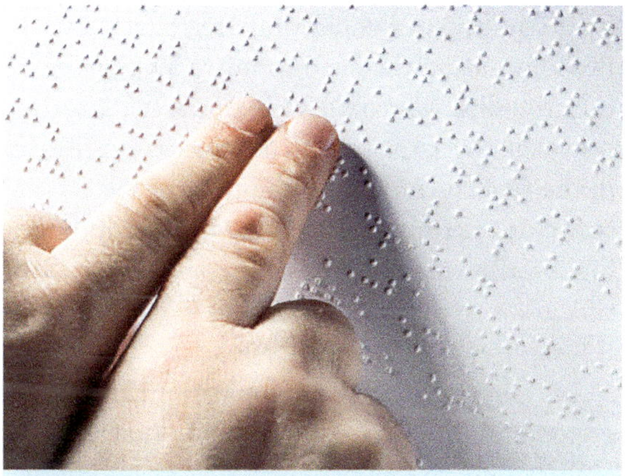

Figure 8.11 Reading Braille is made possible by the cutaneous system

from the source of stimulation; these responses may be accompanied by a facial grimace. When children respond to kisses, hugs, and playful tickling, they are generally exhibiting *approach behaviors*. In fact, these approach behaviors are essential for the human bonding process early in life and are also important later in life when the individual engages in intimacy and human sexual interactions.

Which of these three possible reactions to tactile stimulation will be exhibited depends on many factors. Some of these factors include mood state (awake or sleeping), area of stimulation (body area), gender, and level of maturity. For example, an absence of the palmar, plantar, and Babkin reflexes have been noted during periods of quiet sleep, but these reflexes were sometimes observed during active sleep and nearly always when the infants were quietly awake. Regarding gender, girls have been found to habituate to vibrotactile stimulation at an earlier age than boys (Leader, Baillie, Bahia, & Elsebeth, 1982). This is believed to be a result of girls' greater level of nervous system maturity.

Many experts believe the cutaneous system is the first functional sensory system to develop. For example, Humphrey (1964) has demonstrated the functional capacity of this system's receptors as early as 7.5 weeks of fetal age. More specifically, Humphrey notes that light stroking of the perioral area elicits a neck flexion causing the head to move away from the stimulus. Approximately one week later, however, the same stimulus on occasion results in the fetus turning the head toward the stimulus, accompanied by opening the mouth and swallowing. This is believed to be a precursor to the feeding reflex seen at birth (Humphrey, 1970).

Initially, sensitivity to tactile stimulation is greatest in those parts of the body that children use to explore their ever-changing world. These regions include the mouth, lips, and tongue. One only has to observe a newborn infant for a short period to witness this fact. When a child comes in contact with an object, the first response is generally to place the object into the mouth for exploration. This point is highlighted by Lipsitt's (1978) observation:

> The importance of such tactual stimulation, and the low threshold of the newborn for response to it, can be demonstrated by rotating the finger completely around the lips in a circle, and noting the precise following of such stimulation which many newborns can demonstrate.
>
> (p. 499)

The cutaneous receptors play an important role in both motor development and motor control. For example, as mentioned previously, infants initially use this sense to explore objects within their new world. (See also the discussion of haptic perception in Chapter 11.) Nevertheless, perhaps persons with **Romberg's sign disease** best illustrate the importance of the cutaneous system. Individuals with this disease have varying degrees of damage to the sensory receptors, usually those in the soles of their feet. As a result, they experience difficulty in maintaining balance, especially if their eyes are closed. Furthermore, if the sensory receptors are damaged in the hands, fine motor manipulations with the hands or fingers are extremely difficult when vision is not available, and even impossible if the receptors are completely destroyed. Just think how often you have held an object in your hand only to have it start to slip. When this happens, most individuals are capable of quickly grasping the object to keep it from falling. In fact, Johansson and Westling (1988) report that the process of recognizing that an object is slipping from our grasp and then tightening our grasp quickly only takes about 80 milliseconds. This research indicates the rapidity with which individuals can respond to cutaneous stimulation.

SUMMARY

- A sharp visual image results when light entering the eye converges on the part of the retina called the macula. Accommodation is the process that maintains a clear retinal image in the presence of varying light conditions.
- The eye develops as an outgrowth of the forebrain and remains an inseparable component of the central nervous system throughout the lifespan. Like the brain, the eye achieves most of its growth prior to birth.
- The eye is functionally immature at birth. Visual acuity steadily improves during the first 4 to 5 years, as do depth perception and field of vision. These visual attributes correlate positively with selected motor tasks.
- After about 40 years of age, changes occur in functional vision. These changes become noticeable because the amount of light reaching the eye's retina is reduced and focusing near objects frequently becomes difficult. Also with advancing age comes the risk of developing age-related eye diseases. The four major AREDs are age-related macular degeneration, glaucoma, cataracts, and diabetic retinopathy.
- The effects of blindness on motor development depend on the age of onset and the degree of residual vision remaining, if any. Blindness exerts its most devastating effects on motor development and motor performance when a newborn is totally blind. Because visual curiosity typically elicits movement, children without sight are not visually motivated to explore their unseen world. If these infants are to develop typically, another sensory modality (usually sound) must be substituted for vision.
- Vision is not the only sensory modality known to influence motor development and motor performance. Three other important sensory systems are the proprioceptive system, the auditory system, and the cutaneous system. The proprioceptive system receives sensory input from joint receptors, muscle spindles, and the Golgi tendon organs. Each of these types of specialized receptors monitors the stretch and/or force being placed on a muscle and its tendons. The vestibular system, an element of the proprioceptive system, provides information regarding changes in the body's position in space and the location of the body's limbs in space without visual reference to them. The primary components of the vestibular system include the semicircular canals and the otolith organs. The auditory system allows sounds to be received, selected, organized, and interpreted. The cutaneous system, which provides tactile sensitivity, is a specialized system that receives information regarding pressure, temperature, and pain.

key concept review

accommodation
age-related macular degeneration (AMD)
Amsler grid
auditory perception
binocular vision
blindness
cataracts
ciliary muscle
coincidence-anticipation
cones
crossed-lateral dominance
cutaneous system
diabetic retinopathy
drusen
dynamic visual acuity
eye dominance
glaucoma
Golgi tendon organs
hyperopic
macula
mechanoreceptors
motion hypothesis
muscle spindles
otolith organs
peripheral vision
presbyopia

proprioceptive system
retina
rods
Romberg's sign
saccadic eye-movement system
semicircular canals
senile miosis
senile ptosis
smooth ocular-motor pursuit system
Snellen eye chart
static visual acuity
strabismus
tracking
unilateral dominance
vestibular apparatus
visual acuity
visual cliff

questions for reflection

1. Can you draw an illustration of the human eye and describe how the human eye is very much like a camera?
2. Can you outline the timing of development for key physical eye structures including the following: rods, cones, lens, ciliary muscles, and dilatory muscles of the pupil?
3. How are static and dynamic visual acuity assessed in children and adults? What are the typical values of static visual acuity for individuals at birth, 1 year, and 3 years of age?
4. Can you describe research regarding the relationship between visual acuity and skilled motor performance?
5. What changes in vision occur with aging?
6. Can you describe and illustrate why binocular vision is necessary for depth perception?
7. What is the typical course of development leading to mature depth perception? Support your answer by describing Gibson and Walk's classic 1960 study.
8. Can you identify the typical range of lateral and vertical fields of vision in children and adults?
9. What are eye dominance, unilateral dominance, and crossed-lateral dominance? What are the research findings associated with each of these concepts?
10. Can you identify and explain each of the two eye-movement systems?
11. Can you describe the development of visual tracking behavior, paying attention to coincidence-anticipation?
12. Can you describe the motor development of children with visual impairments and contrast their play behavior with the play behavior of children with sight?
13. What are the specialized receptors of the proprioceptive system?
14. Draw an illustration of the human ear and describe the development of auditory perception.
15. What are the four skin senses? How is the cutaneous system important for both motor development and motor performance?

online resources

Age-Related Macular Degeneration: What You Should Know, www.nei.nih.gov/health/maculardegen
American Academy of Otolaryngology, www.entnet.org
American Optometric Association, www.aoa.org
Foundation Fighting Blindness, www.blindness.org
National Eye Institute, www.nei.nih.gov
National Federation of the Blind, www.nfb.org
National Institute of Deafness and Other Communication Disorders, www.nidcd.nih.gov
Vestibular Disorder Association, www.vestibular.org
Vision and Eye Health, www.vision-and-eye-health.com

REFERENCES

Adelson, E., & Fraiberg, S. (1976). Sensory deficit and motor development in infants blind from birth. In Z. S. Jastrzembska (Ed.), *The effects of blindness and other impairments on early development*. New York: American Foundation for the Blind.

Alex, S., Petersen, S., Lieberman, L., Beach, P. S., & Brian, A. (2019). Teaching strategies to improve object control development for children with visual impairments in physical education. *Palaestra*, *33*, 34–39.

American Academy of Ophthalmology (2018). Sunglasses: Your prescription for eye health. Retrieved from www.aao.org/newsroom/news-releases/detail/sunglasses-your-prescription-eye-health.

American Academy of Ophthalmology (2019). Eye disease statistics. Retrieved from www.aao.org/eye-disease-statistics.

American Optometric Association (2017). *Evidence-based clinical practice guideline: Comprehensive pediatric eye and vision examination*. St. Louis, MO: American Optometric Association.

Ang, B. (2015). *Visual field*. Retrieved from www.vision-and-eye-health.com.

Bastawrous, A., Rono, H., Livingstone, I. A. T., Weiss, H. A., Jordan, S., Kuper, H., et al. (2017). The development and validation of a smartphone visual acuity test (Peek Acuity) for clinical practice and community-based fieldwork. *Ophthalmology*, *133*, 930–937.

Beals, R. P., Mayyasi, A. M., Templeton, A. E., & Johnson, W. L. (1971). The relationship between basketball shooting performance and certain visual attributes. *American Journal of Optometry and Archives of American Academy of Optometry*, *48*, 585–590.

Bhootra, A. K., & Sumitra, M. D. (2008). *Elite sports and vision*. New Delhi, India: Jaypee Brothers Medical Publishers.

Boron, W. F., & Boulpaep, E. L. (2009). *Medical physiology*. 2nd ed. Philadelphia, PA: Saunders Elsevier.

Bottomley, J. (2010). *Geriatric rehabilitation*. Thorofare, NJ: SLACK Incorporated.

Brady, C. J., Eghrari, A. O., & Labrique, A. B. (2015). Smartphone-based visual acuity measurement for screening and clinical assessment. *JAMA*, *314*, 2682–2683.

Caputo, R., Tinelli, F., Bancale, A., & Campa, L., Frosini, R., Guzzetta A., et al. (2007). Motor coordination in children with congenital strabismus: Effects of late surgery. *European Journal of Paediatric Neurology*, *11*, 285–291.

Celeste, M. (2002). A survey of motor development for infants and young children with visual impairments. *Journal of Visual Impairment & Blindness*, *96*(3), 169–174.

Corbin, C. B. (1980). *A textbook of motor development*. 2nd ed. Dubuque, IA: Brown.

Crocetta, T. B., Guarnieri, R., Antunes, T. P. C., Massetti, T., deAbreu, L. C., Fabian, P., et al. (2018). Instruments for studying coincidence-anticipation timing task: An updated systematic review. *Journal of Physical Education and Sports Management*, *5*, 37–52.

Davids, K. (1987). The development of peripheral vision in ball games: An analysis of single- and dual-task paradigms. *Journal of Human Movement Studies, 13*, 175–284.

Eser, I., Durrie, D. S., Schwendeman, F., & Stahl, J. D. (2008, September). Association between ocular dominance and refraction. *Journal of Refractive Surgery*, 685–689.

Garvey, K. A., Dodson, V., Messer, D. H., Miller, J. M., & Harvey, E. M. (2010). Prevalence of strabismus among preschool, kindergarten, and first-grade Tohono O'odham children. *Optometry*, *81*(4), 194–199.

Gibson, E. J., & Walk, R. D. (1960). The visual cliff. *Scientific American*, *4*, 67–71.

Gorusupudi, A., Nelson, K., & Bernstein, P. S. (2017). The age-related eye disease 2 study: Micronutrients in the treatment of macular degeneration. *Advances in Nutrition*, *8*, 40–53.

Haibach, P. S., Wagner, M. O., & Lieberman, L. J. (2014). Determinants of gross motor skill performance in children with visual impairments. *Research in Developmental Disabilities*, *35*, doi: 10.1016/j.ridd.2014.05.030.

Hatton, D. D. (1995). Developmental growth curves of young children who are visually impaired. Unpublished doctoral dissertation, University of North Carolina, Chapel Hill.

Heiting, G. (2019). *How your vision changes as you age*. Retrieved from www.allaboutvision.com/over60/vision-changes.htm.

Held, R., & Hein, A. (1963). Movement-produced stimulation in the development of visually guided behavior. *Journal of Comparative and Physiological Psychology, 56*, 872–876.

Humphrey, T. (1964). Some correlations between the appearance of human fetal reflexes and the development of the nervous system. *Progress in Brain Research, 4*, 93–133.

Humphrey, T. (1970). The development of human fetal activity and its relation to postnatal behavior. In H. Reese & L. Lipsitt (Eds.), *Advances in child development and behavior.* Vol. 5. New York: Academic Press.

Ikeda, M., & Takevchi, T. (1975). Influence of foveal load on the functional visual field. *Perception and Psychophysics, 18*, 255–260.

Isaacs, L. D. (1983). Coincidence-anticipation in simple catching. *Journal of Human Movement Studies, 9*, 195–201.

Isaacs, L. D. (1984). Players' success in T-baseball. *Perceptual and Motor Skills, 59*, 852–854.

Isaacs, L. D. (1987). Modifying the Bassin anticipation timer. *Journal of Human Movement Studies, 13*, 461–465.

Isaacs, L. D. (1990). Effects of angle of approach on coincidence-anticipation timing within a two-target display. *Journal of Human Movement Studies, 19*, 171–179.

Johansson, R. S., & Westling, G. (1988). Programmed and triggered actions to rapid load changes during precision grip. *Experimental Brain Research, 71*, 72–86.

Kuhlman, J. S., & Beitel, P. A. (1997). Development/learning of coincidence-anticipation. NASPSPA Abstracts. *Journal of Sports and Exercise Psychology, 19*, S76.

Laborde, S., Dosseville, F., Pascale, L., & Margas, N. (2009). Interaction of hand preference with eye dominance on accuracy in archery. *Journal of Perceptual and Motor Skills, 108*, 558–564.

Laby, D. M. & Kirschen, D. G. (2017). The refractive error of professional baseball players. *Optometry and Vision Science*, *94*, 564–573.

Laby, D. M., Kirschen, D. G., Rosenbaum, A. L., & Mellman, M. F. (1998). The effects of ocular dominance on the performance of professional baseball players. *Ophthalmology, 105*(5), 864–866.

Laby, D. M., Rosenbaum, A. L., Kirschen, D. G., Davidson, J. L., Rosenbaum, L. J., Strasser, C., & Mellman, D. (1996). The visual function of professional baseball players. *American Journal of Ophthalmology*, *122*(4), 476–485.

Leader, L., Baillie, P., Bahia, M., & Elsebeth, V. (1982). The assessment and significance of habituation to repeated stimulus by the human fetus. *Early Human Development, 7*, 211–219.

Levtzion-Korach, O., Tennenbaum, A., Schnitzer, R., & Ornoy, A. (2000). Early motor development of blind children. *Journal of Pediatrics and Child Health, 36*, 226–229.

Li, C., Beaumont, J. L., Rine, R. M., Slotkin, J., & Schubert, M. C. (2014). Normative scores for the NIH toolbox dynamic visual acuity test from 3 to 85 years. *Frontiers in Neurology, 5*, 223.

Lieberman, L. J., Ponchillia, P., & Ponchillia, S. (2013). *Physical education and sport for people with visual impairments or deafblindness: Foundations of instruction.* New York: American Federation of the Blind Press.

Lipsitt, L. P. (1978). Sensory and learning processes of newborns: Implications for behavioral disabilities. *Allied Health Behavior Science, 1*, 493–522.

Macfarlane, A., Harris, P., & Barnes, I. (1976). Central and peripheral vision in early infancy. *Journal of Experimental Child Psychology, 21*, 532–538.

Magill, R. A., & Anderson, D. (2013). *Motor learning: Concepts and applications.* 10th ed. Boston: McGraw-Hill.

Morris, G. S. (1980). *Elementary physical education: Toward inclusion.* Salt Lake City, UT: Brighton.

National Eye Institute (2004). Prevalence of open-angle glaucoma among adults in the United States. *Archives of Ophthalmology, 122*, 532–538.

National Eye Institute (2008). Progress in eye and vision research, 1999–2006. Retrieved from https://nei.nih.gov/sites/default/files/nei-pdfs/NEI_ProgressDoc.pdf.

National Eye Institute (2019). Open-angle glaucoma. Retrieved from https://nei/nih.gov/eyedata/glaucoma.

Payne, V. G. (1988). Effects of direction of stimulus approach, eye dominance, and gender on coincidence-anticipation timing performance. *Journal of Human Movement Studies, 15*, 17–25.

Ratnapriya, R., Sosina, O. A., Starostik, M. R., Kwicklis, M., Kapphahn, R. J., Fritsche, L. G., et al. (2019). Retinal transcriptome and eQTL analyses identify genes associated with age-related macular degeneration. *Nature Genetics*, doi: 10.1038/s41588-019-0351-9.

Razeghi, R., Nia, P. S., Bushehri, N. S., & Maleki, F. (2012). Effect of interaction between eye-hand dominance on dart skill. *Journal of Neuroscience and Behavioural Health*, 4(2), 6–12.

Rono, H. K., Bastawrous, A., Macleod, D., Wanjala, E., Di Tanna, G. L., Weiss, A. A., et al. (2018). Smartphone-based screening for visual impairment in Kenyan school children: A cluster randomized controlled trial. *The Lancet*, 6, 924–932.

Sanders, G. (2011). Sex differences in coincidence-anticipation timing (CAT): A review. *Perceptual and Motor Skills, 112*, 61–90.

Sanderson, F. H., & Whiting, H. T. A. (1974). Dynamic visual acuity and performance in a catching task. *Journal of Motor Behavior, 6*, 87–94.

Sanderson, F. H., & Whiting, H. T. A. (1978). Dynamic visual acuity: A possible factor in catching performance. *Journal of Motor Behavior, 10*, 7–14.

Shaffer, D. R. (2001). *Developmental psychology: Childhood and adolescence*. 5th ed. Pacific Grove, CA: Brooks/Cole.

Shea, C. H., Shebilske, W. L., & Worchel, S. (1993). *Motor learning and control*. Englewood Cliffs, NJ: Prentice-Hall.

Suttle, C. M., Melmoth, D. R., Finlay, A. L., Stoper, J. J., & Grant, S. (2011). Eye-hand coordination skills in children with and without amblyopia. *Investigative Ophthalmology & Visual Science, 52*, 1851–1864.

Troster, H., & Brambring, M. (1993). Early motor development in blind infants. *Journal of Applied Developmental Psychology, 14*, 83–106.

Uchida, Y., Kudoh, D., Higuchi, T., Honda, M., & Kanosue, K. (2013). Dynamic visual acuity in baseball players is due to superior tracking abilities. *Medicine and Science in Sports and Exercise*, *45*(2), 319–325.

Wagner, M. O., Haibach, P. S., Lieberman, L. J. (2013). Gross motor skill performance in children with and without visual impairments: Research to practice. *Research in Developmental Disabilities*, *34*, doi: 10.1016/j.ridd.2013.06.030.

Walk, R. D. (1981). *Perceptual development*. Monterey, CA: Brooks/Cole.

Whiting, H. T. A. (1971). *Acquiring ball skill: A psychological interpretation*. Philadelphia, PA: Lea & Febiger.

Wilson, T., & Falkel, J. (2004). *Sports Vision*. Champaign, IL: Human Kinetics.

PART IV

Movement across the Lifespan

9 INFANT REFLEXES AND STEREOTYPIES

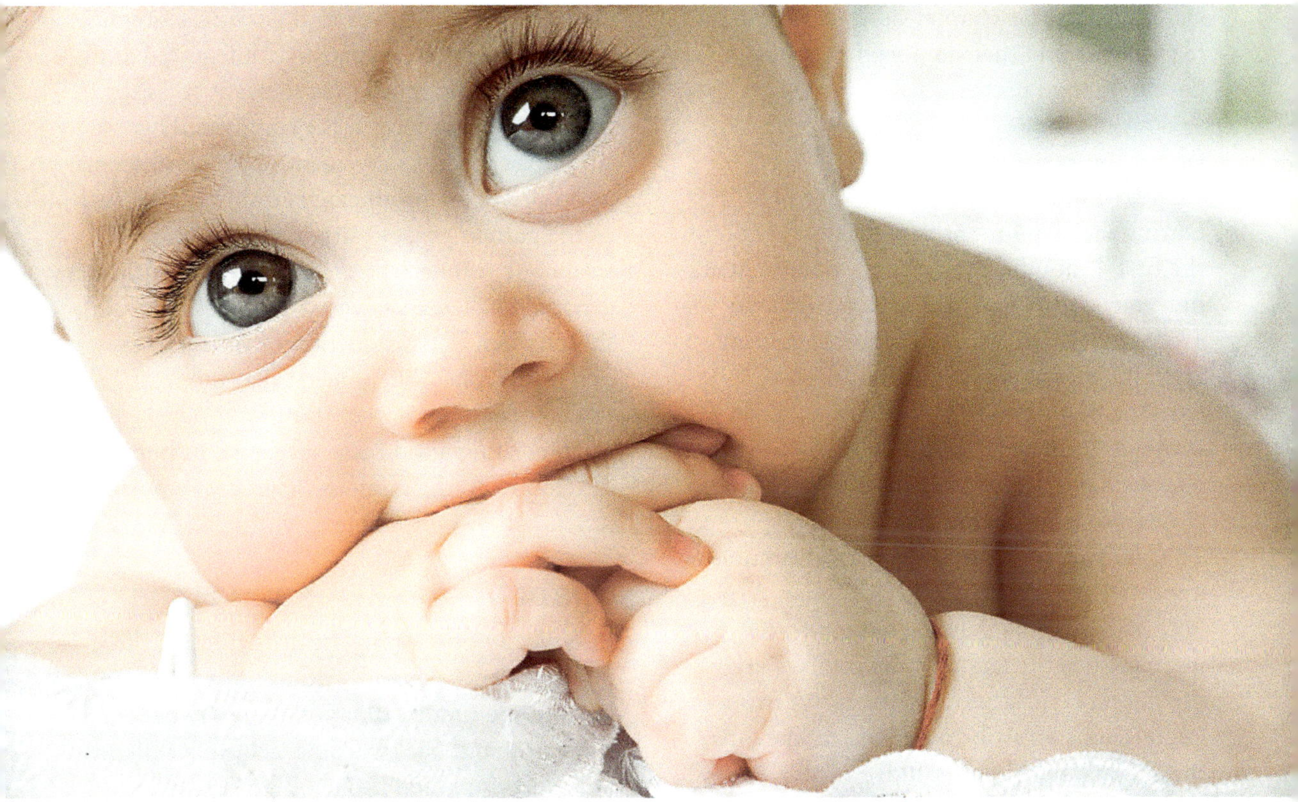

Chapter Objectives

From the information presented in this chapter, you will be able to

- Explain the importance and the role of the infant reflexes
- Pinpoint and explain the number of infant reflexes
- Describe the primitive reflexes
- Describe the postural reflexes
- List and explain some stereotypies

Infancy is one of the most interesting times of life. It is particularly fascinating for motor development because of two types of movements that are characteristic of the first several months of life: infant reflexes and stereotypies. This chapter describes these movements and their importance in the developmental process.

INFANT REFLEXES

During the last 4 months of prenatal life and the first 4 months after birth, a human being's movement repertoire includes movements that are reflexive; that is, each movement is an involuntary, stereotyped response to a particular stimulus. As an example, when a stimulus, such as touching the palm of the infant's hand, is applied, the stimulated hand closes in a routine or stereotypical response. That is, each time the appropriate stimulus is applied, the same, or a highly similar, response occurs (see Figure 9.1). Perhaps even more interesting is the fact that the reflexes are involuntary; these movements result from an unconscious effort by a person, unlike later, more familiar voluntary movements.

Most reflexes also occur **subcortically**, which literally means "below the level of the cortex of the brain," or, more understandably, "below the level of the higher brain centers." Reflexes are processed in such lower brain areas as the brain stem (Malina, Bouchard, & Bar-Or, 2004). Reflexive movements are, therefore, produced without direct involvement of the higher brain centers. The electrical impulse that the stimulus creates travels to the central nervous system. From there, the information is integrated and the appropriate movement message is issued to the muscles involved in the response. This simple method of movement production seems appropriate for producing certain reflexes such as the palmar grasp—although even this seemingly simple reflex is more complex than is generally believed, as we will discuss later in this chapter. The production of the reflexes is one of the many phenomena that interest researchers in human motor development. As an interesting and necessary aspect of human development, the infant reflexes are important to study (see Table 9.1).

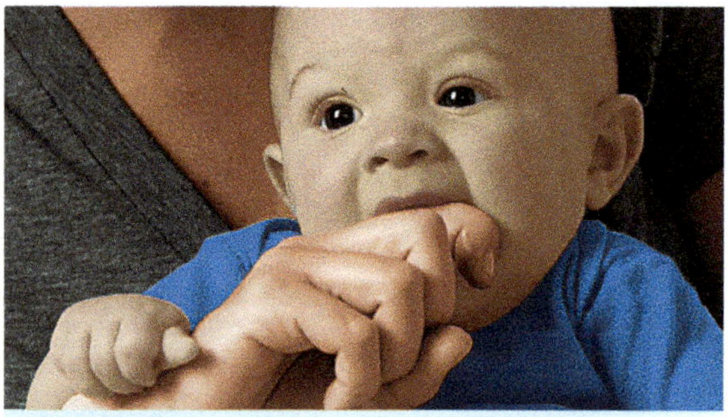

Figure 9.1 The first few months of human motor development are among the most interesting, because they are characterized by involuntary movements called reflexes

Infant Versus Lifespan Reflexes

In typically developing, healthy infants, the infant reflexes generally do not last much beyond the first birthday (the downward, sideward, and backward parachuting reflexes are exceptions; see Table 9.2). Many experts believe, however, that these reflexes do not

Table 9.1 Why study the infant reflexes?

1.	During the last 4 prenatal months and the first 4 postnatal months, reflexive movement is a dominant form of movement in human infants.
2.	In that they secure nourishment and protection, the primitive reflexes are critical for human survival.
3.	The postural reflexes are believed to be basic to more complex, voluntary movements of later infancy.
4.	Though the ages of appearance and disappearance of infant reflexes are somewhat variable, reflexes can provide important information in diagnosing infant health and neurological maturation.

Table 9.2 Expected time of occurrence of selected infant reflexes

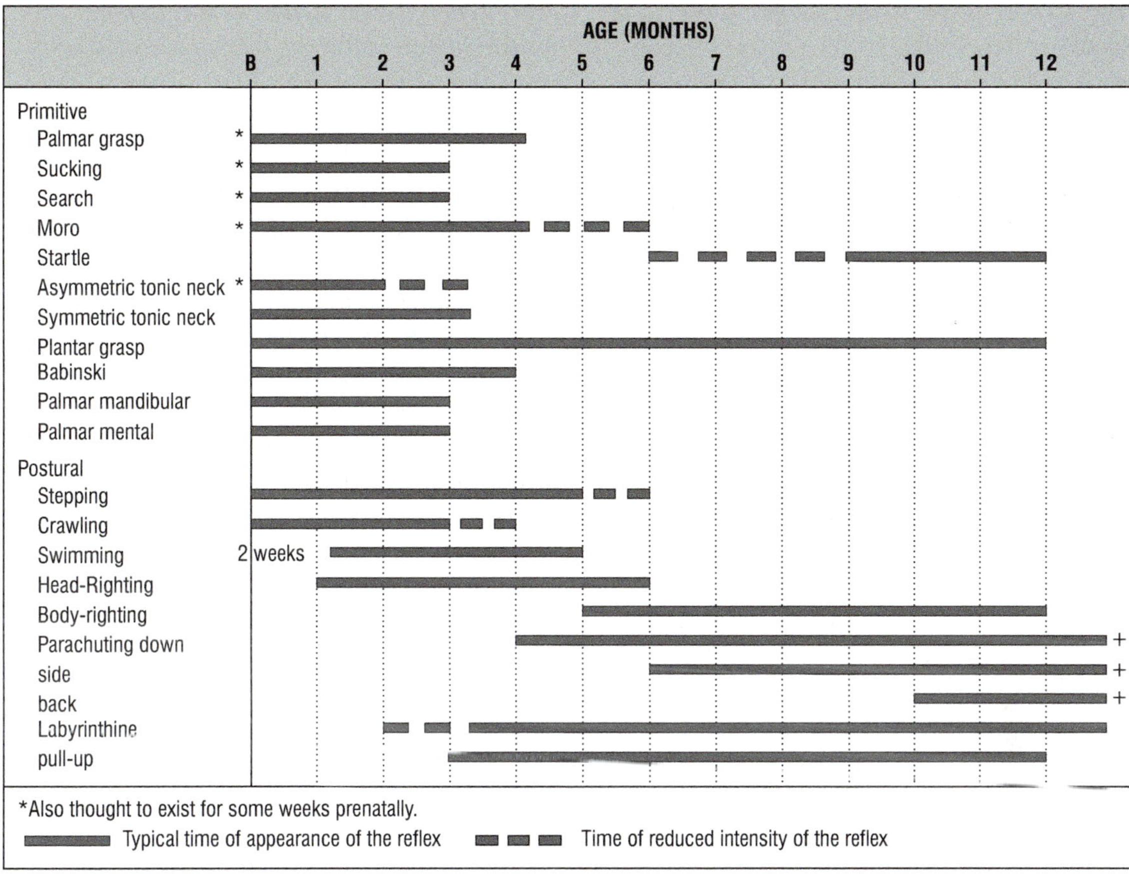

completely disappear. Rather, they are inhibited by the maturing central nervous system and integrated into new movement behaviors. Reflexes that would typically subside after the first year may persist in individuals with damaged or diseased central nervous systems, those under extreme stress, or those using certain drugs (Malina et al., 2004).

Some reflexes typically do persevere past infancy. In fact, in typically developing, healthy individuals, several reflexes last throughout the lifespan. All reflexes that endure throughout the lifespan in typically developing and healthy individuals are called **lifespan reflexes**. For example, most of us have personally experienced the knee-jerk reflex; while we are seated, the physician taps our patellar tendon directly below the patella and our lower leg "jerks," performing a rapid, partial extension. The flexor withdrawal reflex is another example. It exists during infancy yet does not typically cease at the end of the first year of life. In the flexor withdrawal reflex, the arm abruptly flexes upon touching a sharp or hot object. Obviously, this reflex is often quite useful in protecting us from injury. Because this chapter emphasizes the infant reflexes, the lifespan reflexes will not be discussed here.

Primitive Reflexes

A human being is born with few voluntary capabilities and limited mobility. Human neonates are basically helpless and, therefore, highly dependent on their caregivers and their reflexes for their protection and survival. The **primitive reflexes** are the infant reflexes that serve predominantly for protection, nutrition, or survival. The primitive reflexes appear as early as 25 or 26 weeks during gestation (Jaiswal & Morankar, 2017) and are typically suppressed by around 6 months of age in all typically developing newborns.

Here we discuss the stimulus, response, approximate age of emergence and disappearance, and various points of interest concerning many infant primitive reflexes. This section is not an all-inclusive list of the infant reflexes; it discusses the primitive reflexes considered the most interesting, important, or exemplary.

Palmar Grasp Reflex

The **palmar grasp reflex**, one of the best known of all infant reflexes, may also be one of the first to emerge (see Figure 9.2). The palmar grasp reflex generally appears in utero, as early as the fifth month of gestation. As mentioned earlier, evidence indicates that this reflex may be much more complex than is generally believed. The basic palmar grasp reflex is a response to tactile stimulation of the palm of the hand. When the palm is stimulated, all four fingers of the stimulated hand flex or close. Although the thumb does not respond to this stimulus, the grasping response of the reflex can be surprisingly forceful. For example, if an adult simultaneously stimulates both of an infant's palms, the infant may respond with a grasp sufficiently forceful to enable the adult to lift the infant completely off the supporting surface (Futagi, Toribe, & Suzuki, 2012). The palmar grasp reflex typically endures through the fourth month, and it gradually decreases in strength across those first few months (Dionisis, Moraes, Tudella, et al., 2015). A grasping action of the hand will likely persist past the fourth month, but it will be voluntary, not reflexive. In fact, the palmar grasp reflex is believed to play an important role in the acquisition of early forms of voluntary reaching and grasping.

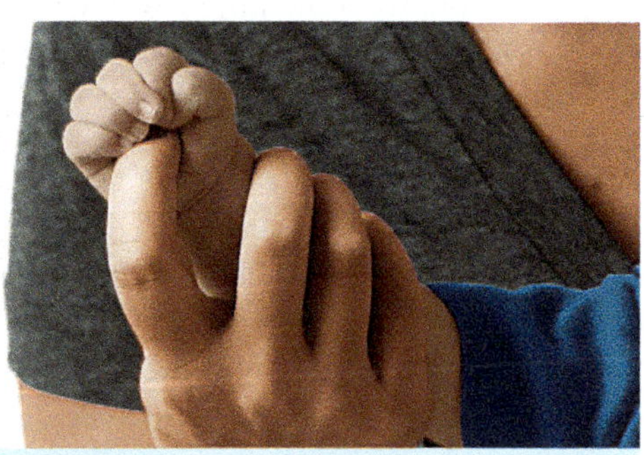

Figure 9.2 The palmar grasp reflex is one of the most noticeable reflexes in infants

This reflex can also be an easy to administer and important part of an infant's neural exam as the outcome can provide key information regarding the baby's motor skill and neural health (Marques-de-Moraes, Dionisio, Tan, & Tudella, 2017). In these exams an excessively strong palmar grasp may be indicative of cerebral palsy while an asymmetric response may indicate damage to the cerebellum, hemiplegia (paralysis on one side) or kernicterus (brain damage associated with severe jaundice and high levels of bilirubin) (Jaiswal & Morankar, 2017).

Interestingly, researchers have found that we may be able to predict handedness in adulthood by using the palmar grasp reflex. Researchers believe that the hand that shows the stronger reflexive grasp in infancy may be likely to become the dominant hand later in life. Furthermore, the palmar grasp reflex is believed to provide an accurate indication of neural health. If the grasp is weak or absent upon birth, or exaggerated after the fifth month of life, this may indicate the presence of a neurological disorder (Dionisis et al., 2015).

Sucking Reflex

Another reflex that appears very early in life is the **sucking reflex**, which is typically present prenatally. The sucking response is elicited when the lips are stimulated, such as by the touch of the mother's breast or a finger (see Figure 9.3). This stimulation actually evokes two sucking-related responses. The first and more obvious response is the creation of a

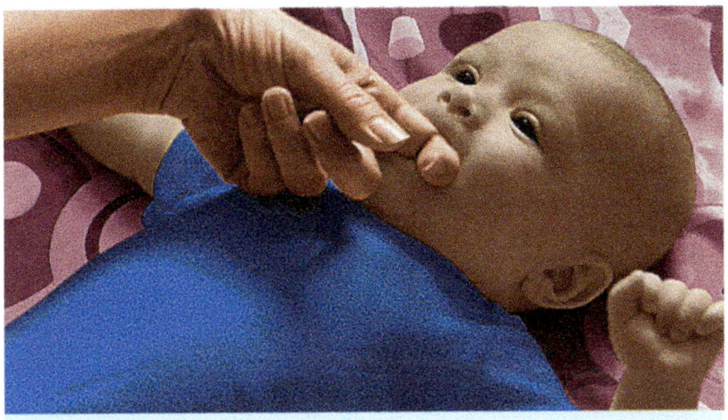

Figure 9.3 The sucking reflex occurs pre- and postnatally

negative intraoral pressure as the sucking occurs. Second, the tongue applies a positive pressure; it presses upward and slightly forward with each sucking action. Following the appropriate stimulation, a series of sucking movements takes place, each movement consisting of the simultaneous application of negative and positive pressure.

As a result of the sucking reflex, babies are often born with blisters or pads on their lips. These minor, self inflicted lesions, which may appear on one or both sides of the lips, result from the baby sucking in utero as early as the 25th week of gestation. It is important that the baby's family and the physician understand the source of these blisters, to avoid unnecessary anxiety upon the baby's birth. It is even recommended that these blisters be used as a screening tool for healthy neuronal function in neonates (Henrik, 2013).

In addition to being a valuable assessment tool, the sucking reflex is important for an infant to be able to ingest nutrition. A neonate is born without the voluntary capacity to ingest food, so the sucking reflex enables the baby to ingest by involuntary means the nutrients essential for survival. Nonnutritive sucking also provides a means of self-soothing for a baby who is distressed. Of course, babies also use their mouths and sucking to explore their environment through touch (Harding, Frank, Dunga, & Colton, 2012). This movement typically remains a reflex through the third month of infancy; thereafter, it will be voluntary.

Search Reflex

Like the sucking reflex, the **search reflex** is believed to exist for some weeks prenatally, and it persists through the third month of infancy in most instances. The search reflex generally can be elicited by softly stroking the area of the face surrounding the mouth. The infant will respond by turning her or his head in the direction of the stimulus (see Figure 9.4; Harding et al., 2012). The sensitive areas surrounding the mouth are sometimes referred to as the cardinal points, so the search reflex is also called the cardinal points reflex (and, as mentioned earlier, the rooting reflex).

The search reflex is often considered in conjunction with the sucking reflex, a logical approach because both reflexes are functionally linked to obtaining food. The search reflex helps the infant locate the source of nourishment, and then the sucking reflex enables the baby to ingest the food. This reflex, however, contributes to more than the baby's nourishment, as the rotation of the neck often elicits other reflexes, including the head- and body-righting reflexes. Failure or persistence of this reflex may be a sign of central nervous system or sensorimotor dysfunction (Sheridan, 2014). Asymmetrical appearance of the reflex

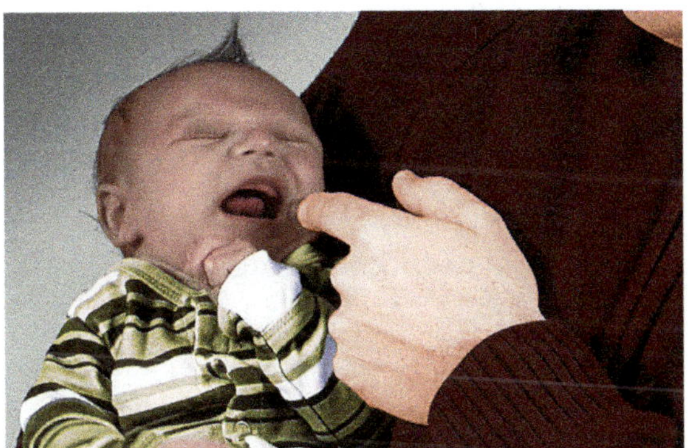

Figure 9.4 The search reflex helps the baby locate nourishment. The baby turns the head toward the food source when the cheek near the mouth is gently stimulated.

PINPOINTING THE NUMBER OF INFANT REFLEXES

The total number of infant reflexes is difficult to determine. Various experts often use different terms to refer to the same reflex. For example, the rooting reflex is also called the search reflex or the cardinal points reflex.

Also, the reflexes themselves are often not clearly defined. The components, as well as the name, of a certain infant reflex may vary, depending on the source. The palmar grasp reflex generally is considered to consist of the four fingers closing when the palm is stimulated. However, as suggested earlier, it may in fact be much more complex. Multiple stimuli and multiple responses appear to be involved in reflexive grasping. Along with the familiar closing of the four fingers when the palm is stimulated, a stimulation between the thumb and forefinger elicits a flexion of just those two digits. During the weeks after the palmar grasp reflex first appears, a similar response can be elicited for each finger individually if the surface of the palm near the base of that finger is stimulated. The question then arises whether these local reactions are distinct infant reflexes or are all part of the palmar grasp. Such questions exist for other reflexes, as well, complicating attempts to number and organize the infant reflexes accurately.

Further complicating categorization of the infant reflexes, infants perform many movements during the early months of life that are most likely reflexes but have never been named or listed anywhere. One example is the stereotypic "elbowing" movement. This movement, which was once postulated to be a primitive reflex, was first noticed by physicians when they performed ultrasound tests in the abdominal region of newborns, just below the ribs. To test the hypothesis that this movement is a reflex, researchers examined 71 healthy, full-term babies from 1 to 3 days of age. All babies were tested every two weeks thereafter through day 86 of life—a total of seven times. The testing involved a complete neurological examination followed by a gentle pressing of the abdomen with a wooden model of an ultrasound probe. Most of the babies responded by rapidly bringing together (adducting) the elbows with the arms flexed. This was followed by extension of the arms and swiping of the abdomen as if to brush away the stimulating object. This response to the stimulus was present in over 70 percent of the babies and was most obvious at about 2 weeks and 1 month of age. The authors speculated that this reflex is a primitive reflex to protect the abdominal area. The authors believe the movement is reflexive because it is involuntary and happens the same way each time the stimulus is applied. Like other infant reflexes, this response becomes increasingly suppressed over time (Saraga, Resic, Krnic, et al., 2007).

may mean an injury has occurred in a facial nerve or muscle or in one side of the brain.

Moro Reflex

The **Moro reflex**, named after Ernst Moro, often exists at birth, and it endures until the infant is approximately 4–6 months old. It is a form of startle, thought to be a protective response to a loss of physical support or a disruption in the body's balance (Brucknerova, Holomanova, Ujhazy, & Mach, 2012). It can be elicited in many ways. One stimulus is to place the palm of the hand under the baby's head and then suddenly, but gently, lower the

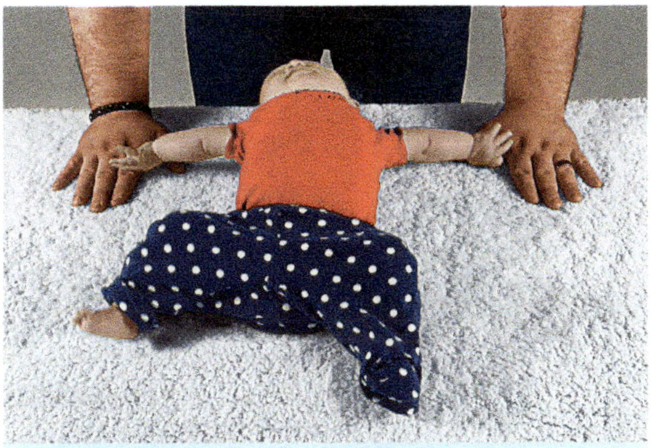

Figure 9.5 The Moro reflex is elicited by the same stimuli that induce the startle reflex. The Moro, however, precedes the startle and causes the arms and legs to extend immediately rather than flex.

head a few inches. This stimulus causes the baby's arms, fingers, and legs to extend (see Figure 9.5) and then flex. The baby is also apt to cry following the application of the stimulus (Rousseau, Matton, Lecuyer, & Lahaye, 2017). The same response occurs if the entire baby is held and suddenly lowered 3 or 4 in (8–10 cm; Gascon, 2012). Occasionally, a slight tremor will accompany the extension of the limbs and a "C" shape will be formed by the semi-flexion of the thumbs and index fingers (Futagi et al., 2012). Also, if the surface on which the baby is lying is struck with the palm of the hand, typically the Moro reflex will occur.

There is some disagreement concerning the role of the legs in the Moro reflex. Most experts agree that the legs extend unless they are already extended, in which case they flex. In both of these situations, a slight tremor or shaking of the legs may occur. Interestingly, the disappearance of this reflex depends on the type of stimulus used; the "head drop" Moro disappears sooner than the other two types. Furthermore, researchers have determined that there is a developmental trend related to how quickly the reflex responds to the stimulus—a form of reaction time. The shortest reaction time was found in 1-month-old infants, with the time increasing through 2 and 3 months of age (Iiyama, Miyajima, & Hoshika, 2002).

The Moro reflex is one of the most useful for diagnosing the infant's neurological maturation. Failure to acquire the Moro reflex by birth may indicate a central nervous system dysfunction; high-risk babies are more likely to display an atypical or absent response. The degree of the response may also vary, with higher-risk babies having a weaker response (Sohn, Ahn, & Lee, 2011). Asymmetry in this reflex (absence or weakness on one side) may indicate hemiplegia, damage to the brachial plexus (group of nerves that stem from the spine and extend down the arm), or even a broken clavicle (Jaiswal & Morankar, 2017). Persistence of the Moro reflex past the expected time of suppression may indicate a sensorimotor problem. In addition, persistence will delay voluntary sitting, head control, and other motor milestones. Asymmetry of the Moro, as we have seen with other reflexes, may indicate an injury to one side of the brain.

Startle Reflex

Similar in many ways to the Moro reflex, the **startle reflex** can be elicited by a rapid change of head position or striking the surface that supports the baby, as well as most any unexpected and abrupt stimulus. However, whereas the Moro causes the limbs to extend immediately, the startle reflex causes the arms and legs to flex immediately. The startle reflex is accompanied by a "flexor response with symmetrical activation of different muscles resulting in a facial grimace, abduction of the arms, flexion of the neck, trunk, elbows, hips, and knees" (Dreissen, Bakker, Koelman, & Tijssen, 2012, p. 35). Furthermore, the Moro normally disappears at 4–6 months of age, but the startle may not appear until 2–3 months after the Moro disappears. The startle reflex in this form is typically suppressed by 1 year of age, although less severe startle responses are elicited throughout the lifespan.

Asymmetric Tonic Neck Reflex

The **asymmetric tonic neck reflex**, sometimes referred to as the bow and arrow or fencer's position, is commonly seen in premature babies but may not be noticeable in full-term infants. This reflex can be elicited when the baby is prone or supine. When the head is turned to one side or the other, the limbs on the face side extend while the limbs on the opposite side flex (Hamer & Hadders-Algra, 2016; see Figure 9.6). Although the asymmetric tonic neck reflex is rare in newborns, it occasionally can be elicited in infants up to 3 months old. This reflex is believed to facilitate the development of an awareness of both sides of the body, as well as helping to develop eye-hand coordination.

Symmetric Tonic Neck Reflex

In the asymmetric tonic neck reflex, the right-side limbs respond differently from the left-side limbs, but this is not the case in the **symmetric tonic neck reflex**. As the term implies, in this reflex the limbs move symmetrically. This symmetrical response can be elicited by placing the baby in a supported sitting position. If the infant is tipped backward far enough, the neck eventually extends, which is the stimulus for a corresponding extension of the arms and flexion of the legs. However, if the baby is tipped forward until the neck is fully flexed, the arms flex and the legs extend (Bruijn et al., 2013; see Figure 9.7).

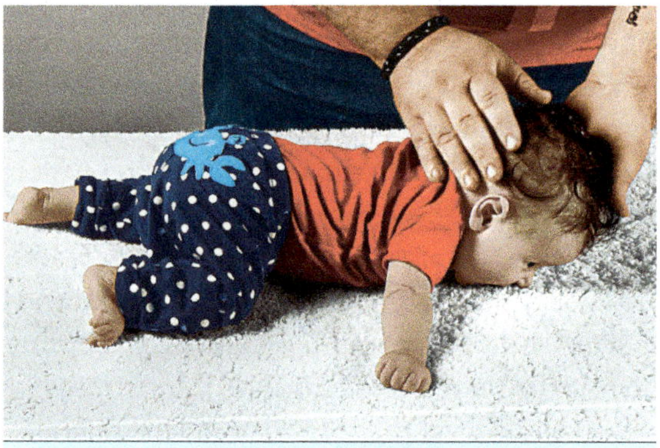

Figure 9.6 The asymmetric tonic neck reflex causes flexion on one side of the body and extension on the other

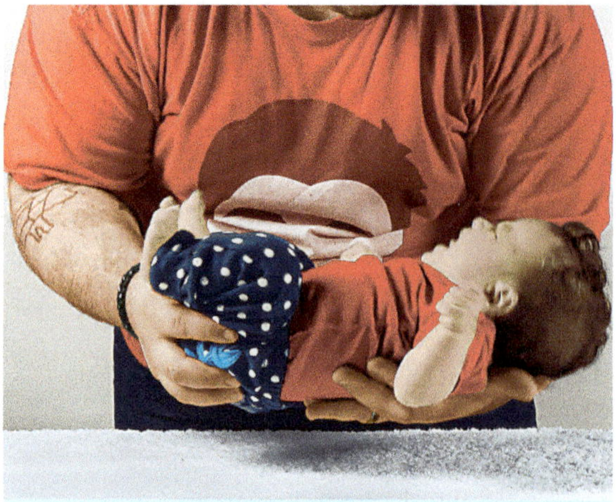

Figure 9.7 The symmetric tonic neck reflex is often observable during the first few months of life

The symmetric tonic neck reflex is often noticeable from birth through approximately 3 months of age. Persistence in this reflex can cause serious problems. For example, persistence may impede voluntary head lifting when the infant is in a prone or supine position. It will also inhibit reaching and grasping, unsupported sitting, balance for walking, and virtually all major motor milestones.

Plantar Grasp Reflex

The **plantar grasp reflex** typically can be elicited from birth through the first year of infancy. This reflex is easily evoked by applying slight pressure, usually with the fingertip, to the ball of the foot, causing all the toes of that foot to flex. The toes curl around the stimulating object as if attempting to grasp, as in the palmar grasp reflex of the hand (Hamer & Hadders-Algra, 2016; see Figure 9.8).

According to Futagi and Suzuki (2010), the plantar grasp reflex is important clinically as a weak or absent plantar grasp at the expected time of appearance could indicate spasticity,

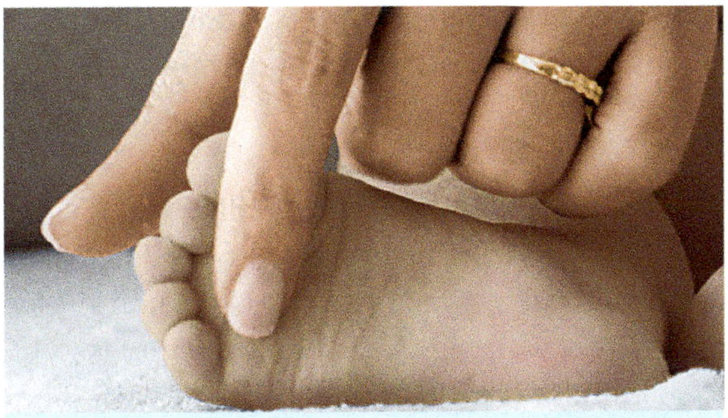

Figure 9.8 In the plantar grasp reflex, the toes appear to be attempting to grasp

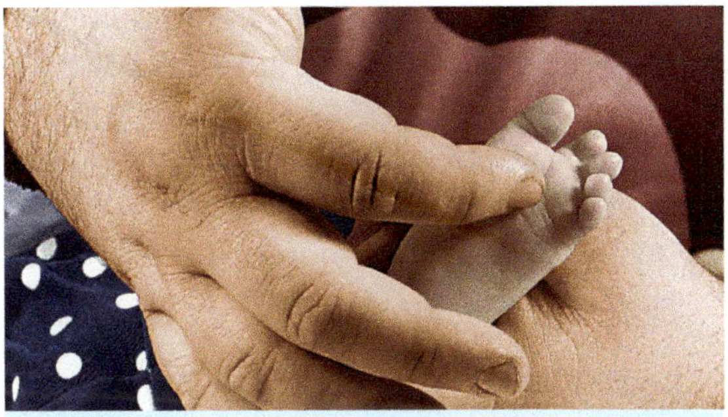

Figure 9.9 The Babinski reflex elicited by a stimulus somewhat similar to that of the plantar grasp reflex, but the response is different

mental delays or impediments, or even cerebral palsy. The extended appearance of the reflex beyond the expected period of delay can have similar clinical significance. The plantar grasp must be suppressed before the child can stand erect, stand alone, or walk. Parents will find it difficult to put shoes on a child who still exhibits an active plantar grasp reflex.

Babinski Reflex

The **Babinski reflex** was discovered by Joseph Babinski in 1896. Like the plantar grasp reflex, this reflex is typically evident from birth, and it remains present for the first several months of life in typically developing babies. To elicit a response, the bottom or lateral portion of the foot is stroked (see Figure 9.9) when the lower limb is fairly relaxed, resulting in a dorsiflexion (elevation) of the great toe and sometimes all the toes of the stimulated foot. In infants, the Babinski reflex is typical, but its appearance in adults is an important indicator of possible upper motor neuron lesions and associated dysfunction; it is also seen in some children with learning or behavioral disorders (Ambesh, Paliwal, Shetty, & Kamholz, 2017). Interestingly, it is being detected more commonly in older adults and is thought to be a sign of declining neural function (Pauc, 2011).

Palmar Mandibular Reflex

The **palmar mandibular reflex**, or Babkin reflex, is another infant reflex typically present

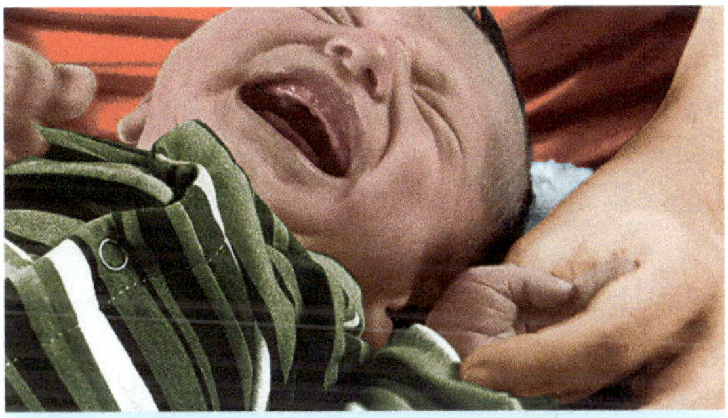

Figure 9.10 The palmar mandibular reflex is one of the most unusual reflexes because it makes the eyes close, the mouth open, and the head tilt forward

at birth. The Babkin is elicited by applying pressure simultaneously to the palm of each hand, eliciting all or one of the following responses: the mouth opens, the eyes close, and the neck flexes, tilting the head forward (Futagi, Yanagihara, Mogami, et al., 2013; see Figure 9.10). The Babkin response also occurs if the hand of a human neonate is lightly stimulated by hair. This reflex typically disappears by 3 months. Interestingly, some experts believe that this reflex links the human to animals lower on the phylogenetic scale, because it often helps young animals cling to their mother when feeding. Like many of the infant reflexes, the palmar mandibular reflex has clinical significance as abnormalities in its appearance can indicate neurological impairment. The reflex tends to be more likely to be elicited when the baby is awake and alert, not sleepy, though significant variations in response can exist, especially in babies born preterm. In more typical cases, according to Futagi and associates (2013), it gradually fades into voluntary movements of the eyes, hands, and mouth to enable the coordination required for feeding.

Palmar Mental Reflex

The **palmar mental reflex**, like the Babkin, elicits a facial response; it occurs when the base of the palm of either hand is scratched. This stimulus causes the lower jaw to open and close (see Figure 9.11). The actual response is, thus, a series of contractions of the jaw muscles. Like the Babkin, the palmar mental reflex is first observable at birth and typically ceases by the third month.

Postural Reflexes

Reflexes believed to be related to the development of later voluntary movement are known as postural reflexes. **Postural reflexes** are thought to be a basis for voluntary movements such as crawling, standing, or walking.

Here we discuss the details of the postural reflexes. As with our examination of the primitive reflexes, this discussion is not meant to be comprehensive but rather to highlight important points about these reflexes. Generally, the postural reflexes occur later in infancy than the primitive reflexes, although a few exist earlier, such as the stepping and crawling reflexes (Malina et al., 2004).

Stepping Reflex

The **stepping reflex** is sometimes called a walking or placing reflex and is considered to be a forerunner to an important voluntary movement, walking. The stepping reflex is elicited by holding the infant upright with the feet touching a supporting surface; the pressure on the bottom of the feet causes the legs to lift and then descend (see Figure 9.12). This leg action often occurs alternately and, therefore, resembles a crude form of walking (Gascon, 2012). It is more irregular than voluntary walking and lacks the controlled upright positioning. It has the appearance of "exaggerated marching with flexed legs, high foot lift, and flatfooted touch-down . . . ground forces are less accurately controlled, and newborns exert more vertical than horizontal force" in their movement (Lacquaniti, Ivanenko, & Zago, 2012, p. 823). Although this reflex is also called the walking reflex, there is none of the hip stability or accompanying arm movement that occurs with voluntary walking. The stepping reflex generally can be elicited within the first few

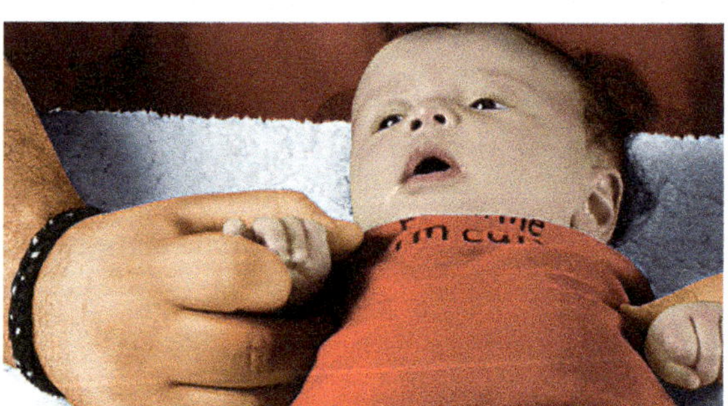

Figure 9.11 The palmar mental reflex is elicited by scratching the base of either palm

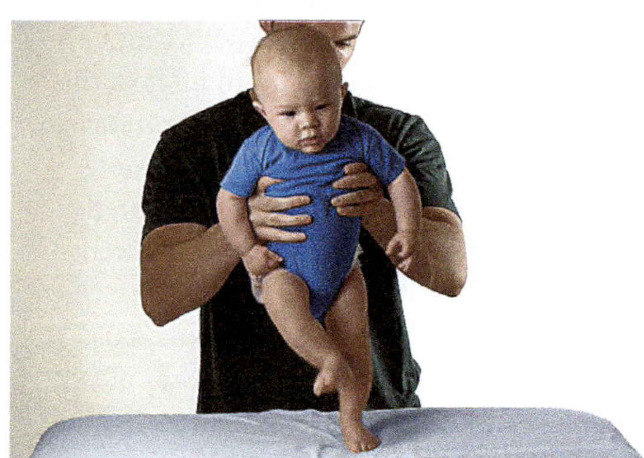

Figure 9.12 The stepping reflex can be elicited within the first few weeks following birth, even though unassisted voluntary walking may not occur until the first birthday

weeks following birth and persists through the fifth or sixth month. The stepping reflex generally disappears around 2 months of life, but it reappears a few months later before seeming to evolve gradually into voluntary walking.

Interestingly, researchers have observed developmental changes across the first several months of this reflex. These include excessive coactivation or simultaneous contraction of the mutual antagonist muscles during the stance phase of the pattern (when both feet are touching the ground) during the first month (Okamoto, Okamoto, & Andrew, 2001). However, during the second month of this reflex's existence, the contraction patterns become more cooperative or reciprocal, despite a slight forward-leaning posture and slightly flexed legs. The researchers believe these changes to be a function of gradual improvements in balance, postural control, and strength that ultimately lead to the phasing out of the reflex as complete voluntary control of walking sets in.

Crawling Reflex

The **crawling reflex** is another example of an infant reflex that is considered a precursor to later voluntary movement. This reflex can be observed from birth through the first 3 to 4 months. To elicit this reflex, the baby is placed prone on the floor or table. The soles of the feet are stroked alternately, causing the legs and arms to move in an action similar to crawling (see Figure 9.13). The crawling reflex disappears about 3 months before more voluntary creeping begins. This reflex is believed to further development of sufficient muscular tone for future voluntary creeping.

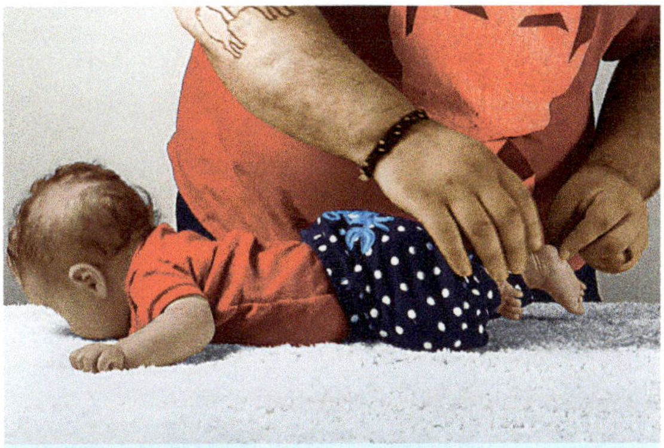

Figure 9.13 The crawling reflex is believed essential to the development of future voluntary creeping

Swimming Reflex

One of the most unusual infant reflexes is the **swimming reflex**. Involuntary swimming-like movements can be elicited days after birth. This reflex was originally noted by the early developmentalist, Myrtle McGraw (1939). She placed neonates face-down in the water and noticed swimming like movements. Hence, the reflex was deemed the swimming reflex. This may have been something of a misnomer, however, as it was later noted that babies of a similar age would also perform these same movements when held horizontally over a solid surface, such as a tabletop or a floor, or over the surface of water (Langendorfer, 2007). The response to the stimulus of being held horizontally is the movement of the arms and legs in a well-coordinated swimming-type (or crawling-like) action (see Figure 9.14). These movements are observable as early as the second neonatal week and typically endure through the fifth month of infancy. Recognition of this reflex has contributed substantially to the popularity of infant swim programs. Proponents of such programs assume that early stimulation of this reflex will positively affect voluntary swimming later in life though, as discussed in Chapter 5, there is little scientific evidence to support this view.

Head- and Body-Righting Reflexes

The **head- and body-righting reflexes** are two similar infant reflexes believed to be related to

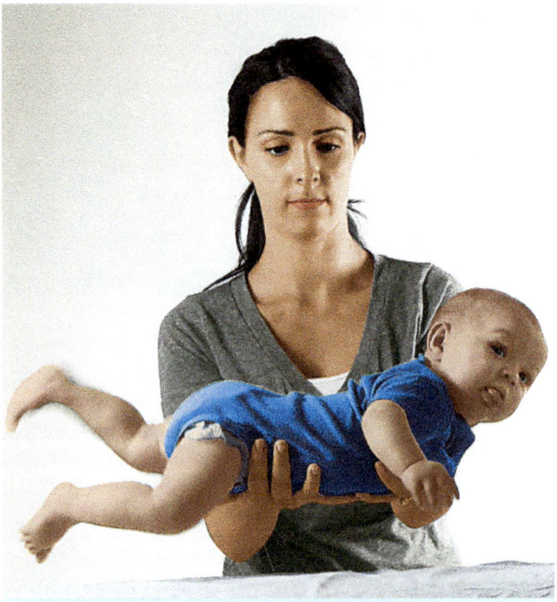

Figure 9.14 The swimming reflex is characterized by the baby's swimming-like movements when held in a horizontal position

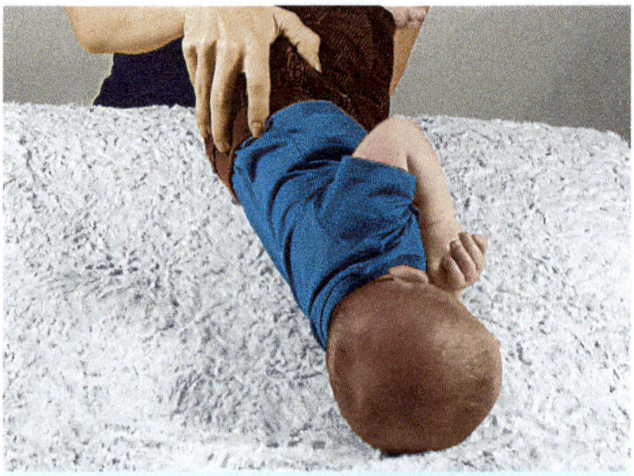

Figure 9.15 In the head-righting reflex, the head "rights" itself with the body when the body is turned to one side

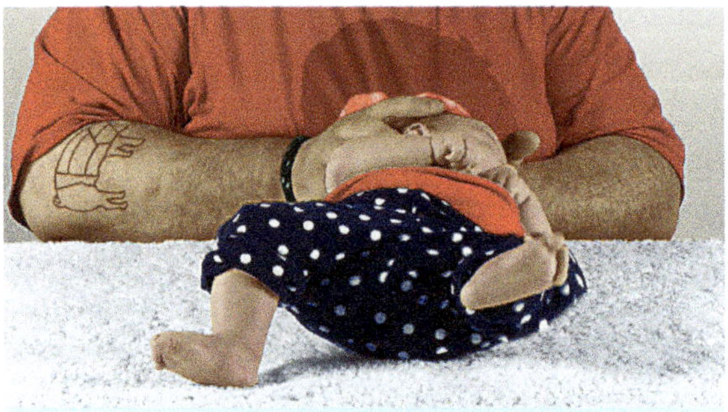

Figure 9.16 In the body-righting reflex, the body "rights" itself with the head when the head is turned to one side or the other

the attainment of voluntary rolling movements. The head-righting reflex can be observed as early as the first month of infancy. This reflex is elicited by turning the baby's body in either direction when the infant is supine. The head responds by "righting" itself with the body; in other words, the head returns to a front-facing position relative to the shoulders (see Figure 9.15). This reflex typically disappears by the age of 6 months.

In contrast to the head-righting reflex, the body-righting reflex involves the head turning and the body "righting" itself (see Figure 9.16). If the infant is placed supine and the head gently turned to one side or the other, the body follows. That is, the body rotates in the direction the head is turned to regain the front-facing relationship between the head and the shoulders. This rotation of the body is not segmental; the body responds by rotating as a single unit. Unlike the head-righting reflex, the body-righting reflex may not be evident until the fifth month of infancy. It frequently lasts throughout the first year of life.

Parachuting Reflexes

The **parachuting reflexes** (or propping reflexes) appear to be related to the attainment of upright posture. These reflexes occur when the infant is tipped off balance in any direction. Becoming off balance when in an upright position stimulates a protective movement in the direction of the potential fall. For example, when the infant is tilted forward, the arms make a propping movement, extending toward the front as the fingers extend and separate. This reflex occurs as early as 4 months of age. These propping movements appear to be conscious attempts to break a fall, but, like all infant reflexes, they are actually involuntary (see Figure 9.17).

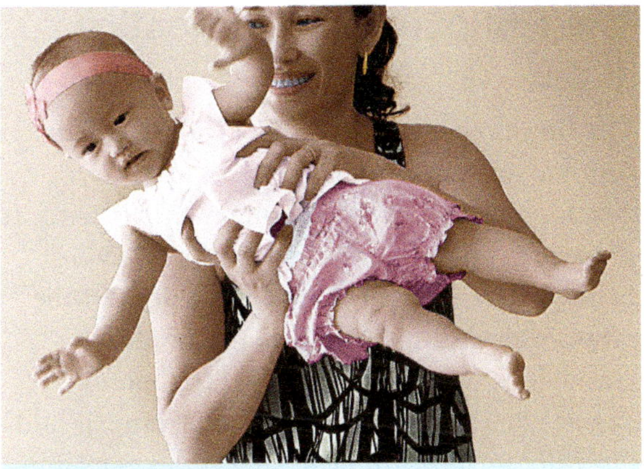

Figure 9.17 Parachuting reflexes appear to occur consciously in an effort to break a potential fall, but, like all reflexes, they are really subcortical

These propping movements can also occur downward, sideward, and backward. The downward parachuting reaction can be elicited as early as 4 months if the child is suddenly lowered 2 to 3 feet when held upright. The infant's legs suddenly extend and spread, and the feet rotate slightly outward. The sideward propping movements are observable after approximately 6 months of age and are most easily elicited by placing the infant in a sitting position and then gently tilting him or her to one side. As in the forward parachuting reflex, the arms and fingers extend, in this case toward the side of the potential fall. The backward propping movement may not occur until 10 months of age and, like the other parachuting reflexes, typically causes a propping movement in the direction of the potential fall. However, the backward propping reflex may also cause the body to rotate, apparently to avoid falling backward. All of the propping reflexes frequently persist past the first year of life.

In a study conducted specifically on the parachuting and lateral propping reflexes of preterm infants, researchers determined that these reflexes existed in approximately 8 percent of babies at 6 months but in nearly 90 percent by 9 months of age. As a result, these researchers concluded that lateral and parachuting reflexes can be assessed in preterm children and may be viable markers of neurological development (Ohlweiler, da Silva, & Rotta, 2002). Children with cerebral palsy may not exhibit this reflex, or it may appear in an abnormal form. In children with hemiplegia, it would appear asymmetrically (Jaiswal & Morankar, 2017).

Labyrinthine Reflex

The **labyrinthine reflex** generally appears at approximately 2 to 3 months of age and lasts throughout the first year of life. It is a protective reflex that is crucial for survival. If an infant is placed in a prone position, breathing may be inhibited to the point of suffocation. The helpless neonate has insufficient voluntary capabilities to raise or turn the head to improve breathing. However, the involuntary labyrinthine reflex enables the infant to "right" or elevate the head, thus moving the head to a position more conducive to breathing and allowing the baby to survive.

Although the labyrinthine reflex is a protective function, this reflex, like the parachuting reflexes, may be related to the attainment of upright posture. The labyrinthine is also characterized by the head's tilting in a direction opposite the direction the body is tilted (see Figure 9.18). For example, if the infant is held at the waist and tilted forward, the neck extends to enable the head to maintain its original upright position. If the baby is tilted backward, the neck again extends to enable the head to maintain the upright position. A similar response occurs when the baby is tilted to either side.

Pull-Up Reflex

The **pull-up reflex**, sometimes called the pull-to-sit maneuver (Hamer & Hadders-Algra, 2016), may be another reflex related to the attainment of upright posture. Like the

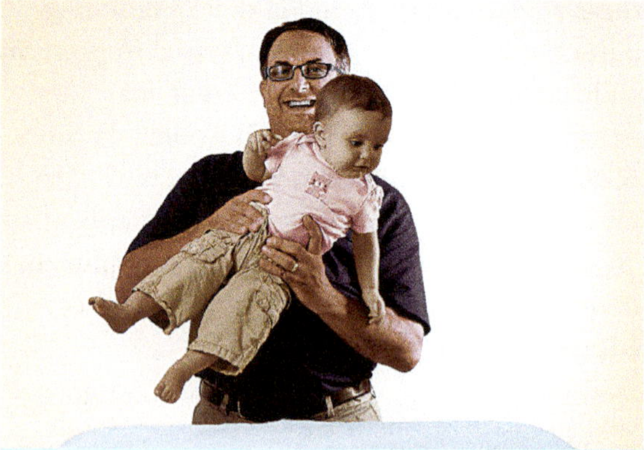

Figure 9.18 The labyrinthine reflex endures throughout most of the first year and apparently is related to the attainment of upright posture

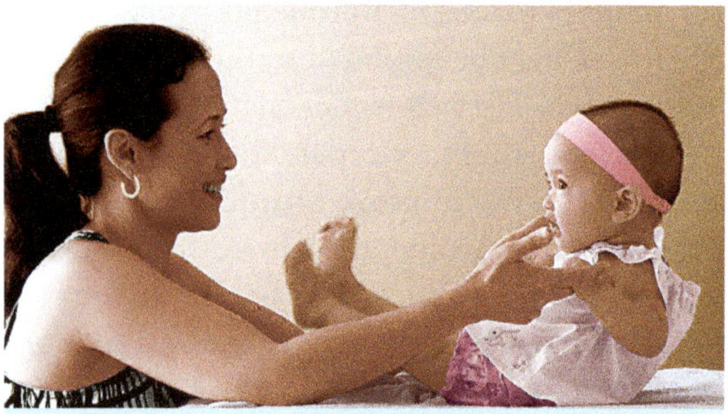

Figure 9.19 In the pull-up reflex, when the baby is tipped backward, the arms flex in an effort to maintain the upright position

labyrinthine reflex, the pull-up reflex may not be observable until the third month of infancy. This reflex is most easily elicited by placing the infant in a supported standing or sitting position. Holding the baby's hands, one carefully tips the child in any direction; this stimulus makes the supporting arm(s) flex or extend in an apparent effort to maintain the upright position (see Figure 9.19). For example, if the baby is tipped backward, the arms flex to pull the child toward the supporting person and into an upright position. If the infant is tipped forward, the arms extend to push her away from the supporting person and back toward the initial upright position. The pull-up reflexes generally disappear by the first birthday.

The Reflexes as Diagnostic Tools

The infant reflexes are crucial for the infant's survival and seem to be related to the development of future voluntary movements as these early, involuntary forms of movement behavior are also important indicators of the infant's level of neurological maturation (Jaiswal & Morankar, 2017). Thus, many experts believe an infant's neural exam should typically include a test of their reflexes as one means of diagnosing abnormalities (Marques-de-Moraes et al., 2017). Although the age at which each infant reflex emerges and disappears varies with each child, knowledge of the typical timeline can help in diagnosing problems. Reflexes are age-specific in typically developing, healthy infants and are, therefore, viable indicators of neurological maturity. Thus, any severe deviations from expected time frames may indicate neurological immaturity or dysfunction. If the reflex in question is lacking, excessively weak, asymmetrical (appearing more forcefully on one side of the body than the other), or persisting past the typical age of disappearance, the examining health professional is alerted to a need for additional testing or for intervention. Using the infant reflexes as diagnostic tools can lead to the early identification of abnormalities that, in turn, can lead to earlier referrals, diagnosis, treatment, and better long-term health for the individual (Jaiswal & Morankar, 2017). Infant reflexes that persevere past the normal time of extinction can have adverse effects on typical motor development while affecting effective sensory processing of the brain. The inhibition of the infant reflexes within the typical or expected time frame allows for typical motor development as the infant more frequently interacts with the surroundings in more complex ways. In short, perseveration can have a negative impact on future development and may be an indicator of neurological dysfuntion (Chinello, Di Gangi, & Valenza, 2018).

Diagnosis, treatment, and prognosis for conditions such as cerebral palsy are often determined by several factors. These include the infant's performance on classic neural exams, motor milestones the child has achieved at a given age, and her or his performance on various primitive reflexes. Therefore, pediatricians should possess a fundamental knowledge of these reflexes. Clinical knowledge of the infant reflexes is relatively easily acquired, easy to incorporate into exams, and quite useful in diagnosis. In fact, the assessment of infant reflexes is one of the simplest and most frequently employed tools in infant examinations (Sohn, Ahn, & Lee, 2011).

Reflexes should be tested carefully and only by trained professionals. Some parents become frantic when they cannot elicit a particular reflex, assuming that their child has an impaired neurological system when, in fact, the parents' incorrect application of the stimulus or the baby's temporary behavioral state is responsible for the lack of response. Usually, for any infant reflex to be elicited there must be a state of quiet. If the baby is restless, crying, sleepy, or distracted, she or he may not respond to the applied stimulus; this lack of response certainly should not be considered an indication of a neurological aberration.

Many infant reflexes are tested during routine physical examinations of the baby. As mentioned earlier, one of the reflexes most commonly used to detect neurological dysfunction is the Moro reflex, which may signify a cerebral birth injury if it is lacking or asymmetrical. Gascon (2012) considers the Moro reflex to be the most important reflex for neural examination of infants. The asymmetric tonic neck reflex is another commonly used diagnostic tool for infants. If this reflex perseveres past the expected time of disappearance, cerebral palsy or other neural damage could be indicated. These reflexes are two examples of the many infant reflexes that help healthcare professionals determine an infant's neurological state. The Milani Comparetti Neuromotor Developmental Examination is an evaluation instrument that uses several infant reflexes. This test was designed to evaluate the neurological maturity of children from birth to 24 months of age.

ROLE OF INFANT REFLEXES IN DEVELOPING FUTURE MOVEMENT

Some reflexes are believed to be directly integrated, modified, and incorporated into more complex patterns to form voluntary movements. The stepping reflex is one of the most obvious examples of a postural reflex, that is, a reflex that would seem to facilitate later voluntary movement. If an infant 1 or 2 months old is held upright with the feet touching a supporting surface, the pressure on the feet stimulates the legs to perform a walking action. This movement is, of course, reflexive; the infant makes no conscious effort to produce this movement—the movement occurs involuntarily and subcortically. This early, involuntary, walking-like movement appears to be a critical antecedent to the development of voluntary walking, which appears in the months to follow.

However, the link between postural reflexes and later voluntary movement has come into question. The reflexes that are believed to be linked to voluntary behavior often disappear before the onset of the "related" voluntary movement, and this occurs with the stepping reflex. This reflex is noticeable soon after birth, but around the sixth month of life the reflex ceases. Application of the appropriate stimulus no longer evokes the walking-like actions in the legs and 4 to 8 months may then elapse before the child can walk voluntarily. This certainly raises the question how something that disappears can be critical to development. The rather long time that passes between the disappearance of the reflex and the onset of the related voluntary movement has led researchers to question the role of the infant reflexes in the development of later voluntary movements.

The overwhelmingly prevalent view, however, is that the reflexes provide a form of practice that assists in the attainment of future movements. They evolve into voluntary patterns of movement and are necessary for initiating movement and the establishment of muscle tone, which is critical to the performance of future voluntary movements.

Research has been conducted to gain scientific insight into this controversy. In one study, infants whose stepping reflex was regularly stimulated began to walk at an earlier age than their nonstimulated counterparts (Zelazo, 1976). This research was undertaken with the assumption that if stimulation of the stepping reflex preceding the disappearance phase affects the rate of emergence of voluntary walking, there must be a link between the pre- and postdisappearance movements. Bower (1976) conducted a similar study in which infants were subjected to "intensive practice" in reaching movements during the involuntary phase of reaching behavior. As in the Zelazo study, Bower found that the predisappearance stimulation expedited the emergence of the postdisappearance voluntary movement. In fact, in some cases, those children who were given practice experienced no disappearance phase whatsoever (Bower, 1976). "Such results pointed to the possibility that the reason abilities disappear is that they are not exercised" (p. 40). More important, these results can be interpreted as demonstrating a link between the predisappearance involuntary reaching and grasping and the postdisappearance voluntary reaching and grasping movements.

Later, Zelazo, Zelazo, Cohen, and Zelazo (1993) examined the effects of practicing reflexes on 32 male infants 6 weeks of age. After only 7 weeks of practice, infants who received elicitation of the stepping reflex stepped more on their own than did a control group of infants who received no extra practice. The researchers speculated that this occurred as a result of several factors. The practice may facilitate the ability of the baby to initiate the stepping pattern, or it may indirectly facilitate the baby's equilibrium. Yet another explanation posited by the researchers was that the practice could have enhanced the baby's muscle strength. Regardless of the explanation, the researchers believed that demonstrating this practice effect is important because it will caution us to use care in interpreting established norms for motor achievement. Clearly, from this research, babies who are in homes where more practice occurs might not fall within expected ranges of development, rendering the charts somewhat fallible. In addition, this study determined that even small amounts of practice caused significant effects. This may contradict claims that early physical therapy will have only minimal effects on neuromotor development of children at this age (Zelazo et al., 1993).

This standardized method of examining reflexive movement presents an opportunity to observe children's motor patterns and the patterns' appropriateness for the children's age. The overall objective of the test is to develop a profile of a child's movement in relation to what is typically expected for children of a specific age. This examination is useful in monitoring motor function during routine checkups and is especially valuable for use with children suspected of a motor delay. The test is based on infant observation and is administratively efficient, taking approximately 10–15 minutes (Yildirim, Aydinli, Ekici, et al., 2012).

Although infant reflexes are often used in infant diagnosis, are generally associated with infant motor development, and typically disappear around the first birthday, research has shown them to reappear occasionally in adults. In a study of just under 500 adults ranging in age from 25 to 82 years, participants were initially tested neurologically and intellectually and then retested 3 and 6 years later. Some primitive reflexes (e.g., sucking, rooting) became more prominent with increasing age and with the onset of chronic neurological conditions such as Parkinson's disease. The researchers believed that the reappearance of these primitive reflexes may indicate how quickly the disease is progressing and how severely the patient is affected. As the disease runs its course and gradually increases its damage to the neural networks, reflexes are more likely to reappear. However, even in presumably healthy participants, 47 percent of men from 25 to 45 years of age exhibited one or more primitive reflexes. That number increased to 73 percent for men 65 to 85 years of age. For women, the numbers were slightly higher, with 51 percent and 75 percent, respectively, exhibiting at least one primitive reflex. These observations led the researchers to conclude that the presence or reappearance of some primitive reflexes increases with age in healthy individuals, though this should not be considered an indication of overall intellectual decline (van Boxtel, Bosma, Jolles, & Vreeling, 2006).

STEREOTYPIES

The infant reflexes are the most studied form of human movement during the first few months of life. Much less attention has been paid to another group of movements also characteristic of infancy. These movements, known as **stereotypies**, were studied more than a half century ago by Lourie (1949). In examining the rhythmic patterns of more than 100 typically developing children, Lourie established several hypotheses about their function. He believed that these somewhat unusual movements are inherent and crucial to the life of a healthy child, as he found increasing numbers of stereotypies in children who had delayed control over their movement. Among their purposes, Lourie posited, was to decrease tension and anxiety, as he noticed increasing amounts of stereotypies during periods of higher anxiety. The stereotypies seemed to calm the child. Lourie also believed that these movements provide stimulation for further development, offer considerable sensory stimulation, and may even serve as a bridge to eventual development of more advanced voluntary movement. Thus, Lourie encouraged these movements as beneficial to later development.

In later work by Thelen (1979), stereotypies were described as rhythmical, patterned (happen the same way each time), and seemingly centrally controlled movements. They are believed to be relatively intrinsic because they do not appear to be behaviors infants learn by imitation. In addition, these stereotyped movements do not seem to serve a purpose and are often invariant (Lewis, Gluck, Bodfish, et al., 1996; Sprague & Newell, 1996), as they are not regulated by the sensory system.

They generally include movements that are among the most simple, patterned actions for the muscle group involved. Stereotypies are often simple flexions, extensions, or rotations that are repeated in nearly identical, often alternating fashion.

Interestingly, this type of movement is common among insects, birds, and fish. Among primates, such as zoo animals, repetitive, patterned movements are often considered pathological. Even for the human being, during any other time of life such movement would be considered a sign of atypical development; indeed, such behavior is often seen in people with mental or emotional disorders (see below; secondary stereotypies). In the human infant, however, stereotypies are considered typical behavior that provide evidence of functional maturation of the neurological system. However, they are not a form of voluntary, goal-oriented movement behavior.

In her research, Thelen (1979) observed many different stereotypies. She found that all 20 infants she observed exhibited stereotypies. In fact, during the periods when stereotyping behavior was most common, the infants often spent as much as 40 percent of each hour exhibiting stereotypies.

Stereotypies of the legs and feet were among the most common and earliest forms of rhythmical and patterned behavior Thelen observed. Rhythmical kicking was the first noticed and was evident for months to follow. These stereotypies of the legs and feet most commonly occurred when the babies were prone or supine. Examples of the leg and feet stereotypies Thelen observed were simultaneous leg kicking, alternate leg kicking, feet rubbing together, single leg kicks of various kinds, and a sharp flexing of the backs of the legs. Stereotypies of the legs were the most common form of stereotyped movement Thelen noted. They also began earlier than the other types, as early as 4 weeks of age. These rhythmical, patterned movements of the legs and feet seemed to reach their peak occurrence at around 24 to 32 weeks of age, becoming much less common by 44 to 52 weeks (Thelen, 1979).

Thelen found that the legs and feet were not the only parts of the body to become involved in stereotyped movement. She categorized other stereotypies by their location of occurrence: several stereotypies occurred in the region of the hands and arms, including arm waving while holding an object, and one arm, as well as two arms, banging against a surface. Thelen also noted several patterned, repetitive hand movements, such as total hand flexion and rotation, as well as individual finger flexion. The peak occurrence for arm and hand stereotypies was 34 to 42 weeks. However, the arm stereotypies generally appeared as early as 4 to 12 weeks, whereas the hand movements typically were not evident until 14 to 22 weeks. The finger stereotypies, like the movements of the arms, occurred as early as 4 to 12 weeks but reached their peak at 24 to 32 weeks.

Thelen placed another group of stereotypies into what she termed the "torso" category. Included were such movements as arching the back and rocking when in an "all fours" or a creeping-like position, rocking and bouncing when in an unsupported sitting position, and bouncing while standing. In general, these movements first appeared as early as 14 to 22 weeks of age and often reached their peak later than the movements of the legs and feet and of the arms and hands (Thelen, 1979).

Thelen's final category of stereotyped movements of infancy was the head and face. This grouping included some of the most interesting stereotypies. Compared with other such movements, the stereotypies in this category were considered somewhat rare. Examples of head and face stereotypies were head nodding, head shaking as if indicating "no," in and out tongue protrusions, and nonnutritive sucking. Thelen (1979) also noted small rhythmical mouthing movements.

The most common stereotypies were the single leg kick, two-leg kick, alternate leg kick, arm wave, arm wave with an object, arm banging against a surface with and without an object, and finger flexion. Thelen concluded that these, as well as the other stereotyped forms of behavior she noted, are apparently developmentally significant. She reached this conclusion on noticing that, for example, stereotyped kicking precedes voluntary use of the legs and stereotyped finger flexion precedes voluntary attempts at grasping. However, stereotypies have not been absolutely determined to be precursors of more mature motor behavior (Thelen, 1979).

The number of different stereotypies increases throughout the first year. The frequency of occurrence also increases throughout the first year, peaking at approximately 24 to 42 weeks of age. Throughout the first year, many stereotypies cease and new ones emerge. During the last 2 to 3 months of the first year the occurrence of stereotypies exhibits a major decline (Thelen, 1979).

In a more recent examination of stereotypies, Temudo and Melo (2015) categorized stereotypies into a primary or secondary class. The **primary stereotypies** are most similar to what we have described so far and occur commonly as a part of typical development during infancy. They occur early in life and routinely disappear as a part of the typical developmental sequence. Secondary stereotypies are those experienced by children, or adults, with various atypical maladies like autism, sensory impairment, or neurodevelopmental disorders. These stereoptypies can be simple, according to these researchers, like tapping or clapping, or they can be complex where sequences of movements are linked and always performed in the same way and in the same order. **Secondary stereotypies** are more common when the individual is under stress, tired, or just plain bored. While the primary stereotypies will dissipate with typical development, the secondary type are more difficult to suppress and may impair more typical motor development if they persevere. Many theories have been derived to explain the secondary stereotypies with some experts believing they are learned behaviors that persist as a result of some form of ongoing reinforcement. Others believe that they may be a function of an immature neurological system and exist to modulate excess arousal (Temudo & Melo, 2015).

SUMMARY

- During the last 4 months in utero and the first 4 months of postnatal life, infant reflexes and stereotypies are the dominant form of human movement. An infant reflex is an involuntary and routine response to a particular stimulus.
- The infant reflexes are extremely important to human development for several reasons. Many of the reflexes are protective; the sucking reflex, for example, enables babies to ingest food. Other reflexes help the baby avoid injury.
- The infant reflexes are considered crucial for the development of subsequent voluntary movements. Reflexes such as crawling, labyrinthine, palmar grasp, and stepping are essential to the attainment of voluntary crawling, upright posture, voluntary grasping, and voluntary walking, respectively.
- Other infant reflexes are important as indicators of the child's neurological development and for diagnosing atypical development. The ages of onset and disappearance of the infant reflexes typically follow a predictable timeline. Deviations from that timeline sometimes indicate neurological damage. Also, an excessively weak, lacking, asymmetrical, or persistent

reflex can indicate a variety of neurological problems.

- Stereotypies are another form of movement observable during infancy. Primary stereotypies are patterned, stereotyped, highly intrinsic, and apparently involuntary movements of the legs and feet; arms, hands, and fingers; torso; and head and face. Like reflexes, these stereotypies are believed to be important in the development of more advanced voluntary movements in later life. They are typical and expected and dissipate as a part of the typical development sequence. Secondary stereoptypies are similar, but are common in individuals with various disabilities like autism. In this case, these repetitive movements that can be as simple as kicks or taps or more complex sequences of movements, can impede typical developmental progression and may not dissipate without appropriate therapeutic intervention.

key concept review

asymmetric tonic neck reflex
Babinski reflex
crawling reflex
head- and body-righting reflexes
labyrinthine reflex
lifespan reflexes
Moro reflex
palmar grasp reflex
palmar mandibular reflex
palmar mental reflex
parachuting reflexes
plantar grasp reflex
postural reflexes
primary stereotypy
primitive reflexes
pull-up reflex
search reflex
secondary stereotypy
startle reflex
stepping reflex
subcortical
sucking reflex
swimming reflex
symmetric tonic neck reflex

questions for reflection

1. What is a reflex? What is an infant reflex?
2. What is the difference between primitive and postural reflexes?
3. Is there any practical value in knowing and understanding the infant reflexes? Give three examples.
4. What are the characteristics of a primitive reflex? Give five examples of a primitive reflex and concisely explain each.
5. What are the differences between a startle and a Moro reflex?
6. Explain five different postural reflexes with emphasis on how each would be elicited.
7. How would one elicit the search reflex? Can you think of any reasons this reflex is important to human development?
8. What are the differences between the asymmetric and symmetric tonic neck reflexes?
9. What is a stereotypy? Is it different from an infant reflex, how? How is it similar to an infant reflex? Give five examples of stereotypies.
10. What are the differences between primary and secondary stereotypies?

REFERENCES

Ambesh, P., Paliwal, V.K., Shetty, V., & Kamholz, S. (2017). The Babinski sign: A comprehensive review. *Journal of the Neurological Sciences*, doi.org/10.1016/j.jns.2016.10.041.

Bower, T. G. R. (1976, November). Repetitive processes in child development. *Scientific American*, 38–47.

Brucknerova, I., Holomanova, A., Ujhazy, E., & Mach, M. (2012). Sixty year anniversary of the Apgar scoring system and 100 year anniversary of the "Moro" reflex. *Neuroendocrinology Letters, 33*, 729–731.

Bruijn, S. M., Massaad, F., MacLellan, M. J., Van Gestel, L., Ivanenko, Y. P., & Duyens, J. (2013). Are effects of symmetric and asymmetric tonic neck reflexes still visible in healthy adults? *Neuroscience Newsletter, 556*, 89–92.

Chinello. A., Di Gangi, V., & Valenza, E. (2018). Persistent primary reflexes affect motor acts: Potential implications for autism spectrum disorder. *Research in Developmental Disabilities*, doi.org/10.1016/j.ridd.2016.07.010.

Dionisis, J., Moraes, M., Tudella, E., Carvalho, W., & Krebs, V. (2015). Palmar grasp behavior in full-term newborns in the 1st 72 hours of life. *Physiology and Behavior*, *139*, 21–25.

Dreissen, Y. E. M., Bakker, M. J., Koelman, J. H. T. M., & Tijssen, A. J. (2012). Exaggerated startle reactions. *Clinical Neurophysiology*, *123*, 34–44.

Futagi, Y., & Suzuki, Y. (2010). Neural mechanisms and clinical significance of the plantar grasp. *Pediatric Neurology*, *43*, 81–86.

Futagi, Y., Toribe, Y., & Suzuki, Y. (2012). The grasp reflex and Moro reflex in infants: Hierarchy of primitive reflex responses. *International Journal of Pediatrics*. Retrieved from www.ncbi.nil.gov/pmc/articles/pmc3384944/.

Futagi, Y., Yanagihara, K., Mogami, Y., Ikeda, T., & Suzuki, Y. (2013). The Babkin reflex in infants: Clinical significance and neural mechanism. *Pediatric Neurology*, *49*, 149–155.

Gascon, G. (2012). Clinical approaches to infants, children, and adolescents with neurologic problems. In A. Y. Elzouki, H. A. Harfi, H. M. Nazer, E. B. Stapleton, W. Oh, & R. J. Whitley (Eds.), *Textbook of clinical pediatrics*. 2nd ed. New York: Springer.

Hamer, E.G., & Hadders-Algra, M. (2016). Prognostic significance of neurological signs in high-risk infants: A systematic review. *Developmental Medicine and Child Neurology*, doi.org/10.1111/dmcn.13051.

Harding, C., Frank, L., Dunga, C., & Colton, N. (2012). The use of nonnutritive sucking to facilitate oral feeding in a term infant: A single case study. *Journal of Pediatric Nursing*, *27*, 700–706.

Henrik, H. D. (2013). Sucking-pads and primitive sucking reflex. *Journal of Neonatal-Perinatal Medicine*, 6, 281–283.

Iiyama, M., Miyajima, T., & Hoshika, A. (2002). Developmental change of Moro reflex with a three-dimensional motion analysis system. *No to Hattatsu* [Brain and Development], *34*(4), 307–312.

Jaiswal, M., & Morankar, R. (2017). Understanding primitive reflexes and their role in growth and development: A review. *International Healthcare Research Journal*, doi: 10.26440/IHRJ/01_08/123.

Lacquaniti, F., Ivanenko, Y. P., & Zago, M. (2012). Development of human locomotion. *Current Opinion in Neurobiology*, *22*, 822–828.

Langendorfer, S.J. (2007). The developmental perspective, the swimming reflex, and the velveteen rabbit. *International Journal of Aquatic Research and Education*, *1*, 93–100.

Lewis, M. H., Gluck, J. P., Bodfish, J. W., Beauchamp, A. J., & Mailman, R. B. (1996). Neurobiological basis of stereotyped movement disorder. In R. L. Sprague & K. M. Newell (Eds.), *Stereotyped movements: Brain and behavior relationships* (pp. 37–67). Washington, DC: Hafner.

Lourie, R. S. (1949). The role of rhythmic patterns in childhood. *American Journal of Psychiatry*, *105*(9), 653–660.

Malina, R. M., Bouchard, C., & Bar-Or, O. (2004). *Growth, maturation, and physical activity*. 2nd ed. Champaign, IL: Human Kinetics.

Marques-de-Moraes, M. V., Dionisio, J., Tan, U., & Tudella, E. (2017). Palmar grasp reflex in human newborns. *Pediatrics and Therapeutics*, doi:10.4172/2161-0665.1000309.

McGraw, M. B. (1939). Swimming behavior of the human infant. *The Journal of Pediatrics*, doi.org/10.1016/S0022-3476(39)80003-8.

Ohlweiler, L., da Silva, A. R., & Rotta, N. T. (2002). Parachute and lateral propping reactions in preterm children. *Arquivos de Neuro-psiquiatria*, *60*(4), 964–966.

Okamoto, T., Okamoto, K., & Andrew, P. D. (2001). Electromyographic study of newborn stepping in neonates and young infants. *Electromyographic and Clinical Neurophysiology, 41*(5), 289–296.

Pauc, R. (2011). The Babinski sign in sickness and in health. *Clinical Chiropracice*, *14*, 122–126.

Rousseau, P. V., Matton, F., Lecuyer, R., & Lahaye, W. (2017). The Moro reaction: More than a reflex, a ritualized behavior of nonverbal communication. *Infant Behavior and Development*, 46, 169–177.

Saraga, M., Resic, B., Krnic, D., Jelavic, T., Krnic, D., Sinovcic, I., et al. (2007). A stereotypic "elbowing" movement: A possible new primitive reflex in newborns. *Pediatric Neurology*, *36*(2), 84–87.

Sheridan, M. (2014). *Mary Sheridan's from birth to five years: Children's developmental progress*. New York: Routledge.

Sohn, M., Ahn, Y., & Lee, S. (2011). Assessment of primitive reflexes in high-risk newborns. *Journal of Clinical Medicine Research*, *3*, 285–290.

Sprague, R. L., & Newell, K. M. (1996). *Stereotyped movements: Brain and behavior relationships*. Washington, DC: American Psychological Association.

Temudo, T., & Melo, C. (2015). Stereotypies: From normal to pathological. *Journal of Pediatric Neurology*, doi: 10.1055/s-0035-1559805.

Thelen, E. (1979). Rhythmical stereotypies in normal human infants. *Animal Behavior*, *27*, 699–715.

van Boxtel, M. P., Bosma, H., Jolles, J., & Vreeling, F. W. (2006). Prevalence of primitive reflexes and the relationship with cognitive change in healthy adults: A report from the Maastricht Aging Study. *Journal of Neurology*, *253*(7), 935–941.

Yildirim, Z. H., Aydinli, N., Ekici, B., Tatli, B., & Caliskan, M. (2012). Can Alberta infant motor scale and Milani Comparetti Motor Development Screening Test be rapid alternatives to Bayley Scales of Infant Development-II at high risk infants? *Annals of Indian Academy of Neurology*, *15*, 196–199.

Zelazo, N. A., Zelazo, P., Cohen, K. M., & Zelazo, P. D. (1993). Specificity of practice effects on elementary neuromotor patterns. *Developmental Psychology*, *29*(4), 686–691.

Zelazo, P. (1976). From reflexive to instrumental behavior. In L.P. Lipsitt (Ed.), *Developmental psychobiology: The significance of injury*. Hillsdale, NJ: Erlbaum.

10 VOLUNTARY MOVEMENTS OF INFANCY

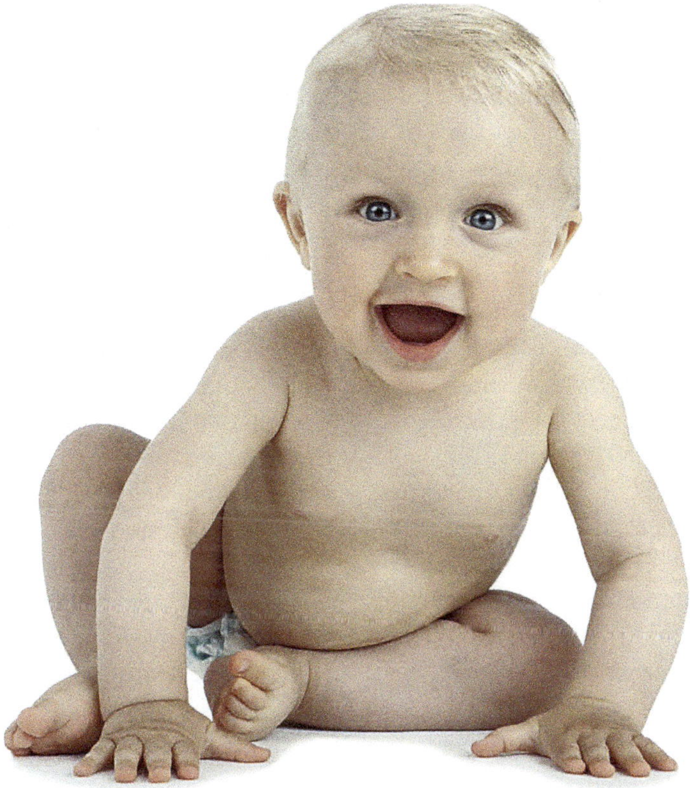

Chapter Objectives

From the information presented in this chapter, you will be able to

- List and categorize the voluntary movements of infancy
- Describe the development of head control during infancy
- Describe the development of general body control during infancy
- Describe the development of prone locomotion during infancy
- Describe the development of upright locomotion during infancy
- Describe the development of stair climbing
- Describe the development of reaching during infancy

As discussed in Chapter 9, reflexive movement is the first dominant form of human movement. The reflex is a unique form of movement that is involuntary and subcortical; it is performed without conscious effort and without stimulation from the higher brain centers. At about the fourth postnatal week, however, cortically controlled **voluntary movement** begins to appear. The first signs of voluntary movement are slight: movements of only the head, neck, and eyes. Nevertheless, after these first cortically controlled movements appear, the voluntary movements become increasingly prevalent and instrumental in enabling children to move in their environment. Cerebral cortical control slowly assumes command of movement production as the subcortically produced reflexes gradually disappear. The diameters of the nerve dendrites, which carry the electrical stimulation to induce movement, slowly increase, accelerating the velocity of the stimulation and, thus, more efficiently facilitating the motor nerve cell activity necessary for producing voluntary movement.

The disappearance of the early reflexes occurs as a result of the brain's cortex beginning to inhibit reflexes from the lower brain areas, such as the brain stem—a major behavioral event in a child's first year. The process of the higher brain center slowly assuming command is gradual, but by the end of the first year, there is almost complete voluntary control of movement (Bilbilaj, 2014). A few of the infant reflexes discussed in Chapter 9 may endure past the child's first year, but most disappear. Voluntary movement becomes the dominant form of human movement midway through that first year. These early voluntary movements are the first, slight beginnings of the more advanced movements that typically follow. Increasing scientific attention has been paid to these early voluntary movements and their relationship to the overall health and well-being of the child. These movements are integral to the child's development in many ways beyond motor development. They are influential in the child's full and healthy development motorically, but also perceptually, socially, and cognitively. Simple examples, that will be discussed in more detail later in the chapter, include the impact of achieving upright posture (e.g., sitting and standing) on expanding the child's visual repertoire or the influence of evolving locomotor skills (e.g., crawling and walking) on a child's ability to actively engage in social interactions (Libertus & Hauf, 2017).

The developmental sequences in these movements are not always orderly, as high degrees of individuality are common between one infant and another. Locomotion is an example; we often see a progression from some form of belly locomotion (such as crawling) to a more elevated crawling on all fours. Similarly, sitting is followed by standing and then cruising around furniture. Subsequently, with the appropriate experiences, instruction, and opportunities, a child learns to walk independently. However, we see wide variations in these common sequences. Some babies scoot on their bottom, rather than crawl; some prefer to roll to move from place to place; others skip belly crawling completely and move right to a more elevated form of crawling on the hands and knees. Many factors, such as experience, affect the sequence and age of acquisition of these behaviors. In fact, regarding when these behaviors will emerge, the child's level of experience may often be a better predictor than age (Adolph & Joh, 2007). Researchers have also sought to determine whether or not the rate of development for various voluntary movements of infancy have changed over the years. A study conducted in Canada, using Canadian norms derived from the Alberta Infant Motor Scale, compared scores from two decades earlier. This cross-sectional study involved over 600 infants, closely divided between males and females, averaging approximately 6 months of age. The onset of major gross motor milestones was found to be quite similar across the 20-year period, though the authors caution that the results of Canadian children may not be applicable to other cultures (Darrah, Bartlett, Maguire, Avison, & Lacaze-Masmonteil, 2014).

Clearly, many of these sequences of development appear somewhat predictably and sequentially as the voluntary movements of infancy progress into the more recognizable movement forms of later life. These progressions and the factors that affect them will be discussed throughout this chapter.

CATEGORIZING THE VOLUNTARY MOVEMENTS OF INFANCY

For ease of organization and discussion, the voluntary movements of infancy are often grouped into three major categories. Depending on the source, the terminology for the three categories varies somewhat. According to Gallahue and colleagues (2012), the three major categories of early voluntary movement are stability, locomotion, and manipulation. **Stability** includes a wide range of voluntary movements, from head control to the eventual attainment of upright posture. **Locomotion** includes such movements as creeping and crawling and all their variations.

Finally, **manipulation** involves the voluntary use of the hands, such as the entire progression of movements leading to the attainment of a mature reaching, grasping, and **releasing** ability. These and all the other important voluntary movements of infancy are discussed on the following pages, in the order of their appearance when possible. This pattern cannot be relied upon absolutely, however, because often the infant acquires more than one motor ability at the same time.

STABILITY MOVEMENTS

Head Control

Because the human being typically develops movement ability cephalocaudally, as discussed in Chapter 1, acquisition of the ability to make voluntary movements begins at the head and progresses down the body (Rachwani, Santamaria, Saavedra, & Woollacott, 2015). At birth, a baby has virtually no voluntary control over the head or neck, although reflexive movement may be evident, as in the head-righting reflex discussed in Chapter 9 (when the body is turned to one side or the other, the head rights itself with the shoulders). One of the first major milestones of motor development is the ability to raise the head while prone (see Figure 10.1). This is a particularly significant achievement given the large size of the baby's head relative to its body. It is also important because raising the head is critical to the development of other behaviors, such as visually scanning the environment and reaching and grasping for surrounding objects.

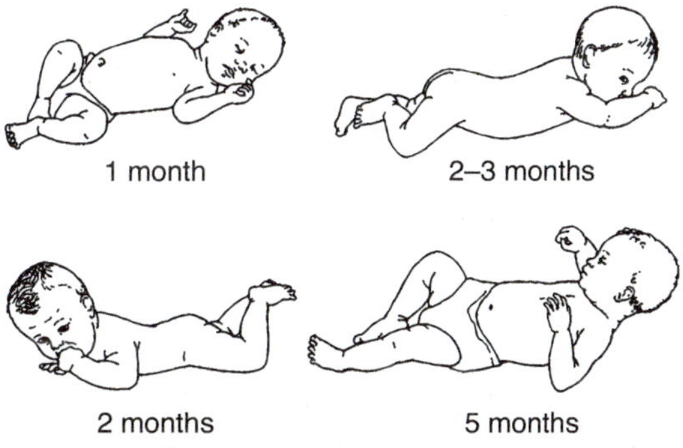

MONTHS	
1	Minimal voluntary control of the head
2	Elevates head when prone with effort
2–3	Positions head from left to right or right to left when prone
5	Elevates head when supine

Figure 10.1 Voluntary control of the head

Although some success at this movement may occur earlier, infants typically start to raise their head at 2 months of age (Figure 10.1). At 3 months, most will be able to extend their neck when they are prone. The achievement of this ability leads to the eventual raising of the chest by pushing up with the arms. At this same age, the infant is typically able to hold the head upright when in an upright position (e.g., standing, sitting). Approximately 2 months later, at 5 months of age, the baby will be able to raise the head when in a supine position (Figure 10.1; Piek, 2006). Thus, the complex process of attaining upright posture has begun.

Body Control

In the cephalocaudal pattern of development, control of the uppermost areas of the body follows attainment of head control. Then, gradually, lower areas of the body also gain voluntary control. This cephalocaudal progression in body control begins at about 2 to 3 months of age, when the child gains the ability to elevate the head along with a slight elevation of the chest. The infant executes this maneuver by applying pressure to the supporting surface with the upper arms. This does not indicate particularly useful control of the arms, however, because the forearms and hands play a minimal role in this effort. Later in this chapter we discuss the development of reaching behavior and, to some extent, grasping behavior; however, the grasp following the reach will be emphasized in Chapter 11, "Fine Motor Development." Control of the arms, hands, and fingers is more thoroughly discussed in that chapter.

Rolling

Gaining voluntary control of body movement is particularly important during the first few postnatal months because these early forms of movement are crucial for attaining more advanced movements. One of the most important forms of body control evident after chest elevation is the child's attempt to roll from a supine to a prone position. The acquisition of this movement skill at approximately 5 months enables the child to attain the proper position for more advanced forms of locomotion (e.g., crawling) (Kobayashi, Watanabe, & Taga, 2016). A form of rolling generally is noticeable earlier (i.e., body righting reflex), but that movement is reflexive, not voluntary.

Most studies indicate that infants can roll voluntarily from prone to supine (belly to back) prior to supine to prone and can perform these rolling actions initially without segmenting the body (head turning first, followed by the shoulders, trunk, and hips). Most studies indicate that the prone-to-supine action can be achieved by approximately 4 months of age and the supine-to-prone action soon thereafter, at approximately 5 months. In both cases a rotation of the trunk is incorporated to complete the rolling action approximately 1 month after the onset of the rolling behavior. Nelson, Yu, Wong, and colleagues (2004) report that considerable variations have been seen in rolling behaviors across cultures. They speculate that bulkier clothing used in some cultures slows the onset of rolling behaviors. How much the people in a given culture tend to carry their babies could also affect the onset of rolling behavior, as being carried would allow for less experience or practice of the activity (Nelson et al., 2004).

In a study of Japanese babies and their rolling behavior, Kobayashi and colleagues (2016) studied babies aged from 5 to 7 and 8 to 10 months. The younger group had just begun to roll (supine to prone), whereas the older group was more experienced. In this research, all babies started in the supine position (on their backs) and were encouraged to roll by their parents. Major differences that were observed between groups included greater use of the lower limbs and faster overall movements in the older infants. The younger group also rolled from a starting position with a wider base of support. The older group was more likely to initiate the roll from an unstable position as rolling is most efficiently initiated from an unstable position. The older infants also demonstrated greater overall control of body segments and were more likely to roll in both directions than the younger babies. These researchers also noted that over half of infants aged 5 to 6 months and almost all (i.e., 90 percent) of 9-month-olds have the ability to roll over.

Upright Posture

Another important voluntary movement that indicates children's constantly expanding repertoire of movement is the attainment of an upright posture (e.g., sitting and standing). Upright posture is important because it frees the hands for more selective reaching, grasping, and releasing (see Figure 10.2). While supine or prone, the child has limited use of the arms and hands. In fact, these body parts are often occupied with maintaining or changing the horizontal body position and, therefore, are unavailable for selective attempts to obtain or manipulate objects in the child's environment. In addition to positioning the baby for a number of subsequent movements, upright posture is critically important to perceptual, social, physical, and cognitive development. This is exemplified by sitting that is discussed in the next section.

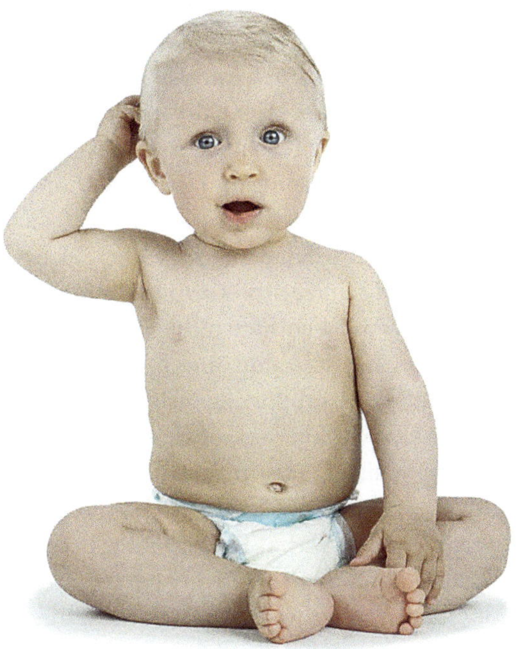

Figure 10.2 Ability to maintain upright posture frees the hands and arms for reaching and grasping

Sitting

Sitting is a major motor milestone. It frees the hands for exploration while placing the baby in a position for, literally, a broader visual view of the world. Babies who can sit independently have demonstrated greater manipulative skill, more advanced object exploration, improved perception, and longer-term effects like enhanced cognitive and academic ability (Karasik, Tamis-LeMonda, Adolph, & Bornstein, 2015).

Most of what has been learned about motor development, including sitting, has been gleaned from research on babies in western cultures. Experience is believed to be a primary predictor of a baby's ability to maintain posture while sitting. Experience is variable from one culture to another, and researchers have determined that babies from a number of cultures typically sit before babies in western cultures. Examples include babies from certain Caribbean and African countries. Approximately a fourth of babies from western cultures have been found to sit at 5 and a half months with almost all of them sitting by 7 months. By comparison, Ugandan infants typically sat by 4 months while 5 months was typical for babies from the West Indies. Japanese, Taiwanese, and Brazilian babies sat somewhat later than babies from the western cultures. Other research found that babies in the U.S., Oman, Norway, Ghana, and India averaged 5.9 for the onset age of independent sitting, but the range was substantial at just under 4 months to just over 9 months of age. These kinds of differences may be a function of cultural expectations. For example, in the U.S., mothers are often expected to stay close when their infants are sitting as a safeguard for falling, especially, if the baby is sitting in an elevated area. Other cultures are less strict in this area and allow babies the greater challenge of sitting independently and with less postural support. Thus, the babies of these less restrictive cultures were more generally proficient at sitting earlier than babies from cultures with more restrictive parental ideals (Karasik et al., 2015).

As mentioned earlier, learning to sit is instrumental to the attainment of an array of other movement abilities. Rochat (1992) conducted one of the most detailed studies of the impact of an infant's ability to "self-sit" on the development of early eye-hand coordination. Rochat's subjects were two groups of infants 5 to 8 months old. Half were able and half were unable to sit on their own. Each infant was presented with a variety of displays while in four different positions: seated, reclined, prone (75 degrees to the floor), and supine. Overall, the nonsitters contacted the objects in the display 89 percent of the time, and sitters made contact 98 percent of the time. All infants were found to have the least amount of success while in the supine position. Furthermore, the nonsitters exhibited significantly more two-handed reaches overall. However, when seated, the nonsitters' incidence of two-handed responses decreased, compared with other positions. Overall, the sitters tended to reach more with one hand in all positions, whereas the nonsitters tended to use one hand only when seated. Rochat believed these findings demonstrate the importance of self-sitting for early eye-hand coordination. Specifically, infants' ability to sit appears to be linked to the use of the hands in reaching activities.

In one of the first studies to examine the interaction of learning to sit and reaching behavior, Harbourne, Lobo, Karst, and Galloway (2013) studied infants from the time they began to sit with some degree of support until they sat independently (no arm support). The babies studied were initially between 4 and 5 months of age and were able to sit by supporting themselves by propping themselves with their own arms. The researchers determined that sitting emerges around 4 to 5 months of age once babies have developed the ability to control their head and have developed a reasonable degree of trunk support. Generally, over the next 3 to 4 months, babies transition to fully independent sitting. This occurs through three stages, according to these researchers. The first stage involves supporting oneself with the arms, followed by, in stage two, sitting with brief and intermittent support of the arms. The last stage is fully independent sitting with no need for arm support.

Sitting in general and especially stage three sitting have been strongly associated with the development of object manipulation. Sitting increases the baby's opportunities to locate objects visually, places the baby in a positive upright position for reaching, and frees the hands to enable reaching and manipulation of objects. In Harbourne and colleagues' (2013) study, successful reaching increased as sitting ability matured. In earlier stages of sitting, babies are often faced with a dilemma when presented with a desirable object (e.g., a toy): do they move the supporting arm and reach for it, thus risking falling over, or do they maintain their upright sitting posture and forgo the toy? In the initial stages of sitting, reaching may be constrained as infants at this age appear to understand that an attempted reach may result in toppling over. However, in this study, the researchers found that the infants were persistent in their reaching attempts, even when they knew they might topple over. Thus, these researchers contended that the relationship between sitting and reaching is reciprocal, especially once the infant has some experience in both skills. Then, independent sitting facilitates reaching and grasping behavior; the desire to reach also challenges, or perturbs, the efforts to sit independently. This, they said, creates a "complex dual sit-reach behavior that enhances the development of both skills while expanding the baby's overall interaction with the environment" (Harbourne et al., 2013, p. 438).

Standing

The progression in attaining upright posture does not end with sitting. One of the most commonly known movement landmarks is achieving complete upright posture, an unsupported standing position. This movement ability, like the others discussed earlier, is critical to future development. An upright posture enables children to walk; walking lets children expand their exploratory range and, therefore, facilitates cognitive, social, and motor development. The onset of the standing progression generally occurs at about 9 months, when children begin to exhibit the ability to pull themselves up from a sitting to a standing position. For the child to attain the standing position, an external object such as a piece of furniture is required for support (Atun-Einy, Berger, & Scher, 2012). Following a period of experimentation to "test" his or her balance, the child can stand beside furniture, occasionally reaching out for support. This standing position is characterized by a wide base of support and a "high guard" arm position. In other words, the feet generally are a considerable distance apart and the hands held high. By the age of 1 year, the child often can stand unassisted (see Figure 10.3) and, soon thereafter, even "cruise" around furniture, occasionally releasing touch support, maintaining balance, and continuing movement around the supporting object (Atun-Einy et al., 2012).

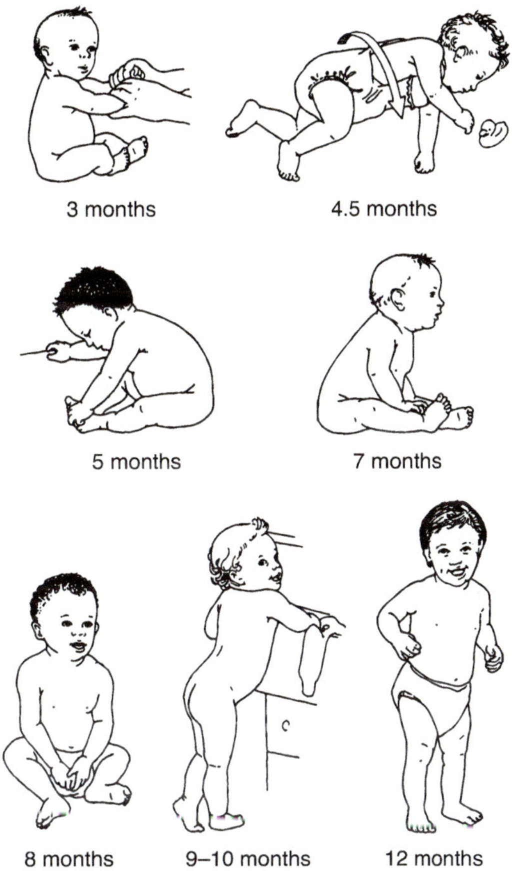

MONTHS	
3	Tries to roll from supine to prone position; maintains sitting position when assisted
4.5	Rolls from supine to prone position
5	Sits when holding external supporting object
7	Achieves sitting position from prone or supine position
8	Sits alone
9–10	Pulls self to standing position, briefly maintains stand while holding external supporting object
12	Stands unassisted

Figure 10.3 Voluntary control of the body

LOCOMOTION MOVEMENTS

Locomotion is moving the body from one point in space to another. Many believe it to be one of the greatest accomplishments of infancy.

Clearly, it is no simple task. It requires a fundamental ability to overcome gravitational forces. It also requires adjusting to the increasing demands of balance, as well as an awareness of the physical and motor requirements of propelling oneself through a changing environment, all while continually adjusting to the gradually changing dimensions of one's own body. Early forms of locomotion, such as crawling, are important individually but also contribute greatly to many other advances in human development. The development of crawling has been linked to improvements in cognitive ability, language and social development, and the growing ability to be self-directed and initiate many social and explorative activities that were previously impossible (Kretch, Franchak, & Adolph, 2014).

Prone Locomotion

As mentioned, the acquisition of body control during infancy facilitates the development of other movements. Locomotion evolves from children's gaining the ability to position their bodies for movement from one location in space to another. Initially, children position themselves pronely. From the onset of voluntary attainment of the prone position to the end of the child's first year, several transformations take place in a child's prone locomotion. Semblances of crawling occur prior to 7 months of age, but these movements are reflexive rather than voluntarily controlled. The next 6 months are the most important in voluntary locomotion; during this time the child becomes adept at movements in the prone position. This is a valuable movement acquisition because locomotion, even in the prone position, enables the child to explore the surrounding environment more thoroughly.

Like all the voluntary movements of infancy, locomotion develops in a somewhat predictable progression. However, although the progression generally is similar for all children, the rate at which these movement skills are acquired may vary considerably. The rate of acquisition for *all* voluntary movements during infancy may vary, but the differences among children for attaining prone locomotor movements are especially great.

Crawling and **creeping** are the two locomotion movements that have received the most attention among both the general populace and motor developmentalists. Unfortunately, a consensus does not exist as to the specific meanings of the two terms. To many parents and laypeople, creeping is a precrawling movement consisting of inefficient, highly variable arm and leg movements intended to propel the body forward. According to many contemporary references, however, that description is more accurate for crawling, where crawling actually precedes creeping in the progression of movement acquisition for prone locomotion (Piek, 2006). For our purposes, we will use the term *crawling* for the less mature of the two forms of locomotion, regardless of the popular use of the term.

Crawling

Crawling usually begins between approximately 7 and 8 months of age (this time may vary considerably, depending on the child and the environment). In the child's first attempts at locomotion, the trunk is minimally elevated off the supporting surface (see Figure 10.4). This movement is often termed belly crawling. The infant tries to travel by thrusting the arms forward and then subsequently flexing them. The flexion of the arms may eventually lead to a slight forward thrust. Initially the legs are minimally involved; eventually they play an extremely important role in the more advanced forms of prone locomotion. Soon after the initial attempts at forward progress, the child may flex a leg or both legs up to or under the body. This flexion may cause the body to move toward the rear

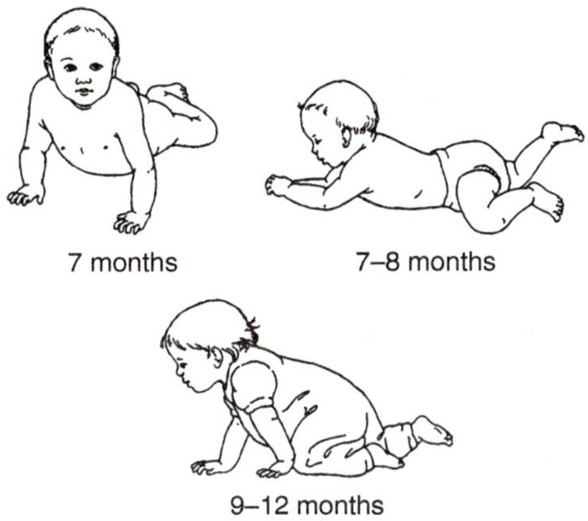

MONTHS	
7	Slightly elevated trunk; forward arm extension and flexion create occasional forward movement; leg flexion occasionally creates backward crawling
7–8	Initial crawling
9–12	Creeping; creeping up stairs

Figure 10.4 Prone locomotion

and produce a backward crawling. This somewhat counterproductive form of locomotion is temporary, however, because the child soon begins to use the legs more efficiently to help move forward. The child flexes the legs and then re-extends them for propulsion. This action may initially involve extending both legs simultaneously in a vigorous motion that causes the body to move forward in short and abrupt actions.

In a longitudinal study on the development of crawling (Adolph, Vereijken, & Denny, 1998), 28 babies were followed from their first attempt to crawl until they began to walk. The researchers focused specifically on how age, body dimensions, and experience affected crawling development. Major findings are summarized in Table 10.1. Generally, these researchers found that "each subsequent posture marked a small triumph over gravity in an orderly march toward erect locomotion" (p. 1299). Gradual, continuous improvement in both crawling proficiency and speed were

Table 10.1 Keys in learning to crawl

1.	"No strict progression of obligatory, discrete stages" (p. 1299) appears to exist in the development of prone locomotion.
2.	Multiple crawling postures are often exhibited in the development of crawling/creeping.
3.	Many babies crawl on their bellies prior to hands-and-knees crawling, but many skip belly crawling and proceed directly to hands and knees.
4.	The amount of experience that a child gains in early forms of crawling seems to predict the speed and efficiency of later forms of crawling/creeping.
5.	Babies who belly crawl are more proficient on their hands and knees than those who do not.
6.	The first form of mobility for many babies is often a bellydragging form of crawling.
7.	Smaller, slimmer, more naturally proportioned babies crawl earlier than do larger, chubbier babies.
8.	The last milestone preceding walking is always either hands-and-knees creeping or shifting from a prone position to sitting.

Source: Adolph, Vereijken, and Denny (1998).

noted as most babies, but not all, displayed "stages" on their way to walking. Some babies skipped a stage completely, and several were found to "straddle" stages. For example, nearly half of the babies skipped belly crawling altogether. Nevertheless, notable individual patterns in the developmental sequence included lifting the head and chest off the ground, pivoting in circles while on the belly, pulling forward with the abdomen dragging on the ground, hopping forward on the belly with the belly alternately on and off the ground, and rhythmical rocking on the hands and knees.

Although strict stages were not found to exist, a consistent trend was observed. For example, all babies studied demonstrated at least one "clumsy" precursor to prone progression before actually beginning hands-and-knees creeping. These "clumsy" attempts

CREEPING OR CRAWLING? WHICH COMES FIRST?

Most parents consider creeping to be the lower, less mature forerunner to crawling, but many experts reverse the terms. Regardless of the term used, the sequence of development stays the same, from an initial, inconsistent, somewhat inefficient, low form of locomotion to a more elevated, consistent, and highly efficient form of locomotion on all fours.

included movements such as pivoting and rocking. All in all, 25 unique combinations of body parts were used for propulsion and balance, with all involving both arms and at least one leg (Adolph et al., 1998).

Creeping

Gradually, the infant elevates the body from the supporting surface. As the elevation of the body increases, the legs can be flexed into a position beneath the body, increasing the infant's ability to locomote and leading to the more sophisticated movement form known as creeping. Crawling is a form of locomotion in which the body is, in a sense, dragged or "slid" along the supporting surface, whereas creeping is an elevated, highly efficient form of locomotion. In fact, many children who have learned to walk often revert to creeping when they have a desire to make speedy progress.

Once the body is elevated from the supporting surface, a variety of limb movements are evident in creeping. Initially, the child will move only one limb at a time, which is obviously an inefficient, slow form of beginning creeping that has yet to be perfected. Eventually, the child develops a **contralateral** or a **homolateral** creeping pattern. The homolateral pattern is characterized by the limbs on the same side simultaneously moving forward or backward; for example, as the right leg goes forward, so does the right arm. Most children creep contralaterally; that is, the movements of the limbs oppose each other. For example, as the right leg moves forward, the right arm moves back. Rather than the arm and leg on the same side moving simultaneously, the arm and leg on opposite body sides work together.

An efficient form of creeping, contralateral or homolateral, may begin to appear as early as 9 months of age. However, most children do not creep efficiently until their second year. Once children begin to creep, they rapidly become so efficient that they can creep up stairs. This form of creeping is almost identical to creeping on a flat surface but initially may cause frustration because most likely the child will be unable to descend the stairs.

Upright Locomotion

Many experts consider upright locomotion, which includes walking, the culmination of the infant's acquisition of a series of voluntary movements. Learning to walk is a lengthy and complicated process and requires many months to achieve a relatively functional and adaptable form. Like other movements discussed in this chapter, it is also paramount to other apsects of motor development in addition to being complementary to cognitive, social, perceptual, and physical development (Looper & Chandler, 2013).

Walking

Of obvious importance, walking is the result of the progression of movement skills described to this point. Like crawling, walking is important in itself while being influential in the many other important developmental processes. For example, the onset of walking, as we indicated in Chapter 2, has been strongly associated with language development (Walle & Campos, 2014).

Although there is no question of the value of upright locomotion, many parents place too much significance on the age at which their offspring start walking. The acquisition of any skill—motor, cognitive, or social—is enough to excite many parents, but they often place extreme emphasis on the age of acquisition of unassisted walking. Contrary to the belief of many parents, there is little evidence that early walking accelerates or refines skill performance later in life.

Before a child walks unassisted, a predictable movement progression generally occurs. If assisted with considerable support, a child can walk as early as 7 months of age, although this varies considerably (Piek, 2006).

In fact, children occasionally walk independently at 8 months of age, but this is rare. At approximately 10 months, a child can walk with much less support. Generally, by this time a strong handhold is enough to enable the child to "cruise" laterally around furniture or other supporting objects. By 11 months, children have typically progressed to a level of proficiency enabling them to walk when led by another person. Finally, by approximately one year of age or slightly after, the child typically walks unassisted, though, again, considerable variability exists among children (Merens, 2015). See Figure 10.5.

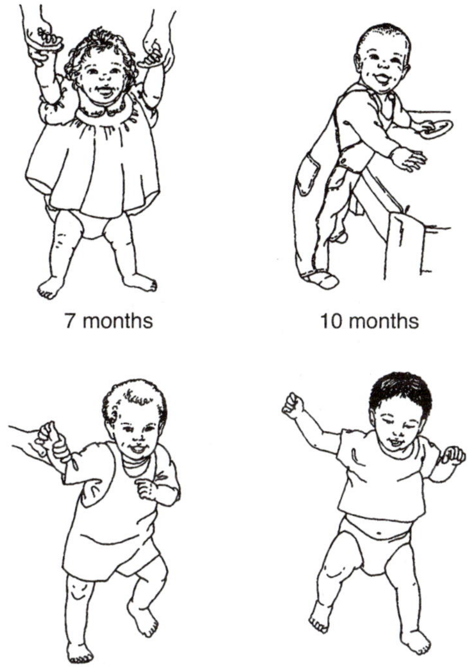

MONTHS	
7	Walks with considerable support or assistance
10	Walks laterally around furniture using handhold for support
11	Walks when led with slight handhold to maintain balance
12	Walks unassisted

Figure 10.5 Upright locomotion

Regardless of when a child begins to walk independently, the initial upright locomotion is far from a mature walking pattern. Each step in the progression to a mature walking pattern is characterized by many immature walking techniques. For example, the infant often assumes a wide stance. The knees maintain a flexed position, and the toes point out slightly. The length of the steps is highly inconsistent. (The more advanced forms of walking are discussed in Chapter 12.)

Bisi and Stagni (2015) studied 20 infants over a 6-month period aged from 10 to 16 months. Regardless of the infant's age, these researchers found that after approximately two months of walking independently a developmental shift or trend occurs. This shift, that the researchers attributed to improved postural control, was characterized by faster walking as a result of longer, rather than faster, steps. They also found that stride time was shorter for the first two months of walking, but increased for the next four months. The stride rate, or cadence, was also found to increase for the first two months, but slowed for the duration of the six months of observation. Throughout the six months, stride and step rate were found to be highly variable and not indicative of any particular trend (Bisi &

Stagni, 2015). Looper and Chandler (2013) conducted a similar investigation of young walkers. They found that these infants, at first, spent substantial time in the double support phase of walking (e.g., when both feet are in contact with the ground) to assist with balance. However, this decreases considerably by five months of walking as they gain greater ability to maintain the trunk and head in an upright position. This enables them to take longer strides whereas walking speed was increased in the younger walkers by taking faster, not longer, strides. Looper and Chandler (2013) indicated that the first several months are notable for the rapid change in walking characteristics as toddlers learn to control their posture and are more capable of controlling their balance and avoiding a fall.

In another study, Adolph, Cole, Komati, and colleagues (2012) observed 12- to 19-month-old children and found that infant walking generally occurs during exploration or interaction with a caregiver. It is rarely continuous as young walkers frequently increase their speed, then slow, and then perhaps speed up again. Their walking involves swerving and frequent falls. With practice and age, older infants begin to walk faster, go farther, and take longer, narrower strides. They also fall less frequently. These researchers believed that infants are motivated to walk because it delivers them to their destination faster than other methods of locomotion. They further believed that infants master walking by "accumulating massive amounts of practice" (Adolph et al., 2012, p. 1393). For the 12- to 19-month-old infants in this study, practice included well over 2,000 steps per day and an average of 17 falls per hour.

Interestingly, Theveniau and colleagues (2014) examined the effect of a baby's clothing on walking development. They compared healthy babies divided into three clothing groups: (1) a diaper with trousers; (2) a diaper with tracksuit pants (more stretchy than regular pants); and (3) a diaper with underwear. Overall, the walking speed and length of steps increased as all babies gained experience. During that same period the step width decreased for all. Walking with the trousers slowed the walk and decreased the length of the step compared to the underwear condition which was attributed to the trousers being somewhat stiff and restrictive. The tracksuit condition also reduced the step length compared to the diaper condition. Thus, the longer pants seem to have the greater effect on walking characteristics of young walkers especially for those who had been walking for more that six months. The researchers concluded that the stiffness and cut of clothing do impact walking development and can lead to a less mature form of walking in young toddlers (Theveniau, Boisgontier, Varieras, & Olivier, 2014).

Stair Climbing

Despite the common presence of stairs in American homes, very little research has been conducted over the years to examine **stair climbing** by infants and young children and the typical sequence of development in this important form of locomotion. In the first "comprehensive examination" (p. 37) of infants' stair climbing, Berger, Theuring, and Adolph (2007) sought to describe the progressions for ascending and descending stairs, as well as provide insight into the strategies infants use. Toward this end, the researchers interviewed parents regarding their children's stair-climbing development. The average age of their infant children was just over 1 year (12.53 months).

The youngest group of infants, ranging in age from 8 to 9 months, did not ascend or descend the stairs. At 13 months, most could ascend and nearly half were able to descend (see Figure 10.6). Nearly 90 percent of the infants learned to descend after learning to ascend the stairs; 12 percent learned to do both on the same day.

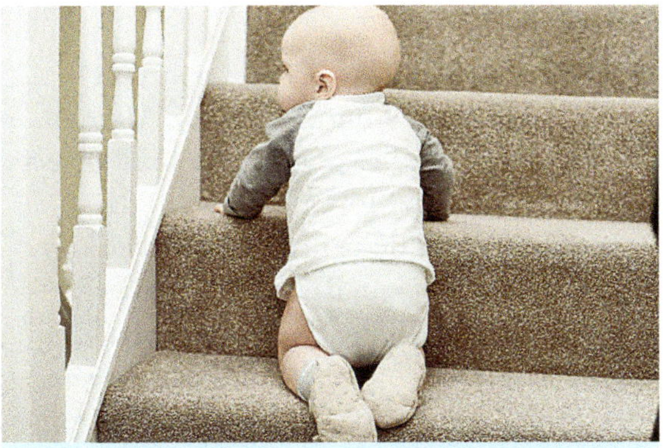

Figure 10.6 By just over 1 year of age, most children are able to ascend stairs, usually by crawling on their hands and knees or, sometimes, on the hands and feet

In addition, most of the infants were able to crawl and cruise before they could ascend stairs without assistance, though they could ascend the stairs prior to being able to walk independently. Almost all of the infants first approached their ascent up the stairs by crawling, using their hands and knees or, in some cases, their hands and feet. A very small number, 6 percent, first attempted the ascent by walking up, with most using a handhold for support. Coming down the stairs, the infants used many more variations in strategies. Over 75 percent of the infants crawled down with the feet leading; some slid down the stairs feet first. Somewhat surprisingly, nearly 10 percent walked down while grasping a handhold, such as a banister, and approximately 13 percent scooted down the stairs in a seated position. A few, approximately 2 percent, crawled or slid down the stairs on their belly with the face leading (Berger et al., 2007).

The technique employed for the descent appeared to be affected by the infant's age at the time. Younger infants more commonly crawled, rather than walked, down stairs. Interestingly, the youngest participants, who were approximately 11 months of age, attempted the descent by crawling down with the face leading. Those who led with the feet were as much as a month older than the face-first descenders. Yet, even older groups (approximately 13.5 months) tended to scoot down on their bottoms, or they walked down by using a handhold (over 14 months). Nearly 90 percent of the infants who could walk crawled up the stairs during their first ascent; being able to walk appeared to affect their strategy for descending, as well. Those who had the least walking experience were most likely to crawl down face-first, whereas those who had greater experience walking were more likely to opt for scooting down on their rear end or walking down with a handhold. The authors found no significant differences between the girls and the boys in the age of stair ascending or descending milestones. In general, most of the infants were able to ascend the stairs a few months after they learned to crawl and a few weeks before they could descend (Berger et al., 2007).

Children who had greater access to stairs were found to crawl or walk up stairs earlier than those who did not. However, having stairs in the home did not seem to affect the age of ascent for those who ascended on their belly, and it did not affect the age of descent. The authors concluded that parents can facilitate their children's stair climbing through instruction and offering experiences on stairs. Berger and colleagues stated that they consider stair climbing to be an excellent example of how numerous factors come together in children's attainment of motor milestones. In this case, factors include the child's physical and cognitive ability, parental support in terms of providing opportunities and instruction, and the presence of stairs in the home (Berger et al., 2007).

MANIPULATION MOVEMENTS

Parents and others are familiar with many of the voluntary movements of infancy discussed so far. The child's first successful and unsupported stand is frequently a highlight of infancy that parents eagerly anticipate. Creeping, and especially walking, are similarly awaited. But early voluntary use of the hands generally is not anticipated as much as other voluntary infant movements. Parents readily cite the date of the child's first unassisted walk, but generally they are much less aware of the baby's initial attempts to reach, grasp, and manipulate nearby objects, even though these are extremely important aspects of the child's motor development. Use of the hands enables children to gather information about their environment in a new way (see Figure 10.7). Manipulation enables increased and more varied exploration; this new mode of exploration lets the child discover properties of objects and use the objects as implements in achieving goals.

As explained in Chapter 9, the child's first forms of manipulation are reflexive. The palmar grasp reflex is not intentional manipulation, but it does give the child an involuntary means of grasping an object during the first few postnatal months. Although reaching and grasping are virtually inseparable, for the purposes of organization, we will emphasize reaching in this chapter and grasping in Chapter 11, where we discuss fine motor development.

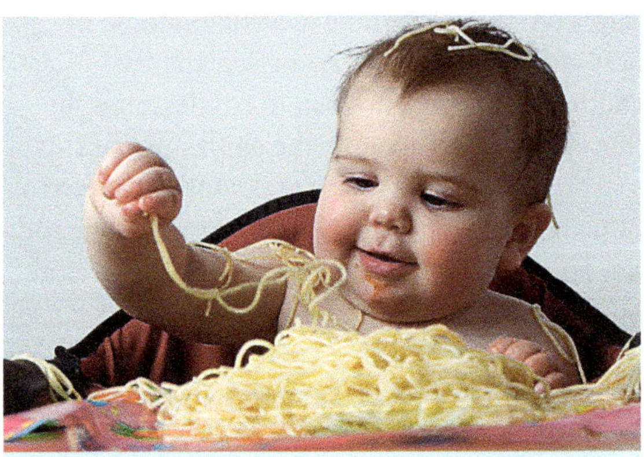

Figure 10.7 Use of the hands enables infants to learn about their world in new and different ways

Reaching

Reaching is another incredibly important motor skill acquired during infancy. After all, the reach is integral to attaining desired objects in our environment. It is a movement that, throughout life, is done many times each day (Rouse, Mazurek, Liu, Rivlis, & Schieber, 2019). Ultimately, it enables us to feed and groom ourselves, communicate, write, create art projects, and perform more advanced movement related activities, games, and sports. It is among the first functional movements to be acquired and evolves through a series of complex developmental steps that often vary considerably from one child to the next. A child's attainment of adequate reaching ability can be predictive of future motor and cognitive disorders (Karl, Sacrey, & Whishaw, 2019). While reaching is often a key part of a reach, grasp, and withdraw series of movements, in this section the main focus will be on reaching with grasping being given greater emphasis in Chapter 11 where the focus is specifically on fine motor acquisition.

Reaching starts before the baby is born, with signs of reaching the hand to the face and withdrawing the arm as early as three months of gestation. At just under five months of gestation babies have been seen placing their thumbs in their mouths, and newborns spend significant time exploring their face (usually the mouth) with their hands. Even at such a young age, reaching accuracy is found to improve with maturity. Reaching can consume as much as 20 percent of the baby's time while awake. They spend a great deal of time performing "movement babbling" with the arms. This involves arm movements that appear to be haphazard and unintentional, though they may be essential to exploring and learning the extent of one's reaching and manual capabilities (Karl et al., 2019).

As learned in Chapter 9 about infant reflexes, many of these early arm movements may be involuntary, though they will become increasingly voluntary (under cortical control) with time. Throughout the first few months of life many reaches to nearby objects and self-touches can be observed. The self-touches are believed to be critical in increasing self and body awareness. Through these self-touches babies develop an increased awareness and understanding of qualities like shape and texture in addition to learning the bodies' capabilities and limitations. Across the initial five months of life the self-touches evolve. Initially, they are propelled by the shoulder with little flexion in the elbow and a closed hand. The reach is still stiff and somewhat uncontrolled, and corrective movements of the arm can be observed. Gradually, the trunk begins to participate in the motion as more elbow flexion and finger extension are experienced. As early as 2 months of age the baby can be seen making more fingertip and palm contacts with the body parts like the feet, legs, and torso. Nevertheless, successful acquisition of the target object is rare until around 6 months of age when the reach becomes more coordinated with other parts of the body. At approximately 3 to 4 months of age, reaches are mainly just extended to touch, but do not really attain the target object. In fact, even making contact may be accidental. A bit later, somewhere between 4 and 6 months, the infant can effectively reach, grasp, and withdraw, but it is still quite immature. From 4 to 8 months, researchers believe that infants learn to rely on their own somatosensory (related to senses like pain, pressure, or cold rather than specific senses like vision) feedback to help accurately direct the reach, grasp, and withdrawal. Thus, they use haptic perception more than their own vision to direct the reach and grasp. Haptic perception, as we discuss in more detail in Chapter 11, is using the hands to hold and explore objects to learn about object characteristics like texture, size, shape, and weight. By 8 months, and into the 9th month of life, babies use their own sense of vision to facilitate the accuracy of their reach, knowing when to open and close their hand prior to touching the target object and even to assist in the withdrawal of the arm (Karl et al., 2019).

Corbetta, Wiener, and Thurman (2019) have also expored reaching in infancy. As suggested above, these researchers claim that the role of vision becomes increasingly important as the baby matures. At birth, however, visual acuity is lacking, though by the end of the first year of life it generally reaches adult levels and continues to evolve through 12 or 13 months of life. According to Corbetta and colleagues, stereopsis is also critical to reaching success. Stereopsis involves the alignment of the eyes and their ability to focus on the same point in space and integrate the two views into one. Clearly, stereopsis affects depth perception. This phenomenon typically evolves around 3 months of age and its full function is often demonstrated by the baby focusing for longer periods on nearby objects and more general arm activity (Corbetta et al., 2019).

According to Adolph and Robinson (2015), "goal-directed" reaching generally appears from 3 to 6 months of age. The wide range of ages for the onset of intentional reaching, they say, is a function of the complexity and difficulty in this task. The reach is characterized by reductions, with maturity, in variability between babies as well as more consistency in each reach. Upon initial attempts, infants attempt to simplify the movement by fixing the elbow joint, making the movement more of a gross, often jerky, whole arm movement with highly variable speed. Soon thereafter, the elbow flexion and extension are evident, enhancing the accuracy of the movement. Over the first couple of years of life the reach gradually appears more mature (i.e., adult-like) as it gets smoother and more consistent (e.g., fewer changes in direction). Adolph and Robinson indicate that, eventually, two more mature phases ensue. The first is characterized by a faster acceleration of the hand to the target. The second generates a slower progression toward the object, allowing for adjustments in the actual grasp immediately before contact with the object (Adolph & Robinson, 2015). Like Adolph and Robinson (2015), Corbetta et al. (2019) see the development of reaching as a two-phase process. **Phase I** lasts from approximately 3 to 5 to 7 to 8 months. According to these researchers, it is a transport phase where reaching ability improves by adjusting the speed of the reach in various reaching situations. It is also characterized by exploratory swipes at objects and considerable trial and error. With maturity, both the reach and the grasp are gradually adjusted based on the physical characteristics of the target object. Initially, this is all done with stationary objects, though within a few weeks babies may attempt to intercept moving objects as well. At first, in this phase, contacts with the target object may be unsuccessful. If contact is made, it is with varying parts of the hand with no actual grasp. Within a few weeks, however, most infants will be able to fully grasp the target object. Their perception as to which objects are within reach also improves. The reach, in general, is greatly facilitated at this time by the acquisition of the ability to self-sit. Once they can control the upright posture, the trajectory and range of the reach can be expanded and improved (Corbetta et al., 2019).

Phase II, as proposed by Corbetta and colleagues, occurs at approximately 7 to 8 months of age. In this phase the infant shows signs of having a pre-plan for the reach and grasp as the process becomes a means to achieve a goal, rather than being a goal in itself. This is demonstrated by the infant showing signs of greater haptic awareness of the object and uses this information to adjust the reach and grasp (Figure 10.8). For example, decisions may be made to use two hands rather than one based on the size or perceived weight of the object, or the hand may open wider based on the perceived larger size of the object (Corbetta et al., 2019). See Table 10.2.

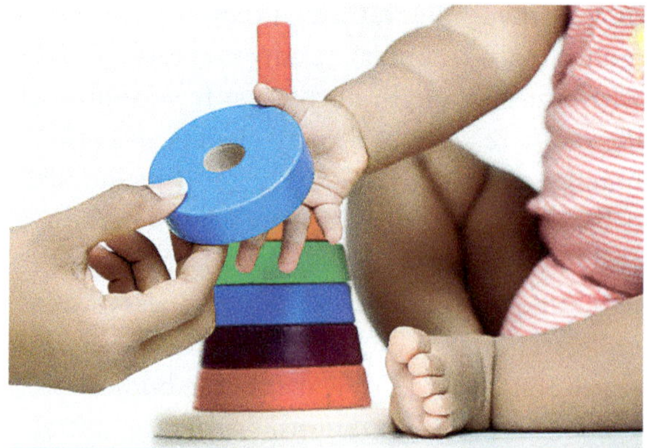

Figure 10.8 As the role of vision in infancy increases in importance for the reach, it begins to diminish in importance for the grasp

Bimanual Control

Many cognitive and psychomotor skills are necessary for optimal manual control. So far we have dealt predominantly with one-handed reaching. However, in many practical instances, movement of both of the arms and hands must be integrated.

Atun-Einy, Berger, Ducz, and Scher (2014) examined the development of two-handed, or bimanual, reaching. These researchers agreed that purposeful reaching starts around 4 months but lacks clear control at that time. It is often characterized by more flailing than directed reaching and is typified by numerous corrective actions. Interestingly, it is also frequently characterized by the use of the two hands together, rather than just one. This may be a limiting factor, because most infants cannot yet sit or stand independently in a position that leaves both hands free. Thus, they need external support to perform the two-handed reach or are limited to reaching when

Table 10.2 Approximate ages of occurrence and highlights of reaching behavior

Age	Characteristics
3 months of gestation	Reaching to hand/face
5 months of gestation	Placing thumb in mouth
At birth	Exploring face/mouth and movement babbling
1st few months	Attempted reaching to nearby objects/self-touching
3 months	Functional stereopsis
3–4 months	Reaching to touch, not obtain
4–6 months	Effective reaching, but still immature technique
4–8 months	Using somatosensory/haptic perception to direct reach and grasp
6 months	More successful attainment of target object
3–5 to 7–8 months	Phase I – transport phase, exploration, trial and error, grasp and speed adjusted for object, upright sitting
7–8 months	Phase II – pre-planning, greater haptic awareness, initial interception of moving objects

lying supine. One-handed reaching becomes dominant a month or two later when babies begin to differentiate between larger and smaller objects. When they perceive a larger object, they will employ two hands in their reach; they will use one hand for smaller objects. At around 7 months of age the reach pattern becomes much less variable, with infants demonstrating an ability to adapt their reach to the requirements of the situation. By this time, most infants have achieved the ability to sit independently, which enhances their opportunities to reach, as the hands are freed to operate in front of the body.

At around 1 year of age, when upright and independent locomotion begins to emerge, the babies in this study switched back to the use of bimanual reaching. This increased use of both hands for reaching was not seen when the babies could only pull themselves to a stand alongside a piece of furniture, for example. However, as soon as a baby could locomote, or cruise, around the furniture with touch support, bimanual reaching began to re-emerge (Atun-Einy et al., 2014).

In classic research on bimanual reaching, Jerome Bruner (1970) examined several specific manipulative circumstances, including complementary use of the hands. In examining the progression of reaching and grasping behavior, Bruner specifically investigated infants' control of several objects simultaneously. Subjects who were 4 to 17 months old were handed one toy and then, immediately, a second toy. The second toy was handed to the side of the child's body that was already occupied by the first toy. If the infant did not take the second toy within 15 to 20 seconds, the toy was moved to the infant's midline. If the child took the toy at any time, he or she was handed a third and possibly a fourth toy.

The 4- to 5-month-old infants in this research exhibited varying abilities. Some could not receive any of the toys; others could receive the toys but were unable to maintain control thereafter. None of the subjects in this youngest of the age groups could deal with more than one toy at a time.

The 6- to 8-month-old subjects displayed a more developed ability. They easily received the first toy and generally received a second. To facilitate this process, they transferred the first toy to the opposite hand for storage while receiving the second toy on the side to which it was offered. To manage three objects, however, appeared to be beyond the ability of the infants in this group.

The 9- to 11-month-old group exhibited another new skill. Most subjects at this age could receive three objects, although this task was troublesome initially. To manipulate three objects, the children frequently positioned the initial toy(s) in their lap or on a nearby chair to free one hand for receiving the next toy. By 12 months of age, the infants often handed the initial toys to an experimenter or a nearby parent for safekeeping. By this age, Bruner noted, subjects could cross the midline in handing the toys to a nearby person, a skill usually not exhibited in younger age groups. In addition, children in the two oldest age groups, the 12- to 14-month-olds and the 15- to 17-month-olds, could all handle three or more objects successfully. However, the oldest subjects consistently used a storage method, whereas the 12- to 14-month-old group used a variety of techniques. Even among these two groups of older subjects, the children stored the toys on their lap or on the chair or handed them to a nearby person rather than storing them in the other hand. An important point in this research was that infants as young as 6 to 8 months showed complementary use of the two hands to achieve a purposeful goal, storing a toy in one hand to free the receiving hand for a second toy.

Bruner performed additional research to examine bimanual control more specifically. In this research, a child was presented with a box with a toy visible inside. To obtain the toy, the child had to slide open a wooden lid, keep the lid open, and grasp and withdraw the toy with the other hand. For this research, Bruner used the same subjects who were studied in the previous investigation, with the exception of the 4- to 5-month-old group. Bruner found that although the younger children succeeded in this endeavor only approximately 20 percent of the time, the older children did so 90 percent of the time. A common progression was noted. Younger subjects often simply struck the box. A second strategy, also unsatisfactory, was closing the door immediately after opening it. These children then used a successful but still single-handed approach: they opened and released the lid to free the hand for grabbing the toy. Once the lid was released, the children slowly slipped their hand into the box to obtain the toy. This technique was commonly used by the subjects in the 12- to 14-month-old group and occasionally by older subjects. In approximately 16–17 percent of all trials, the subjects in the 12- to 14-month-old group used both hands. However, Bruner describes these movements as inefficient and characterized by poor timing.

The complementary use of two hands increased in the two older age groups. In fact, these children used two hands over 30 percent of the time. Bruner concluded from this research that the bimanual control necessary for success in this task, although well structured and differentiated by 18 months of age, still could not be considered mastered.

Relationship of Reaching and Postural Control and Their Role in Child Development

Atun-Einy and colleagues (2014) examined two-handed, or bimanual, reaching and its relationship to the development of upright locomotion, such as cruising or walking. As stated previously, these researchers found that when upright and independent locomotion began to emerge at around 1 year of age, the babies in their study reverted to a more common use of bimanual reaching. The researchers noted that the abilities to attain and maintain upright posture and to walk seemed to be linked to the expanded use of two hands.

As this research indicates, a strong relationship appears to exist between reaching behavior and upright posture, whether sitting or standing. Soska and Adolph (2014) examined this relationship and found that improved postural control did assist in reaching and, therefore, grasping, releasing, and even general exploration and learning. Visually guiding the arm, they found, requires a stable trunk. Once initial truncal support is gained, reaching evolves from two-handed reaching (as seen in Atun-Einy and colleagues' 2014 study) to a more common use of one hand, where accuracy in the reach becomes more necessary. In short, these researchers concluded that postural control is a vital element and facilitator of significant changes in human development; it enhances exploration, learning in general, and social interaction as infants develop more ways to engage with objects and people in their environment.

In similar work, Rachwani and his research team (2015) found infants to have much less stability when provided with pelvic (hip region) versus thoracic (trunk region) support. Thus, reaching was found to be more direct, smoother, and more efficient when babies were provided with thoracic support, rather than pelvic support, when reaching. This, according to the researchers, indicated a very strong correlation between reaching behavior and postural control. In fact, the researchers considered these to be "inter-related milestones" (p. 1).

In addition, like Soska and Adolph, these researchers believed that postural support and reaching are critical to the development of a number of advancing perceptual, intellectual, and social skills. Of course, these authors are quick to remind us that many factors affect the reach, including visual perception, neuromuscular factors, biomechanical factors (e.g., arm length, weight), and proprioceptive or haptic information received via the body or the target object. Neck stability, for example, generally enables a 4-month-old to reach fairly accurately as a stable head enables accurate vision of the target object. Successful reaching, in many ways, requires "whole body engagement" (p. 2) as the arms, the support of the trunk and head, and the vision are just a few examples of the bodily elements that must work together to produce a successful reach (Rachwani et al., 2015).

SUMMARY

- By the end of the first few postnatal months, infant reflexes have begun to be replaced by cortically controlled voluntary movements. These voluntary movements develop in a fairly predictable sequence, although the rate of acquisition of the movement skills may vary considerably from child to child.
- Voluntary movement follows a cephalocaudal pattern of development: the head is the first body part to come under voluntary control. This is an important movement acquisition because it enhances the child's ability to scan the environment visually.
- Body control is gained soon after control of the head. The child gains control of the upper body first, with lower portions gradually acquiring voluntary movement. Control of the body enables the child to position appropriately for the eventual acquisition of locomotion and to position the body in such a way as to free the hands for reaching and grasping.
- Locomotion is an important contributor to the child's cognitive development because it permits the experience of many new environments. Initial crawling is slow, inefficient, awkward, and characterized by an extremely low to the ground prone position. Soon the child develops a more elevated and efficient form of locomotion known as creeping.
- Independent walking is preceded by several assisted forms of upright locomotion. Cruising laterally around furniture, while maintaining a handhold for balance, and assisted walking are both significant forms of locomotion because they contribute to the

emergence of independent walking and, later, running in the locomotor progression.

- When climbing stairs, infants younger than 1 year may not be able to ascend stairs at all, whereas those at 13 months and older often ascend and descend, usually learning to ascend prior to descending. Infants do not necessarily need to be walking to ascend stairs. Most infants learn to locomote in a prone position, and most initially ascend in a prone position, though a small number make their first attempt in an upright position with a handhold. When descending, infants of less than 1 year of age tend to crawl down, often face-first, while older infants often attempt the descent by scooting on their bottom or walking with a handhold. Access to stairs and parental instruction can facilitate this behavior, according to Berger et al. (2007).
- According to recent research, reaching behavior emerges in two phases. Phase I is characterized by exploration, trial and error reaching, and gradual adjustments of the speed of the reach. Phase II involves more pre-planning, greater haptic awareness and the initial interception of moving objects. Increasing control of the arms and hands is particularly important for children because it allows increased manual exploration and facilitates daily routine activities. Upright posture and locomotion facilitate the emergence of reaching abilities. Upright positioning frees the hands for more frequent use; locomotion enables the child to move to objects of interest to manipulate them.

key concept review

contralateral
crawling
creeping
homolateral
locomotion
manipulation
Phase I reaching
Phase II reaching
releasing
stability
stair climbing
voluntary movement

questions for reflection

1. What are the three categories of voluntary movement during infancy? Describe each category and give three examples of movements within each.
2. How does infant head control evolve from birth to approximately 5 months of age?
3. How does infant upright posture evolve from birth to approximately 8 months of age?
4. Does culture affect the onset of sitting ability? How?
5. Describe the body position of an infant in the early stages of standing.
6. Which occurs first, crawling or creeping? Describe each and explain the difference between the two. What is meant by contralateral creeping?
7. What does the term *proximodistal* mean? Give two examples of this principle.
8. What are the characteristics of Phase I and Phase II reaching?
9. Generally describe the developmental sequence in the development of reaching.
10. What is bimanual control? Give two examples of this concept and generally describe the developmental sequence of bimanual control.

REFERENCES

Adolph, K. E., Cole, W. G., Komati, M., Garciaguirre, J. S., Badaly, D., Lingeman, J. M., et al. (2012). How do you learn to walk? Thousands of steps and dozens of falls per day. *Psychological Science, 23*, 1387–1394.

Adolph, K. E., & Joh, A. S. (2007). Motor development: How infants get into the act. In A. Slater & M. Lewis (Eds.), *Introduction to infant development*. Oxford: Oxford University Press.

Adolph, K. E., & Robinson, S. R. (2015). Motor development. In R. M. Lerner (Ed.), *Handbook of child psychology and developmental science*, vol. 2. 7th ed. New York: Wiley.

Adolph, K. E., Vereijken, B., & Denny, M. A. (1998). Learning to crawl. *Child Development*, *69*(5), 1299–1312.

Atun-Einy, O., Berger, S. E., Ducz, J., & Scher, A. (2014). Strength of infants' bimanual reaching patterns is related to the onset of upright locomotion. *Infancy*, *19*, 82–102.

Atun-Einy, O., Berger, S. E., & Scher, A. (2012). Pulling to stand: Common trajectories and individual differences in development. *Developmental Psychobiology*, *52*, 187–198.

Berger, S. E., Theuring, C., & Adolph, K. E. (2007). How and when infants learn to climb stairs. *Infant Behavioral Development*, *20*, 36–49.

Bilbilaj, S. (2014). The importance of babies' movement in the first year of life. *Journal of Education and Social Research*, *4*, 381–389.

Bisi, M.C., & Stagni, R. (2015). Evaluation of toddlers' different strategies during the first six-months of independent walking: A longitudinal study. *Gait & Posture*, doi.org/10.1016/j.gaitpost.2014.11.017.

Bruner, J. S. (1970). The growth and structure of skill. In K. J. Conolly (Ed.), *Mechanisms of motor skill development*. New York: Academic Press.

Corbetta, D., Wiener, R.F., & Thurman, S.L. (2019). Learning to reach in infancy. In D. Corbetta & M. Santello (Eds.), *Reach-to-grasp behavior: Brain, behavior, and modeling across the lifespan* (pp. 18–41). New York: Routledge.

Darrah, J., Bartlett, D., Maguire, T. O., Avison, W. R., & Lacaze-Masmonteil, T. (2014). Have infant gross motor abilities changed in 20 years? A re-evaluation of the Alberta Infant Motor Scale normative values. *Developmental Medicine & Child Neurology*, doi.org/10.1111/dmcn.12452.

Gallahue, D. L., Ozmun, J. C., & Goodway, J. (2012). *Understanding motor development: Infants, children, adolescents, adults*. 7th ed. New York: McGraw-Hill.

Harbourne, R. T., Lobo, M. A., Karst, G. M., & Galloway, J. C. (2013). Sit happens: Does sitting development perturb reaching development, or vice versa? *Infant Behavior and Development*, *36*, 438–450.

Karasik, L. B., Tamis-LeMonda, C. S., Adolph, K. E., & Bornstein, M. H. (2015). Places and postures: A cross-cultural comparison of sitting in 5-month-olds. *Journal of Cross-Cultural Psychology*, doi-org.libaccess.sjlibrary.org/10.1177/0022022115593803.

Karl, J. M., Sacrey, L. R., & Whishaw, I. Q. (2019). Multiple motor channel theory and the development of skilled hand movements in human infants. In D. Corbetta, & M. Santello (Eds.), *Reach-to-grasp behavior: Brain, behavior, and modeling across the lifespan*. New York: Routledge.

Kobayashi, Y., Watanabe, H., & Taga, G. (2016). Movement patterns of limb coordination in infant rolling. *Experimental Brain Research*, *234*, 3433–3445.

Kretch, K. S., Franchak, J. M., & Adolph, K. E. (2014). Crawling and walking infants see the world differently. *Child Development*, *85*, 1503–1518.

Libertus, K., & Hauf, P. (2017). Motor skills and their foundational role for perceptual, social, and cognitive development. *Frontiers in Psychology*, doi.org/10.3389/fpsyg.2017.00301.

Looper, J., & Chandler, L. S. (2013). How do toddlers increase their gait velocity? *Gait & Posture*, doi.org/10.1016/j.gaitpost.2012.09.009.

Merens, T. A. (2015). The toddler gait—normal or not. *Pediatric Annals*, doi.org/10.3928/00904481-20150512-04.

Nelson, E. A. S., Yu, L. M., Wong, D., Wong, H. Y. E., & Yim, L. (2004). Rolling over in infants: Age, ethnicity, and cultural difference. *Developmental Medicine and Child Neurology*, *46*, 706–709.

Piek, J. P. (2006). *Infant motor development*. Champaign, IL: Human Kinetics.

Rachwani, J., Santamaria, V., Saavedra, S. L., & Woollacott, M. (2015). The development of trunk control and its relation to reaching in infancy: A longitudinal study. *Frontiers in Human Neuroscience*, doi: 10.3389/fnhum.2015.00094.

Rochat, P. (1992). Self-sitting and reaching in 5- and 8-month-old infants: The impact of posture and its development on early eye-hand coordination. *Journal of Motor Behavior*, *24*(2), 210–220.

Rouse, A. G., Mazurek, K. A., Liu, Z., Rivlis, G., & Schieber, M. H. (2019). How separate are reaching and grasping? In D. Corbetta, & M. Santello (Eds.), *Reach-to-grasp behavior: Brain, behavior, and modeling across the lifespan*. New York: Routledge.

Soska, K. C., & Adolph, K. E. (2014). Postural position constrains multimodal object exploration in infants. *Infancy*, *19*, 138–161.

Soska, K. C., Robinson, S. R., & Adolph, K. E. (2015). A new twist on old ideas: How sitting reorients crawlers. *Developmental Science*, *18*, 206–218.

Theveniau, N., Boisgontier, M. P., Varieras, S., & Olivier, I. (2014). The effects of clothes on independent walking in toddlers. *Gait & Posture*, doi.org/10.1016/j.gaitpost.2013.08.031.

Walle, E. A., & Campos, J. J. (2014). Infant language is related to acquisition of walking. *Developmental Psychology*, *50*, 336–348.

11 FINE MOTOR DEVELOPMENT

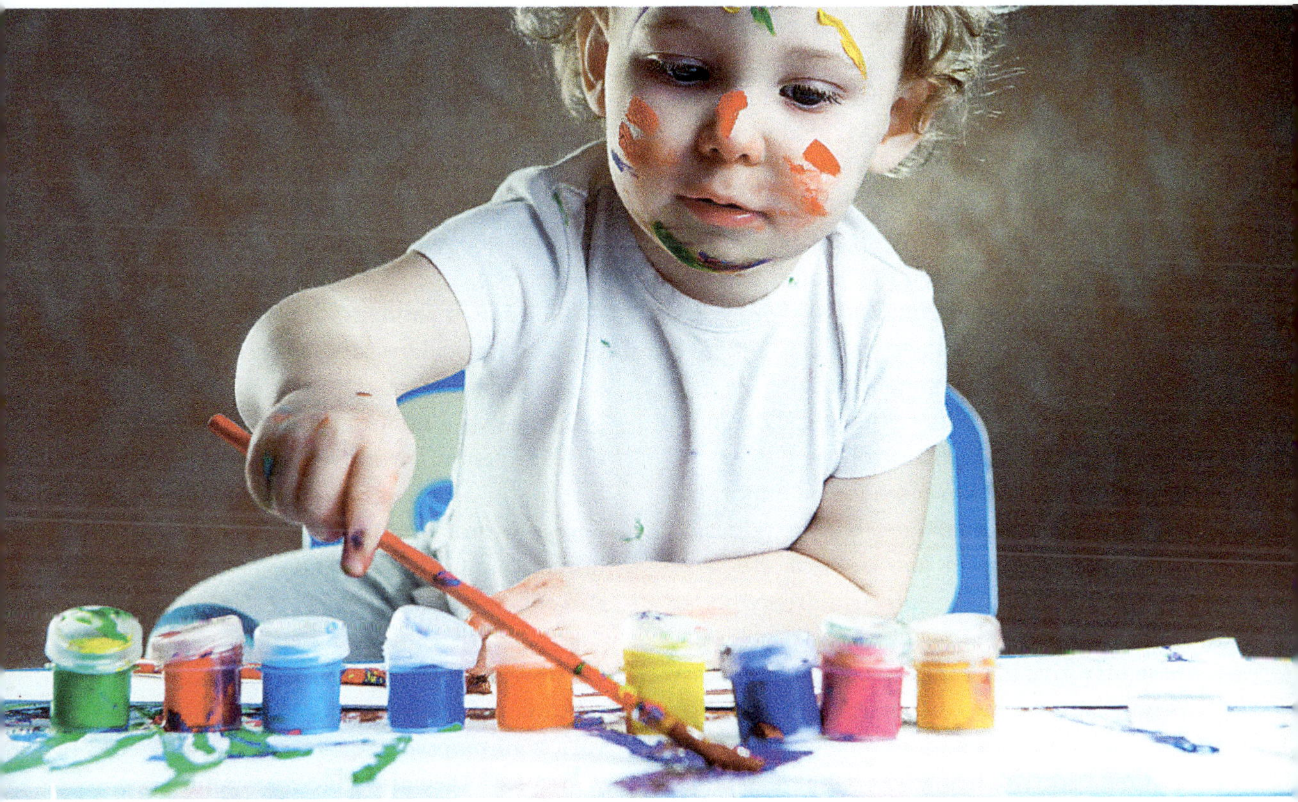

Chapter Objectives

From the information presented in this chapter, you will be able to

- Describe the development of prehension
- Explain an alternate view of the development of prehension
- Explain exploratory procedures and the development of haptic perception
- Describe the development of holding a writing implement
- Explain the dynamic tripod from 6–14 years of age
- Describe the development of handwriting in adulthood
- Describe the movement products of handwriting and drawing development across the lifespan
- Describe the impact of the development of keyboarding versus handwriting skills on writing

The term **fine motor** generally refers to those movements predominantly produced by the smaller muscles or muscle groups of the body. As discussed in Chapter 1, we use the terms *fine* and *gross motor* generally to categorize types of movement. Running and walking are functions predominantly of the larger muscle groups of the body, so we usually think of these as gross motor movements. Manual activity, such as sewing, sculpting, drawing, and playing most musical instruments, involves smaller muscle groups of the body, so such movements are, therefore, considered fine motor.

Fine movements are integral to motor development in general, as well as to other areas of human development, such as academics and social development. Fine motor skills—printing, writing legibly, or keyboarding, for example—can be important for transmitting ideas. Grooming activities, such as brushing one's hair or teeth, are considered fine movements. Children who lag in fine motor development in areas such as these may give the appearance of being messy or unkempt, which, of course, can affect their social relationships and ultimately how these children perceive themselves (Gaul & Issartel, 2016). Fine movements can also be instrumental in sports, games, exercise, and recreational activities that we generally associate with gross movement. For example, though throwing is generally considered a gross movement, it certainly has fine movement characteristics. The small adjustments made by the hand or fingers are critical to the accuracy of the throw, just as the small adjustments made at the ankle and foot are critical to accuracy in kicking. Hence, fine movement control can enhance overall movement performance. That, in turn, can contribute to improved levels of physical fitness, enhanced personal hygiene and appearance, more mature movement ability, and more successful interactions in movement activities. Skill in playing games has been shown to be one of the best indicators of a child's social status (Piek, Baynam, & Barrett, 2006).

Fine movement can also be essential to academic success as studies show that between 30 and 60 percent of an elementary school day can be comprised of fine movement activities, and 80 percent of those involve pencil- or pen-based activities. Hence, children with better fine motor skills have been shown to be more prone to academic success, especially in the areas of math and reading development in the early grades (Gaul & Issartel, 2016).

Out of a concern for the developmental proficiency of children's fine motor ability, Gaul and associates studied second, fourth, and sixth graders in Ireland to determine their proficiency, comparing years past with current developmental norms. When tested on several fine motor aspects of the Bruininks-Oseretsky Test of Motor Proficiency, participants were found to improve with age, but fell below more current expected norms. These authors speculated that this could be because children are now being exposed to more passive technological activities as opposed to the variety of more active movement experiences of years past. They also note that culture is a contributing factor as children from Hong Kong have been found to perform better on fine motor tasks than American children of a similar age. Similar differences have been found when comparing children from Belgium to Australian children. Thus, these authors cautioned that care must be taken when comparing norms from one country to another (Gaul & Issartel, 2016).

While parents are often aware of gross motor milestones and any delays that may occur, fine movements are more subtle and less easily tracked. Thus, research in this area can be useful. In a study to explore children's fine movement and their relationship to environmental influences. Comuk-Balci and associates (2016) examined the effects of factors such as gender, the mother's age and education, socioeconomic status, or the size of the family, by testing over 3,000 boys and girls from birth to just under 7 years of age on the fine motor components of the Denver II Developmental Screening Test. Environmental factors were found to be instrumental. For children over two years of age, gender, older mothers, and more maternal education were associated with greater success on fine motor tasks. For younger children, the family's higher socioeconomic status was found to have a positive association with fine movement ability. Like other similar studies, girls were found to begin earlier on many fine movements and have been found to perform better than boys on previous tests of eye-hand coordination, manual control, and tracing tasks. The researchers involved with this investigation believe all of these findings are important in helping experts determine where fine motor intervention may be necessary. Improving fine movement at an early age is critical as it affects other areas of development and is related to success in school (Comuk-Balci, Bayoglu, Tekindal, Kerem-Gunel, & Anlar, 2016).

During the latter part of life, discussed later in the chapter, some aspects of fine motor ability have been shown to decline. When, and if, these abilities deteriorate, activities of daily life (e.g., buttoning a shirt, unlocking a door, handwriting) can become more difficult. Thus, minor, or in some cases major, challenges may arise in an individual's daily activities (Hoogendam, van der Lijn, Vernooij, et al., 2014).

THE DEVELOPMENT OF PREHENSION

Manipulation is the general term referring to hand use, mostly reaching and grasping. As discussed in Chapter 10, the reach is that part of the arm and hand movement that delivers the hand to the desired target. This movement is performed with more or less accuracy, depending on the individual's development in this movement. The grasp follows the reach and involves the opening and closing of the hand once it is delivered to the appropriate location (Karl & Whishaw, 2014). Grasping is a skill that is integral to our daily lives. We use it to acquire objects, of course, but we also use it to explore, manipulate, and reshape the world around us. Immediately after birth, we begin to extend our arms toward desirable objects. By a few months of age, the skill has become sufficiently honed to allow successful grasps (Daum & Gredeback, 2011). **Prehension** is a term that applies specifically to the act of grasping, and it includes approaching, grasping, and releasing objects. Prehension is critical to the development of a multitude of hand movements used throughout the lifespan.

Although reaching and grasping work in conjunction, most of our discussion regarding reaching appeared in Chapter 10, where we discussed the development of voluntary movement. This chapter will place greater emphasis specifically on the action of grasping and the use of the hand and fingers in this movement.

Halverson's Stages of Grasping Development

One of the most frequently cited studies in the area of prehension was completed nearly 90 years ago. Halverson's work (1931) is a classic study in the area of early manipulation because of the depth of the conclusions and the importance of the subject. However, the findings of this research have been questioned, as we will discuss later in the chapter.

Halverson's aim was to examine the development of prehension, particularly the grasp, in children 16–52 weeks old. Halverson presented each child with a 1-in (2.5 cm) red cube, filmed the child's response, and then described the developmental progression for the grasp of the cube. Generally, Halverson noted that the total process of prehension—early reaching, grasping, and releasing behavior—involved four steps: (1) the object is visually located; (2) the object is approached; (3) the object is grasped; (4) the child disposes of the object by releasing it.

Halverson (1931) also noted that there were three basic methods of reaching. The most immature method involved sweeping the hand and arm in a backhand manner toward the object. Eventually, this mode of reaching evolved into a more mature sweeping or scooping approach. Despite the advanced nature of this method relative to the backhand style, this second method was indirect or "circuitous" and involved approaches from a variety of angles. Finally, the children in the study developed the direct reach that is common in slightly older, more motorically advanced children.

The brunt of Halverson's investigation concerned the actual grasp of the object. Overall, Halverson noted that younger children had not yet developed the ability to oppose the fingers with the thumb. When these children reached for the red cube, the thumb's position during the reach often indicated the likelihood of the thumb being used in opposition to the fingers. If the thumb was inward when the hand approached the cube, thumb opposition was likely to occur. However, a thumb positioned downward or curled under the hand indicated an upcoming grasp that was less mature than the thumb-opposition grasp (Halverson, 1931).

Halverson also found a relatively specific progressive sequence of grasping behavior in his 4- to 13-month-old subjects. Initially, at 4 months of age, the children were totally incapable of making contact with the object. Next, at 5 months, children could contact crudely but could not actually acquire the object. The third step in the developmental sequence of grasping, known as the "primitive squeeze," was also characteristic of children very near 5 months of age. In this case, the child generally thrust the hand beyond the desired object and then scooped or corralled the object inward until the object was actually squeezed against the body or the other hand. The hand performed no real grasping action. In the fourth step, at approximately 6 months of age, a grasp of sorts did occur. The child performed this "squeeze grasp" by approaching the object laterally with the hand until contact was made; then, the fingers closed around the object and pressed it against the palm of the hand. This system of acquiring the cube was the first sign of an actual grasp and was typically clumsy and unsuccessful (Halverson, 1931).

The fifth type of grasping, the "hand grasp," occurred at approximately 7 months. This grasp was somewhat similar to the squeeze grasp, except that the child bridged the hand down over the cube. The child maintained the thumb in a position parallel to the fingers, which curled down over the side of the cube. Once that position was attained, the fingers pressed the cube against the heel of the hand. The sixth level of grasping ability was similar to the fifth and was also common in infants at approximately 7 months. In the "palm grasp," the hand was again placed down over the cube. However, as the fingers curled down over the side of the cube, so did the thumb. This appeared to be an initial sign of the thumb's ability to oppose the movement of the fingers (Halverson, 1931).

The opposition of the thumb became increasingly apparent in the seventh level of grasping. At approximately 8 months, the child performed the "superior palm grasp" by placing the hand, radial side down, on the cube. The thumb then pressed on the near side of the cube as the first two fingers curled down onto the far side and applied opposing pressure. This system was similar to the grasp observed in level 8, the "inferior forefinger grasp," which appeared at 9 months. The thumb and forefinger opposition noted in level 8 once again was evident, but the child initiated it by wrapping the fingers around the cube pointing medially rather than downward. As in the seventh level, the cube, once acquired, was controlled and maintained near the palm area of the hand (Halverson, 1931).

At 13 months of age, in the next to last (ninth) level of grasping that Halverson observed, the child finally controlled and maintained the cube with the fingertips of the first three fingers, which were opposed by the thumb. To attain this control, the child stabilized the hand on the tabletop during the initial contact and grasp of the cube. This hand stabilization differentiated level 9, the "forefinger grasp," from level 10, the "superior forefinger grasp," which also became common among infants at approximately 13 months of age. Otherwise, the superior forefinger grasp was similar to the level 9 grasp (Halverson, 1931). Generally, Halverson noted a proximodistal progression, as discussed in Chapter 1, such that movement ability progressed in a direction away from the core of the body. Although the child's initial efforts at obtaining an object through reaching and grasping consisted of crude shoulder and elbow movements, the finer movements of the hand, and finally of the fingertips, eventually attained control. In addition, Halverson noted a gradual increase in the movements' speed and efficiency as these children aged from 16 to 52 weeks. The movement abilities that Halverson described are likely to emerge earlier today than in previous years as a result of enhanced standards of living, improved nutrition, greater awareness of the importance of early motor experiences, and increasingly early use of electronic devices by young children. As with most voluntary movements of infancy, the specific times at which the various grasping-related skills emerge continue to be quite variable from person to person.

An Alternate View of the Development of Prehension

As discussed, Halverson (1931) viewed the development of prehension as an ordered, relatively fixed sequence of grip patterns predictably evolving with increasing age and maturity. However, according to Newell, Scully, Tenenbaum, and Hardiman (1989), this view may have resulted from the narrow range of constraints imposed in Halverson's research. In that study, the young subjects were offered cubes of only one size to grasp, and this may have affected the outcome.

Newell and his associates (1989) sought to examine the effects of using various sizes of objects that had been scaled to the hand size of the preschool-age and adult subjects. The researchers used 10 cube sizes to examine which hand was employed, the number of fingers used with the thumb in contacting objects, the depth of finger contact, and type of grip (side, top, and so forth). Some differences were noted. For example, adults used one hand 60 percent of the time (two hands 40 percent of the time), while children used one hand 38.6 percent of the time. Older child subjects were found to demonstrate slightly more use of the right hand, indicating that hand dominance may not yet be firmly established by the age of 4 years, though Scharoun and Bryden (2015) found a "strong pattern of handedness" and "reliable use of a preferred hand" (p. 1) emerging by the ages of 7 to 10 years. Newell and his research team found the object-to-hand-size ratio to be a significant factor related to the subject's use of one or two hands. When objects were scaled to the subject's hand size, the overall trend for grasping was quite similar for adult and child subjects. One finger and the thumb were used for small objects. Two or three fingers were used with the thumb for intermediate-sized objects, and four fingers and the thumb were used for large objects. The size of the object that seemed to create a shift to a new pattern of grasping differed among age groups. However, when the object was scaled to the subject's hand size, the "shifting point" was quite similar among the groups.

According to Newell and associates (1989), more than 1,000 combinations of finger-thumb grips are possible, but the subjects tended to use only a fraction of those. Adult subjects regularly employed 14 combinations, and children used 22. Even with regard to preferred grips, certain choices appeared to dominate. Five grips accounted for 62 percent of the grips used by children and 89 percent of the grips used by adults (see Figure 11.1). The authors noted that eliminating the "playful behavior" of the child subjects would have increased the percentage of times that the children used the five most common grips.

Based on the results of their research, Newell and associates concluded that task constraints, in this case, object size, play a major role in grip patterns for children and adults. Furthermore, contrary to traditional views of grip-pattern development (i.e., Halverson's), children and adults use similar patterns for objects of similar size relative to their hand size. In short, developmental progressions may be considerably more "flexible" than those Halverson described (Newell et al., 1989). In fact, Halverson's work may be "a reflection of the narrow range of constraints tested rather than a rigid sequence of biological or cognitive prescriptions for action" (p. 819).

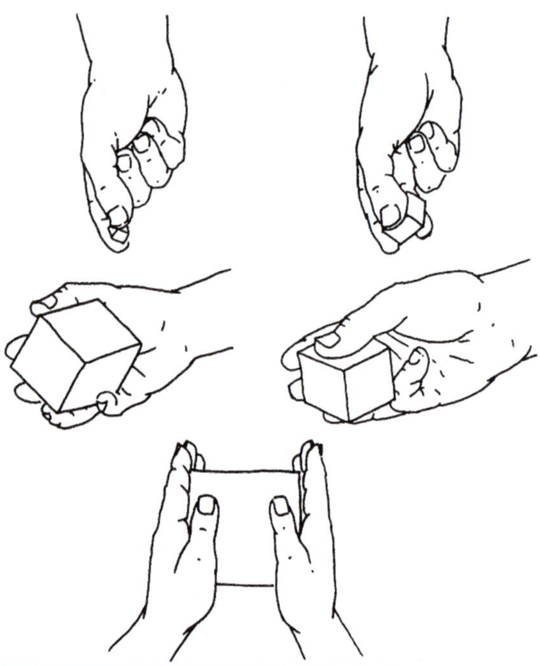

Figure 11.1 The five most common grip patterns encountered by Newell, Scully, Tenenbaum, and Hardiman (1989) in their research on child and adult grip patterns

To gain further insight into the development of prehension, Newell and his colleagues conducted additional studies. Their subjects were 4- to 8-month-old infants, and in one study the children were compared with adult subjects. One aim of the research was to determine if the size of the hand in relationship to the size of the object would "define" the grip patterns of children when compared with adults.

In the study comparing infants with adults, all subjects were asked to grasp inverted cups that had been scaled to hand size. For both the infants and the adults, the grip pattern varied systematically with the cup size: the subjects used more fingers when the cup size increased. When the cup was scaled to hand size, many similarities were noted in the grasping patterns of the infants and the adults. Subjects were generally found to use two hands more commonly with larger objects than with small. According to the authors, this indicated an ability to differentiate one- and two-handed grasps and object size among children as young as 4 months. All subjects in this study, even the 4-month-olds, exhibited an ability to differentiate finger use based on object size. However, the younger subjects exhibited more variability in finger combinations. The number of fingers employed was also influenced by the object's shape. In addition, for the infants, approximately 50 percent of the one-handed grasps occurred with the right hand (or the left hand). Apparently, hand dominance had not yet begun to evolve in the young children (Newell, McDonald, & Baillargeon, 1993).

In the study of infants only, as in Newell's previous research, five-finger configurations accounted for most grips. In addition, as we might expect from the research cited earlier, minimal age differences were noted in the grasping of 4- to 8-month-olds, though the younger subjects required more haptic information to differentiate grip configurations, whereas 8-month-olds were more likely to use visual information (Newell, Scully, & McDonald, 1989).

Adjustment to Task Constraints in Grasping

More recently, researchers have focused on grasping during infancy and how the forces applied depend on task constraints. Sgandurra, Cecchi, Serio, and colleagues (2012) studied this specific movement every two weeks in infants from 18–41 weeks of age. They found that purposeful gripping developed after purposeful reaching, increased significantly in force from 18 to 30 weeks, and plateaued thereafter. They also determined that infants seemed to differentiate the size and shape of objects as early as 4 months of age, as they employed various grip configurations for different objects. Hand closure, for example, varied, based on the size of the target object. The younger infants in the study often touched the object repeatedly before deciding on a grip force.

In a lengthier longitudinal study, Lee, Liu, and Newell (2006) also examined the development of infant grasping. Infants were, again, tested every two weeks, starting at 9 weeks of age and concluding at just over 3 years of age. During the testing, the infants were seated and presented with balls and cups. Both hard and soft red balls of varying sizes were used. The cups were presented to the infants in both up and down positions. At 9 to 17 weeks of age the infants exerted minimal "goal-directed" effort to grasp the objects. This increased to a maximal amount of activity by the time the infants reached 29–37 weeks of age. However, the type of object (cup or ball) that was presented to the infants was significant. The type of grip that the infants employed also changed across the nearly 3 years of the investigation. From about 3 months of age, the infants began to adjust their grip according to the task constraints or the situation's requirements. Early on, from about 9–15 weeks, the child's hand movements rarely resulted in actually touching the object presented. However, presentation of the cups resulted in more touches than grasping the balls. The authors noted that the infants' visual awareness of the objects being presented to them seemed to increase from about 4 months onward. At that time, the number of reaches toward the objects began to increase, and general hand movements and contacts with the objects also increased.

By approximately 5 months the number of actual grasps, especially involving the soft balls, increased significantly. Hence, the size and texture of the object presented to the infants affected the grasping movement, and this effect increased as the children grew older. For example, the sequence of development when the soft balls were presented appeared to evolve from no touch at all to a one-hand touch and, eventually, a one-hand grasp. During that same time period, when the hard balls were presented, the lack of a touch evolved to a touch but not to the one-hand grasp. Such differences were also noted when balls of various sizes were presented to infants at approximately 5 months of age and older. The smallest ball (2 in/5 cm in diameter) was grasped at 19 weeks for the soft ball but not until over 30 weeks for the hard ball. A similar phenomenon was seen with the cups: placing the cup opening up or down affected the likelihood of the infant's grasping the cup.

Notably, however, the cup seemed to elicit a finger-and-thumb opposition grasp that did not appear when the balls were presented. Again, this clearly indicates that object constraints affect the development of early grasping behavior. In other words, the child's developmental sequence depends on the exact nature of the task at hand. The researchers noted that individual infants in some cases devised their own strategies that differed from those of the group as a whole, demonstrating the individual nature of the development of many of the voluntary movements of infancy (Lee et al., 2006).

Anticipation and Object Control in Reaching and Grasping

Being able to anticipate the spatial characteristics and orientation of target objects is essential to successful reaching and grasping. This is particularly important given the wide variety of sizes, shapes, textures, and positioning of potential target objects (Ransburg, Reiser, Munzert, Jovanovich, & Schwarzer, 2017).

Classic and innovative research designed to examine this phenomenon was conducted by Mounoud and Bower (1974). The study was conducted to specifically study infants' awareness of the properties of objects and its effect on their reaching and grasping behavior. As is the case with many movement behaviors, the infants' reaching and grasping showed a distinct progression. Mounoud and Bower determined that prior to 9 months of age, the child's application of force in the reach and grasp was unrelated to the weight of the object. Regardless of the object's weight, the child applied the same force in both the arm movement and the subsequent grasp. The researchers determined this by observing that their subjects' arms suddenly rose or fell when they grasped a series of objects of varying weights. Mounoud and Bower gained additional information by placing force transducers on the objects, which indicated the magnitude of the force being applied during the grasp.

By 9 months of age, most of the subjects had developed the ability to adjust to the weight of the object after they had grasped it. However, they showed limited anticipatory abilities. This inadequacy diminished by 1 year of age as the infants developed skill in adjusting their arm and hand tension when they were repeatedly presented with the same object. The children initially made errors, but if the same object was presented repeatedly, the errors were eliminated. However, this held true only for the familiar objects—the knowledge the infants gained from their repeated experiences with one object did not positively affect their performance on the first few trials with new objects (Mounoud & Bower, 1974).

By the age of 18 months, the children exhibited anticipation. Upon repeated presentations, they displayed an awareness of the same object weighing the same. Furthermore, the subjects seemed to follow the "rule" that objects similar to a familiar one weigh more or less than the familiar object, based on length. Therefore, although anticipation was evident, it was not always accurate because longer objects are not always heavier. Nevertheless, Mounoud and Bower concluded that, by the age of 18 months, their subjects had developed the ability to perform two critical skills: to anticipate and to differentiate their reaching and grasping responses.

In more recent research on infant anticipation and grasping, Ransburg and fellow researchers studied 10-month-old infants compared to college students. Cylindrical objects of varying sizes were used, so they could be presented to the grasper horizontally and vertically. All participants were seated during their grasping trials with the infants in high chairs. Hand positions were analyzed

HAPTIC PERCEPTION AND EXPLORATORY PROCEDURES

Haptic perception involves the active use of the hands in holding and exploring an object to acquire information about the object (Reuter, Voelcker-Rehage, Vieluf, & Godde, 2012). Examples of properties that can be haptically perceived include temperature, size, texture, hardness, weight, and shape. Haptic sensitivity seems to emerge in a predictable sequence. Infants often demonstrate the capability to discriminate between the hardness and softness of objects.

The majority of research on haptic perception has involved texture or shape distinction and subjects over 6 months of age. Only infants over 6 months old have been studied concerning haptic perception of temperature; however, children much younger than 6 months withdraw their hands from heat and cold. Children over 6 months can perceive and discriminate hardness; little is known concerning younger children's perception of hardness and softness. Children under 6 months are not believed to possess the ability to perceive texture, though those between 6 and 12 months do. Similar findings exist for the perception of weight, though this ability begins a few months later, at around 9 months. Shape perception evolves later yet, around 12 to 15 months. In short, a consistent order of emergence for haptic perception appears to exist (Bushnell & Boudreau, 1993).

Case-Smith, Bigsby, and Clutter (1998) focused on younger children in a study examining the effect of haptic attributes of objects on infants' grasping patterns. Two- to 6-month-old infants were presented with three different objects varying in haptic characteristics. Grasping was found to vary significantly by age, and it also varied based on the haptic characteristics of the object. More mature skills were noticed in the infants when the haptic characteristics of the object were closely matched to the infant's level of skill. The researchers' overall conclusions were that haptic characteristics do affect infants' movement patterns and that the influence changes with age. This finding was thought to be particularly important as it suggested that caregivers could potentially facilitate children's grasping development by attempting to match objects' haptic features with the infants' skill level.

In a similar study, Paulus and Hauf (2012) studied 11-month-old infants to determine their object preferences based on texture and weight and found that infants are able to differentiate objects visually and tactilely based on texture and weight. Previous research had shown that, generally, infants demonstrate a preference for novel objects over ones they have seen previously; they tend to prefer lighter objects over heavier ones; based on visual information exclusively, they prefer to look at complicated patterns or objects; and when they choose among objects based on vision alone, versus vision and reaching, they again prefer complicated-looking objects. To understand these phenomena more comprehensively, Paulus and Hauf sought to determine if infants would prefer to reach for an object made of wood (with a smooth texture) or for objects made of sponge. To examine further the effect of an object's weight, the researchers adjusted the objects for weight and used objects of the same overall size and shape. The infants demonstrated a clear preference for the spongy texture regardless of its weight. Thus, in this study, texture seemed to be a stronger determinant of preference than weight. The authors concluded that the infants' object choices resulted from a combination of visual and haptic information and that various senses interacted to influence the infants' choices about reaching and grasping. In addition, toward the end of their first year of life, these infants already demonstrated unique preferences relating to characteristics such as texture and weight.

The emergence of haptic perception appears to be closely linked to the child's ability to perform certain types of hand movements, called **exploratory procedures**. An example of an exploratory procedure is lateral, alternate rubbing motions across an object's surface to detect its texture (Lederman & Klatzky, 1987). Another example is "unsupported holding," when the child holds an object and alternately raises and lowers it to assist in the perception of weight. Figure 11.2 illustrates these and other exploratory procedures. Any restriction of these hand movements may inhibit a child's ability to learn about an object. Thus, an inability in any of the exploratory procedures may reduce certain forms of haptic sensitivity.

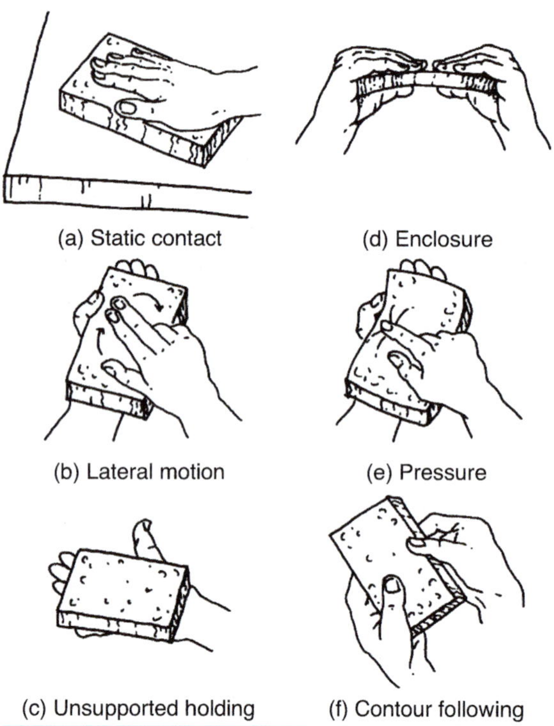

Figure 11.2 The optimal hand movement patterns for acquiring the object properties of (a) temperature; (b) texture; (c) weight; (d) volume/size; (e) hardness; and (f) shape

Source: Lederman & Klatzky (1987). Used with permission from Academic Press, Inc.

immediately before and during the grasp using a motion capture system. Both infants and adults were found to adjust their wrists, thumbs, and index fingers according to the size and position of the target object. These researchers noted that adults commonly adjust their hand position prior to the contact in anticipation of the grasp and can adjust that hand position based on simultaneous consideration of multiple characteristics of the object. Younger infants, however, may only make adjustments after making initial contact with the object, whereas at around 9 months of age babies can begin to anticipate the horizontal or vertical positioning of the target object by orienting the back of their hands sideways for vertically positioned objects and palms up for horizontal positions (Ransburg et al., 2017).

Infant-Childhood Object Manipulation Development

According to Bushnell and Boudreau (1993), infants' object manipulation develops in three phases. In the first phase, from birth to 3 months, babies simply clutch objects in the fist.

This action is largely influenced by the palmar grasp reflex, discussed in Chapter 9. At this age, the child holds the object with one hand, occasionally brings it to the mouth or to the body's midline, and holds it with both hands. The fingers may not open and close much while the child holds the object, but if they do, the fingers create a kneading motion. Exploratory procedures at this age may be sufficient for the child to detect haptic properties of temperature, size, and hardness. According to Bushnell and Boudreau, the available research suggests that the child's ability to detect haptic properties typically emerges in this order.

The second phase of infants' object manipulation begins at approximately 4 months of age, when children begin to evidence a wider variety of hand movements. Visual control of manipulation and more varied and differentiated movements are noticeable. These movements include poking, scratching, rubbing, waving, and banging objects. Infants also move objects from hand to hand and perform some unsupported holding (see Figure 11.2). As Bushnell and Boudreau indicated, once these manipulatory capabilities are exhibited, the capabilities seem to facilitate the development of haptic abilities, as haptic sensitivity to hardness emerges around 6 to 7 months of age. Haptic sensitivity to texture typically emerges around 6 months, but sensitivity to weight may not occur until after 9 months. In short, throughout the middle of the child's first year, several manipulatory capabilities emerge that appear to be similar to those necessary for perceiving haptic properties.

By 9 to 10 months, infants enter a third phase of object manipulation, when their ability to sit makes two-handed manipulation easier. In complementary bimanual activities, one hand positions an object while the other manipulates and explores it. Around this time, children exhibit contour following: one hand maintains hold on the object while the other hand smoothly passes over the object's outline. This gradually evolving manipulatory ability appears to contribute to the infant's ability to perceive configurational shape, which, according to Bushnell and Boudreau, emerges around 12 to 15 months in most infants.

Gonzalez and Nelson (2015) further addressed bimanual hand use in infants by creating what they called a "blueprint" for studying this complex skill. In this article, they indicate that infants begin to manipulate objects using **role-differentiated bimanual manipulation** (RDBM). RDBM involves one hand holding, or stabilizing, the target object while the other hand moves the object as desired. During infancy they may display a preference for one hand over the other as the manipulator versus the stabilizer. However, this may vary based on the characteristics of the target object. With increasing age, the two hands will more commonly perform increasingly different tasks with the two hands and one object. Nevertheless, at 1 year of age, only about half of all infants will perform RDBM in what Gonzalez and Nelson refer to as "fully differentiated." By 18 months of age their skills will be fully differentiated in over 70 percent of cases and in almost all cases by the age of 2 years. Examples of RDBM skills that are often seen at around 1 year of age include removing or inserting objects using the two hands. By a year and a half or 2 years, many babies can unscrew or unzip objects using the two hands working together. Hand preferences, they say, emerge at around 1 year of age with a general preference for using the right hand (Gonzalez & Nelson, 2015).

Generally, children's manipulatory capabilities seem to determine the order in which their haptic perceptions emerge. One possible exception may be weight perception, which appears to emerge several months after the child develops the ability to perform

OBJECT MANIPULATION AND INFANTS' BODY POSITIONS: THE FIRST TWO YEARS

In a study to determine how object manipulation develops across the first two years of life, especially in light of the other rapidly developing movement changes, Lobo, Kokkoni, de Campos, and Galloway (2014) studied babies from birth to 24 months. These researchers were especially interested in how the infants' body positions (i.e., supine, prone, and sitting) affected object manipulation.

Clearly, infants' ability to interact with objects in their environment is present from very early after birth and undergoes significant change over the first 6 months of life. Holding and touching their own body is a common and expected behavior among newborns. The researchers postulate that this behavior may be a continuation of several weeks or months of prenatal activity, when tactile self-exploration (e.g., umbilical cord) is common. Over the first several months of postnatal life babies progress to a very high level of interaction with environmental objects. This includes interacting with objects with one and both hands, banging objects, mouthing them, and exchanging them from one hand to the other. During these first few months of life, according to the researchers, babies shift quickly among many different movements and combinations of movements designed to help them learn about objects (Lobo et al., 2014).

The researchers described the development of the babies' exploratory movements as somewhat predictable. They noted that body touching was common and peaked very early, decreasing as other abilities emerged. Mouthing objects was less common soon after birth and became most common at approximately 6 months of age; among children around 2 years of age, mouthing objects was rare. Visual exploration of objects was uncommon prior to 3 months of age but gradually increased thereafter. From 3 to 6 months of age, infants commonly mouthed objects, banged them, and transported them into the line of sight; Lobo and colleagues speculated that the increase in these movements was related to the children's improving ability to reach and control their hands. In the last half of the infants' first year, "increased fingering, rotating, manipulation, and squeezing" (2014, p. 344) of objects were common. Again, the researchers speculated that these behaviors were made possible by continuing improvements in the infants' reaching and grasping abilities.

When these researchers examined object manipulation behaviors among these babies relative to body positioning, interesting findings emerged. For example, the infants performed far fewer manipulatory behaviors and performed them less frequently when in the prone position, a position in which the hands are somewhat constrained against the floor. When children are supine or sitting, their hands are free from such constraint and well positioned to acquire and manipulate objects. Lobo and associates found the quantity of manipulatory activity to be similar when infants were supine and seated. Though other researchers had speculated that, because of gravitational constraints, these behaviors would be less common when infants were supine, Lobo and colleagues posited that they occurred as frequently because of the babies' past experience, that is, because a great deal of object manipulation occurs when the infant is in the supine position during the first few months following birth.

In short, these researchers concluded that active and even intense exploration of objects starts in the first few weeks of life. The most significant developmental change was seen during the first 6 months, though babies continued to expand their repertoire of manipulatory behaviors to accommodate the object and the situation across their first two years.

unsupported holding (around 4 months of age). Though research is contradictory as to when the haptic ability to perceive weight emerges, Bushnell and Boudreau believed it may not be until around 9 months of age. In spite of this possible exception, manipulation appears to be integral to the emergence of haptic ability because the child cannot discriminate object properties that correspond to exploratory procedures that have not yet evolved. Thus, an infant's manipulatory ability appears to be a constraint to the perception of certain object properties.

By school age, the haptic ability may still not be fully developed, and it may not be until middle childhood or early adolescence. Researchers have posited that the ability to discriminate an object's size and orientation may not be fully developed (adult-like ability) until 8 to 12 years of age (Gori, Squeri, Sciutti, et al., 2012). By the time people have reached adulthood, they have generally become highly effective in determining objects' properties through haptic perceptions and in utilizing that information (Jao, James, & James, 2014).

Adulthood Fine Movement and Touch Perception

A decline in the performance of fine motor tasks, especially use of the hands, in later adulthood is often viewed as one of the most troubling aspects of getting older. Obviously, a loss of skill in this area can severely affect daily functioning, including work-related and self-care activities. As a result, the overall quality of life can be impacted as functional independence wanes. Despite these views, the nature of these declines is variable and dependent upon factors like age, health, and gender, to name a few. To examine this phenomenon, Skrzek and colleagues (2015) studied nearly 500 Polish and Czech women over the age of 60 years on hand dominance and performance on a series of fine motor tasks like aiming, inserting pins, and hand tapping. Most measures were found to decline with age as the researchers indicated that fine movements became less synchronized and smooth. Interestingly, the dominant hand, usually the right, appeared to show greater decline than the non-dominant hand. These authors noted that these changes may relate to numerous age-related modifications affecting the hands as one ages. For example, skeletal muscle may atrophy, reducing muscle strength and endurance. The peripheral nervous system may also decline, hampering nerve conductivity and the perception of senses like touch. Slower motor activation and poorer eye-hand coordination may also be factors that impair fine motor ability in later life (Skrzek et al., 2015).

In additional research on fine movement and touch perception among adults, Reuter and colleagues (2012) studied three groups of workers aged 18 to 65 (young, middle-aged, and older adults). Noting that declines in touch perception and manual dexterity are related and that both frequently show declines in later adulthood, these researchers sought to understand the relationship between work experience and touch and haptic perception. What is the influence of work experience on touch perception, and does work experience slow the decline in touch perception that we expect to see with age? The researchers subdivided the three groups of subjects into subgroups based on the individuals' level of work experience involving manual dexterity. The subjects were all tested on a series of tasks related to touch and haptic ability. On the tactile-related tests, which simply tested the sense of touch, the younger and middle-aged adults performed better than the older adults. The younger adults showed no significant differences from the middle-aged adults, but the middle-aged adults differed significantly from the older adults. Age-related declines appeared to begin around the age of 45 years, with more severe declines occurring later in life. Thus, overall results indicated that performance in the tactile tasks declined with age in later adulthood. In addition, work-related experience did not seem to offset the tactile declines demonstrated in this research (Reuter et al., 2012).

However, this study found no age-related differences in performance on the haptic tasks (involving object and pattern discrimination) that were more dependent on a cognitive element to determine object properties. This finding was similar to the results of previous research in which older adults, through their mid-eighties, were shown to perform haptic tasks, such as object and pattern discrimination as well as young adults, with minimal differences in accuracy and precision.

One explanation for this difference in the older adults' performance on the two types of tasks may be that cognitive awareness (which was perhaps enhanced in individuals with more experience) was more important on the haptic tests than on the tests based more exclusively on the sense of touch. The researchers were somewhat surprised that related manual work experience did not seem to offset the tactile declines seen in this study (Reuter et al., 2012).

HANDWRITING AND DRAWING

Handwriting and drawing are complex fine motor skills that involve the manual formation of numbers, letters, and various characters or designs. Handwriting, in particular, is critical to our communication and essential to academic success. Nevertheless, studies have found that from 10 to nearly 50 percent of children may initially face difficulties in learning this process with boys often facing greater obstacles than girls. Poor handwriting has been associated with poorer academic success and, therefore, negative labeling of some children. This, of course, can eventually affect self-esteem. On the other hand, handwriting proficiency has been positively associated with both length and quality of compositions prepared by young writers (Feng, Lindner, Ji, & Joshi, 2019). So, in spite of the emergence of computer technology, handwriting remains an important mode of communication and a necessary tool for the completion of many daily tasks, and for children, it is critical to academic success. For example, errors in handwriting, among kindergartners, are highly correlated with success in writing and math up to the sixth grade. According to Maldarelli and colleagues, handwriting proficiency can be measured by the written product (i.e., what it looks like) or by the process or technique employed by the writer. Either way, success is dependent upon one's perceptual and intellectual capabilities (Maldarelli, Kahrs, Hunt, & Lockman, 2015). Both handwriting and drawing simultaneously involve the intellectual thought process, visual and perceptual processing, and movement control (Dinehart, 2014). If any one of these processes is limited, illegible or incomplete handwriting can occur (van Drempt, McCluskey, & Lannin, 2011b), and drawings may not be recognizable. In extreme cases, an individual may not be able to perform a writing or drawing task at all.

Handwriting and Drawing Development

Handwriting begins with simple scribbling on a page. This early form of drawing serves as "an apprenticeship" (Feder & Majnemer, 2007, p. 313) for what will become a more recognizable and intentional form of handwriting as the child develops the ability to create shapes, which evolve into letters. Printing letters often begins as children attempt to reproduce geometric shapes, starting with vertical strokes, around 2 years of age. Horizontal strokes follow approximately 6 months later, and full circles are often noted by the third year of age. Children will attempt to recreate crosses by 4 years of age, squares by 5 years, and triangles by 5.5 years. The ability to draw these geometric shapes is often viewed as an indicator of a child's readiness for writing.

Gender plays an important role in the development of handwriting, especially over the age of 7 years, when girls tend to show a significantly higher quality of writing and a faster handwriting speed. Overall, handwriting quality generally develops rather rapidly in first grade in the United States, but it is found to plateau slightly in second grade. Development continues in third grade as handwriting becomes a more "automatic" operation, becomes clearly more organized, and comes to be seen as an important means of organizing thoughts and ideas. Legibility and speed are considered the most important components of handwriting. Handwriting speed increases throughout the primary grades, and the overall quality of handwriting continues to increase through middle school (Feder & Majnemer, 2007).

Palmis and associates (2017) examined handwriting in 5- to 12-year-old children and adults and noted that thousands of hours and many years of practice may occur before one can write a word series fluently. From 5 to 7 years of age, children often experience a transition from "ballistic," short-quick motions followed by pauses in their writing to examine for errors. As little as two years later, writing may still lack the automation experienced by adults, though children are often capable of integrating information gleaned visually and proprioceptively to assist in their writing process. The size of the letters formed will have typically decreased, though their velocity may still be slow in comparison to an adult writer. By 9 to 10 years of age, writing has generally been mastered as children begin to personalize their own style of writing as they are capable of writing with less detailed attention to the task. The significant differences in handwriting between the ages of 7 and 10 years has been attributed, in part, to the advancing ability of one's memory of the required movement program that enables the child to write with less focus on the actual movement process. Thus, it becomes more automatic (Palmis, Danna, Velay, & Longcamp, 2017).

External factors have been found to be critical elements in children's handwriting performance. Their sitting position, the chair or desk configuration, the type of writing implement, environmental factors such as lighting and noise levels, and the type of instruction and amount of practice a child has received all can have significant effects on the individual's performance.

The Development of Grasping Position

Development in early childhood. Prior to developing a mature grasp of a writing implement, the child passes through a series of rather predicable stages of handwriting technique with regard to grasping. After examining children who were 1.5 to 7 years old, Rosenbloom and Horton (1971)

TECHNOLOGY AND THE STUDY OF HANDWRITING AND DRAWING

Technological advances have changed the ways we can study handwriting and drawing movements. We can now describe more parameters related to the development of handwriting and drawing and describe them more accurately using more technologically advanced equipment.

In a study on the handwriting kinematics of children and youth (Accardo, Genna, & Borean, 2013), subjects approximately 8 through 14 years of age were asked to write on force-sensitive tablets, as fast as they could in one case and as accurately as possible in the other. Overall, as expected, older participants wrote faster on the timed task and more accurately in less time in the accuracy task compared to their younger counterparts. Older subjects also wrote smaller letters and demonstrated an enhanced "letter arrangement" (p. 144). The researchers also determined that, for older subjects, the number of hand strokes required for each letter was reduced, indicative of continued improvement in motor control in the writing process. With regard to writing speed, the velocity of horizontal movements increased along with the subjects' age, but the vertical speed remained fairly constant across ages. In short, these researchers concluded that handwriting development within this age group showed evolution across a number of parameters. Specifically determining the parameters that indicate developmental change is important for handwriting diagnostics, which will be especially helpful for individuals who demonstrate a significant deficit in handwriting ability.

In another study employing force-sensitive tablets, Accardo et al. (2013) examined first- through fifth-grade children's drawing movements. As expected, fine motor proficiency was found to improve along with the subjects' age. A number of factors evidenced this improvement, including an increase in drawing speed and a decrease in fine motor variations when the children drew circles. The researchers determined the speed of drawing by measuring "in air" and "on paper" times during the drawing tasks (p. 171). The on-paper time was totaled to determine total drawing time. The researchers concluded that the older participants drew faster because they had generally become more mature and proficient in their drawing skills. Drawing speed was seen as an important variable as it affects a child's ability to keep pace with classroom demands. Though the researchers measured the pressure applied to the writing implement while drawing, this measure was not found to characterize development as it fluctuated across grades. It may be more a function of the drawing task than any developmental progression (Lin, Luo, Wu, et al., 2015).

determined that the earliest grasp of a writing implement usually involves the entire hand. In the **supinate grasp**, all four fingers and the thumb wrap around the pencil to form a fist. This immature grasp, pictured in Figure 11.3, is typically replaced by the **pronate grasp**, which consists of a palm-down hand position (see Figure 11.4).

Once the child begins to use the pronate grasp, the thumb and fingers commence to play

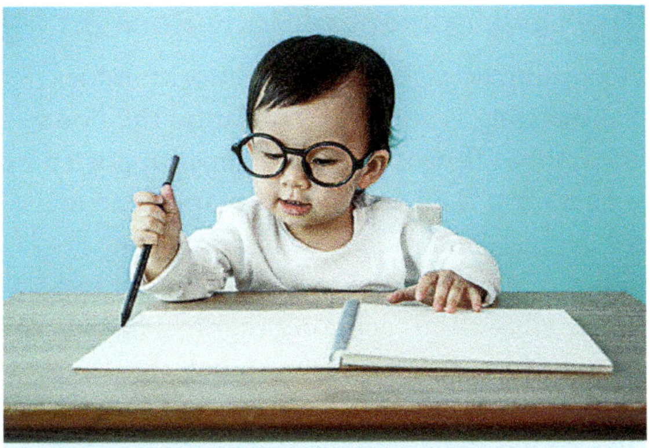

Figure 11.3 The supinate grasp is the first stage in holding a writing or drawing implement

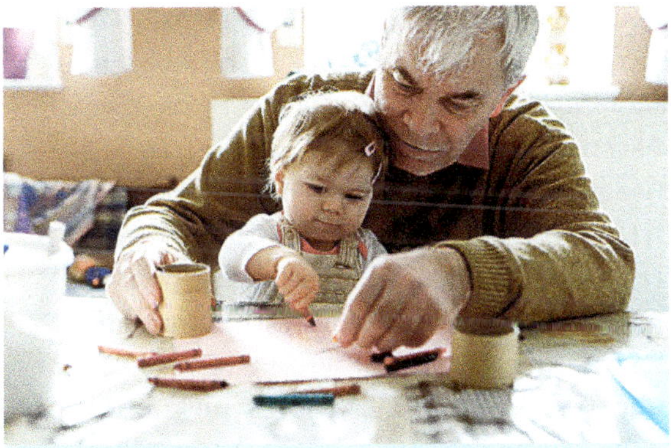

Figure 11.4 In the pronate grasp the hand is held with the palm down

an increasingly important role in the development of the child's handwriting or drawing technique. For example, very young children often use their nonwriting hand to adjust the writing implement. However, as the child's control over the fingers and thumb improves, that action becomes less important because the child can adjust the implement by using the fingers and thumb of the writing hand.

Generally, from 2 to 6 years of age, as the child's writing ability develops, the hand moves progressively closer to the tip of the pencil. Initially, a child holds the pencil a considerable distance from the tip as the movements emanate from the shoulder. Later, the elbow produces the movement necessary to propel the pencil. Finally, in proximodistal fashion, the fingers and thumb gain sufficient control and the child's pencil control improves. This improved level of movement technique, characterized by minute flexions and extensions of the hand joints involved in forming the tripod (discussed in the next section), emerges in most children when they are 4 to 6 years old. In most cases, the child has developed a rather mature dynamic tripod by 7 years of age (Rosenbloom & Horton, 1971).

The development of the dynamic tripod from 6 to 14 years of age. The mature grasp of the pencil or crayon is referred to as the **dynamic tripod.** This is a finger posture in which the thumb, middle finger, and index finger function as a tripod for the writing implement, enabling the child to perform small, highly coordinated movements of the implement. Figure 11.5 illustrates the dynamic tripod. This writing or drawing hand position typically develops from the simple tripod, in which the hand is positioned correctly but the small, coordinated movements common to the more mature dynamic tripod are lacking. The dynamic tripod is usually present by 7 years of age.

Few investigations have been conducted on fine motor development beyond childhood,

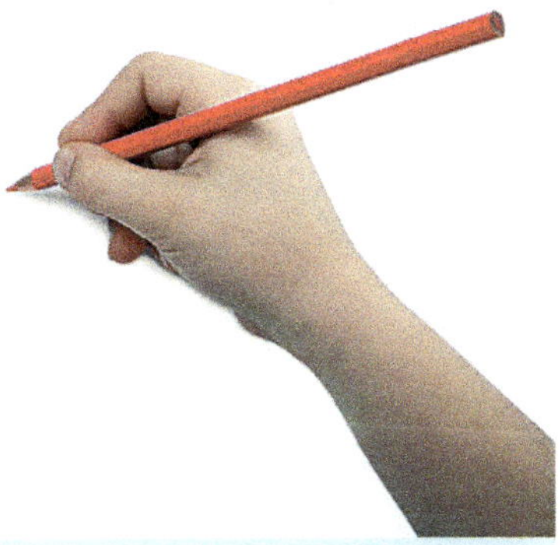

Figure 11.5 The dynamic tripod, the third and final stage of holding a writing or drawing implement. The thumb, middle finger, and index finger form a base for the implement

including the development of the dynamic tripod. Ziviani (1983) conducted one such study, examining the refinement of the dynamic tripod technique in children aged 6–14 years old. The researchers photographed subjects while they were writing and then rated them on four characteristics. The degree of flexion of the interphalangeal joint (large knuckle) of the writing forefinger was noted: if the flexion exceeded 90 degrees, the subject was assigned a score of 1; if the angle was less than 90 degrees, a score of 2 was assigned. The angle of forearm pronation/supination was also deemed a critical factor. If the forearm was supinated at less than 45 degrees, the subject was assigned a 1; a 2 was assigned for any other condition. Third, if any finger in addition to the index finger was used on the shaft of the pencil, the subject received a 1. If the thumb and index finger gripped the pencil and the pencil rested on the radial aspect (thumb side) of the middle finger, the subject was assigned a 2. Finally, if the fingers did not form a pad-to-pad opposition around the pencil, a 1 was assigned; if they did, a 2 was assigned.

With this method, Ziviani determined that for both index finger flexion and forearm pronation/supination, younger subjects had a significantly greater likelihood of scoring a 1 than their older counterparts. In other words, the younger subjects would be more likely to flex the index finger and to supinate the forearm excessively. The age of changing from the immature to mature characteristics on both the finger flexion and the forearm positioning was found to be approximately 10 years. The number of fingers that subjects used on the pencil and the pad-to-pad opposition were not found to be significantly age-related. In general, Ziviani concluded that the dynamic tripod does continue to be refined between the ages of 6 and 14 years.

The Development of Body Position

According to experts, an ideal position for handwriting is with the feet flat on the floor, the lumbar (lower) back and hips supported by a back rest, the knees flexed at approximately 90 degrees, and the elbow and forearm supported on the desktop, with a slight bend at the elbow. Intervention programs have been found to be effective at improving the legibility of writing (Feder & Majnemer, 2007).

De Ajuriaguerra, Auzias, Coumes, and associates (1979, as cited by Blote, 1988) determined that young children show clear developmental trends for body position while handwriting. For example, posture becomes more upright, and the position of the trunk becomes more stable. This stability reduces the need for support by distal body parts, which frees those parts for more mature writing-related movements. The hand also becomes more stable, and children learn to hold the hand below the line of writing instead of on the line. Children also increasingly position the hand in line with the forearm. Generally, children were found to become more economic in their writing style and to display a visible proximodistal trend. In other words, movements close to the body decreased in number and movements farther from the body became more common.

Additional research on the writing posture and writing movements of children from 5.5 to approximately 7.5 years of age found considerable, non-gender-related variations in children's writing development. However, as they aged, children generally tended to develop a mature arm and hand position. Table 11.1 gives percentages of children exhibiting specific handwriting characteristics. Interestingly, between the ages of about 6.5 and 7.5, children were also found to increase the amount of muscle tension in their writing. An extreme low, forward-leaning position also became

Table 11.1 Percentage of children 5.5 to 6.5 years old exhibiting certain handwriting characteristics

Characteristic	Percentage
Whole forearm on table	75
Upright body	81
Body not turned	80
Shoulders horizontal	85
Wrist in line with forearm	52
Wrist slightly extended	41
Paper perpendicular	51
Paper turned counterclockwise	30
Very low grip on pencil	53
Tripod grip	56
Proximal joint of index finger less than 90 degrees	53
Thumb opposing index finger	82
Pencil rests on:	
Third phalanx of middle finger	91
Second phalanx of middle finger	9
Tip of middle finger does not rest on shaft of pencil	87
No recurrent lifting of hand	90
No recurrent lifting of forearm	80

Source: Blote, Zielstra, and Zoetewey (1987).

prominent in many children. This position may allow improved visual inspection of the writing product and is believed to be related to an increased effort to improve the writing. Only one characteristic was found to be significantly gender-related: excessive flexion of the index finger was more common among boys than girls (Blote & van Der Heijden, 1988; Blote, Zielstra, & Zoetewey, 1987).

Drawing and Writing: Movement Products

As described earlier in the chapter, a sequential development occurs in children's technique for the manipulation of a pencil or any writing or drawing implement. This development is universal; only the rate of acquisition of the stages of this movement ability varies. This movement ability is called the *movement process*, and the result of the movement process is known as the *movement product*. This section examines the development of the movement product.

Drawing: The Product

Children typically "draw" before they attempt to form the letters necessary for handwriting. For that reason, early drawing is often considered a "prewriting phase" (Lin et al., 2015, p. 164). Like handwriting, drawing has served as a diagnostic tool for determining fine motor disorders. Drawing ability has been deemed partly a function of children's mental age, with rapid improvements generally occurring across the early school years. Most children initiate their drawing development as early as 15 to 20 months by producing scribbles that have no apparent organization or intended goal. In fact, the child's first attempt at scribbling may occur by accident. Upon being reinforced by the resulting scribbles, the child usually does additional scribbling but often shows signs of hesitancy. The scribbles soon become bolder as the child gains confidence. They also become less spontaneous, and the child begins to draw more slowly, attempting to control the movement of his or her hand visually while also pondering exactly what to create.

Following the collection and in-depth study of paintings by children, Kellogg (1969) proposed that drawing is a four-step process. The **scribbling stage** is the first step to acquisition of the hand-eye coordination necessary for drawing (see Figure 11.6). Step 2, according to Kellogg, is the creation of figures and combinations of figures. This **combine stage** begins with the construction of basic geometric shapes, such as spirals and simple crosses (see Figure 11.7). An example of the combine stage is the 2-year-old's drawing of a series of spiral figures or spirals and circles. The child then slowly develops sufficient understanding and motor control to create more precise figures, such as squares, rectangles, and triangles. Furthermore, the child becomes capable of drawing these shapes in combination with other shapes to form such things as simple houses and other familiar objects.

Step 3 in the development of the drawing product is what Kellogg (1969) refers to as the **aggregate stage** (see Figure 11.8). The child not only combines figures and shapes but does so in combinations of three or more. Of course, the increasing number of combinations of figures enables the child to create more complex drawings. This increasing ability culminates in the **pictorial stage** (see Figure 11.9), which is characterized by the increasing precision and complexity of the child's pictures. An example of this increasing complexity is the drawing of a human figure by an 8- or 9-year-old child who has learned to

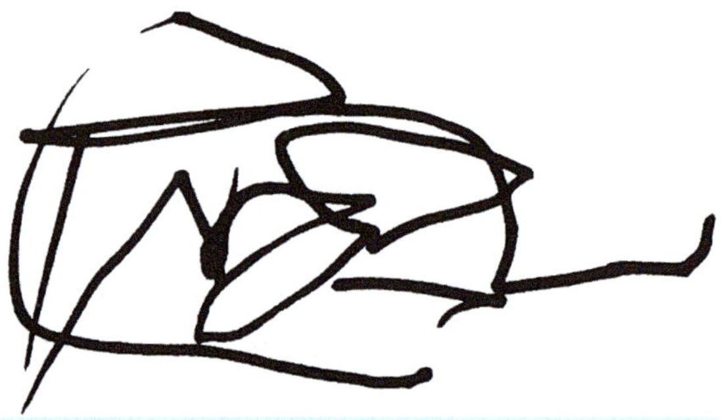

Figure 11.6 Scribbling stage: the first stage of drawing

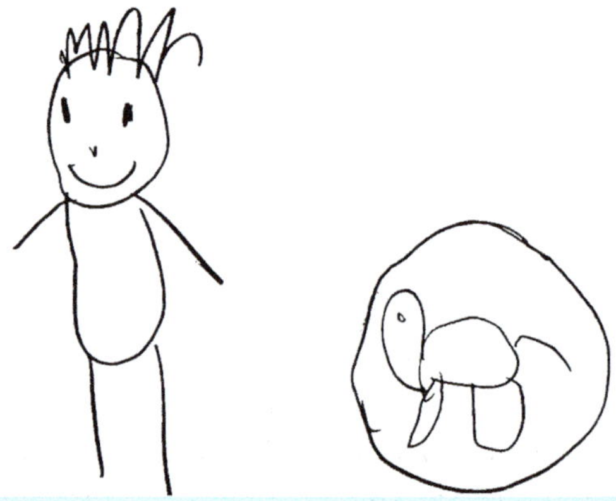

Figure 11.8 Aggregate stage: the child continues to combine figures, but in increasing numbers of combinations

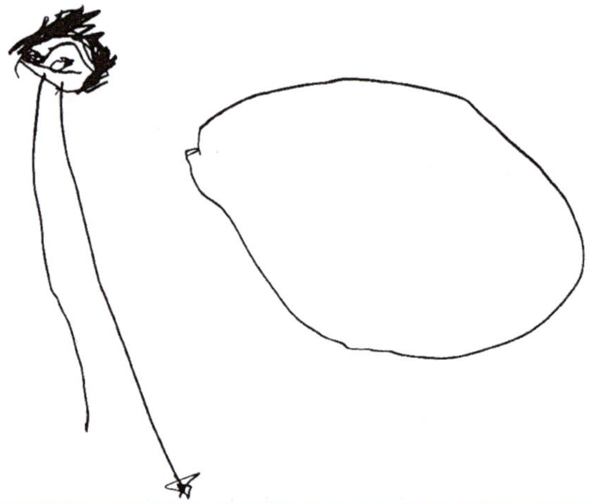

Figure 11.7 Combining stage: the child combines figures and shapes

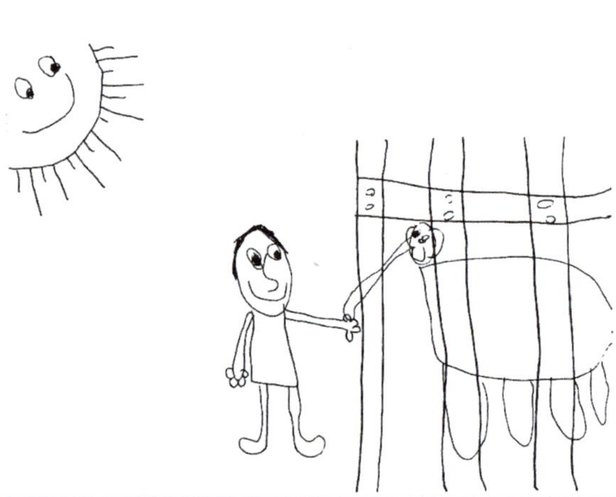

Figure 11.9 Pictorial stage, the last stage of drawing: The child draws with more precision and complexity

draw the figure with depth rather than as a stick figure, as in earlier artwork.

As Kellogg (1969) describes them, these four major stages form a progression that most children follow, but specific age norms for drawing are difficult to determine because a multitude of variables tremendously affect drawing. One of the most important of these is the home environment: children with a home environment conducive to drawing develop skills at an earlier age than average. Particularly notable components of the positive home environment are opportunities to observe other people drawing and availability of the necessary implements.

Children's drawing development has been extensively examined, and much research has explored the development of a specific type of children's drawing: design copying. Typically, this type of research requires children to reproduce a particular design. For example, Birch and Lefford (1967), in one of the most comprehensive examinations of design copying, asked children 5 to 11 years old to reproduce triangles and diamonds by tracing them, drawing them on a line grid, or drawing them freehand. In each case, the products improved and became more consistent as the subjects increased in age. A particularly dramatic increase in ability occurred from 5 to 6 years of age; the magnitude of improvement equaled that which occurs in most children between 6 and 11 years.

Generally, the children involved in this research found tracing to be the least difficult task. Next in order of increasing difficulty was drawing with the line grid, and freehand drawing was the most difficult task. The researchers concluded that tracing of triangles and diamonds was "mature" at 6 years of age for most subjects. Maturity in the line grid tasks occurred at 9 years of age, and freehand drawing of the triangle continued to improve through age 9. Freehand drawing of the diamond continued to improve through age 11, which was the highest age in the research.

Handwriting: The Product

Children at 4 years of age are usually capable of printing recognizable numbers or letters but often fail to organize them purposefully on the page (see Figure 11.10). Typically, the letters or numbers are randomly scattered over the page; they may also be written sideways or with an extreme slant.

By 5 or 6 years, however, the child has generally mastered name printing. The 5-year-old typically writes in large, irregularly shaped uppercase letters that become larger toward the end of the name. The letters of 5-year-old children generally are 0.5 to 2 in (1 to 5 cm) high. The 6-year-old may include the surname or pertinent initials but still writes in uneven uppercase letters, which are occasionally reversed. The letters the 6-year-old produces continue to be large, although they tend to be smaller than those most 5-year olds produce. By age 7, the child's letters have typically decreased in height to approximately 0.25 in (0.5 cm).

Children generally master the production of uppercase letters and name printing in the second grade, but the smaller lowercase letters continue to be difficult for many third-graders.

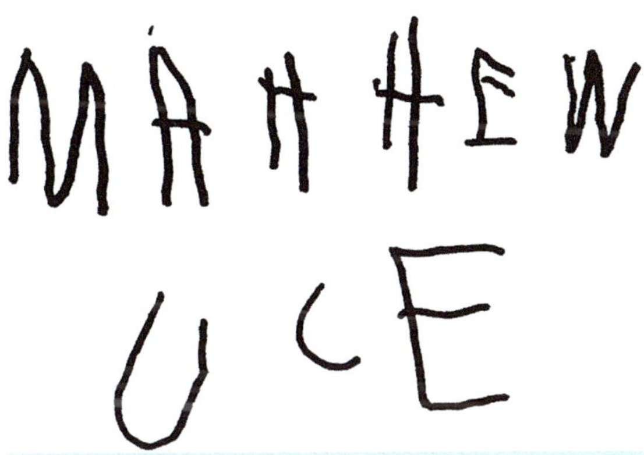

Figure 11.10 The letters a child forms when approximately 4 years old are often uppercase, large, and unorganized on the page

Children through third grade typically find single-stroke letters, such as *I, c*, and *s*, easier to form than multiple-stroke letters, such as *f, k*, and *t*. Also, letters formed from horizontal and vertical strokes, such as *E, T*, and *H*, are easier to write than letters that combine slants or curves with vertical or horizontal strokes, such as *K, B*, and *Z*. Finally, most children also find it difficult to space letters correctly, and this task often remains unmastered until children are approximately 9 years old (Cratty, 1986).

HANDWRITING AND DRAWING IN ADULTHOOD

Because the handwriting and drawing processes and products change so dramatically across the early childhood years, most research has focused on that development period. In fact, studies examining these processes in healthy adults are rare (van Drempt, McCluskey, & Lannin, 2011a). However, research interest in changes during adulthood has been increasing. In addition, though many technological advances have decreased people's general dependence on handwriting, this skill is still important for most adults for recording data and ideas, for communication, and even sometimes for creative expression. Unfortunately, as a result of declining health, the process of handwriting is often found to decline in later adulthood, especially with the onset of various neurological conditions (Dettrick-Janes, McCluskey, Lannin, & Scanlon, 2015).

In a review of adult handwriting development, Dettrick-Janes and colleagues (2015) studied the legibility of writing in healthy adults from 60 to 99 years of age. Participants were asked to write sentences, shopping lists, and transcribe a message taken over the phone. Whereas the quality of the legibility differed somewhat between writing tasks and as a result of the health of the individual, age did not seem to be higly correlated with the quality of the written product. The researchers noted that writing may become somewhat less "tidy," but it was not less legible. Interestingly, printing, rather than cursive style writing was employed in approximately one in ten particpants. In addition, a similar quality of writing was determined whether the participant used a pen or a pencil although pens yielded faster writing speed. Importantly, and in contrast to common beliefs, most declines in writing legibility are believed to be associated with medical conditions and not healthy aging (Dettrick-Janes et al., 2015). In a related study, another group of researchers examined handwriting in healthy people over the age of 65 years. The researchers used a questionnaire, digitized recordings of handwriting, and handwriting logs kept by participants. Although the participants rated the importance of handwriting as being high, they only wrote about three times per day on average with about 18 words per episode. The most common writing activities included note writing, working on puzzles, and list making. In almost all cases, when they wrote, they were seated. Participants showed significant variability in their handwriting, but it was almost always legible. Nearly 20 percent of the participants wrote quire clearly and most employed a writing style that included aspects of both printing and cursive style writing (van Drempt, McCluskey, & Lannin, 2011b).

Hoogendam and colleagues (2014) also examined drawing in a study involving nearly 2,000 Dutch adults ranging in age from their late forties to their mid-nineties, with the average age being just over 77 years. The researchers employed a drawing test to examine the relationship between age and fine movement ability. The participants were asked to trace a spiral drawing on an electronic tablet that recorded a number of important fine motor characteristics. Generally, older age was found to be strongly related to poorer performance on the tracing task. This was particularly notable in the participants who were 75 years old or older, where more substantial deviations from the drawing were noted. One exception was in the movement time: older tracers drew faster and completed the task in less time. Perhaps, this speed contributed to the older participants' number of errors. Like Reuter and colleagues' 2012 study on adults' fine movement and touch perception, Hoogendam's study demonstrated a notable decline in performance later in life. However, in this study, performance remained relatively stable to nearly 75 years of age, when the decline steepened.

KEYBOARDING

Considerable research has been conducted over the years on handwriting and drawing behaviors. However, handwriting is declining as keyboarding is increasing even among our youngest students, preschoolers. Though it is difficult to determine the exact extent of the decline, survey research has indicated that most adult respondents did not handwrite anything in the 41 days prior to taking the survey. Clearly, communication modes such as email and texting are gradually replacing handwritten notes and letters. Several states have even eliminated cursive writing (writing by using flowing strokes and connected letters) in their core educational curriculum. This move is somewhat controversial as many educational experts believe that writing taps a unique cognitive process that improves the efficient recognition of letters and ultimately facilitates learning to read (Chemin, 2014).

Much of the research regarding the impact of keyboarding on human development focuses on comparing keyboarding and handwriting. Berninger, Abbott, Augsberger, and Garcia (2009), for example, compared keyboarding to handwriting as modes of transcribing written information. Specifically, second-, fourth-, and sixth-graders performed three transcribing tasks by using both keyboarding and handwriting. The tasks included transcribing alphabet letters, sentences, and essays. In a 15-second timed test, all of the children produced more alphabet letters by keyboard than by handwriting. However, in a test that timed the production of all 26 alphabet letters, the second-graders required more time to produce the letters when they used the keyboard versus handwriting them, whereas the fourth- and sixth-graders produced the 26 letters faster by using the keyboard. All age groups took longer to transcribe the sentences and essays when they used the keyboard. Sentences that the fourth- and sixth-graders transcribed were found to be more complete when they were written by hand. Children from all three grades transcribed essays faster when they used a pen. In short, the keyboard was faster only for transcribing letters of the alphabet in a short timed test, and even then the second-graders began to require more time with the keyboard than with a pen as the number of letters to be transcribed increased.

In similar research conducted by Connelly, Gee, and Walsh (2007), 300 fifth- and sixth-grade schoolchildren showed a high degree of correlation between their keyboarding and handwriting speeds, with handwriting being consistently faster across both grades. Interestingly, the compositional quality of their written products was also determined to be superior when they were handwritten. These researchers further determined that a 2-year developmental delay existed in the quality of the subjects' keyboarded compositions when compared to their handwritten compositions. This was considered to indicate a need for more and better instruction in keyboarding.

In a study of individuals 16 years of age and older, Chen, White, McCloskey, and colleagues (2011) examined the effect of keyboarding versus handwriting on various writing responses. Their findings were quite similar to those reported in research with younger participants: better performance—including the actual quality of the content of the responses, as well as the speed of producing the responses—was seen overall when the subjects used handwriting versus keyboarding. Younger participants, however, who were generally found to be more experienced in computer use than their older counterparts, showed less negative impact when they used the computer keyboard versus handwriting, leading the researchers to conclude that the poorer overall performance on the keyboard may have been a function of the students' general lack of familiarity with the keyboard. If this is the case, we would expect to see these disparities between keyboarding and handwriting diminish over time as computer use continues to become more common for all age groups. As technology continues to provide alternatives to handwriting (e.g., touch screens, soft touch pads, and so forth), we can expect to see research on the characteristics of the specific movements involved and how these characteristics change from one age group to another.

SUMMARY

- *Fine movement* refers to those movements that are produced predominantly by the small muscles or small muscle groups of the body. These movements are important in and of themselves, but they also can impact children's academic performance, grooming, self-esteem, and communication.
- Manipulation, or use of the hands, is one of the most critical of the fine movements because individuals perform hundreds of manipulative movements each day. Reaching is the movement of the arm that delivers the grasping hand to the desired location. Grasping follows the reach and involves the opening and closing of the hand to acquire the desired object.
- In a frequently cited study, Halverson (1931) described the early reaching and grasping of 4- to 13-month-old infants. Halverson set forth three basic stages of development for reaching and defined a 10-stage progression for grasping. Generally, he noted a proximodistal progression.
- Research by Newell and associates (1989; 1993) has led to questioning of the "classic" work of Halverson. Newell's research examined adults' and children's reaching and grasping when the object size was scaled to the size of the subject's hand. The overall trend for grasping was quite similar for adult and child subjects, though some differences were noted. Object size was found to play a major role in the selection of grip patterns by both children and adults.
- Bushnell and Boudreau (1993) examined haptic perception, or the ability to glean information from objects via the hands. Properties that can be haptically perceived include temperature, size, texture, hardness, weight, and shape. Bushnell and Boudreau found that haptic perception is apparently a function of early ability in manipulation. The emergence of exploratory procedures, such as poking or unsupported holding of an object, was found to be linked to the development of haptic abilities. Thus, any early restriction of an infant's hand movements may restrict the infant's ability to learn about an object's properties. Once haptic abilities are achieved, they remain stable until quite late in life, when declines may occur. Declines in tactile sensing begin to occur

around age 45, with more severe declines seen later in life.

- The development of the hand position for holding a writing implement has been one of the most widely researched areas of fine movement. The first hand position that a child uses for grasping a pencil or crayon is usually a supinate grasp: a fist around the implement. This typically evolves into a pronate grasp, which is a palm-down position in which the fingers curl around the implement, with the index finger extending the length of the pencil or crayon and pointing toward the point. Finally, usually by 7 years of age, the child develops the dynamic tripod, a hand position that permits highly coordinated finger movements.
- Extensive studies by Kellogg (1969) led to the formulation of four major stages of drawing development, determined by the product of the act of drawing. Initially, children go through the scribbling stage, in which they simply scribble with no apparent objective in mind. In the combine stage, children create figures and combinations of figures. The third stage, the aggregate stage, is characterized by combinations of three or more figures. Finally, the pictorial stage is typified by pictures drawn with complexity and precision.
- As with drawing, the development of handwriting can be described by the product of the action. Researchers in this area have noted that recognizable letter writing is generally evident by 4 years of age, although there is little organization of the letters. By 5 or 6 years, children can print their name in large uppercase letters. By 7 years, children write much smaller letters and can effectively print lowercase letters.
- Though most handwriting research has been conducted on children, research interest in adults has been increasing. Older adults have been found to write less legibly than younger adults, and women tend to write faster than men. Adult writers exhibit a variety of hand positions, most of which generate legible and efficient writing. Adults demonstrate considerable variability in their handwriting product; many use a mixture of cursive and printing. The slowest handwriting was exhibited by adults over the age of 65 years. Research on adult drawing found performance in tracing tasks to remain relatively stable across age, up to the age of 75 years. For participants older than 75, age correlated to poorer performance in tracing.
- Although keyboarding is pervasive and replacing handwriting in many aspects of communication, much of the research to this point has focused on comparing keyboarding to handwriting as methods of transcribing information. As technology provides alternatives to keyboard use, further research will be needed on the movement involved with these alternatives.

key concept review

aggregate stage
combine stage
dynamic tripod
exploratory procedures
fine motor
haptic perception
manipulation
pictorial stage
prehension
pronate grasp
role-differentiated bimanual manipulation (RDBM)
scribbling stage
supinate grasp

questions for reflection

1. Explain the term *fine motor.*
2. Summarize the early work of Halverson. According to this researcher, how do reaching and grasping evolve over the first few years of life?
3. What is meant by "an alternative view of the development of prehension?" What are the key factors that make it "alternative?"
4. Summarize Lee, Liu, and Newell's (2006) longitudinal study on infant grasping.
5. What is haptic perception? Describe how it evolves over the first year of life.
6. What is the dynamic tripod? How does it differ from a supinate grasp or a pronate grasp? In which order do these positions typically appear during the first few years of life?
7. Describe the development of drawing as proposed by Kellogg. What are the stages of drawing development, and how would you describe each stage?
8. What is the difference between the drawing product and the drawing process? Give examples of each.
9. What do we know about handwriting development in adulthood?
10. What are some characteristics of drawing in later life?
11. What has research discovered about the differences in students' writing when they used keyboarding versus handwriting? How did the differences vary between younger and older students?

REFERENCES

Accardo, A. P., Genna, M., & Borean, M. (2013). Development, maturation and learning influence on handwriting kinematics. *Human Movement Science, 32*, 136–146.

Berninger, V. W., Abbott, R. D., Augsberger, A., & Garcia, N. (2009). Comparison of pen and keyboard transcription modes in children with and without learning disabilities. *Learning Disability Quarterly, 32*, 123–141.

Birch, H. G., & Lefford, A. (1967). Visual differentiation, intersensory integration, and voluntary motor control. *Monographs of the Society for Research in Child Development, 32.*

Blote, A. W. (1988). *The development of writing behavior.* Personal monograph.

Blote, A. W., & van Der Heijden, P. G. M. (1988). A follow-up study of writing posture and writing movement of young children. *Journal of Human Movement Studies, 14*, 57–74.

Blote, A. W., Zielstra, E. M., & Zoetewey, M. W. (1987). Writing posture and writing movement of children in kindergarten. *Journal of Human Movement Studies, 13*, 323–341.

Bushnell, E. W., & Boudreau, J. P. (1993). Motor development and the mind: The potential role of motor abilities as determinants of aspects of perceptual development. *Child Development, 64*, 1005–1021.

Case-Smith, J., Bigsby, R., & Clutter, J. (1998). Perceptual-motor coupling in the development of grasp. *American Journal of Occupational Therapy*, *52*(2), 102–110.

Chemin, A. (2014, December 16). Handwriting versus typing: Is the pen still mightier than the keyboard? *The Guardian.* Retrieved from www.theguardian.com/science/2014/dec/16/cognitive-benefits-handwriting-decline-typing.

Chen, J., White, S., McCloskey, M., Soroui, J., & Chen, Y. (2011). Effects of computer versus paper administration of an adult functional writing test. *Assessing Writing, 16*, 49–71.

Comuk-Balci, N., Bayoglu, B., Tekindal, A., Kerem-Gunel, M., & Anlar, B. (2016). Screening preschool children for fine motor skills: Environmental influence. *Journal of Physical Therapy Science*, doi: 10.1589/jpts.28.1026.

Connelly, V., Gee, D., & Walsh, E. (2007). A comparison of keyboarded and handwritten compositions and the relationship with transcription speed. *British Journal of Educational Psychology, 77*, 479–492.

Cratty, B. J. (1986). *Perceptual and motor development in infants and children.* 3rd ed. Englewood Cliffs, NJ: Prentice-Hall.

Daum, M. M., & Gredeback, G. (2011). The development of grasping comprehension in infancy: Covert shifts of attention caused by referential actions. *Experimental Brain Research, 208*, 297–307.

Dettrick-Janes, M., McCluskey, A., Lannin, N. A., & Scanlan, J. N. (2015). Handwriting legibility in healthy older adults. *Physical and Occupational Therapy in Geriatrics*, doi.org.libaccess.sjlibrary.org/10.3109/02703181.2015.1037978.

De Ajuriaguerra, J., Auzias, M., Coumes, F., Denner, A., Lavondes-Monod, V., Perron, R., et al. (1979). *Children's handwriting: The development of handwriting and problems in handwriting*. Paris: Delachauz et Niestle.

Dinehart, L. H. (2014). Handwriting in early childhood education: Current research and future implications. *Journal of Early Childhood Literacy*. doi: 10.1177/1468798414522825.

Feder, K. P., & Majnemer, A. (2007). Handwriting development, competency, and intervention. *Developmental Medicine and Child Neurology, 49*, 312–317.

Feng, L., Lindner, A., Ji, X. R., & Joshi, R. M. (2019). The roles of handwriting and keyboarding in writing: A meta-analytic review. *Reading and Writing, 32*, 33–63.

Gaul, D., & Issartel, J. (2016). Fine motor skill proficiency in typically developing children: On or off the maturation track? *Human Movement Science, 46*, 78–85.

Gonzalez, S. L., & Nelson, E. L. (2015). Addressing the gap: A blueprint for studying bimanual hand preference in infants. *Frontiers in Psychology*, doi: 10.3389/fpsyg.2015.00560.

Gori, M., Squeri, V., Sciutti, A., Masia, L., Sandini, G., & Konczak, J. (2012). Motor commands in children interfere with their haptic perception of objects. *Experimental Brain Research*. doiL10.1007/s00221-012-3248-8.

Halverson, H. M. (1931). An experimental study of prehension in infants by means of systematic cinema records. *Genetic Psychology Manuscripts, 10*, 107–286.

Hoogendam, Y. Y., van der Lijn, F., Vernooij, M. W., Hofman, A., Niessen, W. J., et al. (2014). Older age relates to worsening of fine motor skills: A population-based study of middle-aged and elderly persons. *Frontiers in Aging Neuroscience, 6*. doi: 10.3389/fnagi.2014.00259.

Jao, R. J., James, T. W., & James, K. H. (2014). Multisensory convergence of visual and haptic object preference across development. *Neuropsychologia, 56*, 381–392.

Karl, J. M., & Whishaw, I. Q. (2014). Haptic grasping configurations in early infancy reveal different developmental profiles for visual guidance of the reach versus the grasp. *Experimental Brain Research, 232*, 3301–3316.

Kellogg, R. (1969). *Analyzing children's art*. Palo Alto, CA: Mayfield.

Lederman, S. J., & Klatzky, R. L. (1987). Hand movement: A window into haptic object recognition. *Cognitive Psychology*, 22, 421–459.

Lee, M. H., Liu, Y. T., & Newell, K. M. (2006). Longitudinal expression of infants' prehension as a function of object properties. *Infant Behavior and Development*, *29*, 481–493.

Lin, Q., Luo, J. L., Wu, Z., Shen, F., & Sun, Z. (2015). Characterization of fine motor development: Dynamic analysis of children's drawing movements. *Human Movement Science, 40*, 163–175.

Lobo, M. A., Kokkoni, E., de Campos, A. C., & Galloway, J. C. (2014). Not just playing around: Infants' behaviors with objects reflect ability, constraints, and object properties. *Infant Behavior and Development*, *37*, 334–351.

Maldarelli, J. E., Kahrs, B. A., Hunt, S. C., & Lockman, J. (2015). Development of early handwriting: Visual-motor control during letter copying. *Developmental Psychology*. doi: 10.1037/a0039424.

Mounoud, P., & Bower, T. G. R. (1974). Conservation of weight in infants. *Cognition*, *3*, 29–40.

Newell, K. M., McDonald, P. V., & Baillargeon, R. (1993). Body scale and infant grip configurations. *Developmental Psychobiology*, *26*(4), 195–205.

Newell, K. M., Scully, D. M., & McDonald, P. V. (1989). Task constraints and infant grip configurations. *Developmental Psychobiology*, *22*(8), 817–832.

Newell, K. M., Scully, D. M., Tenenbaum, F., & Hardiman, S. (1989). Body scale and the development of prehension. *Developmental Psychobiology*, *22*(1), 1–13.

Palmis, S., Danna, J., Velay, J., & Longcamp, P. (2017). Motor control of handwriting in the developing brain: A review. *Cognitive Neuropsychology*, *34*, 187–204.

Paulus, M., & Hauf, P. (2012). Reaching preferences in 11-month-old infants: The role of objects' material and weight. *International Journal of Developmental Science*, 6, 87–96.

Piek, J. P., Baynam, G. B., & Barrett, C. (2006). The relationship between fine and gross motor ability, self-perceptions and self-worth in children and adolescents. *Human Movement Science*, *25*, 65–75.

Ransburg, N., Reiser, M., Munzert, J., Jovanovic, B., & Schwarzer, G. (2017). Concurrent anticipation of two object dimensions during grasping in 10-month-old infants: A quantitative analysis. *Infant Behavior and Development*, *48*, 164–174.

Reuter, E., Voelcker-Rehage, C., Vieluf, S., & Godde, B. (2012). Touch perception throughout working life: Effects of age and expertise. *Experimental Brain Research*, *216*, 287–297.

Rosenbloom, L., & Horton, M. E. (1971). The maturation of fine prehension in young children. *Developmental Medicine and Child Neurology*, *13*, 38.

Scharoun, S. M., & Bryden, P. J. (2015). Is strength of handedness reliable over repeated testing? An examination of typical development and autism spectrum disorder, *Frontiers in Psychology*, *6*. doi: 10.3389/fpsyq.2015.00017.

Sgandurra, G., Cecchi, F., Serio, S. M., Del Maestro, M., Laschi, C., Dario, P., et al. (2012). Longitudinal study of unimanual grasping forces during infancy. *Infant Behavior and Development*, *35*, 205–214.

Skrzek, A., Pridalová, M., Sebastjan, A., Harásková, D., Fugiel, J., Ignasiak, Z., et al. (2015). Fine motor skills of the hands in Polish and Czech female senior citizens from different backgrounds. *Aging Clinical and Experimental Research*, *27*, 491–498.

van Drempt, N., McCluskey, A., & Lannin, N. A. (2011a). A review of factors that influence adult handwriting performance. *Australian Occupational Therapy Journal*, *58*, 321–328.

van Drempt, N., McCluskey, A., & Lannin, N. A. (2011b). Handwriting in healthy people aged 65 years and over. *Australian Occupational Therapy Journal*, *58*, 276–286.

Ziviani, J. (1983). Qualitative changes in dynamic tripod grip between seven and fourteen years of age. *Developmental Medicine and Child Neurology*, *25*, 778–782.

12 FUNDAMENTAL LOCOMOTION SKILLS OF CHILDHOOD

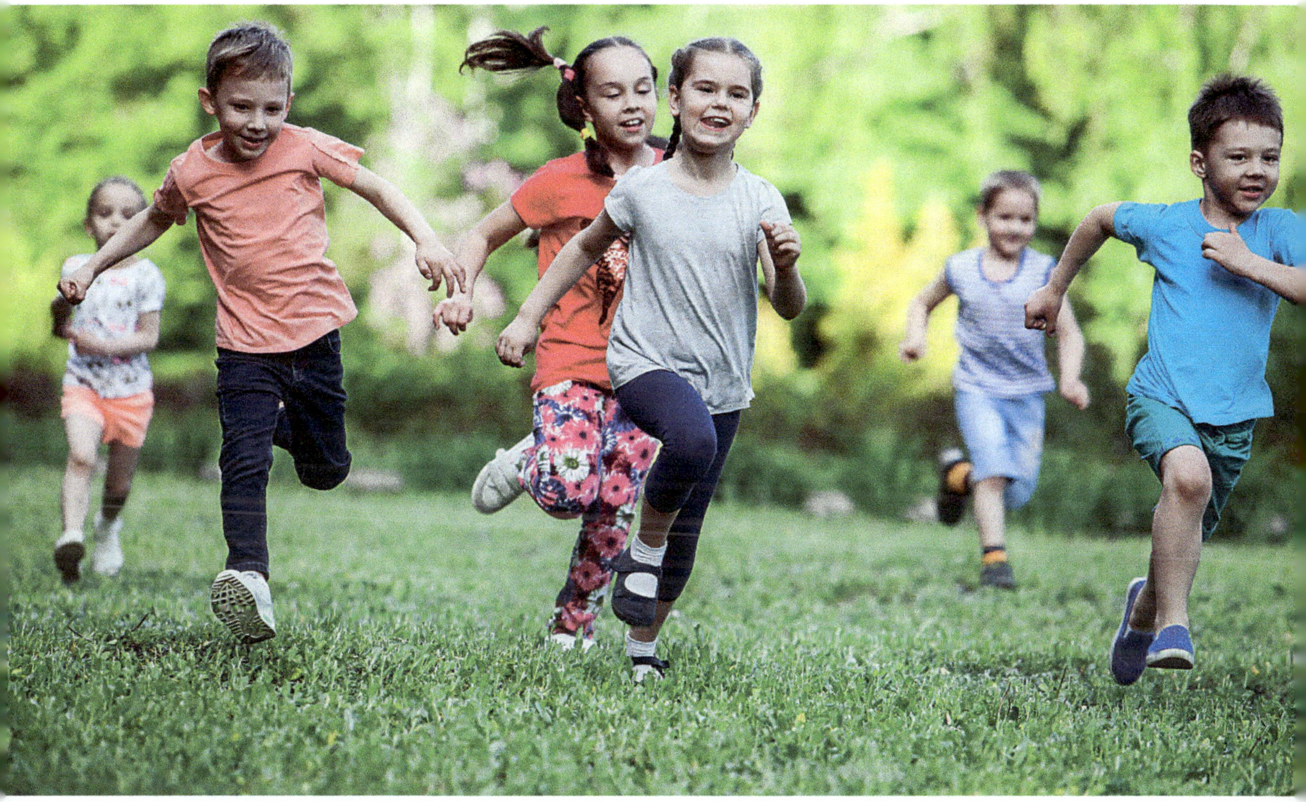

Chapter Objectives

From the information presented in this chapter, you will be able to

- Describe the developmental milestones associated with both immature and mature independent walking
- Describe the developmental milestones associated with both immature and mature running
- Describe the developmental milestones associated with jumping, including the standing long jump, vertical jump, and hopping
- Describe the mature combination of movements that results in the development of galloping, sliding, and skipping
- Describe the constraints that influence the development of the fundamental locomotion skills of walking, running, and jumping

Children's motor repertoires greatly expand during the second year of life. At this time, children no longer have to rely on rudimentary motor behaviors to locomote, explore, and manipulate objects in their environment. They begin to develop and use fundamental locomotion skills that include walking, running, jumping, and hopping. In addition, when several of these skills are combined, galloping, sliding, and skipping emerge. These skills can be thought of as the building blocks of the more specific skills developed later in childhood.

At the end of the first year or at the beginning of the second year, children are capable of walking without support, and soon thereafter running is evident. In turn, as soon as children are capable of momentarily propelling themselves through space, as running requires, they will also be capable of performing some type of jumping and hopping maneuver. As their strength, balance, and motor coordination improve, combination patterns will appear. These combination patterns include galloping, sliding, and skipping.

This chapter reviews the development of these fundamental skills of locomotion and explores factors that may affect this development.

WALKING

The onset of independent **walking** or **upright bipedal locomotion** has far-reaching ramifications for infants. As soon as infants can walk alone, their hands are free to explore. This new posture also allows infants to see the world differently (Kretch, Franchak, & Adolph, 2014) as they can cover more space and better interact in their environment and with their caregivers (Adolph & Tamis-LeMonda, 2014).

This form of locomotion is characterized by a progressive alternation of the leading leg and continuous contact with the supporting surface. The walking cycle or **gait cycle** is the distance covered by two heel strikes of the same foot and consists of two distinct phases: a **swing phase** and a stance or **support phase**. The swing phase begins when the foot or toes of one leg leave the supporting surface and ends when the heel or foot of the same leg recontacts the ground. The time when balance is maintained on only one foot is the support phase. Thus, while the right foot is in the swing phase, the left foot is in the support phase. When both feet are in contact with the supporting surface, the walker is in a **double support phase**.

Developmental Aspects of Walking

Even though walking is one of the most highly automatized motor acts that adults perform, the same is not true for the walking infant. An infant's initial attempt at unsupported walking has little in common with typical adult walking because to achieve independent walking, the infant must overcome two major constraints. Not only must infants have sufficient leg strength to support the body's weight, but they must also be capable of maintaining a state of equilibrium. Both of which are influenced by changes in body dimensions experienced during physical growth (Adolph & Avolio, 2000). Hence, many of the observable characteristics of initial walking occur to increase stability and leg strength (Adolph, Vereijken, & Shrout, 2003); Table 12.1 provides additional information regarding selected concepts in balance development.

The initial movement pattern of independent walking is characterized by short, quick, rigid steps; the toes point outward, and the infant assumes a wide base of support. In addition, the infant makes a flat-footed contact with the ground instead of the heel-toe contact of an adult gait. In a further attempt to maintain stability, the infant carries the arms in a high guard position. Also, the infant keeps the arms rigid; they do not swing freely in opposition to the legs. This independent walking pattern is

Table 12.1 Selected concepts in balance development

∞ **Balance**, sometimes referred to as **postural control**, is a state of equilibrium.
∞ There are two types of balance. **Static balance** is the ability to maintain a desired body posture when the body is stationary. If the body is in motion, balance is referred to as **dynamic balance**.
∞ Balance is task-specific and affected by a multitude of variables (body position, body dimensions, and so forth); thus, it cannot accurately be assessed by any one test.
∞ Balance is affected by somatic developmental changes such as foot length, width of base of support, and height of center of mass above the base of support.
∞ Static balance has been found to be strongly related to the ability to perceive and process visual information important to balance (Hatzitaki, Zisi, Kollias, & Kioumourtzoglou, 2002).
∞ One study found that balance was correlated negatively with body fat as measured by body weight, body mass index, percentage fat, and total fat mass. This may explain, in part, why performers who are overweight often have poorer balance than do those with a healthy weight (Goulding, Jones, Taylor, et al., 2003).

Table 12.2 Selected walking characteristics and their ages of appearance

Characteristic	Appearance*	Range*
Heel strike	22.6	3–50
Base within lateral dimensions of trunk	17.5	5–43
Synchronous movement of upper extremities	21.6	6–43
Double knee lock	27.2	8–55

Note: *Weeks after the onset of independent walking.

Source: Based on Burnett and Johnson (1971).

apparent in most children by 12 months of age, and the typical range is from 9 to 17 months. Table 12.2 summarizes certain walking characteristics and their ages of appearance. During the next two to six years, many gradual changes occur within each gait parameter as the child progressively assumes a more adult-like style of walking (Adolph et al., 2003).

Dynamic Base

To maintain balance during initial walking attempts, the infant places the feet apart to widen the base of support (see Figure 12.1). As balance improves, the child brings the feet closer together. This base of support is brought within the lateral dimensions of the trunk by, on average, 17.5 weeks after the onset of independent walking (Burnett & Johnson, 1971). Bril and Breniere (1992) report that the average stepping width is 9 in (23 cm) at the start of independent walking; this narrows to 6 in (15 cm) about 6 months later. The width continues to narrow until it reaches 4 in (10 cm) by the end of the second year of independent walking.

Foot Angle

Foot angle is the amount of toeing-out or toeing-in. In general, the degree of toeing-out decreases during the first four years of life and then remains fairly stable during the teens. In contrast, toeing-in is rare and considered atypical.

Walking Speed

Walking speed, another gait parameter, is determined by the length of the stride and the speed of the stepping movements. Each measure differs depending on whether the walking movements are performed with or

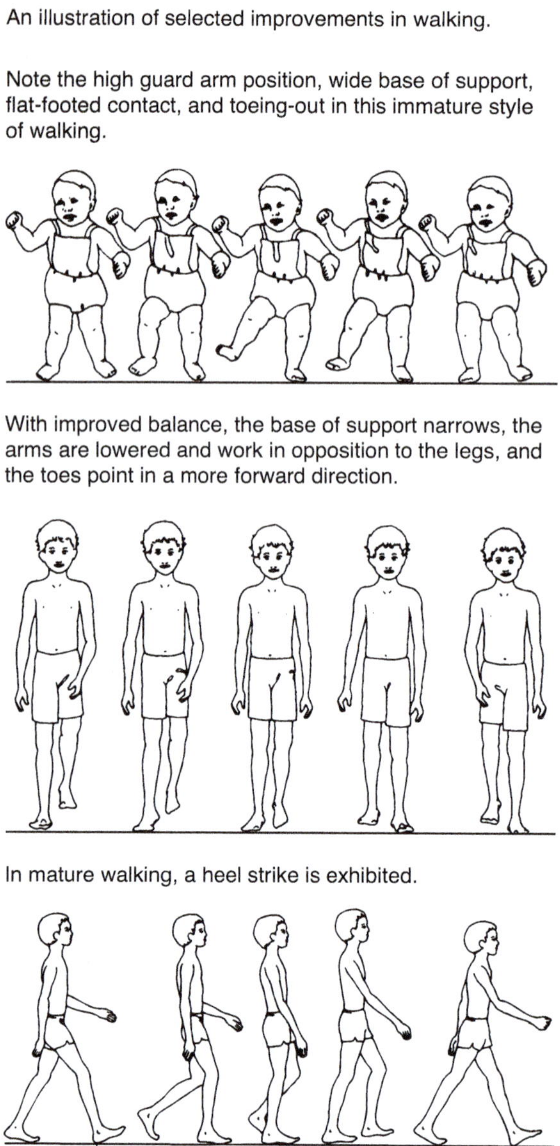

Figure 12.1 An illustration of selected improvements in walking

without support. In fact, when support minimizes their postural requirements, infants show well-coordinated stepping patterns months before the onset of independent walking (Thelen, 1986). Among the seven children Thelen studied, both step frequency and walking speed were greater in independent walking as compared with supported walking, although there was much variability. While observing five children over a two-year period, Bril and Breniere (1992) noted a threefold increase in walking speed in the first six months of independent walking. Furthermore, when these infants first began to walk, increases in their walking speed were attributable mostly to increased step length. This finding had been noted earlier by Phillips and Clark (1987). After five months of independent walking, however, the pattern reversed so that increases in walking speed were attributable primarily to an increased walking cadence. Keogh and Sugden (1985) reported the average cadence for toddlers as 180–200 footfalls per minute, a finding that has been confirmed by Adolph and colleagues (2003). In contrast to the toddler's cadence, a practical adult step cadence is between 100 and 130 footfalls per minute (Tudor-Locke, Aguiar, Han, et al., 2018; Tudor-Locke, Han, Aguiar, et al., 2019). In short, step frequency decreases with advancing age.

Among infants, a lack of neuromuscular control precludes any successful attempt at increasing walking speed by increasing step length. Hence, until the infant gains sufficient neuromuscular control, he or she must take more steps per unit of time to increase walking speed. With age, gains in neuromuscular postural control partly contribute to longer steps.

One older study that illustrates differences in step length, stride length, step frequency, and walking speed was conducted at San Diego Children's Hospital (Sutherland, 1984). Table 12.3 summarizes the findings. Briefly, the researchers concluded that most observable gait changes occur by 3 years of age. In fact, they found little difference between the walking patterns of 3- and 7-year-old children, with the exception of diminished stride length and a fairly high step frequency for younger children. In addition, the average 3-year-old child displayed adult-like joint-rotation characteristics. However, Hausdorff, Zemany, Peng, et al. (1999) have shown that stride

Table 12.3 Selected walking parameters with advancing age

Gait parameter				
Age (years)	Step length (cm)	Stride length (cm)	Steps/minute	Walking speed (cm/s)
1	21.6	43.0	175.7	63.7
2	27.5	54.9	155.8	71.8
3	32.9	67.7	153.5	85.5
7	47.9	96.5	143.5	114.3
Adult (19–40)	65.5	129.4	114.0	121.6

Source: Based on Sutherland (1984).

dynamics mature at different ages and may not be completely mature even in 7-year-old children.

Constraints on the Development of Independent Walking

As described in Chapter 9, shortly after birth the infant is capable of exhibiting leg movements that closely resemble walking. However, independent walking is generally not accomplished until about 12 months of age. The characteristics of early attempts at independent walking—a wide base of support, toes pointing outward, quick and short steps, arms carried in the high guard position, and flat-footed contact with the supporting surface—are all in part results of constraints involving the need to improve both muscular strength and balance. The next sections examine these two major constraints, as well as some of the other most important constraints that have been identified for infant walking.

Muscular Strength

Although the infant is capable of moving the legs in an alternating sequence, the legs, hips, and postural muscles are not initially strong enough to support the body's weight, nor are they strong enough to maintain an upright posture. It is likely that the prone locomotion (creeping and crawling) that precedes independent walking serves in part as a physical conditioning exercise to facilitate the development of strength in these muscle groups. The work of Thelen, Ulrich, and Jensen (1989) suggests that for independent walking to be accomplished, adequate muscular strength must exist in both the trunk and the extensor muscles to maintain an upright posture. Once an upright posture is achieved, then (as compared to prone locomotion) a greater proportion of the body's weight is placed on the legs, especially during the swing phase of independent walking, when the infant must possess enough strength to support the body's weight on one leg alone. Thus, independent walking improves with walking experience because it, in part, services to increase muscular strength (Adolph et al., 2003).

Balance

In addition to the muscular strength needed to support the body's weight and to maintain an upright posture, a lack of balance is also a constraint on the development of independent walking. One study found that during free play, infants between 12 and 19 months of age would fall 17 times per hour (Adolph, Cole, Komati, et al., 2012). With upright locomotion, compared to prone locomotion, the infant is required to operate from a much smaller base of support—from two points of contact (the feet) with the supporting surface, as compared to the four points of contact during prone locomotion. Also, recall from Chapter 6 the discussion of physical growth in bodily proportions. Remember that the infant has a relatively high center of gravity due to the relatively large contribution of the head and trunk to total stature. This high center of gravity, coupled with a small base of support, makes balance very challenging for the infant. The task of walking becomes even more difficult because the child must master dynamic balance in order to transfer its weight from leg to leg during walking. It appears that the prewalking voluntary movement of "walking with handholds" is the infant's way of accomplishing the goal of walking while still in the process of developing dynamic balance.

Walking with External Loads

Researchers have examined the influence of carrying an external load on changes in gait patterns in young children and adolescents (Vaghela, Parekh, Padsala, & Patel, 2019; Whittfield, Legg, & Hedderley, 2005). This line of research has been popularized because of the increasing number of children who complain of back and shoulder pain as a result of carrying heavy backpacks to school, especially backpacks or athletic bags that are carried on only one shoulder. In fact, in one study, 51 percent of the young participants reported back pain (Pascoe, Pascoe, Wang, et al., 1997) and this back pain is more frequent in girls (Cottalorda, Bourelle, & Gautheron, 2004). To examine the influence of external loading and changes in gait patterns during walking, Hong and Brueggemann (2000) required 10-year-old boys to walk on a treadmill while carrying backpack loads of 0 percent (control), 10 percent, 15 percent, and 20 percent of their body weight. Findings indicated that the 20 percent load was responsible for inducing a significant increase in trunk forward lean, an increase in double support and stance durations, and a decrease in trunk angular motion and swing duration. In comparison, the 15 percent load induced a significant increase only in forward lean. No significant differences in gait characteristics were found between the 10 percent and the 0 percent load conditions. As a result, the researchers suggested that backpack weight should not exceed 10 percent of body weight in these young children. This 10 percent of body weight limitation continues to be confirmed in both American and European children (Chen & Mu, 2018; Walicka-Cupry, Skalska-Izdebska, Rachwal, et al., 2015). However, it is alarming that one critical review of 21 studies has found that students on average are utilizing backpacks that generally exceed 15 percent of body weight (Perrone, Orr, Hing, et al., 2018). It appears that the mean backpack weight for children in the United States is approximately 17 percent of mean body weight (Pascoe, et al., 1997); while in Hong Kong it averages 20 percent (Hong, & Grueggemann, 2000).

Researchers in India (Gupta, Kalra, & Iqbal, 2018) have now developed a modified backpack which contains an internal frame designed to evenly distribute the load and allow for greater freedom of movement, all while keeping the load closer to the spine. Preliminary research has found that the use of this modified backpack resulted in a more erect posture, a natural gait, and reduced energy expenditure.

Footwear and Clothing

Footwear is known to influence walking characteristics in both adults and older adults, but little is known of its impact on young children. To examine the influence of footwear on walking characteristics of young children, Ledebt, Rosier, and Savelsbergh (2005) examined the walking of 62 children between 1 and 4 years of age without shoes and with four types of shoes: low cut-supple collar, low cut-stiff collar, high cut-supple collar, and high cut-stiff collar. The authors concluded that walking with shoes of any type caused young walkers to exhibit a more mature walking gait with longer steps and better dynamic balance. Using a meta-analysis design, Wegener and colleagues (2011) concluded that wearing shoes results in faster walking, longer steps, and reduced foot motion in subjects between 2 and 15 years of age. Similarly, clothing, including diapers, underwear, diaper plus trousers, and diaper plus track suit pants, has been found to influence independent walking in toddlers between 6 and 18 months of age (Théveniau, Boisgontier, Varieras, & Olivier, 2014). More specifically, the authors concluded that these types of clothing appear to constrain both step length and walking speed.

RUNNING

Running is sometimes referred to as a natural extension of walking. This form of human locomotion is characterized by an alternate support phase and an airborne or **flight phase**. This flight phase is what most readily distinguishes running from walking (see Figure 12.2).

On average, children begin to exhibit minimal running from somewhere between 6 and 7 months after the onset of independent walking (Whitall & Getchell, 1995), in other words, between the 18th and 19th months of life. As children acquire increased lower-limb strength, improved balance, and, finally, improved motor control, their running pattern becomes more adult-like.

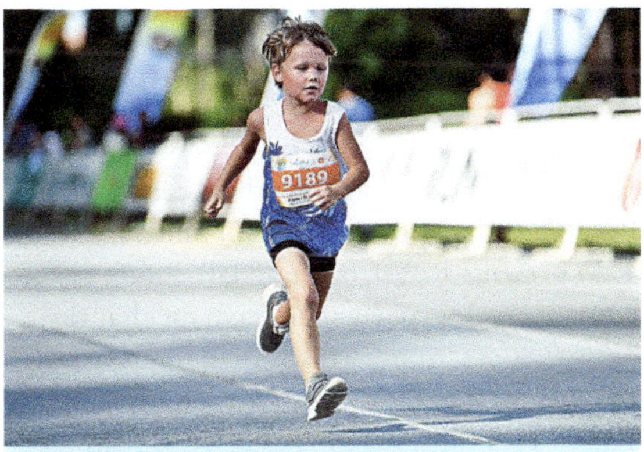

Figure 12.2 Running—the flight phase

Developmental Aspects of the Running Pattern

A close examination of the running pattern reveals that each running cycle consists of three phases: the support phase, the flight phase, and the recovery phase. The arms play an important role. This section examines in detail certain developmental changes that occur in the running cycle.

Support Phase and Flight Phase

In the support phase, the leg absorbs the impact of the striking foot, supports the body, and maintains forward motion while accelerating the body's center of gravity as the leg provides thrust to propel the body forward. The inexperienced runner performs the foot strike with the full sole. As running form improves, the part of the foot that hits the ground moves toward the ball of the foot.

Inexperienced runners are incapable of projecting the body through space for any significant distance because they do not effectively use the thrust leg. The progressive developmental trend of the thrust leg calls for more involvement of the hip, knee, and ankle to provide full extension to generate maximum thrust. This increased extension of the segments of the thrust leg becomes more evident with increasing age.

Recovery Phase

Once the body has been thrust into the air by the vigorous extension of the support leg, the support leg enters a phase of recovery. This leg, which has been projected backward, must be quickly brought forward to repeat its function in the next running cycle. There are obvious developmental trends in how the recovery leg is brought forward.

The experienced runner flexes the knee so the heel of the foot of the recovery leg comes very close to making contact with the buttock. The knee and thigh are then swung forward until the thigh is practically parallel with the running surface. This thigh position is usually reached the moment the support foot leaves the supporting surface. While the body is airborne, the knee of the forward leg is extended, thus allowing the foot to descend toward the running surface. The experienced runner does not place the foot so far in front of his or her center of gravity as to produce a braking effect.

In contrast, the inexperienced runner does not achieve a degree of knee flexion sufficient to bring the heel close to the buttock. Similarly, insufficient hip flexion keeps the thigh from forming a right angle with the body's trunk. In fact, because of this insufficient knee and hip flexion, the inexperienced runner frequently stumbles because there is not adequate clearance between the foot and ground during the recovery phase. Frequently, the inexperienced runner resorts to turning the toes inward or outward to create sufficient foot-ground clearance during the forward swing of the recovery leg.

Arm Actions

The arms play an important role in contributing to running form and performance. During the child's first attempts at running, the arms are flexed in the high guard position to aid balance and do not work in opposition to the legs. In a slightly more adult-like pattern, the arms are lowered and generally hang free but still do not contribute to speed by working in opposition to the legs. Furthermore, when the beginning runner is observed from the front, it is evident that the arms hook or swing across the body's midline, causing inefficient trunk rotation.

In contrast, the experienced runner uses the arms in opposition to the legs. The elbows are flexed at 90 degrees, and a vigorous pumping action of the arms toward but not across the body's midline fosters forward momentum.

Constraints on the Development of Running

As with walking, children must overcome constraints on the development of running, and once again the two most important constraints are muscular strength and balance. Because running requires an airborne or flight phase, the child must possess muscular strength in each leg, enough to propel the child's body through the air. Obviously, excess body weight (body fat) can negatively influence the child's ability to become airborne (Fredriksen, Mamen, Gammelsrud, et al., 2018). Furthermore, additional strength is needed to absorb the force encountered when the airborne foot strikes the landing surface. The magnitude of this impact can exceed three to four times the child's body weight.

At first, running may exhibit many characteristics of an immature walk: a wide base of support, arms held in a high guard position, and flat-footed contact with the supporting surface. Reverting to this immature pattern is the child's way of temporarily improving balance while gaining confidence in performing this new movement.

Developmental Sequences for Running

Researchers have suggested that there are developmental sequences for running. Table 12.4 presents Roberton and Halverson's (1984) component approach analysis. Note that this approach describes changes that are expected to occur within each body segment. In contrast, Figure 12.3 illustrates the total body approach for describing the developmental sequences of running. In this approach, the total body

Stage 1 The arms are extended sideward at shoulder height (high guard position). The stride is short and of shoulder width. The surface contact is made with the entire foot, striking simultaneously. Little knee flexion is seen. The feet remain near the surface.

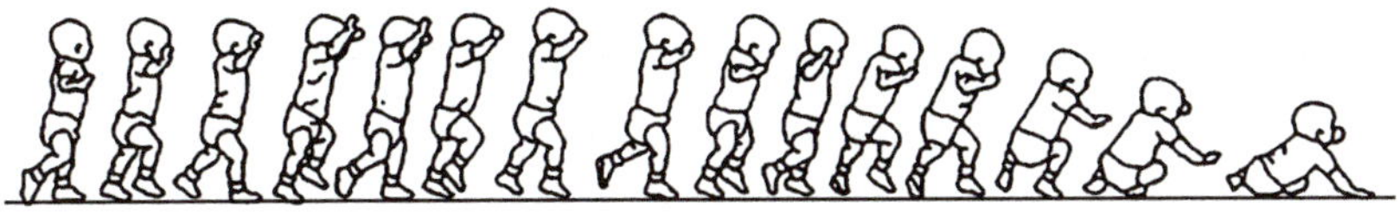

Stage 2 Arms are carried at middle guard position (waist high). The stride is longer and approaches the midsagittal line. The surface contact is usually made with the entire foot, striking simultaneously. Greater knee flexion is noted in the restraining phase. The swing leg is flexed, and the movement of the legs becomes anterior-posterior.

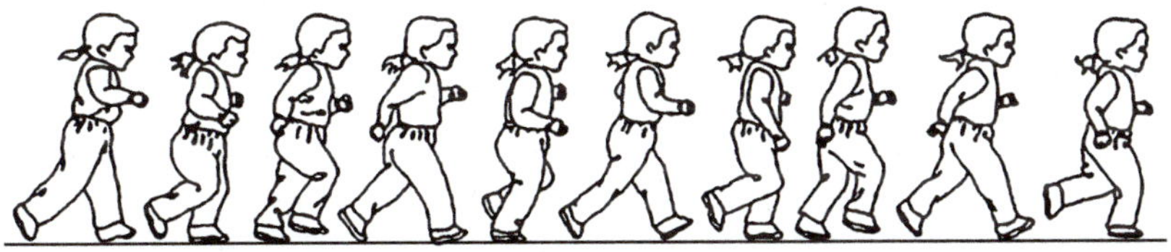

Stage 3 The arms are no longer used primarily for balance but rather are carried below waist level and may flex and assume a counter-rotary action. The foot contact is heel-toe. Stride length increases, and both feet move along a midsagittal line. The swing-leg flexion may be as great as 90°.

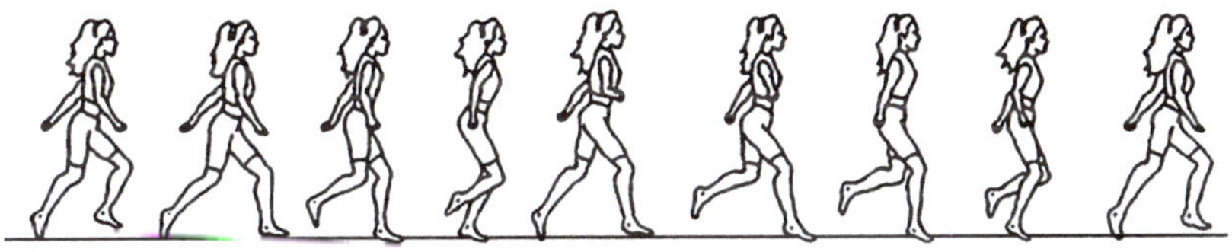

Stage 4 Foot contact is heel-toe at slow or modest velocities but may be entirely on the metatarsal arch while sprinting. Arm action is in direct opposition to leg action. Knee flexion is used to maintain the momentum during the support phase. The swing leg may flex until it is nearly in contact with the buttocks during its recovery phase.

Insufficient movements common to running patterns include inversion or eversion of the foot during the support phase. Inversion results in a medial rotation of the leg and thigh during the support phase and is characterized by an oblique rather than an anterior-posterior pattern as the leg is brought forward in the swing phase.

Eversion of the foot during the support phase results in lateral rotation of the leg and thigh. This pattern is often accompanied by an exaggerated counter-rotary action of the arms in an attempt to maintain a uniform direction.

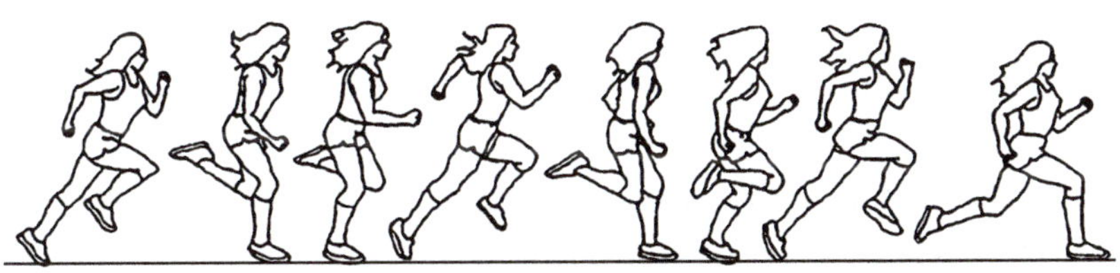

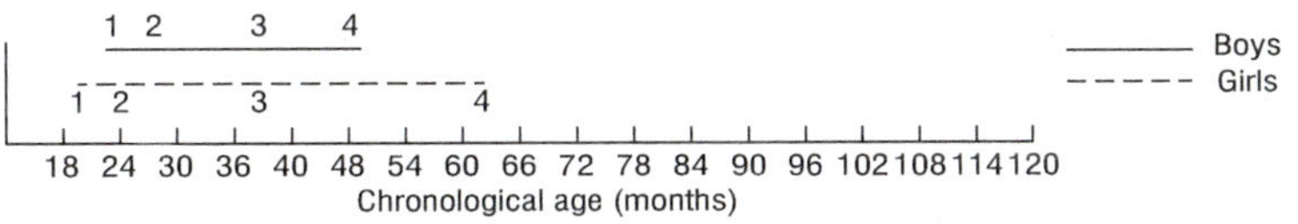

Age at which 60 percent of the boys and girls were able to perform at a specific developmental level for the fundamental motor skill of running.

Figure 12.3 Developmental sequences for running: total body approach

Sources: Fountain, Ulrich, Haubenstricker, and Seefeldt (1981); Seefeldt and Haubenstricker (1982); Seefeldt, Reuschlein, and Vogel (1972). All material used with permission of Dr. John Haubenstricker.

Table 12.4 Developmental sequences for running: component approach

Leg action component	
Step 1:	The run is flat-footed with minimal flight. The swing leg is slightly abducted as it comes forward. When seen from overhead, the path of the swing leg curves out to the side during its movement forward. Foot eversion gives a toeing-out appearance to the swinging leg. The angle of the knee of the swing leg is greater than 90° during forward motion.
Step 2:	The swing thigh moves forward with greater acceleration, causing 90° of maximal flexion in the knee. From the rear, the foot is no longer toed-out nor is the thigh abducted. The sideward swing of the thigh continues, however, causing the foot to cross the body's midline when viewed from the rear. Flight time increases. After contact, which may still be flat-footed, the support knee flexes more as the child's weight rides over the foot.
Step 3:	Foot contact is with the heel or the ball of the foot. The forward movement of the swing leg is primarily in the sagittal plane. Flexion of the thigh at the hip carries the knee higher at the end of the forward swing. The support leg moves from flexion to complete extension by takeoff.
Arm action component	
Step 1:	The arms do not participate in the running action. They are sometimes held in high guard or, more frequently, middle guard position. In high guard, the hands are held about shoulder high. Sometimes they ride even higher if the laterally rotated arms are abducted at the shoulder and the elbows flexed. In middle guard, the lateral rotation decreases, allowing the hands to be held waist high. They remain motionless, except in reaction to shifts in equilibrium.
Step 2:	Spinal rotation swings the arms bilaterally to counterbalance rotation of the pelvis and swing leg. The frequently oblique plane of motion and continual balancing adjustments give a flailing appearance to the arm action.
Step 3:	Spinal rotation continues to be the prime mover of the arms. Now the elbow of the arm swinging forward begins to flex; it then extends during the backward swing. The combination of rotation and elbow flexion causes the arm rotating forward to cross the body's midline and the arm rotating back to abduct, swinging obliquely outward from the body.
Step 4:	The humerus (upper arm) begins to drive forward and back in the sagittal plane independent of spinal rotation. The movement is in opposition to the other arm and to the leg on the same side. Elbow flexion is maintained, oscillating about a 90° angle during the forward and backward arm swings.

Note: These sequences have not been validated. They were hypothesized by Roberton (1983) from the work of Seefeldt, Reuschlein, and Vogel (1972) and Wickstrom (1983).

Source: Roberton and Halverson (1984). Used with permission from current copyright holder, M. A. Roberton.

configuration during performance is described. Figure 12.3 also includes a graph that denotes when 60 percent of girls and boys can perform at each developmental level. This graphed information can be useful to movement specialists when confronted with such questions as "How close to maturity is the child's performance?" or "At what age should the child be expected to perform at a specific level of competence?" This information is also useful for comparing the relative difficulty in achieving the various stages, which roughly corresponds to the time spans between their attainments.

Developmental Performance Trends for Running

Few investigators have studied the kinetics and kinematics of a developmental running pattern in young children. There is, however, no lack of product performance data related to children's running speed. Unfortunately, these data are often difficult to compare because of the different distances the children were required to run and the different types of starts that were used (stationary or running). A comparison of the data suggests overall developmental performance trends. Generally, the data indicate a fairly consistent year-to-year improvement in running speed for both boys and girls.

Branta, Haubenstricker, and Seefeldt (1984) reported an approximate 30 percent increase in running speed in both girls and boys from 5 to 10 years of age. This finding is based on a 30-yard (27.4 m) dash in which a 5-yard (4.6 m) running start was allowed. The running speed for boys between 9 and 17 years of age improved by 20 percent. Girls improved about 8 percent during this time. On average, girls' running speed peaked at about 14 to 15 years of age. Boys' running speed continued to improve beyond 17 years (the top age studied in this research).

Among Slovenian children, Volmut, Pisot, and Simunic (2016) reported finding little improvement in the running speed of girls after 11 years of age, while the boys continued to improve. Likewise, Zavrsnik and colleagues (2016) observed significant gender differences in running speed at 13 years of age, at which time, boys were 10–15 percent faster than girls.

Fountain and colleagues (1981) took a unique approach to studying running speed in young children. These researchers were in part interested in studying the relationship between developmental stage and running velocity. They collected data for three years on a mixed longitudinal sample. Running speed was measured during a 30-yard dash in which a running start was employed (approximately 3 ft/0.9 m). Developmental running stage was assessed by the total body approach. The researchers found developmental stage to account for 19 percent of the variance in total run times for the boys and about 29 percent of the variance in total run times for the girls. In general, the more immature the running pattern, the longer it took the children to complete the 30-yard dash.

When run times were converted to yards/second, it was found that both girls and boys improved by 1.6 yards/sec over the age range studied. By 5 years of age, the boys were running 4.2 yards/sec, and the girls were running 4.0 yards/sec (Fountain et al., 1981).

Running speed in boys has been found to significantly improve as a function of physical maturation. More specifically, Meyers and colleagues have reported that boys become significantly faster during a period of growth just before, through 1.5 years post peak height velocity and that this increase in speed is primarily a function of an increase in stride length (Meyers, Oliver, Hughes, et al., 2015).

JUMPING

Jumping is a fundamental movement that occurs when the body is projected into the air by force generated in one or both legs and the body lands on one or both feet. Jumping can be accomplished in several ways. For example, **hopping** is a form of jumping in which the propelling force is generated in one leg and the landing is accomplished on the same leg. If the landing occurs on the nonpropelling leg, the movement is called a **leap**.

Perhaps the downward leap while descending a step is the child's first experience with jumping. However, a more sensible way to consider the beginning of jumping development is to examine jumping patterns that involve a two-footed takeoff. The two-footed jumping patterns that have received the most attention are the vertical jump and the horizontal or standing long jump. In the **vertical jump**, the body is thrust upward; in the **horizontal jump**, the body is propelled both upward and forward. Regardless of the direction the body is propelled, both two-footed jumping patterns have similar phases, including a preparatory, a takeoff, a flight, and a landing phase.

Phases in Jumping

Preparatory Phase

A great deal of preparatory movement is associated with experienced two-footed jumping. Preparatory movements are necessary to ready the body to spring into action. Such movements include a crouch (flexion of the hips, knees, and ankles) and a backward swing of the arms. Many of these preparatory movements are absent in the inexperienced jumper. For instance, very little if any crouch precedes the jump, and a corresponding arm swing is also absent or minimized.

Takeoff and Flight Phases

Once the preparatory movements have been accomplished, a rapid and vigorous extension of the hips, knees, and ankles along with a vigorous swing of the arms in the direction of desired travel provide the impetus for the body to become airborne. See Figure 12.4. Because the inexperienced jumper does not properly crouch, there is very little extension of the body segments. Furthermore, the inexperienced jumper is not able to integrate the arms with the lower extremities to increase the momentum of the jump. Consequently, only a short distance or height is traversed. Angle of takeoff is also an important factor. The most effective angle of takeoff in horizontal jumping is 45 degrees.

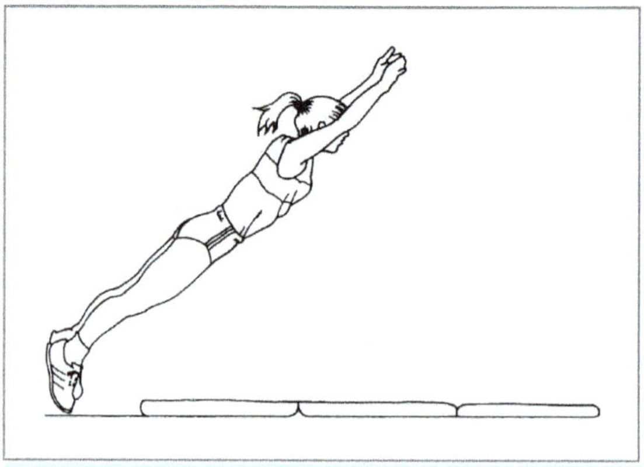

Figure 12.4 The advanced jumper fully extends the body during the takeoff phase

Landing Phase

During the airborne phase of the horizontal jump, the extended legs are brought forward and ahead of the body's center of gravity as the landing is anticipated. Because inexperienced jumpers are unable to gain adequate height and forward momentum, they do not have enough time to get their feet ahead of their center of gravity.

Another obvious characteristic of the inexperienced jumper is the inability to flex the hips, knees, and ankles upon landing. The resulting stiff-legged landing makes the landing look rigid and jolts the jumper. No doubt, this rigid landing can cause injury. Fortunately, Prapavessis, McNair, Anderson, and Hohepa (2003) found that instruction in proper landing technique can significantly lower peak ground reaction forces. The experienced jumper slowly flexes the hips, knees, and ankles to absorb the force of the jump gradually (Figure 12.5).

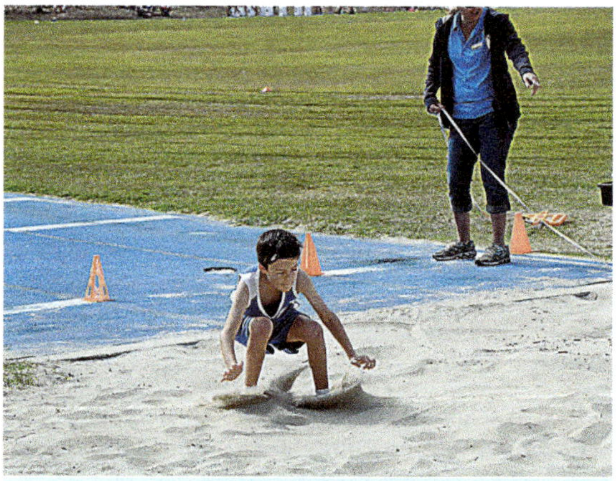

Figure 12.5 The advanced jumper absorbs the landing forces by flexing the knees, hips, and ankles at impact

Constraints on the Development of Jumping

The primary constraint on the development of jumping is the additional strength needed to propel the body into the air. Strength, however, is not the only determining factor. Muscular power is also a necessary component. In the horizontal jump for distance and in the vertical jump for height, the jumper uses both legs to supply the power needed to become airborne. Muscular power is the product of muscular strength and speed of muscular contraction (speed × velocity). The faster the muscle contracts, the greater the amount of power that will be generated. As stated earlier, children who do not possess the muscular strength and power needed to propel the body off the supporting surface are said to be earthbound and do not meet the formal requirement for producing a true jump. Additionally, arm-leg coordination has been found to contribute significantly to vertical jump height (Koren, Pisot, & Simunic, 2016) and when a target is placed overhead, vertical jump performance is enhanced (Poe, 1976). It is possible that the overhead target may contribute to improved utilization of the arms (higher vertical reach), resulting in better arm-leg coordination.

As would be expected, the one-legged hop (a variation of jumping) requires even more muscular strength and power than the two-legged jump, because half the power supply has been removed (a one-legged versus a two-legged takeoff). Additionally, because hopping is generally performed in a sequence of hops, muscular endurance is also a factor in sustained hopping performance.

Developmental Sequences for the Standing Long Jump

Table 12.5 presents a developmental sequence (component approach) for the fundamental motor skill—the standing long jump. Only recently have researchers begun to hypothesize a developmental sequence for the "landing phase" of the standing long jump (Lane, Molina, Tolleson, et al., 2018). Table 12.6 presents this hypothesized sequence. Using a pre-longitudinal screening technique, the researchers were able to demonstrate adequate developmental validity for the proposed sequence, which now must await longitudinal validation.

An alternative developmental sequence (total body approach) is illustrated in Figure 12.6. The latter developmental sequence has withstood preliminary validation on a mixed longitudinal sample (Haubenstricker, Seefeldt, & Branta, 1983). As the graph at the bottom of Figure 12.6 suggests, a developmental stage 1 pattern was found to be most prominent in children under 42 months of age (3.5 years). A stage 2 jumping pattern was found to be most prevalent between 48 and 84 months of age (4 and 7 years), whereas a stage 3 jumping pattern was dominant by 96 months of age (8 years). Only about 10 percent of the older subjects between 102 and 107 months (8.5 and 9 years) were found to exhibit the most mature (stage 4) pattern of jumping.

Developmental Sequences for the Vertical Jump

Unlike horizontal jumping, little scientific inquiry into developmental sequences for vertical jumping has been undertaken. This lack of interest is most likely attributable to several factors. For instance, the horizontal jump is easier to measure than the vertical jump and is included in several popular tests of physical fitness. Nevertheless, following Myers and colleagues (1977), Gallahue, Ozmun, and Goodway (2012) described a developmental sequence for vertical jumping. As noted in Table 12.7 in the next section, the mature form of vertical jumping greatly resembles that of horizontal jumping. More specifically, mature vertical jumpers prepare by taking a

Table 12.5 Developmental sequences for the standing long jump: component approach

Takeoff phase	Flight and landing phase
Leg action component	**Leg action component**
Step 1: Fall and catch. The weight is shifted forward. The knee and ankle are held in flexion or extend slightly as gravity rotates the body over the balls of the feet. Takeoff occurs when the toes are pulled from the surface in preparation for the landing "catch."	Step 1: Minimal tuck. The thigh is carried in flight more than 45° below the horizontal. The legs may assume either symmetrical or asymmetrical configurations during flight, resulting in one- or two-footed landings.
Step 2: Two-footed takeoff; partial extension. Both feet leave the ground symmetrically, but the hips, knees, and/or ankles do not reach full extension by takeoff.	Step 2: Partial tuck. During flight, the hips and knees flex synchronously. The thigh approaches a 20°–35° angle below the horizontal. The knees then extend for a two-footed landing.
Step 3: Two-footed takeoff; full extension. Both feet leave the ground symmetrically, with hips, knees, and ankles fully extended by takeoff.	Step 3: Full tuck. During flight, flexion of both knees precedes hip flexion. The hips then flex, bringing the thighs to the horizontal. The knees then extend, reaching forward to a two-footed landing.
Trunk action component	**Trunk action component**
Step 1: *Slight lean; head back.* The trunk leans forward less than 30° from the vertical. The neck is hyperextended.	Step 1: *Slight lean.* During flight, the trunk maintains its forward inclination of less than 30° and then flexes for landing.
Step 2: *Slight lean; head aligned.* The trunk leans forward less than 30° from vertical, with the neck flexed or aligned with the trunk at takeoff.	Step 2: *Corrected lean.* The trunk corrects its forward lean of 30° or more by hyperextending. It then flexes forward for landing.
Step 3: *Forward lean; chin tucked.* The trunk is inclined forward 30° or more from the vertical at takeoff, with the neck flexed.	Step 3: *Maintained lean.* The trunk maintains the forward lean of 30° or more from takeoff to mid-flight and then flexes forward for landing.
Step 4: *Forward lean; head aligned.* The trunk is inclined forward 30° or more. The neck is aligned with the trunk or slightly extended.	
Arm action component	**Arm action component**
Step 1: *Arms inactive.* The arms are held at the side with the elbows flexed. Arm movement, if any, is inconsistent and random.	Step 1: *Arms winging.* In two-footed takeoff jumps, the shoulders may retract while the arms extend backward (winging) during flight. They move forward (parachuting) during landing.
Step 2: *Winging arms.* The arms extend backward in a winging posture at takeoff.	Step 2: *Arms abducted; lateral rotation.* During flight, the arms hold a high guard position and continue lateral rotation. They parachute for landing.
Step 3: *Arms abducted.* The arms are abducted about 90°, with the elbows often flexed, in a high or middle guard position.	Step 3: *Arms abducted; medial rotation.* During flight, the arms assume a high or middle guard position but medially rotate early in the flight. They parachute for landing.
Step 4: *Arms forward; partial stretch.* The arms flex forward and upward with minimal abduction, reaching incomplete extension overhead by takeoff.	Step 4: *Arms overhead.* During flight, the arms are held overhead. In middle flight, the arms lower (extend) from their overhead flexed position, reaching forward at landing.

Table 12.5 Continued

Takeoff phase	Flight and landing phase
Arm action component	**Arm action component**
Step 5: *Arms forward; full stretch.* The arms flex forward, reaching full extension overhead by takeoff.	

Note: These developmental steps have not been validated. They have been modified by Halverson from the work of Van Sant (1983).

Source: Roberton and Halverson (1984). Used with permission from the current copyright holder, M. A. Roberton.

Table 12.6 Hypothesized developmental sequences for standing long jump landing phase

Shank action	
Level 1	"Acute/Perpendicular": Anterior shank angle at contact is acute or approximately perpendicular to the ground.
Level 2	"Obtuse". Anterior shank angle at contact is clearly obruse relative to the ground.
Foot action	
Level 1	"Asymmetrical Contact": One foot clearly lands before the other; leg configuration during flight is often asymmetrical.
Level 2	"Symmetrical Neutral/Plantarflexed". Two-footed landing; ankle is plantarflexed or neutral just prior to contact resulting in a forefoot or flat-footed landing.
Level 3	"Symmetrical Dorsiflexed": Two-footed landing; ankle is actively dorsiflexed at contact resulting in a distinct heel landing.
Arm action	
Level 1	"No Reach": Arms wing during flight and act only to parachute (i.e., use for balance) during landing.
Level 2	"Slight Forward Reach": Shoulders flex to bring arms in front of the body during flight but the reach is abandoned as shoulders abduct to parachute; often dropped straight in line with the trunk at contact.
Level 3	"Full Forward Reach": Shoulder flexion of > 90 degrees relative to the trunk is observed at foot contact.
Level 4	"Neutral/Hyperextension": Arms are forcefully thrown down and back into full shoulder extension/hyperextension as hips simultaneously flex.

Source: Lane, Molina, Tolleson, et al. (2018). Used with permission.

preparatory crouch and then vigorously swing the arms upward in the desired direction of the jump. In addition, they rapidly extend the hips, knees, and ankles as the body moves upward. Upon landing, the ankles, knees, and hips flex to absorb the impact forces.

In general, mature process characteristics appear in the vertical jump before they appear in the horizontal jump. In fact, adult-like characteristics of the vertical jump have appeared in children as young as age 2 (Poe, 1976), with most children exhibiting mature characteristics by age 5 (Williams, 1983). In comparison, as stated earlier, mature horizontal jumping process characteristics (stage 3 and stage 4) do not predominate until 8 to 9 years of age (Haubenstricker et al., 1983).

Stage 1 Vertical component of force may be greater than horizontal; resulting jump is then upward rather than forward. Arms move backward, acting as brakes to stop the momentum of the trunk as the legs extend in front of the center of mass.

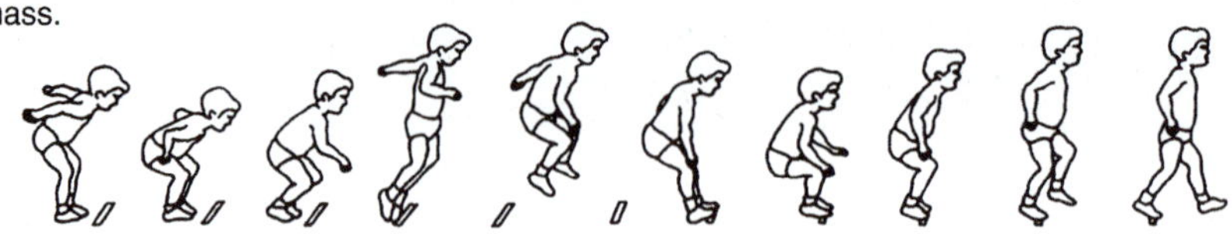

Stage 2 The arms move in an anterior-posterior direction during the preparatory phase but move sideward (winging action) during the in-flight phase. The knees and hips flex and extend more fully than in stage 1. The angle of takeoff is still markedly above 45°. The landing is made with the center of gravity above the base of support, with the thighs perpendicular to the surface rather than parallel as in the reaching position of stage 4.

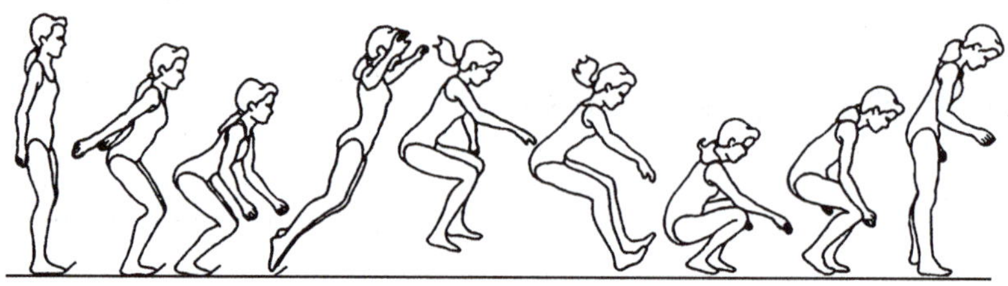

Stage 3 The arms swing backward and then forward during the preparatory phase. The knees and hips flex fully prior to takeoff. Upon takeoff, the arms extend and move forward but do not exceed the height of the head. The knee extension may be complete, but the takeoff angle is still greater than 45°. Upon landing, the thigh is still less than parallel to the surface and the center of gravity is near the base of support when viewed from the frontal plane.

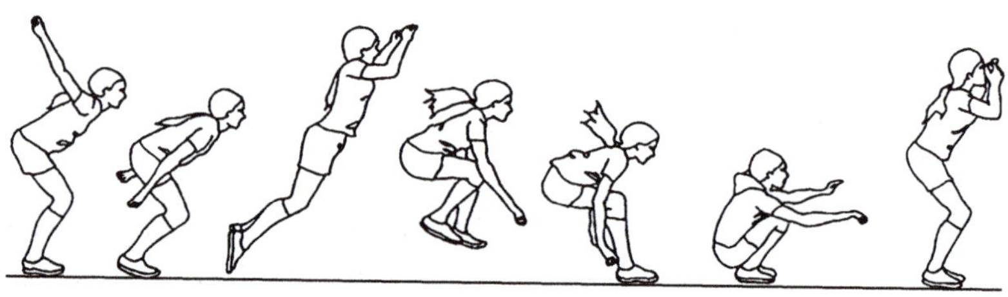

Stage 4 The arms extend vigorously forward and upward upon takeoff, reaching full extension above the head at "liftoff." The hips and knees are extended fully, with the takeoff angle at 45° or less. In preparation for landing, the arms are brought downward and the legs are thrust forward until the thighs are parallel to the surface. The center of gravity is far behind the base of support upon foot contact, but at the moment of contact the knees are flexed and the arms are thrust forward in order to maintain the momentum to carry the center of gravity beyond the feet.

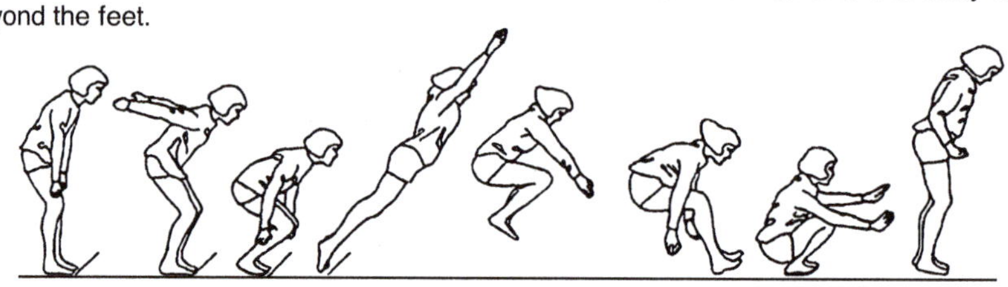

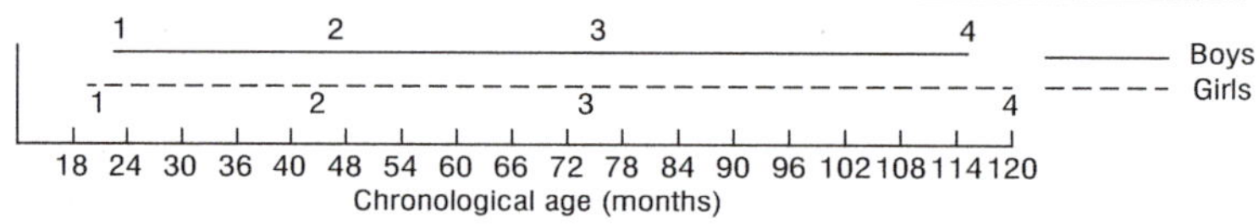

Age at which 60 percent of the boys and girls were able to perform at each developmental level for the fundamental motor skill of the standing long jump.

Figure 12.6 Developmental sequences for the standing long jump: total body approach

Sources: Haubenstricker, Seefeldt, and Branta (1983); Seefeldt and Haubenstricker (1982); Seefeldt, Reuschlein, and Vogel (1972). All material used with permission of Dr. John Haubenstricker.

Table 12.7 Developmental sequence for vertical jumping

Initial stage
Inconsistent preparatory crouch
Difficulty in taking off with both feet
Poor body extension on takeoff
Little or no head lift
Arms not coordinated with the trunk and leg action
Little height achieved
Elementary stage
Knee flexion exceeding 90° angle on preparatory crouch
Exaggerated forward lean during crouch
Two-footed takeoff
Entire body not fully extended during flight phase
Arms attempting to aid in flight and balance
Noticeable horizontal displacement on landing
Mature stage
Preparatory crouch with knee flexion from 60° to 90°
Forceful extension at hips, knees, and ankles
Simultaneous coordinated upward arm lift
Upward head tilt with eyes focused on target
Full body extension
Elevation of reaching arm by shoulder girdle tilt combined with downward thrust of nonreaching arm at peak of flight
Controlled landing very close to point of takeoff

Source: Adapted from Gallahue, Ozmun, and Goodway (2012).

Developmental Performance Trends for Vertical Jumping

Although many studies have examined vertical jumping performance trends in adult populations, few investigators have studied the corresponding developmental trends in children (Isaacs & Pohlman, 2000; Isaacs, Pohlman, & Hall, 2003; Jensen, Phillips, & Clark, 1994; Koren, et al., 2016; Poe, 1976). This is surprising, given the role of the vertical jump in such popular sports as basketball and volleyball. Tables 12.8 and 12.9 summarize vertical jump performance data collected by Isaacs and colleagues (Isaacs & Pohlman, 2000; Isaacs et al., 2003). In these studies, 248 boys and 232 girls aged 7 to 11 (grades 1–5) performed four vertical jumps with a counter-movement and four without one. In the former condition, the child crouched and then immediately jumped vertically, while in the latter the child had to hold the crouched position for 3 seconds before executing the vertical jump. Contrary to findings in adult populations, children performed more poorly with a counter-movement than with none. Apparently, these young children had not yet acquired the neural coordination needed to take advantage of the muscles' plyometric qualities (Focke, Strutzenberger, Jekauc, et al., 2013; Harrison, Ryan, & Hayes, 2007). This assumption has been recently supported in a three-year longitudinal study by Koren, Pisot, and Simunic (2016). These investigators first categorized arm-leg coordination (poor, average, excellent) prior to counter-movement jump performance. They report that the 4- to 6-year-old children with the poorest arm-leg coordination performed worst on the vertical jumping task. At the age of 6 years, 5.9 percent of the boys and 4.4 percent of the girls still exhibited poor arm-leg coordination. An examination of Table 12.7 reveals a large performance spread between the minimum and maximum vertical jump performances for each gender and age. This variability may be due, in part, to differences in arm-leg coordination as described above.

Similar to findings obtained on young American children, studies utilizing European children also report that males tend to jump

Table 12.8 Vertical jump performance variables for children between 7 and 11 years of age (N = 480)*

Male					
Age	**N**	**Mean***	**SD**	**Minimum†**	**Maximum§**
7	39	10.96	1.66	8.5	14.5
8	59	11.03	1.59	8.0	15.5
9	57	11.18	1.86	6.5	15.5
10	53	11.08	2.62	4.0	18.0
11	40	11.93	2.04	7.0	16.0
Female					
Age	**N**	**Mean***	**SD**	**Minimum†**	**Maximum§**
7	33	10.80	1.69	7.0	16.0
8	56	10.97	1.51	8.0	14.5
9	61	10.98	2.11	6.5	16.5
10	42	10.43	2.30	6.5	16.5
11	40	10.33	2.69	5.0	16.5

Notes: †Lowest vertical jump in inches.
§Highest vertical jump in inches.
*Measurement in inches.

Sources: Isaacs and Pohlman (2000); Isaacs, Pohlman, and Hall (2003).

Table 12.9 Selected data on vertical jump performance for children between 7 and 11 years of age (N = 480)*

	Boys					Girls				
Age	**7**	**8**	**9**	**10**	**11**	**7**	**8**	**9**	**10**	**11**
percentile	**Vertical height in inches**					**Vertical height in inches**				
100	14.5	14.5	15.5	18.0	16.0†	16.0	14.5	16.5	16.5	16.5
80	12.5	12.5	12.5	13.0	13.5	16.5	12.5	13.0	12.0	12.5
60	11.5	11.5	12.0	11.5	12.5	11.0	11.5	11.5	11.0	11.0
40	10.5	10.5	11.5	10.5	12.0	10.5	11.0	10.5	9.5	9.0
20	9.5	9.5	9.5	9.0	10.5	9.5	9.0	9.0	8.5	8.5

Notes: *Measurements are rounded to the nearest one-half inch.
†See the discussion of adolescent awkwardness, on p. 173.

Sources: Isaacs and Pohlman (2000); Isaacs, Pohlman, and Hall (2003).

higher than females (Brien, Belton, & Issartel, 2016; Focke et al., 2013) and this gender difference in performance becomes most evident after 7 years of age (Focke et. al., 2013). Focke and colleagues (2013) have determined that boys jump higher than girls because they are capable of producing ground reaction forces over a longer period of time.

Developmental Sequences for Hopping

As discussed earlier, hopping is a form of jumping in which one foot is used to project the body into space and the landing is on the same propelling foot. This fundamental movement is considered more difficult than the two-footed jump because it requires additional strength and better balance.

In a study that employed a prelongitudinal screening technique, Halverson and Williams (1985) provided evidence for the existence of developmental steps in both the leg and the arm components of hopping. The purpose of a prelongitudinal screening is to determine initially if the hypothesized components include all observable behaviors and whether the steps within each component are arranged correctly (Roberton, Williams, & Langendorfer, 1980). After incorporating changes, the researchers were able to describe four steps in the leg component of the hop and five steps in the arm component. Table 12.10 describes each hypothesized step. In each progressive step there is greater extension of the propelling leg and greater involvement of the nonsupport or swing leg to assist projection. The arms are initially inactive but soon become involved, assisting the hop and working in opposition to the legs.

Halverson and Williams (1985) concluded that 5-year-old children were at predominantly low and intermediate developmental levels. In addition, most children used less advanced developmental patterns when hopping on their nonpreferred foot.

Using the total body approach (see Figure 12.7), Haubenstricker, Branta, Seefeldt, and colleagues (1989) produced data that agree with these earlier findings. Namely, children perform hopping better on the preferred foot as opposed to the nonpreferred foot, and most 5-year-old girls and boys have not developed a mature hopping pattern. More specifically, these researchers found 3 percent of the 5-year-old boys and 6 percent of the 5-year-old girls to exhibit a stage 4 hopping pattern (the most mature stage). Over 60 percent of these 5-year-olds were found to exhibit a stage 2 developmental level of hopping. Moreover, 10 percent of the boys and 6 percent of the girls could not hop by 4 years of age.

The stage 1 pattern of hopping was most prevalent in 3-year-old girls and in 3.5-year-old boys. Similarly, girls predominantly exhibited stage 2 characteristics by age 4, and boys were generally displaying these characteristics by age 4.5 (Haubenstricker et al., 1989).

COMBINING FUNDAMENTAL MOVEMENTS

Fundamental motor patterns can be combined to produce new movement patterns. The three most often described patterns are the **gallop**, the **slide**, and the **skip**. As would be expected, these more complex motor patterns do not emerge until sometime after the development of their single-motor-pattern counterparts.

Galloping

Of these three motor patterns, the gallop is the first to be exhibited. The two basic fundamental motor patterns that make up the gallop are: (1) a forward step, followed by (2) a leap onto the trailing foot. By definition, this pattern must be performed in a front-facing direction, and the same leg always leads. Frequently, the gallop begins to emerge shortly

Table 12.10 Developmental steps in two components of hopping: component approach

Leg action component	
Step 1:	*Momentary flight*. The support knee and hip quickly flex, pulling (instead of projecting) the foot from the floor. The flight is momentary. Only one or two hops can be achieved. The swing leg is lifted high and held in an inactive position to the side or in front of the body.
Step 2:	*Fall and catch; swing leg inactive*. Forward lean allows minimal knee and ankle extension to help the body "fall" forward of the support foot and then quickly catch itself again. The swing leg is inactive. Repeated hops are achieved.
Step 3:	*Projected takeoff; swing leg assists*. Perceptible pretakeoff extension occurs in the support leg, hip, knee, and ankle. There is little delay in changing from knee and ankle flexion on landing to takeoff extension. The swing leg now pumps up and down to assist in projection, but range is insufficient to carry it behind the support leg.
Step 4:	*Projection delay; swing leg leads*. The child's weight on landing is smoothly transferred along the foot to the ball before the knee and ankle extend to takeoff. The range of the pumping action in the swing leg increases so that it passes behind the support leg when viewed from the side.
Revised developmental sequence for arm action in hopping	
Step 1:	*Bilateral inactive*. The arms are held bilaterally, usually high and out to the side, although other positions behind or in front of the body may occur. Any arm action is usually slight and not consistent.
Step 2:	*Bilateral reactive*. Arms swing upward briefly and then are medially rotated at the shoulder in a winging movement prior to takeoff. This movement appears to occur in reaction to loss of balance.
Step 3:	*Bilateral assist*. The arms pump up and down together, usually in front of the line of the trunk. Any downward and backward motion of the arms occurs after takeoff. The arms may move parallel to each other or be held at different levels as they move up and down.
Step 4:	*Semi-opposition*. The arm on the side opposite the swing leg swings forward with that leg and back as the leg moves down. The position of the other arm is variable, often staying in front of the body or to the side.
Step 5:	*Opposing assist*. The arm opposite the swing leg moves forward and upward in synchrony with the forward and upward movement of that leg. The other arm moves in the direction opposite the action of the swing leg. The range of movement in the arm action may be minimal unless the task requires speed or distance.

Source: Halverson and Williams (1985). Reprinted with permission from *Research Quarterly for Exercise and Sport, 56*, 37–44.

after running has been accomplished (about 2 years of age). At this time, however, the child will be capable of leading with only the preferred leg. Galloping with the nonpreferred leg as the lead is usually not accomplished until several years later. Figure 12.8 illustrates and describes the developmental sequences for galloping (total body approach).

Sliding

The slide is essentially the same as the gallop, with one exception. Whereas the gallop is a forward movement, the slide is performed sideways. Children's difficulty in performing this more complicated motor pattern arises because they are required to face a different direction from the line of intended movement. More specifically, the child must face straight

Stage 1 The nonsupport knee is flexed at 90° or less, with the nonsupport thigh parallel to the surface. This position places the nonsupport foot in front of the body so that it may be used for support if balance is lost. The body is held in an upright position with the arms flexed at the elbows. The hands are held near shoulder height and slightly to the side in a stabilizing position. Force production is generally limited, so that little height or distance is achieved in a single hop.

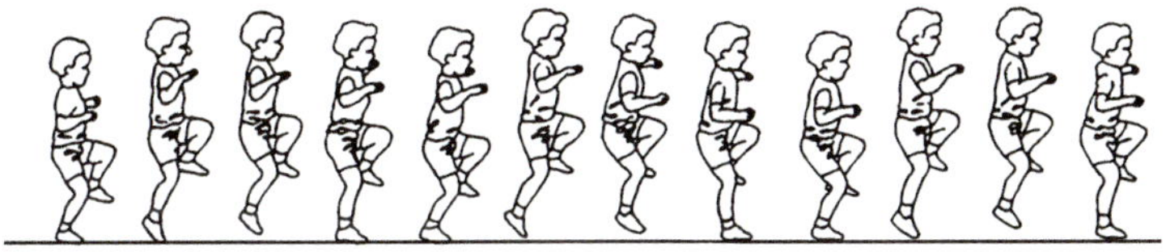

Stage 2 The nonsupport knee is fully flexed, so that the foot is near the buttocks. The thigh of the nonsupport leg is nearly parallel to the surface. The trunk is flexed at the hip, resulting in a slight forward lean. The performer gains considerable height by flexing and extending the joints of the supporting leg and by extending at the hip joint. In addition, the thigh of the nonsupport leg aids in force production by flexing at the hip joint. In the landing, the force is absorbed by flexion at the hips and the supporting knee. The arms participate vigorously in force production as they move up and down in a bilateral manner. Because of the vigorous action and precarious balance of performers at this stage, the number of hops generally ranges from two to four.

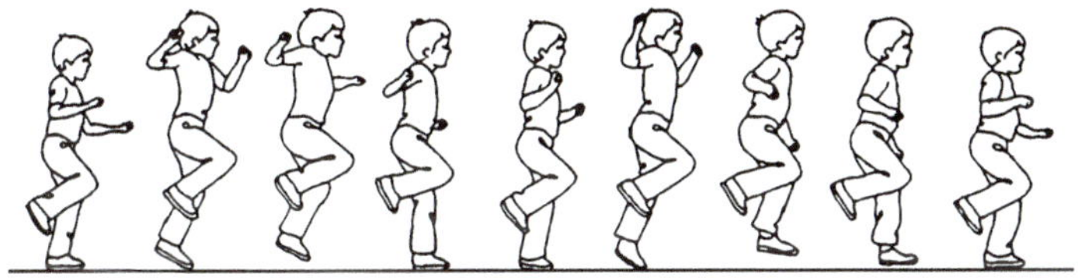

Stage 3 The thigh of the nonsupport leg is in a vertical position with knee flexed at 90° or less. Performers exhibit greater body lean forward than in stage 1 or 2, with the result that the hips are farther in front of the support leg upon takeoff. This forward lean of the trunk results in greater distance in relation to the height of the hop. The knee of the nonsupport leg remains near the vertical (frontal) plane, but knee flexion may vary as the body is projected and received by the supporting leg. The arms are used in force production, moving bilaterally upward during the force-production phase.

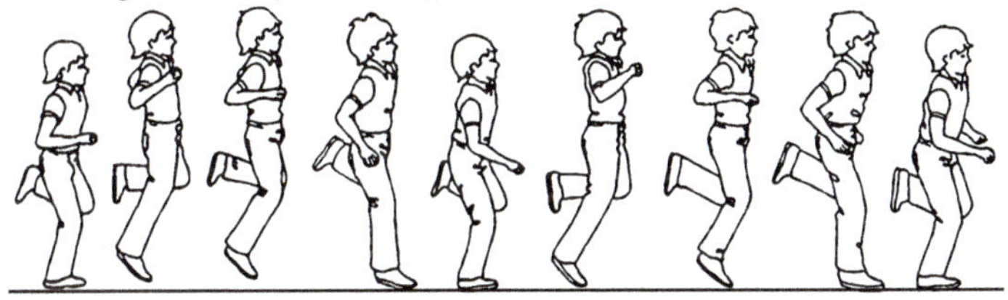

Stage 4 The knee of the nonsupport leg is flexed at 90° or less, but the entire leg swings back and forth like a pendulum as it aids in force production. The arms are carried close to the sides of the body, with elbow flexion at 90°. As the nonsupport leg increases its force production, that of the arms seems to diminish.

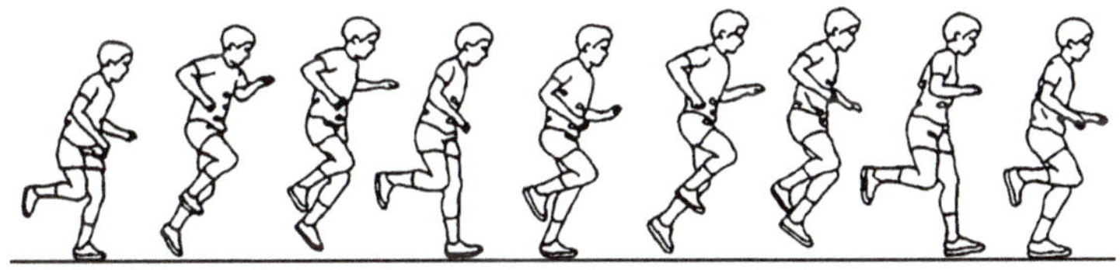

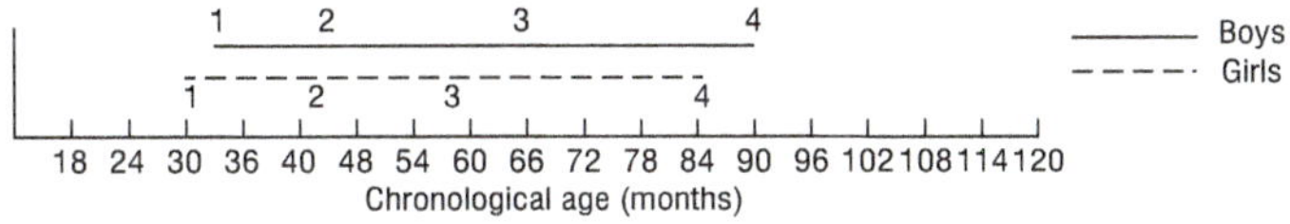

Age at which 60 percent of the boys and girls were able to perform at each developmental level for the fundamental motor skill of hopping.

Figure 12.7 Developmental sequences for hopping: total body approach

Sources: Haubenstricker, Henn, and Seefeldt (1975); Haubenstricker et al. (1989); Seefeldt and Haubenstricker (1974, 1982). All material used with permission of Dr. John Haubenstricker.

Stage 1 The pattern resembles a rhythmically uneven run with the performer often reverting to the traditional running pattern. The tempo tends to be relatively fast and the rhythm inconsistent. The trail leg crosses in front of the lead leg during the airborne phase and remains in front at contact. The trail leg is flexed at ≤45° during the airborne phase. Both feet generally contact the floor in a heel-toe pattern, although either foot may strike the surface flat-footed.

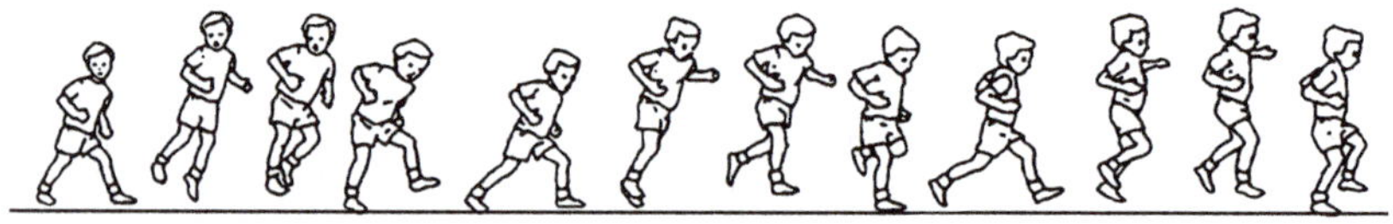

Stage 2 The pattern is executed at a slow to moderate tempo with the rhythm often appearing choppy. The trail leg moves in front of, adjacent to, or behind the lead leg during the airbone phase but is always adjacent to or behind the lead leg at contact. The trail leg is extended during the airborne phase, often causing the trail foot to turn out and the lead leg to flex at ≤45°. The feet usually contact the floor in heel-toe/heel-toe or toe/toe combination. The transfer of weight may appear stiff and exaggerated. The vertical component is often exaggerated as the trunk extends to lift the body up.

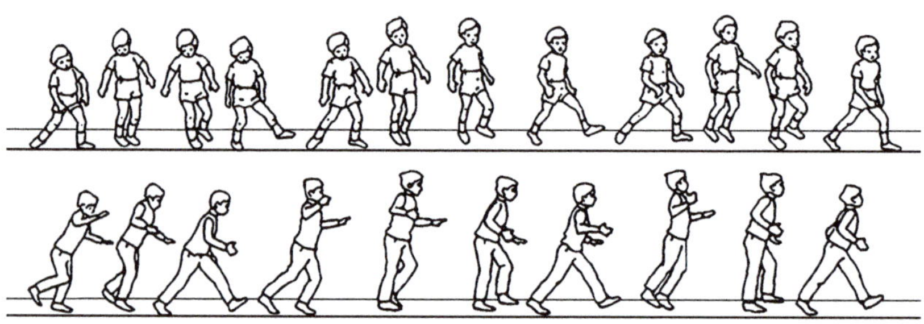

Stage 3 The pattern is smooth, rhythmical, and executed at a moderate tempo. The trail leg may cross in front of or move adjacent to the lead leg during the airborne phase but is placed adjacent to or behind the lead leg at contact. Both the lead and trail legs are flexed at ≤45° with the feet carried close to the surface during the airborne phase. The lead foot meets the surface with a heel-toe pattern followed by a transfer of weight to the ball of the trail foot.

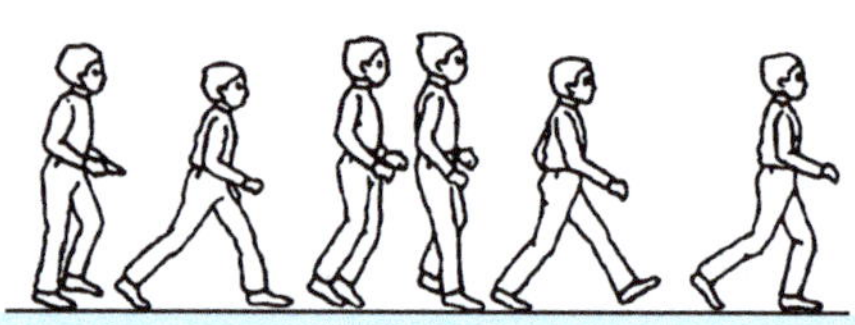

Figure 12.8 Developmental sequences for galloping: total body approach

Source: Sapp (1980). All material used with permission of Dr. John Haubenstricker.

ahead while moving in a sideward direction. As a result, early attempts at sliding frequently start off correctly, but eventually the child begins to point the toe of the leading leg toward the direction of movement, and shortly thereafter the trunk rotates, as well. At this point, the initial slide is converted into the easier motor pattern of galloping. Sliding is an extremely important motor skill for children to acquire because it is used in many types of sporting activities. For example, moving along the baseline in tennis, taking a lead off of a base in baseball, and guarding an opponent in basketball all require sliding.

Skipping

Of the three motor patterns described here, skipping is by far the most difficult. The skip consists of a forward step followed by a hop on the same foot (an uneven rhythmical pattern). In addition, the leading leg alternates. Unlike the gallop and the slide, skipping requires that both motor tasks (step and hop) be

Table 12.11 Developmental sequences for skipping: component approach

Leg action component	
Step 1:	*One-footed skip.* One foot completes a step and hop before the weight is transferred to the other foot. The other foot just steps.
Step 2:	*Two-footed skip; flat-footed landing.* Each foot completes a step and a hop before the weight is transferred to the other foot. Landing from the hop is on the full foot or on the ball of the foot, with the heel touching down before the weight is transferred (flat-footed landing).
Step 3:	*Two-footed skip; ball of the foot landing.* Landing from the hop is on the ball of the foot. The heel does not touch down before the weight is transferred to the other foot. Body lean increases over that found in step 2.
Arm action component	
Step 1:	*Bilateral assist.* The arms pump bilaterally up as the weight is shifted from the hopping to the stepping foot and down during the hop takeoff and flight.
Step 2:	*Semi-opposition.* The arms first swing up bilaterally. During the hop on the right foot, the right arm moves down and back only slightly while the left arm continues to move backward until the step on the left foot. Then, both arms again move forward and upward in a new bilateral pumping action. Now, however, the left arm moves back only slightly while the right arm moves backward until the step on the right foot. Although the arm action has the beginnings of opposition, at some time in the arm cycle both hands are in front of the body.
Step 3:	*Opposition.* The arm opposite the stepping leg swings upward and forward in synchrony with that leg and reverses direction when the stepping leg touches the floor. The arm on the same side as the stepping leg moves backward and down in opposition to the stepping leg. At no time are both hands in front of the body.

Note: These sequences, hypothesized by Halverson, have not been validated. However, efforts are currently underway to validate these sequences (Roberton, 2013).

Source: Roberton and Halverson (1984). Used with permission from the current copyright holder, M. A. Roberton.

accomplished on the same foot before the body's weight is transferred onto the other foot. Obviously, performing dual tasks on a single leg is more difficult than performing a single task per leg, as in galloping or sliding. The child who is first attempting to skip may experience difficulty in maintaining balance. If this balance problem is severe, the child should skip in place while holding on to the back of a chair. With this arrangement, the child can maintain balance while learning this complex motor pattern. Table 12.11 describes both the leg action and the arm action components of the skip from the component approach perspective. Figure 12.9 illustrates and describes the developmental sequences for skipping from the total body approach perspective. As the graph below stage 3 of Figure 12.9 indicates, girls were found to exhibit the stage 3 level about 6 to 7 months before young boys. On average, young boys and girls start to skip sometime between their sixth and seventh birthdays.

SUMMARY

- Walking is a fundamental movement in which there is an alternation of the leading leg and continuous contact with the ground. To maintain balance during initial walking attempts, children spread the feet, point the toes outward, and carry the arms in a high guard position. Most children are capable of independent walking by 12 months; the typical range is from 9 to 17 months.

Stage 1 A deliberate step-hop pattern is employed, an occasional double hop is present, there is little effective use of the arms to provide momentum, an exaggerated step or leap is present during the transfer of weight from one supporting limb to the other, and the total action appears segmented.

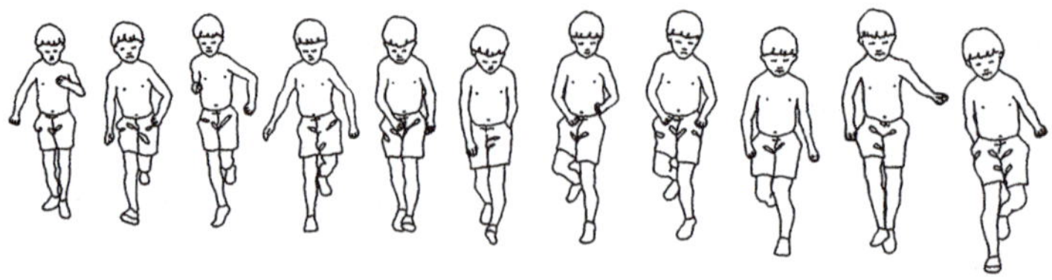

Stage 2 There is rhythmical transfer of weight during the step phase. Increased use of arms in providing forward and upward momentum is seen, as is an exaggeration of the vertical component during the airborne phase—that is, while executing the hop.

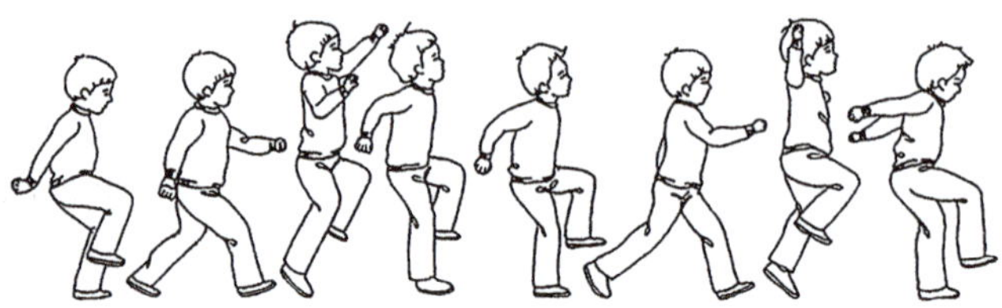

Stage 3 There is rhythmical transfer of weight during all phases and reduced arm action during the transfer-of-weight phase. The foot of the supporting limb is carried near the surface during the hopping phase.

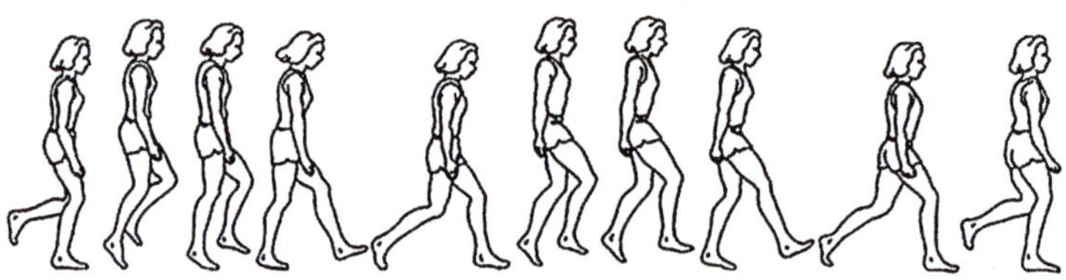

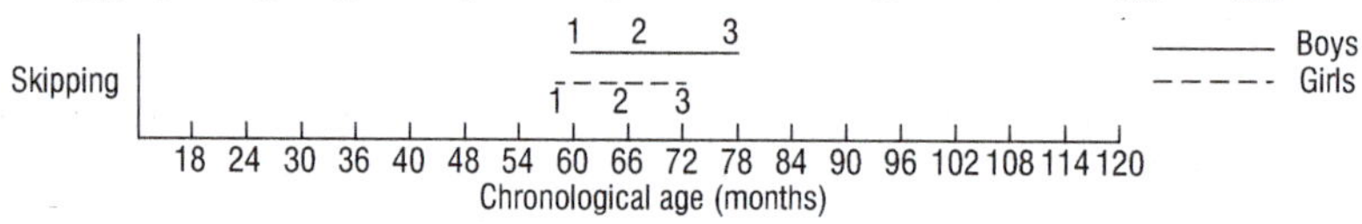

Age at which 60 percent of the boys and girls were able to perform at each developmental level for the fundamental motor skill of skipping.

Figure 12.9 Developmental sequences for skipping: total body approach

Sources: Sapp (1980); Seefeldt and Haubenstricker (1974, 1982). All material used with permission of Dr. John Haubenstricker.

- Running is different from walking in that there is a momentary phase of suspension (flight phase) during which neither foot is in contact with the ground. Most children begin to exhibit minimal running from between 18 and 24 months of age.
- Jumping is propelling the body into the air from force generated in one or both legs and landing on one or both feet. Hopping, vertical jumping, horizontal or long jumping, and leaping are all variations of jumping. Each jumping variation consists of four phases: preparatory, takeoff, flight, and landing. Most children are capable of some form of jumping shortly after acquiring the ability to run.
- After learning to walk, run, jump, and hop, children begin to perform these skills in combination. As a result, new movement skills emerge, including the gallop, slide, and skip. The gallop is a front-facing movement where the child takes a step onto the

forward leg and then a leap onto the rear foot. In galloping, the same leg always leads. Sliding is similar to galloping except that the movement is performed sideways. This skill is more difficult than the gallop because, when sliding, the child must face in one direction (to the front) while moving in a different direction (sideways). Again, the same leg always leads. The most difficult of the three combination skills is the skip. The skip is a step-hop combination where both movements are performed on the same leg before the body's weight is transferred onto the other leg. This dual movement results in an alternation of the leading leg. The skipping pattern is generally first exhibited in both boys and girls sometime between their sixth and seventh birthday.

Table 16.2 summarizes many of the fundamental locomotor skills of childhood from the total body approach (Haubenstricker, 1990).

key concept review

balance
double support phase
dynamic balance
flight phase
gait cycle
gallop
hopping
horizontal jump
jumping
leap
postural control
running
skip
slide
static balance
support phase
swing phase
upright bipedal locomotion
vertical jump
walking

questions for reflection

1. What three phases make up the walking or gait cycle?
2. Can you distinguish between mature and immature foot mechanisms during walking?
3. Can you identify the typical range of time for the onset of independent walking?
4. What are the two primary constraints on the development of independent walking?
5. What are the major phases of running? Identify the typical range of time in which running is first exhibited.
6. What key observational characteristics distinguish mature and immature styles of running for each of the following bodily components: foot strike, heel-buttock relationship, thigh-ground relationship, arm coordination?
7. What are the two primary constraints affecting the development of running? Compare and contrast the differences between these constraints as compared to the constraints on developing independent walking.
8. What is the difference between the two evaluation systems known as the component approach and the total body approach?
9. What is the overall developmental performance trend in running speed for both boys and girls? Identify age ranges associated with the attainment of peak running speed in both boys and girls.
10. What is the association between developmental stage and running speed in both girls and boys?
11. What are the phases associated with horizontal jumping? How do hopping and leaping differ from horizontal jumping?
12. What key observational characteristics distinguish mature and immature styles of horizontal jumping?
13. How is a counter-movement useful during the execution of a vertical jump? In your answer, distinguish between mature and immature styles of vertical jump performance.

14. What are the constraints influencing the development of jumping? In your answer, distinguish between two-legged jumping and the one-legged hop.
15. Can you compare and contrast the gallop and the slide? Why is skipping more difficult than galloping and sliding?
16. Can you describe the general characteristics of skipping performance in young boys and girls? Identify the age range when most young boys and girls begin to skip.

online resources

Gait & Posture Journal, www.journals.elsevier.com/gait-and-posture/

REFERENCES

Adolph, K. E., & Avolio, A. M. (2000). Walking infants adapt locomotion to changing body dimensions. *Journal of Experimental Psychology*, *26*, 1148–1166.

Adolph, K. E., Cole, W. G., Komati, M., Garciaguirre, J. S., Baddaly, D., Lingeman, J. M., et al. (2012). How do you learn to walk? Thousands of steps and dozens of falls per day. *Psychological Science*, *23*, 1387–1394.

Adolph, K. E., & Tamis-LeMonda, C. S. (2014). The costs and benefits of development: The transition from crawling to walking. *Child Development Perspectives*, *8*(4), 187–192.

Adolph, K. E., Vereijken, B., & Shrout, P. E. (2003). What changes in infant walking and why. *Child Development, 74*, 475–497.

Branta, C., Haubenstricker, J., & Seefeldt, V. (1984). Age changes in motor skills during childhood and adolescence. In R. L. Terjung (Ed.), *Exercise and sport sciences review*. New York: Macmillan.

Brien, W. O., Belton, S., & Issartel, J. (2016). Fundamental movement skill proficiency amongst adolescent youth. *Physical Education and Sport Pedagogy*, *21*, 557–571.

Bril, D., & Breniere, Y. (1992). Postural requirements and progression velocity in young walkers. *Journal of Motor Behavior, 24*, 105–116.

Burnett, C. N., & Johnson, E. W. (1971). Development of gait in childhood: Part II. *Developmental Medicine and Child Neurology*, *13*, 207–215.

Chen, Y. & Mu, Y. (2018). Effects of backpack load and position on body strains in male schoolchildren while walking. *PLos One*, 13, doi: 10.1371/journal.pone.0193648.

Cottalorda, J., Bourelle, S., & Gautheron, V. (2004). Effects of backpack carrying in children. *Orthopedics*, *27*, 1172–1177.

Focke, A., Strutzenberger, G., Jekauc, D., Worth, A., Woll, A., & Schwameder, H. (2013). Effects of age, sex and activity level on counter-movement jump performance in children and adolescents. *European Journal of Sport Science, 13*, 518–526.

Fountain, C., Ulrich, B., Haubenstricker, J., & Seefeldt, V. (1981). Relationship of developmental stage and running velocity in children 2.5 to 5 years of age. Paper presented at the Midwest District convention of the American Alliance for Health, Physical Education, Recreation, and Dance, Chicago.

Fredriksen, P. M., Mamen, A., Gammelsrud, H., Lindberg, M., & Hjelle, O. P. (2018). Factors affecting running performance in 6-12-year-olds: The health oriented pedagogical project (HOPP). *Scandinavian Journal of Public Health*, *46*, 61–67.

Gallahue, D. L., Ozmun, J. C., & Goodway, J. (2012). *Understanding motor development*. 7th ed. New York: McGraw-Hill.

Goulding, A., Jones, I. E., Taylor, R. W., Piggot, J. M., & Taylor, D. (2003). Dynamic and static tests of balance and postural sway in boys: Effects of previous wrist bone fractures and high adiposity. *Gait and Posture*, *17*(2), 136–141.

Gupta, I., Kalra, P., & Iqbal, R. (2018). Evaluation of school backpack prototype-based on gait parameters, energy expenditure and posture of students. *Current Science, 115*, 930–936, doi: 10.18520/cs/v115/i5/930-936.

Halverson, L., & Williams, K. (1985). Developmental sequences for hopping over distance: A prelongitudinal screening. *Research Quarterly for Exercise and Sport, 56*, 37–44.

Harrison, A. J., Ryan, W., & Hayes, K. (2007). Functional data analysis of joint coordination in the development of vertical jump performance. *Sports Biomechanics, 6*, 199–214.

Hatzitaki, V., Zisi, V., Kollias, I., & Kioumourtzoglou, E. (2002). Perceptual-motor contributions to static and dynamic balance in children. *Journal of Motor Behavior, 34*(2), 161–170.

Haubenstricker, J. (1990). Summary of fundamental motor skill stage characteristics: Motor performance study—MSU. Unpublished materials, Michigan State University, East Lansing, MI.

Haubenstricker, J., Branta, C., Seefeldt, V., Brakora, L., & Kiger, J. (1989). Prelongitudinal screening of a developmental sequence for hopping. Paper presented at the annual convention of the American Alliance for Health, Physical Education, Recreation, and Dance, Boston.

Haubenstricker, J., Henn, J., & Seefeldt, V. (1975). Developmental sequence of hopping. Rev. ed. Unpublished materials, Michigan State University, East Lansing, MI.

Haubenstricker, J., Seefeldt, V., & Branta, C. (1983). Preliminary validation of a developmental sequence for the standing long jump. Paper presented at the annual convention of the American Alliance for Health, Physical Education, Recreation, and Dance, Minneapolis.

Hausdorff, J. M., Zemany, L., Peng, C. K., & Goldberger, A. L. (1999). Maturation of gait dynamics: Stride-to-stride variability and its temporal organization in children. *Journal of Applied Physiology, 83*, 1040–1047.

Hong, Y., & Brueggemann, G. (2000). Changes in gait patterns in 10-year-old boys with increasing loads when walking on a treadmill. *Gait and Posture, 11*, 254–259.

Isaacs, L. D., & Pohlman, R. L. (2000). Effectiveness of the stretch-shortening cycle in children's vertical jump performance. *Medicine and Science in Sports and Exercise, 32*(5 Supplement), S278.

Isaacs, L. D., Pohlman, R. L., & Hall, T. (2003). Vertical jump performance standards in children: An update. *Strategies, 16*, 33–35.

Jensen, J. L., Phillips, S. J., & Clark, J. E. (1994). For young jumpers, differences are in the movement's control, not its coordination. *Research Quarterly for Exercise and Sport, 65*, 258–268.

Keogh, J., & Sugden, D. (1985). *Movement skill development*. New York: Macmillan.

Koren, K., Pisot, R., & Simunic, B. (2016). Vertical jump height in young children: A longitudinal study in 4- to 6-year-old children. *Annales Kinesiologiae, 7*, 153–170.

Kretch, K. S., Franchak, J. M., & Adolph, K. E. (2014). Crawling and walking infants see the world differently. *Child Development, 85*(4), 1503–1518.

Lane, A. P., Molina, S. L., Tolleson, D. A., Langendorfer, S. J., Goodway, J. D., & Stodden, D. F. (2018). Developmental sequences for the standing long jump landing: A pre-longitudinal screening. *Journal of Motor Learning and Development, 6*, 114–129.

Ledebt, A., Rosier, J. C., & Savelsbergh, G. J. P. (2005). The early development of walking with and without shoes. Unpublished report, Vrije University, Amsterdam.

Meyers, R. W., Oliver, J. L., Hughes, M. G., Cronin, J. B., & Lloyd, R. S. (2015). Maximal sprint speed in boys of increasing maturity. *Pediatric Exercise Science, 27*, 85–94.

Myers, C. B., et al. (1977). Vertical jumping movement patterns of early childhood. Unpublished paper, Indiana University.

Pascoe, D. D., Pascoe, D. E., Wang, Y. T., Shim, D. M., & Kim, L. M. (1997). Influence of carrying book bags on gait cycle and posture of youths. *Ergonomics, 40*, 631–641.

Perrone, M., Orr, R., Hing, W., Milne, N., & Pope, R. (2018). The impact of backpack loads on school children: A critical narrative review. *International Journal of Environment Research and Public Health, 15*. doi: 10.3390/ijerph15 112529.

Phillips, S. J., & Clark, J. E. (1987). Infants' first unassisted walking steps: Relationship to speed. In B. Jonson (Ed.), *International series on biomechanics*. Champaign, IL: Human Kinetics.

Poe, A. (1976). Description of the movement characteristics of two-year-old children performing the jump and reach. *Research Quarterly, 47*, 260–268.

Prapavessis, H., McNair, P. J., Anderson, K., & Hohepa, M. (2003). Decreasing landing forces in children: The effect of instruction. *Journal of Orthopedic & Sports Physical Therapy, 33*, 204–207.

Roberton, M. A. (1983). Changing motor patterns during childhood. In J. Thomas (Ed.), *Motor development during childhood and adolescence*. Minneapolis, MN: Burgess.

Roberton, M. A. (2013). Testing the validity of the Halverson developmental sequences for skipping. *Research Quarterly for Exercise and Sport, 84*, 198–205.

Roberton, M. A., & Halverson, L. E. (1984). *Developing children: Their changing movement*. Philadelphia, PA: Lea & Febiger.

Roberton, M. A., Williams, K., & Langendorfer, S. (1980). Prelongitudinal screening of motor development sequences. *Research Quarterly for Exercise and Sport, 51*, 724–731.

Sapp, M. (1980). The development of galloping in young children: A preliminary study. Unpublished master's project, Michigan State University, East Lansing, MI.

Seefeldt, V., & Haubenstricker, J. (1974). Developmental sequence of hopping. Unpublished materials, Michigan State University, East Lansing, MI.

Seefeldt, V., & Haubenstricker, J. (1982). Patterns, phases, or stages: An analytical model for the study of developmental movement. In J. A. S. Kelso & J. E. Clark (Eds.), *The development of movement control and coordination*. New York: Wiley.

Seefeldt, V., Reuschlein, P., & Vogel, P. (1972). Sequencing motor skills within the physical education curriculum. Paper presented at the American Association for Health, Physical Education, and Recreation, Houston, TX.

Sutherland, D. H. (1984). *Gait disorders in childhood and adolescence*. Baltimore, MD: Williams & Wilkins.

Thelen, E. (1986). Treadmill-elicited stepping in seven-month-old infants. *Child Development, 57*, 1498–1506.

Thelen, E., Ulrich, B. D., & Jensen, J. L. (1989). The developmental origins of locomotion. In M. H. Woollacott & A. Shumway-Cook (Eds.), *Development of posture and gait across the lifespan* (pp. 25–47). Columbia, SC: University of South Carolina Press.

Théveniau, N., Boisgontier, M. P., Varieras, S., & Olivier, J. (2014). The effects of clothes on independent walking in toddlers. *Gait and Posture, 39*(1), 659–661.

Tudor-Locke, C., Han, H., Aguiar, E. J., Barreira, T. V., Schuna, J. M. Jr., Kang, M., et al. (2018). How fast is fast enough? Walking cadence (steps/min) as a practical estimate of intensity in adults: A narrative review. *British Journal of Sports Medicine, 52*, 776–788.

Tudor-Locke, C., Aguiar, E. J., Han, H., Ducharme, S. W., Schuna, J. M. JR, Barreira, T. V., et al. (2019). Walking cadence (steps/min) and intensity in 21–40 year olds: CADENCE-adults. *International Journal of Behavioral Nutrition and Physical Activity, 7*, doi: 10.1186/s12966-019-0769-6.

Vaghela, N. P., Parekh, S. K., Padsala, D., & Patel, D. (2019). Effect of backpack loading on cervical and sagittal shoulder posture in standing after dynamic activity in school age children. *Journal of Family Medicine and Primary Care, 8*, 1076–1081.

Van Sant, A. (1983). Development of the standing long jump. Unpublished paper, Motor Development and Child Study Laboratory, Department of Physical Education and Dance, University of Wisconsin, Madison, WI.

Volmut, T., Pisot, R., & Simunic, B. (2016). The effect of regular sport exercise on muscle contractile properties in children. In F. Eminovic & M. Dopsaj (Eds.), *Physical activity effects on the anthropological status of children, youth and adults* (pp. 41–53). New York: Nova Science Publishers.

Walicka-Cupry, K., Skalska-Izdebska, R., Rachwal, M., & Truszczynaska, A. (2015). Influence of the weight of a school backpack on spinal curvature in the sagittal plane of seven-year-old children. *BioMed Research International*, doi: 10.1155/2015/817913.

Wegener, C., Hunt, A. E., Vanwanseele, B., Burns, J., & Smith, R. M. (2011). Effects of children's shoes on gait: A systematic review and meta-analysis.

Journal of Foot and Ankle Research, 4, doi: 10.1186/1757-1146-4-3.

Whitall, J., & Getchell, N. (1995). From walking to running: Applying a dynamical systems approach to the development of locomotor skills. *Child Development, 66*, 1541–1553.

Whittfield, J., Legg, S. J., & Hedderley, D. I. (2005). Schoolbag weight and musculoskeletal symptoms in New Zealand secondary schools. *Applied Ergonomics, 36*, 193–198.

Wickstrom, R. L. (1983). *Fundamental motor patterns*. 3rd ed. Philadelphia, PA: Lea & Febiger.

Williams, H. G. (1983). *Perceptual and motor development*. Englewood Cliffs, NJ: Prentice-Hall.

Zavrsnik, J., Pisot, R., Volmut, T., Koren, K., Blazun H., Kokol, P., et al. (2016). Lower correlation between biceps femoris contraction time and maximal running speed in children than in adults: A longitudinal study in 9- to 14-year-old children. *Annales Kinesiologiae*, 7, 21–41.

13 FUNDAMENTAL OBJECT-CONTROL SKILLS OF CHILDHOOD

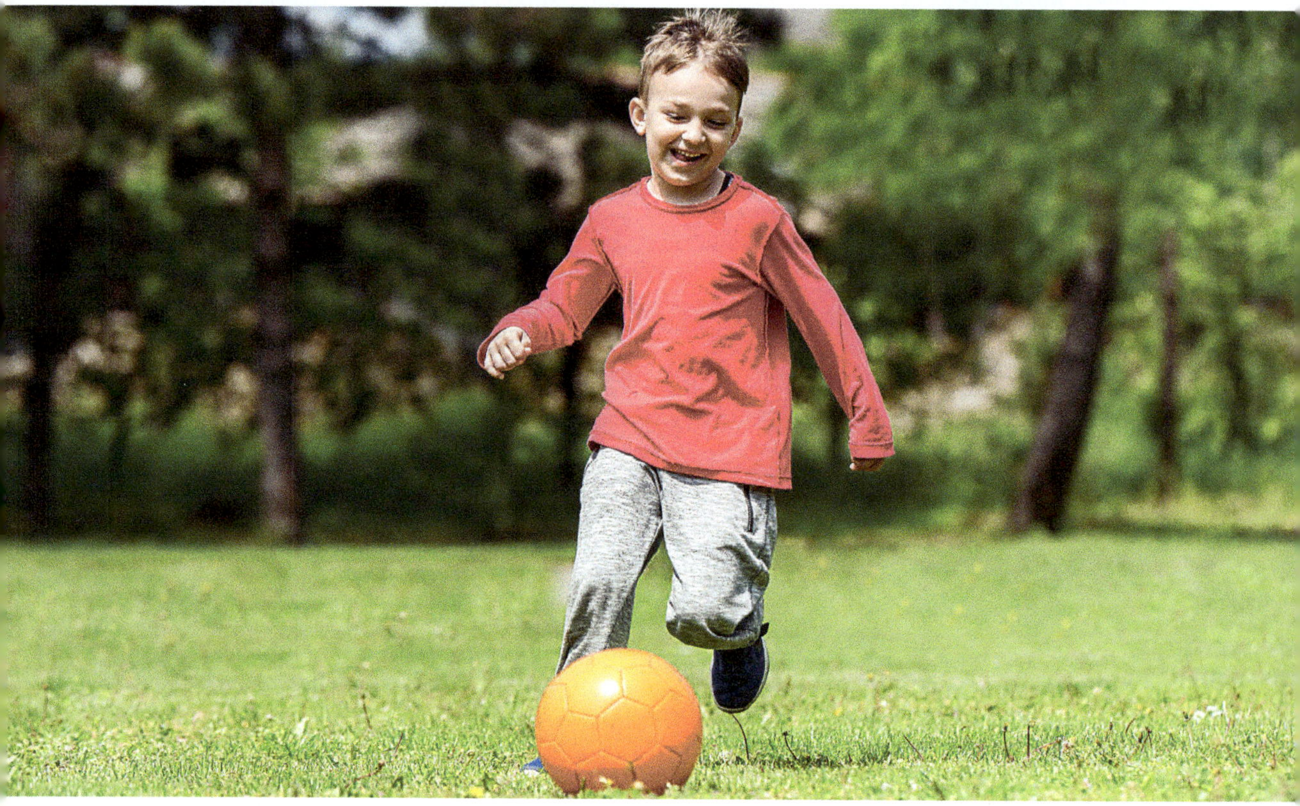

Chapter Objectives

From the information presented in this chapter, you will be able to

- Describe the development of overarm throwing and list the constraints known to influence this development
- Describe developmental aspects of both one- and two-handed catching and list the constraints known to influence catching development
- Describe developmental aspects of ball striking both with external implements (bats, racquets) and without (dribbling, place kicking, punting)

As soon as children can ambulate without assistance, their hands become free to explore the ever-changing environment more effectively. With time, experience, and practice, children's eye-hand and eye-foot coordination dramatically improves. At this time, children will begin to exhibit a category of skills commonly referred to as **object-control skills.** These skills include overarm throwing, both one- and two-handed catching, and striking objects both with and without an implement. Implements that might be used with these object-control skills are racquets and bats. Sport actions that employ these skills without the use of an implement include dribbling, place kicking, and punting.

OVERARM THROWING

Of the fundamental movements discussed in this chapter, **throwing** is perhaps the most complex. There are many different throwing patterns (underarm, sidearm, overarm), but this discussion is limited to one of the most common forms—the one-handed overarm throw. This throw can be conveniently divided into three phases:

1. The *preparatory phase* consists of all movements directed away from the intended line of projection.
2. The *execution phase* consists of all movements performed in the direction of the throw.
3. The *follow-through phase* consists of all movements performed following the release of the projectile (Langendorfer, 1980).

Understanding these three phases will facilitate your comprehension of the following information on throwing.

Developmental Stages of Throwing

Monica Wild (1938) is generally credited with setting the standards for the study of developmental throwing stages. Her classic study, conducted more than 80 years ago, attempted to uncover age and gender characteristics of throwing in children 2 to 12 years of age. As a result of this research, Wild described four developmental overarm throwing stages. Table 13.1 summarizes each stage.

Table 13.1 Wild's four developmental stages of throwing

Stage 1 (2- and 3-year-olds)
Throw is arm-dominated.
Preparatory arm movements involve bringing the arm sideways-upward or forward-upward.
Thrower faces the direction of the intended throw at all times.
No rotation of trunk and hips is evident.
Feet remain stationary during the entire throwing act.
Stage 2 (3.5- to 5-year-olds)
Body moves in a horizontal plane instead of an anterior-posterior plane.
Throwing arm moves in a high oblique plane or horizontal plane above the shoulder.
Throwing is initiated predominantly by arm and elbow extension.
Feet remain stationary, but rotary movement of the trunk is observable.
Stage 3 (5- and 6-year-olds)
Forward step is unilateral to the throwing arm.
Arm is prepared by swinging it obliquely upward over the shoulder with a large degree of elbow flexion.
Arm follows through forward and downward and is accompanied by forward flexion of the trunk.
Stage 4 (6.5 years and older)
Forward step is taken with the contralateral leg.
Trunk rotation is clearly evident.
Arm is horizontally adducted in the forward swing.

Source: Based on findings from Wild (1938).

Within these four stages, two developmental trends are evident. First, movement progresses from an anterior-posterior plane to a horizontal plane; second, the base of support changes from a stationary to a shifting position.

Others have since expanded upon Wild's pioneering work. Langendorfer (1980), for example, studied age-related changes in the arm action components during the preparatory phase of a forceful overarm throw. He proposed a motor development sequence consisting of four hypothesized steps.

- Step 1 is best described as a lack of any preparatory backswing. Once the ball is grasped, it is moved directly forward.
- In step 2, the ball is brought up beside the head by upward humerus flexion and exaggerated elbow flexion.
- Step 3 is subdivided into three options. Option 1 is a circular overhead preparatory movement with the elbow extended. Option 2 is a preparatory movement characterized by a lateral swing backward. Option 3 is a simple vertical lift of the throwing arm.
- Step 4, the most advanced preparatory sequence, is a circular arm action in which the arm moves down and back.

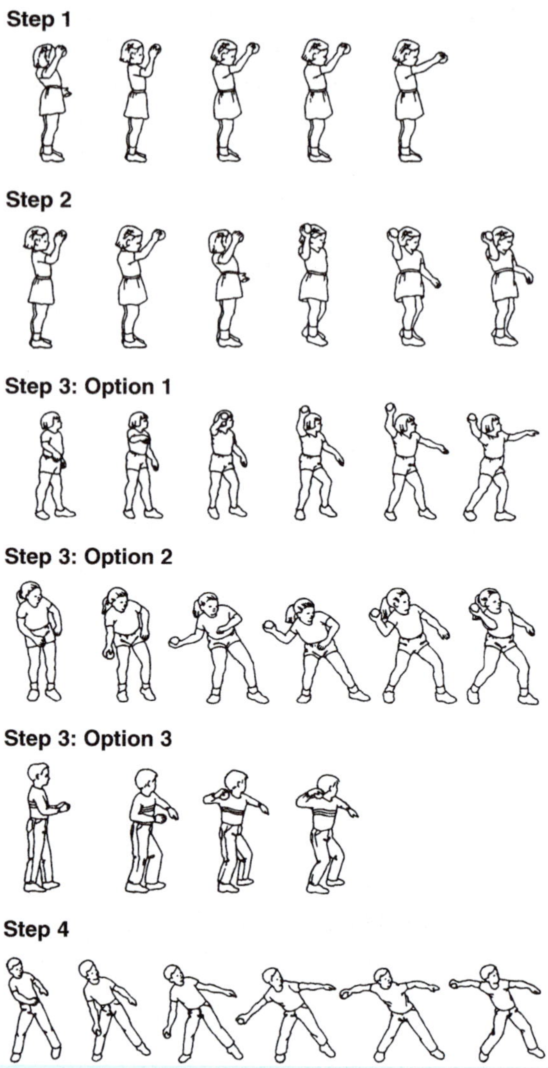

Figure 13.1 The four steps of Langendorfer's hypothesized developmental sequence of the preparatory arm action of the overarm throw. Read all steps from left to right.

Roberton (1978) studied other components related to the forceful overarm throw. She presented longitudinal evidence for developmental stages in the humerus, forearm, and trunk components of the forceful overarm throw. Of particular interest is the following finding:

> Development within component parts may proceed at different rates in the same individual or at different rates in different individuals. For instance, one child might move ahead a stage in his trunk action while another child moved ahead a stage in his arm action. Thus two individuals going through the same stages within each component could look quite different at any one time.
>
> (p. 55)

Roberton also proposed developmental sequences for the backswing in association with Langendorfer and for foot action based on observations by others. Table 13.2 presents Roberton's developmental sequences.

Table 13.2 Roberton's developmental sequences for the trunk, backswing, humerus, forearm, foot action in the overarm throw for force*: component approach

Trunk action	
Step 1:	*No trunk action or forward-backward movements*. Only the arm is active in force production. Sometimes, the forward thrust of the arm pulls the trunk into a passive left rotation (assuming a right-handed throw), but no twist-up precedes that action. If trunk action occurs, it accompanies the forward thrust of the arm by flexing forward at the hips. Preparatory extension sometimes precedes forward hip flexion.
Step 2:	*Upper trunk rotation or total trunk "block" rotation*. The spine and pelvis simultaneously rotate away from the intended line of flight and begin forward rotation, acting as a unit or "block." Occasionally, only the upper spine twists away and then toward the direction of force. The pelvis then remains fixed, facing the line of flight, or joins the rotary movement after forward spinal rotation has begun.
Step 3:	Differentiated rotation. The pelvis precedes the upper spine in initiating forward rotation. The child twists away from the intended line of ball flight and then begins forward rotation with the pelvis while the upper spine is still twisting away.
Preparatory arm backswing component	
Step 1:	*No backswing*. The ball in the hand moves directly forward to release from the original position of the arm when the hand first grasped the ball.
Step 2:	*Elbow and humeral flexion*. The ball moves away from the intended line of flight to a position behind or alongside the head by upward flexion of the humerus and concomitant elbow flexion.
Step 3:	*Circular, upward backswing*. The ball moves away from the intended line of flight to a position behind the head via a circular, overhead movement with elbow extended, an oblique swing back, or a vertical lift from the hip.
Step 4:	*Circular, downward backswing*. The ball moves away from the intended line of flight to a position behind the head via a circular down-and-back motion, which carries the hand below the waist.
Humerus (upper arm) action component during forward swing	
Step 1:	*Humerus oblique*. The humerus moves forward to ball release in a plane that intersects the trunk obliquely above or below the horizontal line of the shoulders. Occasionally, during the backswing, the humerus is placed at a right angle to the trunk, with the elbow pointing toward the target. It maintains this fixed position during the throw.
Step 2:	*Humerus aligned but independent*. The humerus moves forward to ball release in a plane horizontally aligned with the shoulder, forming a right angle between humerus and trunk. By the time the shoulders (upper spine) reach front facing, the humerus (elbow) has moved independently ahead of the outline of the body (as seen from the side) via horizontal adduction at the shoulder.
Step 3:	*Humerus lag*. The humerus moves forward to ball release horizontally aligned, but at the moment the shoulders (upper spine) reach front facing, the humerus remains within the outline of the body (as seen from the side). No horizontal adduction of the humerus occurs before front facing.
Forearm action component during forward swing	
Step 1:	*No forearm lag*. The forearm and ball move steadily forward to ball release throughout the throwing action.
Step 2:	*Forearm lag*. The forearm and ball appear to "lag," i.e., to remain stationary behind the child or to move down or back in relation to the child. The lagging forearm reaches its farthest point back, deepest point down, or last stationary point before the shoulders (upper spine) reach front facing.
Step 3:	*Delayed forearm lag*. The lagging forearm delays reaching its final point of lag until the moment of front facing.

(Continued)

Table 13.2 Continued

Action of the feet[†]	
Step 1:	*No step*. The child throws from the initial foot position.
Step 2:	*Homolateral step*. The child steps with the foot on the same side as the throwing hand.
Step 3:	***Contralateral, short step***. The child steps with the foot on the opposite side from the throwing hand.
Step 4:	***Contralateral, long step***. The child steps with the opposite foot a distance of over half the child's standing height.

*Validation studies (Halverson, Roberton, & Langendorfer, 1982; Roberton, 1977, 1978; Roberton & DiRocco, 1981; Roberton & Langendorfer, 1980) support these sequences for the overarm throw, with the exception of the preparatory arm backswing sequence, which Roberton and Langendorfer (1983) hypothesized from the work of Langendorfer (1980). Langendorfer (1982) felt that the humerus and forearm components are appropriate for overarm striking.

[†]This sequence was hypothesized by Roberton (1983) from the work of Leme and Shambes (1978); Seefeldt, Reuschlein, and Vogel (1972); and Wild (1938).

Source: Roberton and Halverson (1984). Used with permission from the current copyright holder, M. A. Roberton.

Seefeldt, Reuschlein, and Vogel (1972) also hypothesized a developmental sequence for the fundamental motor skill of throwing. Their sequence, which appears in Figure 13.2, has withstood preliminary validation (Haubenstricker, Branta, & Seefeldt, 1983). A close examination of the graph accompanying Figure 13.2 makes apparent the gender difference in throwing development found in this study (Seefeldt & Haubenstricker, 1982). The age at which 60 percent of the boys studied exhibited a stage 5 throwing pattern (most mature) was 63 months (slightly past 5 years of age), and the age at which 60 percent of the girls studied exhibited stage 5 characteristics was 102 months (about 8.5 years).

Developmental Performance Trends for Overarm Throwing

Researchers have used three techniques to study product performance changes in children's throwing performance: (1) throwing for distance; (2) throwing for accuracy; and (3) a measure of throwing velocity. Irrespective of the technique, both genders show annual improvement (Butterfield, Angell, & Mason, 2012; Lorson, Stodden, Langendorfer, & Goodway, 2013; Petranek & Barton, 2011; Roberton & Konczak, 2001).

In most throwing studies where throwing velocity served as a criterion, the data were collected cross-sectionally. A notable exception is the early work of Roberton and colleagues, who longitudinally examined changes in children's overarm ball-throwing velocities. Roberton, Halverson, Langendorfer, and Williams (1979) found that the boys' throwing velocities on average increased 5.04 ft (1.54 m) per second per year (ft/s/yr; range: 5–8 ft/s/yr [1.5–2.4 m/s/yr]), and girls' throwing velocities on average increased 2.94 ft/s/yr (0.9 m/s/yr; range: 2–3 ft/s/yr [0.6–0.9 m/s/yr]). In a follow-up study, 22 boys and 17 girls from the original 54 subjects were reassessed when they reached seventh grade. The results supported the earlier prediction regarding annual units of change for the boys' ball-throwing velocities, but the girls' range of units of change had to be increased to 2–4.5 ft/s/yr (0.6–1.4 m/s/yr).

Runion, Roberton, and Langendorfer (2003) examined 50 boys and girls 13 years of age for

Stage 1 The throwing motion is essentially posterior-anterior in direction. The feet usually remain stationary during the throw. Infrequently, the performer may step or walk just prior to moving the ball into position for throwing. There is little or no trunk rotation in the most rudimentary pattern at this stage, but children at the point of transition between stages 1 and 2 may evoke slight trunk rotation in preparation for the throw and extensive hip and trunk rotation in the follow-through phase. In the typical stage 1, the force for projecting the ball comes from hip flexion, shoulder protraction, and elbow extension.

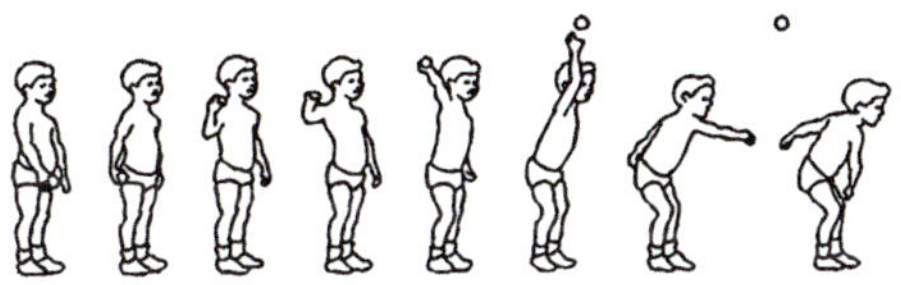

Stage 2 The distinctive feature of this stage is the rotation of the body about an imaginary vertical axis, with the hips, spine, and shoulders rotating as one unit. The performer may step forward with either an ipsilateral or contralateral pattern, but the arm is brought forward in a transverse plane. The motion may resemble a "sling" rather than a throw because of the extended arm position during the course of the throw.

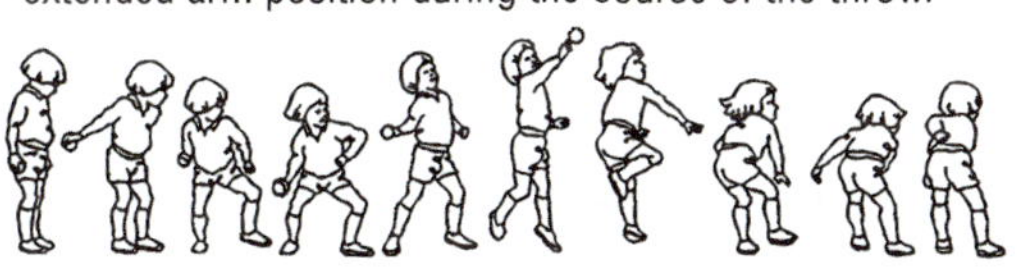

Stage 3 The distinctive pattern in stage 3 is the ipsilateral arm-leg action. The ball is placed into a throwing position above the shoulder by a vertical and posterior motion of the arm at the time that the ipsilateral leg is moving forward. This stage involves little or no rotation of the spine and hips in preparation for the throw. The follow-through phase includes flexion at the hip joint and some trunk rotation toward the side opposite the throwing arm.

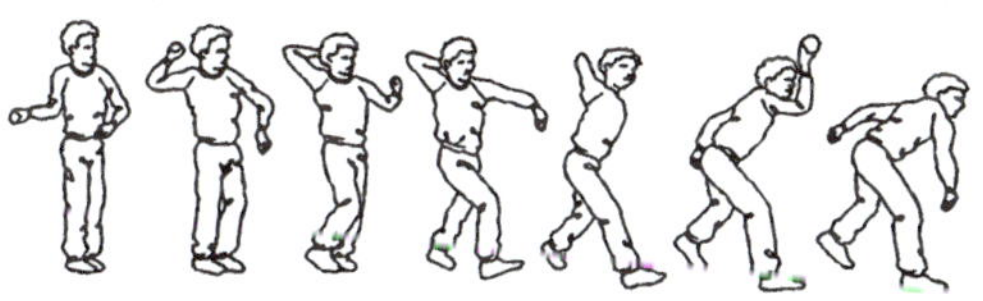

Stage 4 The movement is contralateral, with the leg opposite the throwing arm striding forward as the throwing arm is moved in a vertical and posterior direction during the wind-up phase. There is little or no rotation of the hips and spine during the windup phase; thus, the motion of the trunk and arm closely resembles the motions of stages 1 and 3. The stride forward with the contralateral leg provides for a wide base of support and greater stability during the force-production phase of the throw.

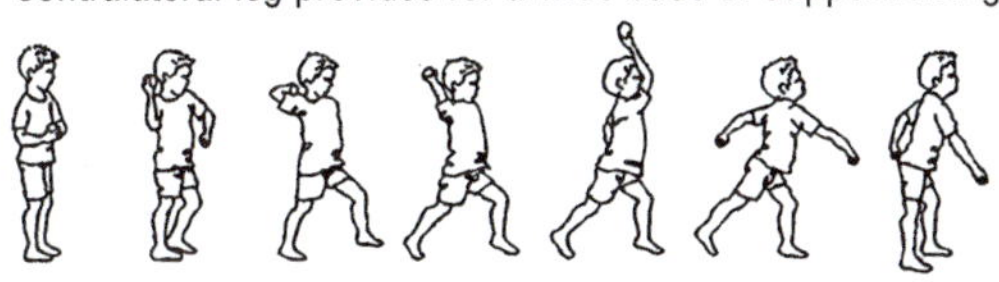

Stage 5 The wind-up phase begins with the throwing hand moving in a downward arc and then backward as the opposite leg moves forward. The concurrent action rotates the hip and spine into position for forceful derotation. As the contralateral toot strikes the surface, the hips, spine, and shoulder begin derotation in sequence. The contralateral leg begins to extend at the knee, providing an equal and opposite reaction to the throwing arm. The arm opposite the throwing limb also moves forcefully toward the body to assist in the equal and opposite reaction.

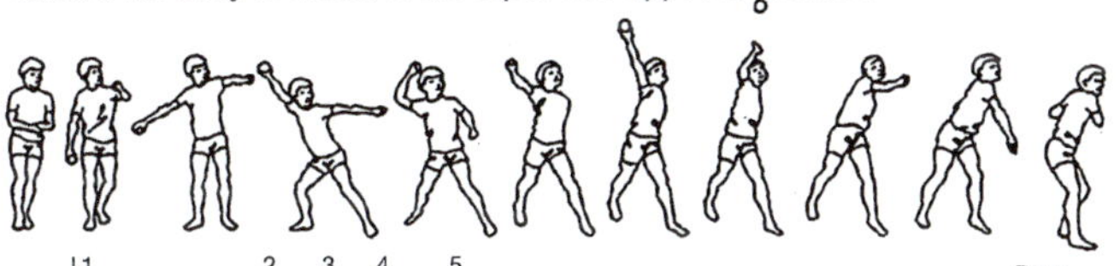

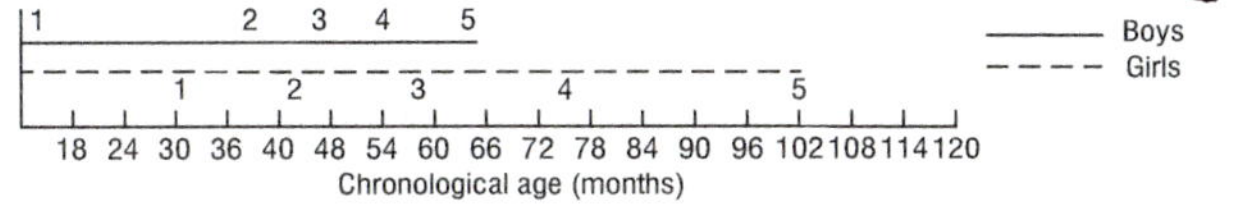

Age at which 60 percent of the boys and girls were able to perform at each developmental level for the fundamental motor skill of throwing.

Figure 13.2 Developmental sequences for throwing: total body approach

Sources: Haubenstricker et al. (1983); Seefeldt and Haubenstricker (1976, 1982); Seefeldt et al. (1972). All material used with permission of Dr. John Haubenstricker.

the purpose of comparing them with a similar cohort of 13-year-olds from 1979. The researchers were particularly interested in determining if the overarm ball-throwing velocity of girls and boys had changed over the intervening 24 years. Findings indicated that the difference in average ball-throwing velocity between the boys and girls had not narrowed during this period. This result seems to indicate that the forceful overarm throw data reported by Halverson, Roberton, and Langendorfer in 1982 remained valid during this period.

Constraints on the Development of Overarm Throwing

A number of structural, task, and environmental constraints have been identified that influence the development of overarm throwing. These constraints can be thought of as factors that help shape the development of the overarm throwing pattern (technique). This section examines selected constraints related to overarm throwing. Additionally, it describes how constraints may help account for gender differences in throwing ability.

Instruction and Instructional Cues

A basic question has been whether instruction can facilitate developmental changes or whether the year-to-year improvement observed in many fundamental skills is attributable more to age (maturation) than to instruction. There are currently two trends of thought. A number of researchers believe that differences in throwing performance, particularly sex differences in throwing performance, are genetically determined and may, therefore, be resistant to instruction (Angell, Butterfield, Loovis, et al., 2018; Lombardo & Deaner, 2018; Thomas, Alderson, Thomas, et al., 2010; Young, 2009). Young (2009) believes the development of throwing may be under the control of an innate motor program; if this is true, then throwing should be resistant to instruction.

Nevertheless, a number of studies have experimentally supported the positive influence of throwing instruction. For example, Halverson and Roberton (1979) examined the influence of throwing instruction and found that instruction was associated with the use of a more advanced throwing form, involving the components of forearm lag, trunk action, stepping action, and range of spinal rotation.

In subsequent studies, the provision of critical instructional cues for throwing has been shown to facilitate both product- and process-oriented performance (Garcia & Garcia, 2005; Lorson & Goodway, 2007). Verbal cues given to participants that have proven to be beneficial include such statements as:

1. Take a long step toward the target with the opposite foot of your throwing arm.
2. Take your arm straight down, then stretch it way back to make an "L" with the arm.
3. Watch the target and release the ball when you see your fingers.

Of these cues, the foot action component reflected the greatest improvement. As a result of this process-oriented improvement, throwing distance was found to increase by as much as 78 in (198 cm; Fronske et al., 1997). This result should be expected because this stepping-forward foot action component of the overarm throw significantly contributes to force-velocity production (Stodden, Langendorfer, Fleisig, & Andrews, 2006a).

Garcia and Garcia (2005) have developed an excellent list of progressive instructional focal points designed to facilitate overarm throwing performance and technique. Focal points have been developed for each of the following body components: stepping, backward arm swing, trunk, forearm, and humerus. The following is an example for the stepping component:

FOCAL POINT	TEACHING CUES AND PHRASES
Stepping	"step on the bug"
Step with contralateral leg	"step with opposite foot" (from throwing arm)
Large step	"make a big step" (forward)
Step and balance on one foot	"lift the stepping foot up—balance on one foot"
Step and balance on one foot leaning	"lift a foot and lean back—the tower of Pisa"
End step with foot pointing to target	"rotate stepping foot toward target before landing"

Most recently, Johnson and colleagues (2019) studied the effects of guided practice instruction toward the improvement of throwing competence in preschool age (3 to 5 years) children. Throwing competence was assessed using both process-oriented assessment techniques (Test of Gross Motor Development-3; Roberton's developmental sequences for throwing) and a product-oriented technique (throwing velocity). The children received 13, 30-minutes instructional sessions over a 7-week period. The researchers found that guided practice volume explained significant improvement in both process- and product-oriented assessments.

Ball Size

As will be discussed later in this chapter, numerous studies have examined the influence of ball size on young children's catching ability, but only a few researchers have examined its influence on throwing performance. Burton, Greer, and Wiese-Bjornstal (1992) examined the influence of ball size on the throwing performance of 40 children (aged 5–6, 7–8, and 9–10) and 20 adults (aged 19–33). The subjects were required to throw six different-sized Styrofoam balls (1.9, 4.1, 5.8, 7.8, 9.6, and 11.6 in [4.8, 10.4, 14.7, 19.8, 24.4, and 29.5 cm] in diameter) as hard as possible. Styrofoam balls were chosen because ball weight can influence throwing performance (van den Tillaar & Ettema, 2011). The researchers evaluated each throwing trial by using Roberton's component approach model for throwing, described earlier in this chapter. This study found throwing technique to be quite stable. More specifically, stable patterns of performance were exhibited 88.4 percent of the time for a selected ball diameter. When patterns of throwing performance became unstable, this marked the beginning of a transition to a new component level 70.6 percent of the time.

In a second study, Burton, Greer, and Wiese-Bjornstal (1993) sought to examine the influence of ball size on grasping patterns, as well as throwing patterns, among individuals in five age categories (5–6, 7–8, 9–10, 13–14, and 19–33 years). The performance task was essentially identical to that of their first study. The researchers witnessed a transition from one-handed grasping to two-handed grasping as the diameter of the ball increased, with adults switching at a significantly larger diameter compared with younger subjects. However, when hand size was taken into consideration, younger subjects were found to switch from a two-handed grasping pattern to a one-handed grasping pattern significantly later than did the adults. Regarding throwing pattern, two-handed throwing was exhibited less than 25 percent of the time and was mostly found among the 5- and 6-year-old girls. These two studies point out the importance of considering both ball size and the relationship between ball size and hand width in assessments of throwing performance.

Selecting equipment that is sized appropriately for the performer's body dimensions is referred to as **body scaling.** As we have seen in the examples presented above, if the ball to be thrown is too large for the performer to grasp with one hand, then the performer will likely have to resort to a more immature throwing pattern of grasping the ball with both hands. Selecting equipment that is appropriately sized for the bodily dimensions of the performer can profoundly improve the performer's movement pattern.

Kinematic Constraints

Another approach to studying developmental changes in overarm throwing involves the examination of quantitative changes. Unlike the study of qualitative changes, research into quantitative changes involves studying possible underlying biomechanical (kinematic) changes in movement. Stodden, Langendorfer, Fleisig, and Andrews (2006a, 2006b) examined selected kinematic variables associated with overarm throwing (e.g., linear and rotational velocities of various body segments). These variables were associated with each of the developmental components of overarm throwing, as defined by Roberton and Halverson (1984) and described earlier in this chapter.

In the first study (Stodden et al., 2006a), the goal was to identify the kinematic variables related to the step and trunk action components of overarm throwing. Increases in kinematic variables were found to be associated with increases in component level. In other words, as increases in kinematic variables were witnessed, associated increases were found in the assessed level of overarm throwing maturity. Specifically, these step and trunk action components included stride length, pelvic and upper torso rotational and linear velocity, degree of trunk tilt, and time from stride foot contact to ball release.

In the second study (Stodden et al., 2006b), the researchers shifted their attention to the kinematic variables associated with upper-extremity actions, specifically the humerus and forearm components. It was found that five of the six humerus kinematic variables and all forearm kinematic variables were potential control parameters and, therefore, represent overarm throwing constraints. The researchers also noted, to no surprise, that improvements in kinematic variables were accompanied by increases in ball velocity.

These studies further support the earlier findings of Roberton and Konczak (2001) in their attempt to answer the question of whether an improvement in movement process (technique) affects the performance outcome. By examining longitudinal data collected over a 7-year period (at 6, 7, 8, and 13 years of age), Roberton and Konczak found that changes in the five components making up the developmental sequence of overarm throwing (see Table 13.2) accounted for 65–85 percent of the variance in children's ball-throwing velocity. Although the components that best predicted ball velocity changed over time, the humerus and forearm action components accounted for a significant portion of the change in the first three age groups studied. Among the oldest subjects (13 years), the stride length (stepping) component accounted for the greatest amount of variance. This finding confirms earlier findings that suggest that advanced throwers step a distance of 80 percent or more of their standing height (Escamilla, Fleisig, Barrantine, et al., 1998). As suggested earlier in the chapter, teachers should attempt to develop and use instructional cues that may influence these developmental components.

Accounting for Gender Differences in Overarm Throwing

Anyone who works regularly with young children will tell you that there is a difference between the overarm throwing of young boys and young girls (Angell, Butterfield, Loovis, et al., 2018; Butterfield, Loovis, & Lee, 2003; Butterfield et al., 2012; Ehl, Roberton, & Langendorfer, 2005; Johnson, Rudisill, Hastie, & Sassi, 2019; Runion et al., 2003). In fact, in a meta-analysis to examine gender differences in 20 motor performance tasks, Thomas and French (1985) found the greatest gender differences in throwing skills, among the skills examined. This finding has led researchers to develop a series of studies designed to uncover why such gender differences may exist. Note that although gender differences in overarm throwing favor boys' performance, many girls involved in sports have exhibited highly advanced throwing patterns (Thomas et al., 2010).

Researchers have speculated that such differences could be accounted for by hereditary and sociocultural factors. A 1986 study by J. D. Nelson, Thomas, K. R. Nelson, and Abraham (1986) supported this view. These researchers found that the throwing performance of 5-year-old girls was 57 percent of that of similar-aged boys. However, when the scores were adjusted for the structural constraints of joint diameters, shoulder/hip ratio, forearm length, and arm and leg muscle mass, the throwing performance of girls improved to 69 percent of that of boys. In a three-year follow-up study involving 26 of the original 100 children (K. R. Nelson, Thomas, & J. K. Nelson, 1991), boys' throwing distance was positively associated with a heredity factor (arm muscle mass) and a sociocultural factor: the presence of a male adult in the home. In contrast, girls who weighed more, were stronger, and had more body fat along with greater joint diameters and more estimated arm and leg muscle mass threw farther than their smaller and weaker female counterparts.

Carlton (1989) investigated how gender-mediated environmental factors could affect differences in boys' and girls' throwing. Using Roberton's five-part component model (see pp. 367–8), Carlton evaluated children aged 3–5. Parents were required to complete an environmental factors questionnaire designed to probe for differences in such factors as the parents' engagement with their children in gross motor play, provision for the use of gross motor toys, participation in recreational activities, attitudes regarding sport participation, participation in movement programs, and the presence of an older sibling. The author concluded that the best predictors of throwing development in girls were participation in sport and movement programs and the presence of an older brother in the household. Barnett and colleagues (2010) suggest that each of these factors could contribute to improved performance through increasing skill practice time. Johnson and colleagues (2019) have also reported a positive association between practice volume and improved overhand throwing performance in young females.

A qualitative evaluation can also be utilized to highlight gender differences in overarm throwing performance. For example, Gromeier, Koester, and Schack (2017) also used Roberton's component approach to assess gender differences in overarm throwing. While the 6- to 16-year-old male and female German handball players demonstrated similar motor patterns involving the humerus and forearm actions, they differed significantly on the trunk, backswing, and stepping actions. A more mature level of performance within these three actions could possibly lead to better female performance. Indeed, among young Japanese children, Roberton's developmental sequence was found to be the best predictor of ball throwing performance (distance; Kasuyama, Mutou, & Sasamoto, 2016).

Finally, Lombardo and Deaner (2018), as well as Angell and colleagues (2018) have determined that factors involving human evolution may account for gender differences in throwing. The authors built their argument on an examination of throwing behaviors believed to be exhibited in early humans. It is believed that, early in human history, throwing was more prevalent among males than females and was probably used during defensive encounters and for hunting. Thus, they view throwing performance as being rooted in human evolution. This view is also supported by research, which notes that while throwing instruction may improve female throwing performance; it does not eliminate the performance gap in favor of males (Angell et al., 2018).

CATCHING

Catching is the action of bringing an airborne object under control by using the hands and arms. In contrast to throwing research, there has been little process-oriented research into developmental stages associated with this fundamental movement pattern. In fact, none of the process-oriented studies for catching described in this chapter has validated its hypothesized stages.

Two-Handed Catching

Developmental Aspects of Two-Handed Catching

Usually, a child's first attempts at stopping or controlling a moving object occur when the child is seated on the floor with the legs spread apart. At first, the child will be successful in stopping a rolled ball by trapping the ball against the legs. With practice, the child will soon be able to trap the ball against the floor by using only the hands, with the palms facing the floor.

A child's first attempts at catching an airborne ball are generally passive. That is, the child stands facing the tosser, who attempts to project the ball into the child's outstretched arms so the child can trap the ball against the body. The palms of the hands face upward, and the child makes no attempt to adjust the body or arms to the oncoming ball.

As their visuoperceptual systems improve, children attempt to adjust their hands and arms to the ball's changing flight characteristics. The child holds the hands with the palms facing one another instead of upward and bends the elbows slightly so that the hands are in front of the face. Still, in most instances, the ball will make initial contact with the arms or body as the child brings her or his arms up toward the face. When the child does manage to retain the ball, this is done by hugging or trapping it against the body. At this stage of development, some children may exhibit fear when the projected ball approaches them. Negative reactions to the tossed ball include turning the head away from the ball, leaning backward away from the ball, and closing the eyes (see Figure 13.3).

At the most advanced level of catching development, the performer adjusts the entire body so as to control the projectile with only the hands. In addition, the catcher with a mature style "gives with the catch." The child absorbs the momentum of the projectile by flexing the elbows at the moment of hand-ball contact; in effect, the elbows work as shock absorbers.

These developmental characteristics are evident in Kay's (1970) classic analysis of the

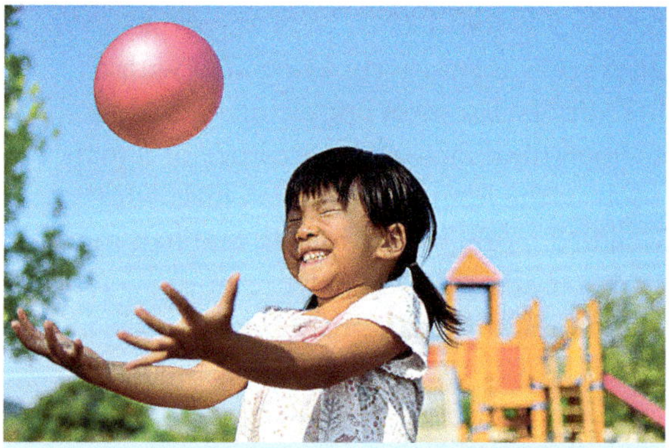

Figure 13.3 This 6-year-old child is showing fear in reaction to the thrown ball

catching styles of 2-, 5-, and 15-year-old children. Kay described the 2-year-old child as approaching the task without any general strategy. Two-year-olds tend to maintain a static position throughout the entire task and focus their eyes on the tosser, not the ball. In short, these young children react too late. As Kay stated, the 2-year-old child is mostly "doing something after it has happened, often very long after, as when she eventually turns to fetch the ball that has fallen" (p. 144).

In contrast, 5-year-old children can anticipate some of the ball's changing flight characteristics, and they focus their eyes on the thrower, the ball, and even their own hands. These children's poor timing and coordination limit their ability to retain the ball. The children's movements are correct but appear to be carried out in slow motion (Kay, 1970).

Finally, 15-year-old adolescents are capable of predicting the ball's flight characteristics, and they carry out preparatory responses well in advance of the ball's arrival. Kay (1970) writes, "The overall impression is one of smoothness and ease. The eyes are concentrated upon the ball; they do not watch the hands, which are controlled entirely from the boy's own awareness of the position of his limbs" (p. 145).

Developmental Sequences for Two-Handed Catching

Table 13.3 presents Roberton and Halverson's (1984) component analysis for the fundamental motor skill of catching. Figure 13.4 illustrates the developmental sequence for catching based on the total body approach. The latter approach has withstood preliminary validation in a mixed longitudinal sample (Haubenstricker et al., 1983).

A close inspection of the graph at the end of Figure 13.4 indicates little difference in the developmental level of catching between boys and girls prior to 48 months of age (4 years). However, at the age of 5, 60 percent of the girls exhibited a stage 4 developmental level of performance, whereas 60 percent of the boys exhibited this level of development at approximately 6 years of age. In another data set, Butterfield and colleagues (2012) found that by 10 years of age 80.5 percent of the boys and girls in their study had achieved a mature catching pattern as measured by the criteria set forth in the Test of Gross Motor Development (see Chapter 16).

One-Handed Catching

Developmental Aspects of One-Handed Catching

A wealth of information exists regarding the development of two-handed catching in young boys and girls, but few studies have examined children's ability to catch with one hand. One of the first studies to examine one-handed catching in young children was conducted by Fischman, Moore, and Steel (1992). The authors were interested in determining performance trends and gender differences in the one-handed catching ability of children between 5 and 12 years of age. In addition, they were interested in studying how the location of the ball toss affects hand orientation and catching success. A tennis ball was tossed from a distance of 9 feet (2.7 m) to one of four locations: waist height, shoulder height, above the head, and out to the side at waist level. As with two-handed catching, performance improved with age for both boys and girls. The success rate among the boys ranged from 17.2 percent at 5 years of age to 95.8 percent at 12 years. For girls, the success rate ranged from 4.2 percent to 92.2 percent at 5 and 12 years of age, respectively. The authors concluded that by age 12 the skill appeared to be essentially mastered, but one could offer an alternate hypothesis; namely, the task may have been too easy for the older children. This was not the case for the younger children. Of the 294 "no contacts" (no part of the body

Table 13.3 Developmental sequences for catching: component approach

Preparation: arm component	
Step 1:	The arms are outstretched with elbows extended, awaiting the tossed ball.
Step 2:	The arms await the ball toss with some shoulder flexion still apparent, but flexion now appears in the elbows.
Step 3:	The arms await the ball in a relaxed posture at the sides of the body or slightly ahead of the body. The elbows may be flexed.
Reception: arm component	
Step 1:	The arms remain outstretched and the elbows rigid. There is little to no "give," so the ball bounces off the arms.
Step 2:	The elbows flex to carry the hands upward toward the face. Initially, ball contact is primarily with the arms, and the object is trapped against the body.
Step 3:	Initial contact is with the hands. If unsuccessful in using the fingers, the child may still trap the ball against the chest. The hands still move upward toward the face.
Step 4:	Ball contact is made with the hands. The elbows still flex, but the shoulders extend, bringing the ball down and toward the body rather than up toward the face.
Hand component	
Step 1:	The palms of the hands face upward. (Rolling balls elicit a palms-down, trapping action.)
Step 2:	The palms of the hands face each other.
Step 3:	The palms of the hands are adjusted to the flight and size of the oncoming object. Thumbs or little fingers are placed close together, depending on the height of the flight path.
Body component	
Step 1:	There is no adjustment of the body in response to the flight path of the ball.
Step 2:	The arms and trunk begin to move in relation to the ball's flight path.
Step 3:	The feet, trunk, and arms all move to adjust to the path of the oncoming ball.

Note: These sequences have not been validated. They were hypothesized by Harper (1979).

Source: Roberton and Halverson (1984). Used with permission from the current copyright holder, M. A. Roberton.

contacted the ball), 269 occurred among the 5- to 8-year-old children. One could speculate that such poor performance was caused by the children's immature temporal and spatial organization (Stone, Maynard, North, et al., 2017). Location of the toss influenced catching success as measured by the number of balls that were correctly retained. Interestingly, when the ball was thrown to certain locations, the children were able to correctly position the arm and hand but could not perform the temporal closing of the hand correctly, especially when the ball was tossed to the shoulder location. Similar findings have been reported in adult populations (Cesqui, Russo, Lacquaniti, & d'Avella, 2016).

Williams (1992a) compared the one-handed and two-handed catching performances of children between 4 and 10 years of age. Catching attempts were classified as being a "cradle" (the hand is flexed to form a cradle into which the ball will passively fall and the

Stage 1 The child presents his or her arms directly in front of the body, with the elbows extended and the palms facing upward or inward toward the midsagittal plane. As the ball contacts the hands or arms, the elbow are flexed and the arms and hands attempt to secure the ball by holding it against the chest.

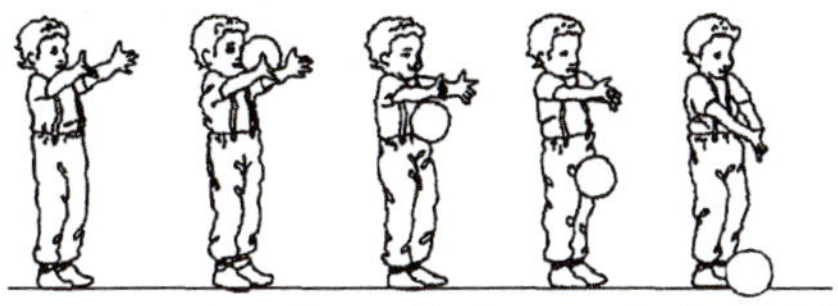

Stage 2 The child prepares to receive the object with the arms in front of the body, the elbows extended or slightly flexed. Upon presentation of the ball, the arms begin an encircling motion that culminates by securing the ball against the chest. Stage 2 also differs from stage 1 in that, in stage 2, the receiver initiates the arm action prior to ball-arm contact.

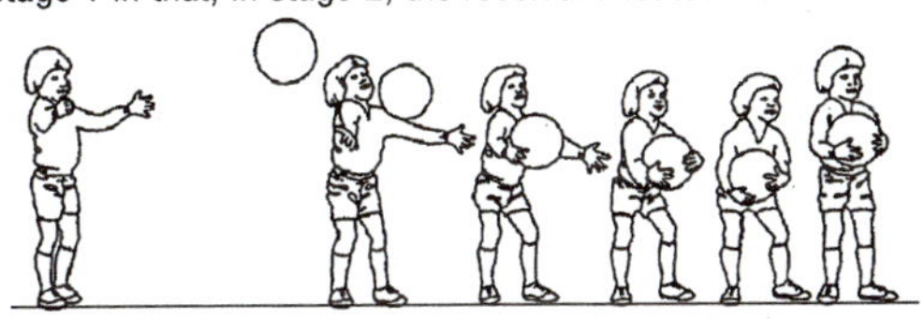

Stage 3 The child prepares to receive the ball with arms that are slightly flexed and extended forward at the shoulder. Many children also receive the ball with arms that are flexed at the elbow and the elbow ahead of a frontal plane.
Substage 1: The child uses the chest as the first contact point with the ball and attempts to secure the ball by holding it to the chest with the hands and arms.
Substage 2: The child attempts to catch the ball with the hands. Upon failure to hold it securely, the child maneuvers it to the chest, where it is controlled by the hands and arms.

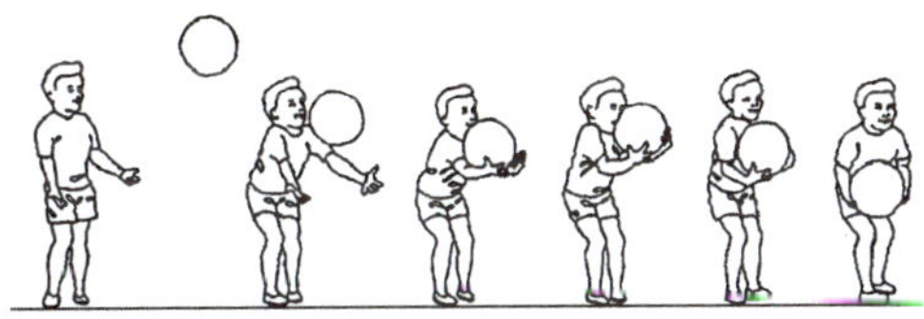

Stage 4 The child prepares to receive the ball by flexing the elbow and presenting the arms ahead of the frontal plane. Skillful performers may keep the elbows at the side and flex the arms simultaneously as they bring them forward to meet the ball. The ball is caught with the hands, without its making contact with any other body parts.

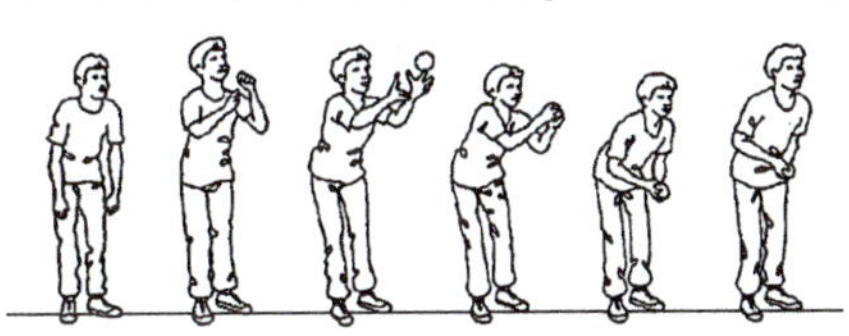

Stage 5 The upper segmental action is identical to stage 4. In addition, the child is required to change the stationary base in order to receive the ball. Stage 5 is included because of the apparent difficulty that many children encounter when they are required to move in relation to an approaching object.

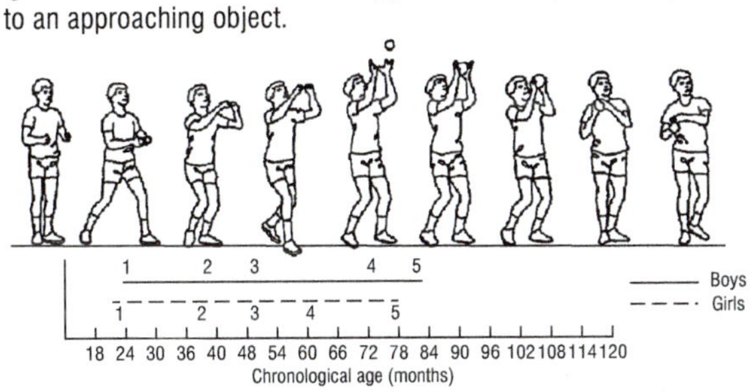

Age at which 60 percent of the boys and girls were able to perform at each developmental level for the fundamental motor skill of catching.

Figure 13.4 Developmental sequences for catching: total body approach

Source: Haubenstricker et al. (1983); Seefeldt (1972a); Seefeldt and Haubenstricker (1982). All material used with permission of Dr. John Haubenstricker.

ball is then trapped against the body), a "clamp" (the hand moves toward the ball, palm facing inward, and as the ball approaches the hand moves underneath the falling ball, which is grasped with the palm of the hand), or a "grasp" (the hand reaches for the oncoming ball with the palm facing the ball, and the flexed fingers grasp the ball well in front of the body). One-handed catching was only one-half as successful as two-handed catching. Although grasping (the most mature technique) was the prominent movement strategy for two-handed catching, the prominent movement strategy for catching with one hand was the cradle (the least mature technique). In fact, grasping declined from 66 percent to 26 percent when one-handed catching was required. This provides further evidence that constraints can contribute to changes in movement patterns.

Constraints on the Development of Catching

There has been no shortage of studies designed to examine factors that may influence catching development. Unfortunately, it is difficult to compare and contrast these studies because they vary as to the major constraint studied (ball size, color of ball and background, vision and viewing time, instruction, knowledge and experience, catching on the run, and catching with a glove) and the type of evaluation system used. Nevertheless, an awareness of these findings can aid future investigative research and provide insight for selecting teaching strategies.

Ball Size

The effects of ball size on an individual's catching ability have received much research attention (Isaacs, 1980; Payne, 1985a; Payne & Koslow, 1981; Strohmeyer, Williams, & Schaub-George, 1991). Initial studies consistently concluded that larger balls improved young children's catching performance. Studies were often based on the premise that young children are far-sighted and would profit from use of the larger ball, which would be easier to track visually. Also, based on neurological considerations, the young children were assumed to have insufficient fine motor control for grasping smaller objects. Most early studies, however, evaluated the children's catching attempts on a pass-fail basis: the child either did or did not retain control of the ball.

Researchers have attempted to eliminate some of the shortcomings of the earlier research by using weighted rating scales to evaluate catching performance beyond the simple pass-fail. These investigations, however, have led to a sharp dissimilarity in findings.

Research has found small balls to be more conducive to successful catching than larger balls (Isaacs, 1980). This research employed a rating scale designed to evaluate the level of maturity the children displayed in their catching technique. As discussed in Chapters 1 and 16, this is a process-oriented method of evaluation. Table 13.3, Figure 13.4, and the scale in Table 13.4 are all examples of process-oriented rating tools for the skill of catching.

Isaacs (1980) found that, generally, a smaller ball tended to elicit a more mature hand catch rather than an arm/chest trap. This research also determined that as the ball size increased, the maturity level in the catching technique regressed. In other words, the child would be more likely to resort to the more immature chest-trap method of catching. This represents another example of the influence of body scaling on motor behavior. Research employing the process-oriented scale found in Table 13.4 was based on the premise that future success in catching depends on the early development of a mature technique, hence the interest in process-oriented evaluation.

In contrast, studies that have found children to be more successful in catching larger relative

Table 13.4 Process-oriented rating scale for the skill of catching

1.	Initial body contact; subject makes no attempt to contact the ball.
2.	Arm and/or body contact, miss: Initial attempt to contact is made on the arms and/or body, and the ball is missed.
3.	Arm and/or body contact, save: Initial contact is on the arms and/or body, and the ball is retained.
4.	Hand contact, miss: Initial contact is made with the hands, but the ball is then dropped immediately or dropped following arm or body contact.
5.	Hand contact, assisted catch: Initial contact is made with the hands. The ball is juggled but retained by using arms and/or body for assistance.
6.	Hand contact, clean catch: The ball is contacted and retained by the hands only. The ball may be brought into the body on the follow-through after control is gained with the hands.

Sources: Hellweg, 1972; Isaacs, 1980.

to smaller balls have generally employed rating scales designed to evaluate the level of control that the child maintained over the ball, regardless of the maturity of the catching technique. These are product-oriented evaluations. The following is an example of a product-oriented rating scale (Payne, 1985a; Payne & Koslow, 1981):

1. Failure to react
2. One hand contacts, ball dropped
3. Two hands contact, ball dropped
4. Uncontrolled catch (bobbled)
5. Controlled catch

This research was based on the premise that children's ability to control the ball is important, as regardless of the maturity of their technique, success in controlling the ball would inspire them to try again.

Clearly, we need more information on this topic. In particular, we need to know what the critical issue is in teaching this or any motor skill. Should we place the premium on early acquisition of a mature technique or on early success in terms of simply controlling the ball (Payne, 1982)? Unfortunately, little scientific information is available to answer this question, which is so critical to the optimal teaching of motor skills to children.

Ball and Background Color

Manipulation of both ball color and background color may provide a way to improve catching performance. Here the most important element is likely the contrast between the approaching ball and its background. It stands to reason that increased contrast would allow for improved visual tracking.

Data that Isaacs (1980) obtained indicate that a child's preferred color may also influence the child's catching performance. In the study, subjects were required to choose their favorite-colored ball before being administered a criterion catch test. Results of this study indicated that irrespective of the balls' specific colors, both the boys and the girls tended to catch their preferred-color ball significantly better than the nonpreferred-color balls. Isaacs speculated that because the children in this study focused their selective attention on the preferred-color ball for a longer time when catching it, they were able to obtain more critical information concerning the ball's flight.

Vision and Viewing Time

Without a doubt, the catcher must rely on visual information to form a strategy that will lead to a successful catch. Research indicates that as viewing time decreases, so does proficiency in retaining the projectile (Nessler, 1973; Whiting, Gill, & Stephenson, 1970). Thus, the teacher should use a ball that moves slowly through space (e.g., beach ball, whiffle ball, sponge ball) when tossing to inexperienced catchers.

Instruction

In an experiment with a single-subject design, Williams (1992b) trained an 8-year-old boy to catch. Training consisted of four assessment sessions and three instruction-plus-practice sessions administered alternately on seven successive days. Each instruction-and-practice session lasted 30 minutes. Following the third instruction-and-practice session, significant changes were observed in the boy's percentage of successful catches and in the level of maturity (technique) he used to retain the projected ball. Williams noted that by the end of the study, this 8-year-old boy's catching ability had progressed from that of a typical 8-year-old to that typical of children who are two years older.

Instruction designed to influence a performer's "focus of attention" during a ball catching task has proven to be a beneficial strategy. More specifically, focus of attention during a ball catching task can take one of two forms. First, an internal focus of attention where the performer is instructed to "concentrate on the hands" and second, an external focus of attention where the performer is instructed to "concentrate on the ball." Using these two focuses of attention instructional strategies, Abdollahipour and Psotta (2017) required 25 elementary school age children (mean = 8.75 yrs) from the Czech Republic to attempt to catch tennis balls projected a distance of 15 meters. Prior to the catching attempts, the young subjects were instructed as to where their attention should be concentrated during the catching attempts. The researchers concluded that catching attempts were most successful when an external focus of attention was employed. Thus, focusing on environmental effects (ball) proved to be more effective than focusing on bodily movements (hands).

Knowledge and Experience

In Chapter 2, we described in some detail the positive relationship between an individual's knowledge of a specific sport and subsequent sport performance. Research suggests that knowledge regarding the specific task of catching may influence catching performance. For example, Kourtessis (1994) studied the influence of procedural and declarative knowledge (see Chapter 2) of ball catching in children (6–12 years old), both with and without physical disabilities. Procedural knowledge, as measured by a 15-task ball-catching hierarchy, was found to be higher in the populations without disabilities than the populations with disabilities. Furthermore, the children who were ambulatory with physical disabilities scored higher than their peers who were nonambulatory with physical disabilities. Declarative knowledge, however, did not differ significantly among the various groups. Thus, it appears that declarative and procedural knowledge do not develop at the same rate and that catching experience may foster the acquisition of procedural knowledge, even though a deficit in declarative knowledge may exist. Similarly, Lefebvre (1996) reported that experience in catching is a crucial factor in a child's ability to predict the flight of a thrown ball. This research suggests that providing children the opportunity to catch thrown balls is, in and of itself, an important instructional strategy.

Catching on the Run

Catching involves adjustments of not only the hands and arms but also the entire body when the ball is projected away from the child. Understandably, a ball projected directly toward the child is easier to catch than a ball that requires the child to move to a new location to intercept it (Keegan, 1989). Therefore, teachers should use caution in, or avoid entirely, pairing up an inexperienced thrower with an inexperienced catcher. The inexperienced thrower's inability to throw the ball directly to the inexperienced catcher will definitely increase the difficulty of the catching task.

Catching with a Glove

In one-handed catching, the performer must not only position the hand in the path of the oncoming ball but also correctly time the closure of the fingers around the ball. It appears that the use of a glove alters the nature of the errors typically observed in bare-handed catching during these two phases. In fact, initial research suggests that the use of a glove improves catching success by reducing the precision necessary for limb-hand positioning and by altering the temporal grasping component (Fischman & Mucci, 1989; Fischman & Sanders, 1991). In other words, gloved catching is easier because the ball has a larger target and is grasped with a larger surface area (see Figure 13.5). At youth baseball games, a common sight is the young participant who mistimes the hand closure around the ball but can still hold on to it. Generally, half of the ball is in the glove and half is out. Without the glove, closing the fingers too late would have resulted in a missed catch. Therefore, instructors should view one-handed glove catching as simpler than bare-handed catching. However, instructors should make sure that participants possess enough hand (grasping) strength to squeeze the glove efficiently. A new, stiff glove or one that is too large may hinder catching if the participant cannot close the glove's fingers.

Catch-Throw: A Dual Task Constraint

Catching and throwing are oftentimes referred to as complementary skills. This is because in many real-world activities, once a ball is caught, the performer is generally required to then throw the ball to a teammate (baseball) or toward a goal (handball), oftentimes under a

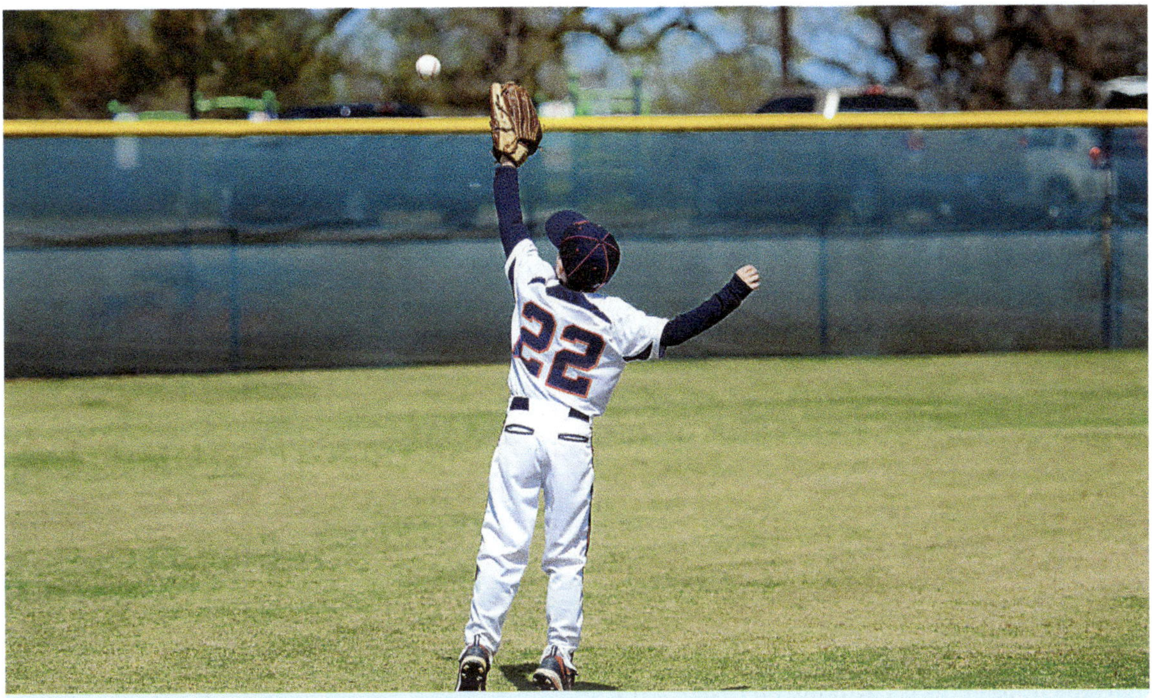

Figure 13.5 Catching performance is improved when a glove is used as it reduces the precision necessary for limb-hand positioning and alters the temporal grasping component of the hand closure

temporal constraint. Is it possible that knowing in advance the need to perform a second task, may have an influence on the movement patterns used to accomplish both tasks? To help answer this question, movement patterns of experienced Japanese baseball players were assessed under two task constraints (Murase, Yokoyama, Fujii, et al., 2016). More specifically, a shoulder and hip segmental analysis was performed using optical motion cameras while both catching a launched ball (catching task) and while catching and then immediately throwing the ball to a human target (catch-throw task). The researchers found that during the simple catching task, there were no changes in the shoulder-hip angles. However, significant rotational changes were uncovered during the catch-throw task. The research team concluded that whenever individuals are required to perform several movements successively, the terminal phase of the first movement and the preparatory phase of the second movement change as a function of the tasks goal. Thus, when teaching successive movement skills, the transition between skills is actually a new skill that must be addressed.

STRIKING

Striking is a fundamental movement in which the performer uses a designated body part or some implement to project an object. Propulsion skills are necessary in many sport activities and can occur in a variety of forms. For example, the bare hand is used as the striking implement in volleyball. The striking pattern can be underhand, as in serving the volleyball, or overhand, as in spiking the volleyball. When an implement is used, such as a racquet or bat, the striking pattern is accomplished with either one or two hands. This section describes the development of movement patterns for striking an object with a body part (hand or foot) and with an implement (racquet or bat).

Developmental Aspects of One- and Two-Handed Striking

The child's initial attempt to strike an object with either the bare hand or some implement is very similar to the overarm throwing pattern young children exhibit. Briefly, at an inexperienced level of development, the child uses an overarm pattern that consists predominantly of flexion and extension of the forearm. The child usually directly faces the object to be struck and may or may not take a forward step. If the child does take a forward step, it is with the **homolateral** leg, the leg on the same side of the body as the striking arm.

Table 13.5 Major characteristics of general striking development

Inexperienced striker	
1.	Striker usually takes no step, but if the striker does, it is with the homolateral leg.
2.	Striker uses an up-down striking motion.
3.	Striker takes little backswing with the striking arm or implement.
4.	The striker's trunk and hips do not rotate and there is no block rotation.
5.	Striker holds the arms rigid with little, if any, wrist snap when swinging a paddle or bat.
Advanced striker	
1.	Striker takes a forward step with the foot opposite the striking arm or striking side.
2.	Striker uses a full backswing.
3.	Striker swings the striking implement horizontally.
4.	Differentiated trunk and hip rotation is present.
5.	In the two-handed striking pattern, the striker's arms are relaxed and there is a noticeable coordinated wrist snap when swinging the bat.

Source: Payne (1985b).

Thus, all of the striking movements are accomplished in the anterior-posterior plane. The child's upward-downward swing pattern gradually "flattens out." Flattening out the swing facilitates the child's ability to contact the ball. Table 13.5 summarizes the major characteristics of striking development.

Developmental Sequence of Striking

Figure 13.6 describes and illustrates a total body approach to the analysis of striking with a bat.

Stage 1 The motion is primarily posterior-anterior in direction. The movement begins with hip extension and slight spinal extension and retraction of the shoulder on the striking side of the body. The elbows flex fully. The feet remain stationary throughout the movement with the primary force coming from extension of the flexed joints.

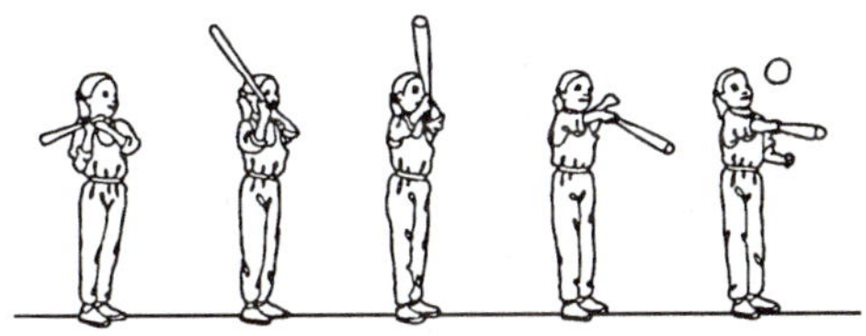

Stage 2 The feet remain stationary or either the right or left foot may receive the weight as the body moves toward the approaching ball. The primary pattern is the unitary rotation of the hip–spinal linkage about an imaginary vertical axis. The forward movement of the bat is in a transverse plane.

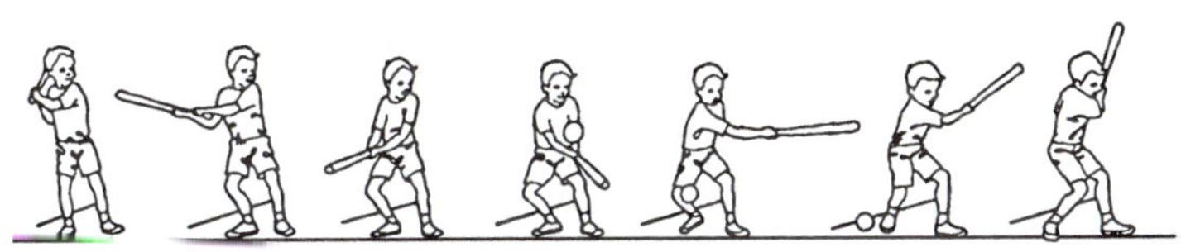

Stage 3 The shift of weight to the front-supporting foot occurs in an ipsilateral pattern. The trunk rotation-derotation is decreased markedly in comparison with stage 2, and the movement of the bat is in an oblique-vertical plane instead of the transverse path seen in stage 2.

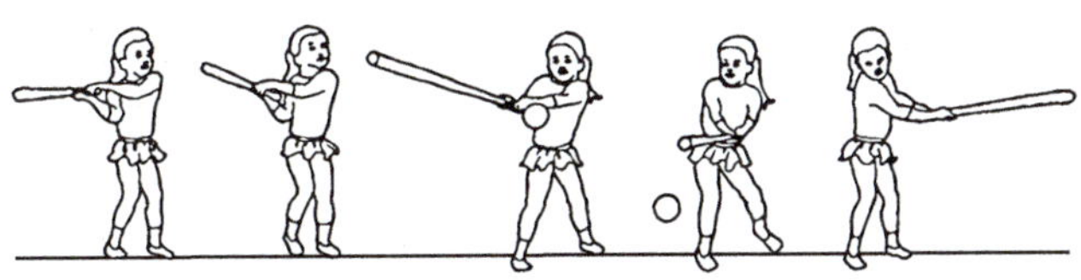

Stage 4 The transfer of weight in rotation-derotation is in a contralateral pattern. The shift of weight to the forward foot occurs while the bat is still moving backward as the hips, spine, and shoulder girdle assume their force-producing positions. At the initiation of the forward movement, the bat is kept near the body. Elbow extension and the supination-pronation of the hands do not occur until the arms and hands are well forward and ready to extend the lever in preparation to meet the ball. At contact the weight is on the forward foot.

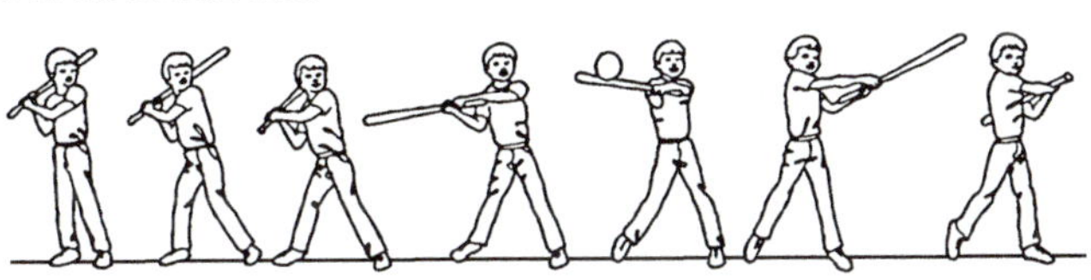

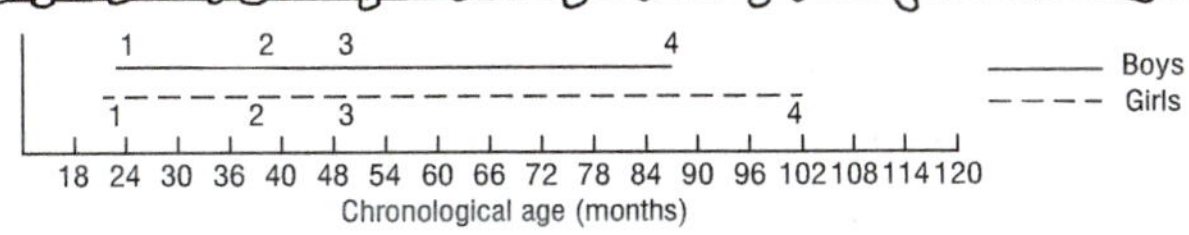

Age at which 60 percent of the boys and girls were able to perform at each developmental level for the fundamental motor skill of striking with a bat.

Figure 13.6 Developmental sequences for striking with a bat: total body approach

Source: Seefeldt and Haubenstricker (1982). All material used with permission of Dr. John Haubenstricker.

OBJECT-CONTROL SKILLS WITHOUT IMPLEMENTS

Stationary Ball Bouncing

Bouncing a ball is a fundamental movement used in many childhood and some adult activities. At an advanced level of development, a person bounces a ball by using the hand to push the ball repeatedly downward, a movement called **dribbling.** At inexperienced levels of performance, a person uses one or two hands to strike instead of push the ball. Thus, striking is one of the developmental stages of ball bouncing.

Initially, the striking pattern resembles a spanking or slapping motion of the hand and wrist (see Figure 13.7). Wickstrom (1980), one of the few researchers to study the acquisition of ball-handling skills in young children, filmed 115 children in kindergarten through second grade to study developmental characteristics in this fundamental movement pattern. He noted that the inexperienced dribbler holds the fingers of the striking hand close together and sometimes slightly hyperextends the fingers at contact. Following contact with the ball, the child quickly retracts the arm, and there is little extension of the elbow. Because their eye-hand coordination is poor, young performers strike the ball in an inconsistent manner. As would be expected, young children have difficulty controlling the direction in which the ball is hit. Timing hand-ball contact is also difficult for the inexperienced performers. It is common to observe an inexperienced performer slapping at the ball when the ball is traveling down and quickly retracting the arm when the ball is rebounding up, thus never making contact with the ball.

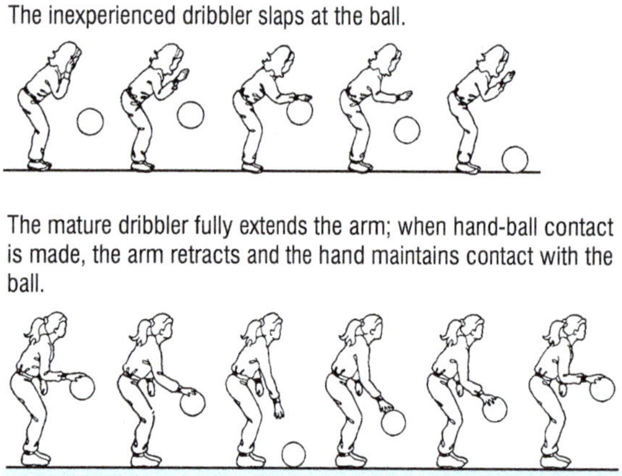

Figure 13.7 An illustration of inexperienced and mature dribbling

In contrast, the experienced dribbler pushes the ball toward the floor so that the elbow is nearly fully extended. The dribbling arm stays extended and recontacts the ball when it bounces, approximately two-thirds of the way up. Once hand-ball contact has been made, the hand retracts slowly, thus enabling the hand to maintain contact with the ball. The ball is once again pushed downward to start another dribbling cycle. The fingers are spread apart throughout the movement.

The transition from inexperienced to experienced performance becomes evident as the individual gradually extends the elbow and delays retracting the forearm. Meeting the ball before it has reached its peak height and "giving" with the ball enable the hand to maintain contact with the ball, so the ball is pushed rather than struck toward the floor.

Kicking

Kicking is another form of striking; here, the foot is used to give impetus to a ball. Two styles of kicking are place kicking and punting.

Place Kicking

In **place kicking,** the ball is placed either on the ground or on a kicking tee.

Developmental sequence for place kicking. In the most mature form of place kicking, the advanced performer will approach the ball with a running start. The last step taken prior to ball-foot contact involves a leap step onto the plant or support foot. Simultaneously, the kicking leg is prepared by flexing the knee and hyperextending the hip. This preparatory backswing will enable the performer to thrust the leg forward vigorously and to project the ball powerfully. After kicking the ball, the kicking leg continues to travel upward—the leg is allowed to follow through. The follow-through should be vigorous enough to cause the support leg to leave the ground. Simply put, the performer hops on the support leg. During this kicking sequence, the kicker's center of gravity is displaced. To maintain balance, the advanced placekicker positions the trunk so it leans slightly backward and uses the arms to oppose the action of the legs.

In contrast, the inexperienced placekicker lacks many of the preparatory movements of the advanced kicker. The child simply pushes the ball away with the foot. In fact, the foot barely leaves the ground, there is no backswing of the kicking leg, the leg remains straight throughout the kicking motion, and there is no follow-through. In addition, the child holds the arms straight by the side of the body rather than using them to maintain balance.

At an intermediate level of place-kicking development, preparatory movements are noticeable. There is less flexion of the knee and hip than in an advanced pattern, but some preparation is evident. The arms are elevated to help maintain balance but still do not work in opposition to the legs. The follow-through of the kicking leg is evident after the kick but is less than what is expected at an advanced level of kicking development. These developmental changes in place kicking are illustrated and presented in more detail in Figure 13.8.

Constraints on place kicking. Researchers have identified potential constraints on kicking performance. One example is "kicking distance," which Mally, Battista, and Roberton (2011) identified as a control parameter in place kicking. Children in their study would spontaneously change their approach to accomplishing the kicking task when told the goal was to kick the ball farther. For this change, the children tended to adopt a more mature pattern of performance. More specifically, when told to kick the ball farther, the children tended to take more steps toward the ball and to use a longer leap step onto the support leg prior to foot-ball contact. Other changes included greater acceleration of the thigh and greater knee flexion. Following foot-ball contact, the body's momentum carried the child forward of the ball's placement instead of backward. Obviously, each of these pattern changes contributes to the production of more bodily force.

Punting

Unlike place kicking, in which one kicks a stationary ball, **punting** involves striking an airborne ball with the foot. Obviously, the complexity of punting greatly exceeds that of place kicking. Table 13.6 describes the hypothesized developmental sequences for punting, based on the component approach (Roberton & Halverson, 1984), and Figure 13.9 describes and illustrates this task from the perspective of the total body approach. Many of the developmental characteristics involved in the place kick are also evident in punting: the punter with an immature style is generally stationary, fails to prepare the kicking leg properly, and fails to follow through with sufficient force. Also, at this immature level of performance there is no leap step prior to ball-foot contact and no hop on the supporting foot following ball-foot contact; both movements would be evident in the most mature level of both kicking and punting performance. In addition, the punter with an immature

Stage 1 *Preparatory phase:* The performer is usually stationary and positioned near the ball. If the performer moves prior to kicking, the steps are short and concerned with spatial relationships rather than attaining momentum for the kick.

Force production: The thigh of the kicking leg moves forward with the knee flexed and is nearly parallel to the surface by the time the foot contacts the ball. Knee-joint extension occurs after contact, resulting in a pushing rather than a striking action. Upper extremity action is usually bilateral but may show some opposition in older performers. (If the performer is too far from the ball as the extremity moves to meet the ball, the knee flexes only slightly and the leg swings forward from the hip in a pushing action.)

Follow-through phase: The knee of the kicking leg continues to extend until it approaches 180°. If the trunk is inclined forward following contact with the ball, the performer will step forward to regain balance. If the trunk is leaning backward, the kicking leg will move backward after ball contact to achieve body balance.

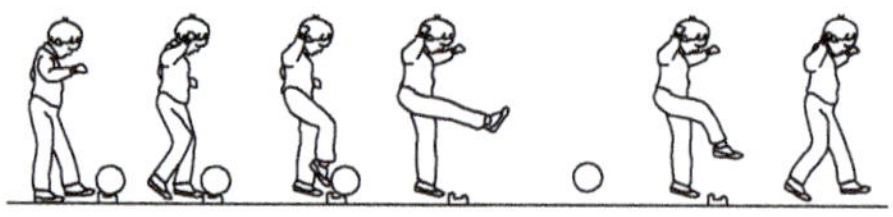

Stage 2 *Preparatory phase:* The performer is stationary. Initial action involves hyperextension at the hips and flexion at the knee so that the thigh of the kicking leg is behind the midfrontal plane. The arms may move into a position of opposition in situations of extreme hyperextension at the hips.

Force production: The kicking leg moves forward with the knee joint in a flexed position. Knee-joint extension begins just prior to foot contact with the ball. Arm-leg opposition occurs during the kick.

Follow-through phase: Knee extension continues after the ball leaves the foot, but the force of the kick usually is not sufficient to move the body forward. Instead, the performer usually steps sideward or backward.

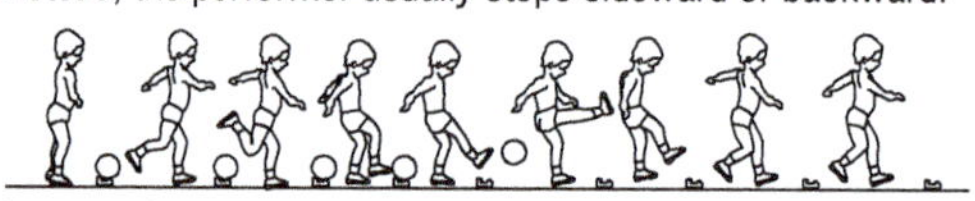

Stage 3 *Preparatory phase:* The performer takes one or more deliberate steps to approach the ball. The support leg is placed near the ball and slightly to the side of it.

Force production: The kicking foot stays near the surface as it approaches the ball, resulting in less flexion than in stage 2. The trunk remains nearly upright, thereby preventing maximum force production. The knee begins to extend prior to contact. Arm–leg opposition is evident.

Follow-through phase: The force of the kick may carry the performer past the point of contact if the approach was vigorous. Otherwise, the performer may remain near the point of contact.

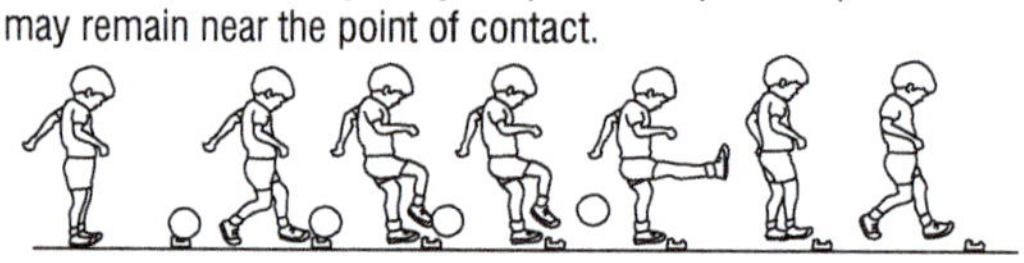

Stage 4 *Preparatory phase:* The approach involves one or more steps with the final "step" being an airborne run or leap. This permits hyperextension of the hip and flexion of the knee as in stage 2.

Force production: The shoulders are retracted and the trunk is inclined backward as the supporting leg makes contact with the surface and the kicking leg begins to move forward. The movement of the thigh nearly stops as the knee joint begins to extend rapidly just prior to contact with the ball. Arm–leg opposition is present as in the previous two stages.

Follow-through phase: If the forward momentum of the kick is sufficient, the performer either hops on the support leg or scissors the legs while airborne in order to land on the kicking foot. If the kicking foot is not vigorous, the performer may merely step in the direction of the kick.

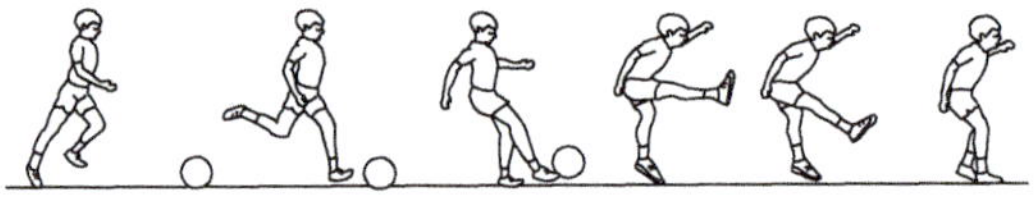

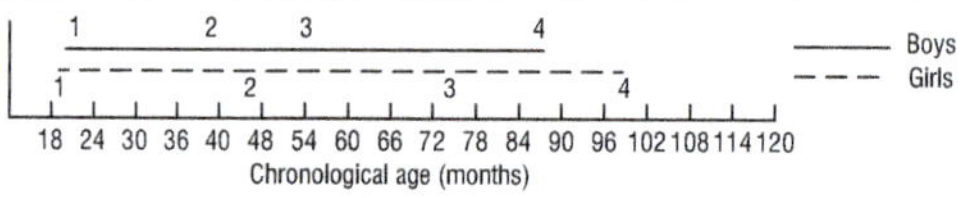

Age at which 60 percent of the boys and girls were able to perform at each developmental level tor the fundamental motor skill of kicking.

Figure 13.8 Developmental sequences for kicking: total body approach

Sources: Haubenstricker, Seefeldt, Fountain, and Sapp (1981); Seefeldt (1972b); Seefeldt and Haubenstricker (1975a, 1982). All material used with permission of Dr. John Haubenstricker.

Table 13.6 Developmental sequences for punting: component approach

Ball release: arm component	
Step 1:	Hands are on the sides of the ball. The ball is tossed upward from both hands after the support foot has landed (if a step was taken).
Step 2:	Hands are on the sides of the ball. The ball is dropped from chest height after the support foot has landed (if a step was taken).
Step 3:	Hands are on the sides of the ball. The ball is lifted upward and forward from waist level. It is released at the time of or just prior to the landing of the support foot.
Step 4:	One hand is rotated to the side and under the ball. The other hand is rotated to the side and top of the ball. The hands carry the ball on a forward and upward path during the approach. It is released at chest level as the final approach stride begins.
Ball contact: arm component	
Step 1:	Arms drop bilaterally from ball release to a position on each side of the hips at ball contact.
Step 2:	Arms bilaterally abduct after ball release. The arm on the side of the kicking leg may pull back as that leg swings forward.
Step 3:	After ball release, the arms bilaterally abduct during flight. At contact, the arm opposite the kicking leg has swung forward with that leg. The arm on the side of the kicking leg remains abducted and to the rear.
Leg action component	
Step 1:	Either no step or one short step is taken. The kicking leg swings forward from a position parallel to or slightly behind the support foot. The knee may be totally extended by contact or, more frequently, is still flexed 90° with contact above or below the knee joint. The thigh is still moving upward at contact. The ankle tends to be flexed.
Step 2:	Several steps may be taken. The last step onto the support leg is a long stride. The thigh of the kicking leg has slowed or stopped forward motion at contact. The ankle is extended. The knee has 20° to 30° of extension still possible by contact.
Step 3:	The child may take several steps, but the last is actually a leap onto the support foot. After contact, the momentum of the kicking leg pulls the child off the ground in a hop.

Note: These sequences, hypothesized by Roberton (1983), have not been validated.

Source: Roberton and Halverson(1984). Used with permission from the current copyright holder, M. A. Roberton.

technique holds the ball with both hands and generally presents it by tossing it upward and slightly forward.

In contrast, the mature punter will move forward rapidly, leaping onto the support foot prior to ball-foot contact. The kicking leg is prepared by hyperextending the hip and flexing the knee. Following ball-foot contact, a vigorous follow-through generally causes a forward hop on the support leg.

SUMMARY

- This chapter describes the development of a group of motor skills collectively referred to as object-control skills. The specific skills described in this chapter included overarm throwing, both one- and two-handed catching, striking with an implement (racquet or bat), and striking with a body part (dribbling, place kicking, and punting).

Stage 1 The performer is stationary as the hands and foot prepare for the punting action. The ball is held with both hands at waist height or higher prior to placing it in position for punting. The ball may be manipulated in a variety of ways for punting: (1) It may be held in both hands as the punting foot is lifted forward and upward with hip and knee flexion. The punting force in this situation represents a push as the ball is contacted by the plantar side of the foot when the knee extends. (2) The ball may be tossed up and forward into the air. The performer then must move forward to get the body into punting position. (3) The performer may bounce the ball and attempt to punt it as it rebounds from the surface. Whatever the mode of placing the ball into a punting position, the primary characteristics of stage 1 are a stationary preparatory position and flexion at the hip and knee of the punting leg, placing these segments in front of the midfrontal plane.

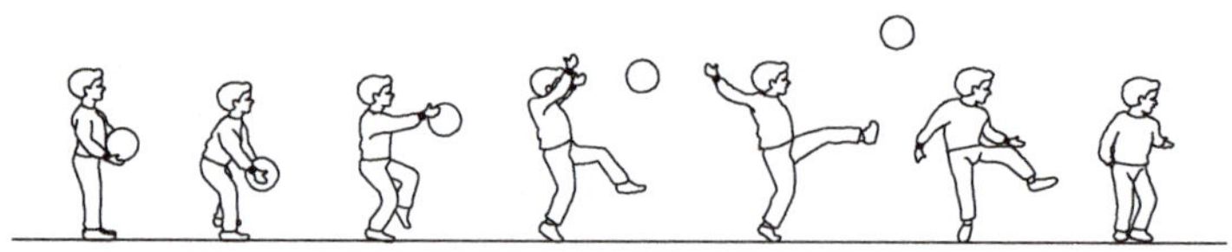

Stage 2 The performer is stationary during the preparatory phase. The ball is held in both hands and may be dropped or tossed forward or upward in preparation for punting it with the foot. The nonsupport leg is flexed at the knee, and the thigh is perpendicular to the surface or behind the midfrontal plane as the leg is placed into punting position. As the punting leg moves forward, its momentum may carry the performer forward tor a step, but generally the force is upward, causing the punter to step backward after striking the ball.

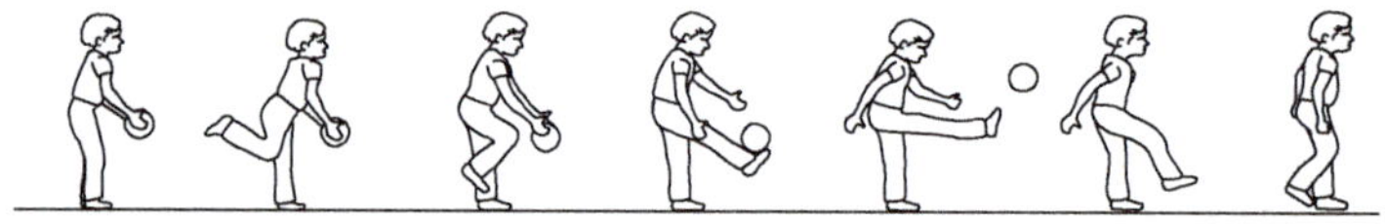

Stage 3 The performer moves forward deliberately for one or more steps in preparation for punting the ball. The ball is generally released in a forward and downward direction. The knee is flexed at 90° or less, but the thigh is farther behind the midfrontal plane than in stage 2 because of the stepping action. The follow-through of the striking leg will generally carry the punter ahead of the point where the ball was contacted.

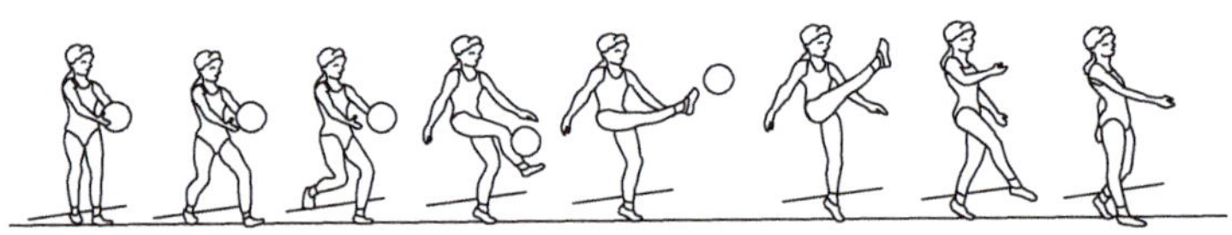

Stage 4 The punter's approach is rapid, usually comprising one or more steps, culminating in a leap just prior to contacting the ball. If the leap does not precede the punt, the punter may enhance forward momentum by taking a large step. The ball is contacted at or below knee height as a result of the ball having been released in a forward and downward direction. The momentum of the swinging leg carries the punter off the surface in an upward and forward direction after the punt.

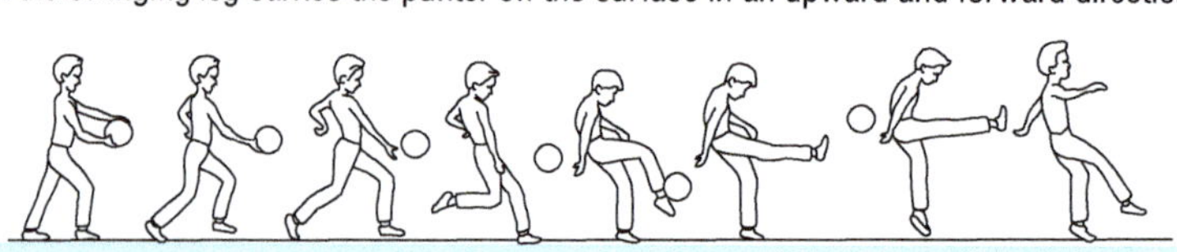

Figure 13.9 Developmental sequences for punting: total body approach

Source: Seefeldt and Haubenstricker (1975b). All material used with permission of Dr. John Haubenstricker.

- One-handed overarm throwing consists of a preparatory phase, an execution phase, and a follow-through phase. Initially, throwing is arm-dominated; in contrast, advanced throwing involves trunk rotation and a forward step with the contralateral leg. Thus, movement progresses from an anterior-posterior plane to a horizontal plane, and the base of support changes from a stationary to a shifting position. There are gender differences in overarm throwing. One study that examined gender performance differences found that, of the 20 skills examined, the greatest difference in performance was for throwing. It appears that both biological and sociocultural constraints contribute to performance differences between the genders.

- Adult-like catching involves using only the hands to bring a moving object under control. The infant's first attempt at stopping a moving object usually occurs when the child is seated and traps a rolled ball against the body. Next, the child stands and attempts to trap a rolled ball against the floor. When they first attempt to catch a thrown ball, some children may exhibit fear. Factors such as ball size, color of ball and background, vision and viewing time, instruction, knowledge and experience, catching on the run, and catching with a glove can all influence children's catching performance.
- Based on the limited amount of research available regarding children's one-handed catching, it appears that children are only about one-half as successful when they attempt to catch with one hand as with two. Children's technique regresses when they attempt to catch with one hand instead of two. As with two-handed catching, one-handed performance improves with age for both boys and girls. It appears that the major difficulty for young children is not hand orientation but the ability to time the closure of the fingers around the approaching ball (grasping).
- Striking is a fundamental movement in which the performer uses a designated body part or implement to project an object. When an implement is used, the inexperienced striker swings the implement up and down in a movement similar to an overarm throwing pattern. In contrast, the experienced striker's swinging motion is sidearm or horizontal. Ball bouncing, place kicking, and punting are examples of fundamental movements in which a body part is used to strike a ball.
- Appendices C.1 and C.2 provide assessments based on summaries of many of the object-control skills of childhood, taking a component approach and total body approach, respectively.

key concept review

body scaling
catching
contralateral
dribbling
homolateral
kicking
object-control skills
place kicking
punting
striking
throwing

questions for reflection

1. What are the three phases associated with overarm throwing?
2. According to Wild, what developmental changes are exhibited across the four developmental stages of overarm throwing? Compare and contrast these stages.
3. What four steps are associated with the preparatory phase of overarm throwing? In your answer describe the three terms that are most often used to describe the most mature technique.
4. What three techniques are used for evaluating overarm throwing performance trends? Which technique is best? Why?
5. Describe the trend in ball-throwing velocity among both girls and boys in relation to overarm throwing performance.

6. What constraints are known to influence overarm throwing development?
7. How do researchers account for gender differences in overarm throwing development and performance? Answer from both biological and sociological standpoints.
8. Can you describe fear reactions to a thrown ball?
9. What constraints are known to influence two-handed and one-handed catching development?
10. How does using a glove influence catching performance?
11. What are the characteristics of general striking development? Distinguish between mature and immature striking performance.
12. What key observational characteristics distinguish mature and immature ball bouncing?
13. How do place kicking and punting differ? Which is more difficult and why?
14. What key observational characteristics distinguish the mature and immature techniques of kickers (place kicking and punting)?

online resources

History of Michigan State University's Motor Development Study, www.education.msu.edu/kin/documents/kin100c4.pdf

REFERENCES

Abdollahipour, R. & Psotta, R. (2017). Is an external focus of attention more beneficial than an internal focus to ball catching in children? *Kinesiology*, *49*, 235–241.

Angell, R. M., Butterfield, S. A., Loovis, E. M., Mason, C. A., & Nightingale, C. J. (2018). Children's throwing and striking: A longitudinal study. *Journal of Motor Learning and Development*, *6*, 315–332.

Barnett, L. M., van Beurden, E., Morgan, P. J., Brooks, L. O., & Beard, J. R. (2010). Gender differences in motor skill proficiency from childhood to adolescence: A longitudinal study. *Research Quarterly for Exercise and Sport, 81*, 162–170.

Burton, A. W., Greer, N. L., & Wiese-Bjornstal, D. M. (1992). Changes in overhand throwing patterns as a function of ball size. *Pediatric Exercise Science, 4*, 50–67.

Burton, A. W., Greer, N. L., & Wiese-Bjornstal, D. M. (1993). Variations in grasping and throwing patterns as a function of ball size. *Pediatric Exercise Science, 5*, 25–41.

Butterfield, S. A., Angell, R. M., & Mason, C. A. (2012). Age and sex differences in object control skills by children ages 5 to 14. *Perceptual and Motor Skills, 114*, 261–274.

Butterfield, S. A., Loovis, E. M., & Lee, J. (2003). Throwing development by children in grades K-8: A multi-cohort longitudinal study. *Journal of Human Movement Studies, 45*, 31–47.

Carlton, E. B. (1989). An investigation of gender-mediated factors in preschool children's overarm throwing development. Unpublished doctoral dissertation, University of California, Berkeley, CA.

Cesqui, B., Russo, M., Lacquaniti, F., & d'Avella, A. (2016). Grasping in one-handed catching in relation to performance. *PLoS ONE, 11*, 1–25.

Ehl, T., Roberton, M. A., & Langendorfer, S. J. (2005). Does the throwing "gender gap" occur in Germany? *Research Quarterly for Exercise and Sport, 76*, 488–493.

Escamilla, R., Fleisig, G., Barrantine, S., Zhen, N., & Andrews, J. (1998). Kinematic comparisons of throwing different types of baseball pitches. *Journal of Applied Biomechanics, 14*, 1–23.

Fischman, M. G., Moore, J. B., & Steel, K. H. (1992). Children's one-hand catching as a function of age, gender, and ball location. *Research Quarterly for Exercise and Sport, 63*, 349–355.

Fischman, M. G., & Mucci, W. G. (1989). Influence of a baseball glove on the nature of errors produced in simple onehanded catching. *Research Quarterly for Exercise and Sport, 60*, 251–255.

Fischman, M. G., & Sanders, R. (1991). An empirical note on the bilateral use of a baseball glove by skilled catchers. *Perceptual and Motor Skills, 72*, 219–223.

Fronske, H., Blakemore, C., & Abendroth-Smith, J. (1997). The effect of critical cues on overhand throwing efficiency of elementary school children. *Physical Educator, 54*, 88–95.

Garcia, C., & Garcia, L. (2005). Developmental and instructional considerations for teaching the overhand throw to young children. *Illinois Journal for Health, Physical Education, Recreation and Dance, 51*, 15–20.

Gromeier, M., Koester, D., & Schack, T. (2017). Gender differences in motor skills of the overarm throw. *Frontiers in Psychology. 8*, Article 212, doi: 10.3389/fpsyg.2017.00212.

Halverson, L. E., & Roberton, M. A. (1979). The effects of instruction on overhand throwing development in children. In G. Roberts & K. Newell (Eds.), *Psychology of motor behavior and sport—1978*. Champaign, IL: Human Kinetics.

Halverson, L. E., Roberton, M. A., & Langendorfer, S. (1982). Development of the overarm throw: Movement and ball velocity changes by seventh grade. *Research Quarterly for Exercise and Sport, 53*, 198–205.

Harper, C. J. (1979). Learning to observe children's motor development: Part III. Observing children's motor development in the gymnasium. Paper presented at the national convention of the American Alliance for Health, Physical Education, and Recreation, New Orleans, LA.

Haubenstricker, J., Branta, C., & Seefeldt, V. (1983). Preliminary validation of developmental sequences for throwing and catching. Paper presented at the annual conference of the North American Society for the Psychology of Sport and Physical Activity, East Lansing, MI.

Haubenstricker, J., Seefeldt, V., Fountain, C., & Sapp, M. (1981). Preliminary validation of a developmental sequence for kicking. Paper presented at the Midwest District convention of the American Alliance for Health, Physical Education, Recreation, and Dance, Chicago.

Hellweg, D. A. (1972). An analysis of perceptual and performance characteristics of the catching skill in 6–7 year old children. Unpublished doctoral dissertation, University of Wisconsin, Madison, WI.

Isaacs, L. D. (1980). Effects of ball size, ball color, and preferred color on catching by young children. *Perceptual and Motor Skills, 51*, 583–586.

Johnson, J. L., Rudisill, M. E., Hastie P. A., & Sassi, J. (2019). The influence of guided practice on overhand throwing competence in preschool children in a mastery motivational climate. *Journal of Motor Learning and Development*, *7*, 64–83.

Kasuyama, T., Mutou, I., & Sasamoto, H. (2016). Development of overarm throwing technique reflects throwing ability during childhood. *Physical Therapy Research*, *19*, 24–31.

Kay, H. (1970). Analyzing motor skill performance. In K. Connolly (Ed.), *Mechanisms of motor skill development*. New York: Academic Press.

Keegan, T. A. (1989). Development of ball catching skills among boys of elementary school age. Unpublished master's thesis, Temple University, Philadelphia.

Kourtessis, T. (1994). Procedural and declarative knowledge of ball-catching in children with physical disabilities. Unpublished master's thesis, McGill University, Montreal.

Langendorfer, S. (1980). Longitudinal evidence for developmental changes in the preparatory phase of the overarm throw for force. Paper presented at the Research Section of the American Alliance for Health, Physical Education, Recreation, and Dance, Detroit.

Langendorfer, S. (1982). Developmental relationships between throwing and striking: A prelongitudinal test of motor stage theory. Unpublished doctoral dissertation, University of Wisconsin, Madison, WI.

Lefebvre, C. (1996). Prediction in ball catching by children with a developmental coordination disorder. Unpublished master's thesis, McGill University, Montreal.

Leme, S., & Shambes, G. (1978). Immature throwing patterns in normal adult women. *Journal of Human Movement Studies, 4*, 85–93.

Lombardo, M. P., & Deaner, R. O. (2018). On the evolution of the sex differences in throwing: Throwing is a male adaptation in humans. *The Quarterly Review of Biology, 93*, 91–119.

Lorson, K. D., & Goodway, J. D. (2007). Influence of critical cues and task constraints on overarm throwing performance in elementary age children. *Perceptual and Motor Skills, 105*, 753–767.

Lorson, K. M., Stodden, D. F., Langendorfer, S. J., & Goodway, J. D. (2013). Age and gender differences in adolescent and adult overarm throwing. *Research Quarterly for Exercise and Sport, 84*, 239–244.

Mally, K. K., Battista, R. A., & Roberton, M. A. (2011). Distance as a control parameter for place kicking. *Journal of Human Sport & Exercise, 6*, 122–134.

Murase, D., Yokoyama, K., Fujii, K., Hasegawa, Y., & Yamamoto, Y. (2016). Baseball catching patterns differ according to task constraints. *Advances in Physical Education, 6*, 151–157.

Nelson, J. D., Thomas, J. R., Nelson, K. R., & Abraham, P. C. (1986). Gender differences in children's throwing performance: Biology and environment. *Research Quarterly for Exercise and Sport, 57*, 280–287.

Nelson, K. R., Thomas, J. R., & Nelson, J. K. (1991). Longitudinal change in throwing performance: Gender differences. *Research Quarterly for Exercise and Sport, 62*, 105–108.

Nessler, J. (1973). Length of time necessary to view a ball while catching it. *Journal of Motor Behavior, 5*, 179–185.

Payne, V. G. (1982). Current status of research on object reception as a function of ball size. *Perceptual and Motor Skills, 55*, 953–954.

Payne, V. G. (1985a). Effects of object size and experimental design on object reception by children in the first grade. *Journal of Human Movement Studies, 11*, 1–9.

Payne, V. G. (1985b). Teaching elementary physical education: Recognizing stages of the fundamental movement patterns (videotape). Northbrook, IL: Hubbard Scientific Publications.

Payne, V. G., & Koslow, R. (1981). Effects of varying ball diameters on catching ability of young children. *Perceptual and Motor Skills, 53*, 739–744.

Petranek, L. J., & Barton, G. V. (2011). The overarm throwing pattern among U-14 ASA female softball players: A comparative study of gender, culture, and experience. *Research Quarterly for Exercise and Sport, 82*, 220–229.

Roberton, M. A. (1977). Stability of stage categorizations across trials: Implications for the "stage theory" of overarm throw development. *Journal of Human Movement Studies, 3*, 49–59.

Roberton, M. A. (1978). Longitudinal evidence for developmental stages in the forceful overarm throw. *Journal of Human Movement Studies, 4*, 167–175.

Roberton, M. A. (1983). Changing motor patterns during childhood. In J. Thomas (Ed.), *Motor development during childhood and adolescence* (pp. 48–90). Minneapolis, MN: Burgess.

Roberton, M. A., & DiRocco, P. (1981). Validating a motor skill sequence for mentally retarded children. *American Corrective Therapy Journal, 35*, 148–154.

Roberton, M. A., & Halverson, L. E. (1984). *Developing children: Their changing movement*. Philadelphia, PA: Lea & Febiger.

Roberton, M. A., Halverson, L. E., Langendorfer, S., & Williams, K. (1979). Longitudinal changes in children's overarm throw ball velocities. *Research Quarterly for Exercise and Sport, 50*, 256–264.

Roberton, M. A., & Konczak, J. (2001). Predicting children's overarm throw ball velocities from their developmental levels in throwing. *Research Quarterly for Exercise and Sport, 72*, 91–103.

Roberton, M. A., & Langendorfer, S. (1980). Testing motor development sequences across 9–14 years. In C. Nadeau, W. Halliwell, K. Newell, & G. Roberts (Eds.), *Psychology of motor behavior and sport—1979*. Champaign, IL: Human Kinetics.

Roberton, M. A., & Langendorfer, S. (1983). Changing motor patterns during childhood. In J. Thomas (Ed.), *Motor development during childhood and adolescence*. Minneapolis, MN: Burgess.

Runion, B., Roberton, M. A., & Langendorfer, S. J. (2003). Forceful overarm throwing: A comparison of two cohorts measured 20 years apart. *Research Quarterly for Exercise and Sport, 74*, 324–330.

Seefeldt, V. (1972a). Developmental sequence of catching skill. Paper presented at the annual convention of the American Association for

Health, Physical Education, and Recreation, Houston.

Seefeldt, V. (1972b). Developmental sequence of kicking. Unpublished materials, Michigan State University, East Lansing, MI.

Seefeldt, V., & Haubenstricker, J. (1975a). Developmental sequence of kicking. Rev. ed. Unpublished materials, Michigan State University, East Lansing, MI.

Seefeldt, V., & Haubenstricker, J. (1975b). Developmental sequence of punting. Unpublished materials, Michigan State University, East Lansing, MI.

Seefeldt, V., & Haubenstricker, J. (1976). Developmental sequence of throwing. Rev. ed. Unpublished manuscript, Michigan State University, East Lansing, MI.

Seefeldt, V., & Haubenstricker, J. (1982). Patterns, phases, or stages: An analytical model for the study of developmental movement. In J. A. S. Kelso & J. E. Clark (Eds.), *The development of movement control and coordination*. New York: Wiley.

Seefeldt, V., Reuschlein, P., & Vogel, P. (1972). Sequencing motor skills within the physical education curriculum. Paper presented at the annual convention of the American Association for Health, Physical Education, and Recreation, Houston, TX.

Stodden, D. F., Langendorfer, S. J., Fleisig, G. S., & Andrews, J. R. (2006a). Kinematic constraints associated with the acquisition of overarm throwing part I: Step and trunk actions. *Research Quarterly for Exercise and Sport, 77*, 417–427.

Stodden, D. F., Langendorfer, S. J., Fleisig, G. S., & Andrews, J. R. (2006b). Kinematic constraints associated with the acquisition of overarm throwing part II: Upper extremity actions. *Research Quarterly for Exercise and Sport, 77*, 428–436.

Stone, J. A., Maynard, I. W., North, J. S., Panchuk, D., & Davids, K. (2017). Temporal and spatial occlusion of advanced visual information constrains movement (re)organization in one-handed catching behaviors. *Acta Psychological, 174*, 80–88.

Strohmeyer, H. S., Williams, K., & Schaub-George, D. (1991). Developmental sequences for catching a small ball: A prelongitudinal screening. *Research Quarterly for Exercise and Sport, 62*, 257–266.

Thomas, J. R., Alderson, J. A., Thomas, K. T., Campbell, A. C., & Elliott, B. C. (2010). Developmental gender differences in overhand throwing in Aboriginal Australian children. *Research Quarterly for Exercise and Sport, 81*, 432–441.

Thomas, J. R., & French, K. E. (1985). Gender differences across age in motor performance: A meta-analysis. *Psychological Bulletin, 98*, 260–282.

van den Tillaar, R., & Ettema, G. (2011). A comparison of kinematics between overarm throwing with 20% overweight, regular, and 20% overweight balls. *Journal of Applied Biomechanics, 27*, 252–256.

Whiting, H. T. A., Gill, E. B., & Stephenson, J. M. (1970). Critical time intervals for taking in flight information in a ball-catching task. *Ergonomics, 13*, 265–272.

Wickstrom, R. L. (1980). Acquisition of a ball-handling skill. Paper presented at the Research Section of the American Alliance for Health, Physical Education, Recreation, and Dance, Detroit, MI.

Wild, M. (1938). The behavior pattern of throwing and some observations concerning its course of development in children. *Research Quarterly, 9*, 20–24.

Williams, J. G. (1992a). Catching action: Visuomotor adaptations in children. *Perceptual and Motor Skills, 75*, 211–219.

Williams, J. G. (1992b). Effects of instruction and practice on ball catching skill: Single-subject study of an 8-year-old. *Perceptual and Motor Skills, 75*, 392–394.

Young, R. W. (2009). The ontogeny of throwing and striking. *Human Ontogenetics 3*, 19–31.

14 YOUTH SPORTS

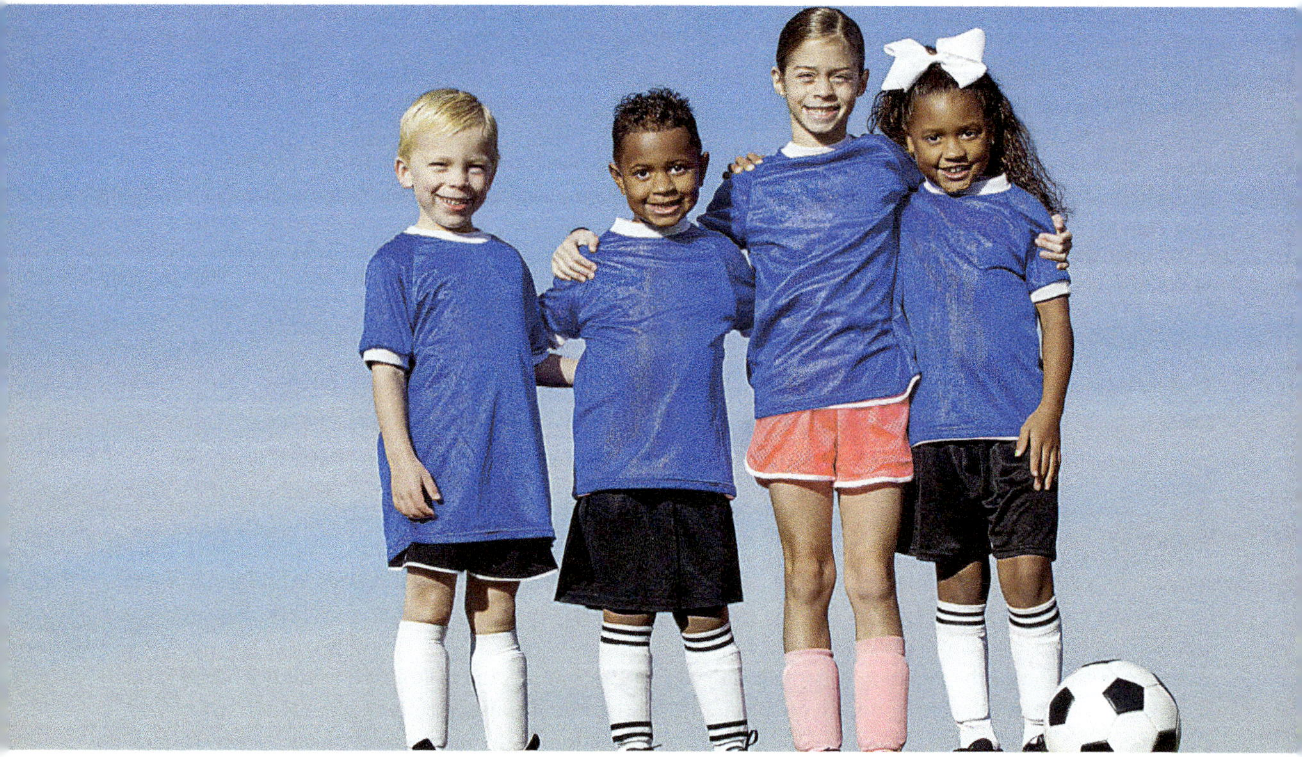

Chapter Objectives

From the information presented in this chapter, you will be able to

- Describe specific categories of youth sports and account for the explosion in the number of children and youths participating in organized youth sport programs
- Describe the 10 most important reasons given for participating in youth sports
- Explain competence motivation theory and describe how this theory influences children's participation in youth sports
- Explain the 11 most important reasons why children and young adults stop playing a particular sport
- Describe both the medical and psychological issues surrounding youth sport participation
- Describe characteristics of the volunteer coaching profession and the arguments about the mandatory certification of coaches
- Describe the role of parental education in curbing youth sport violence toward parents, officials, coaches, and players
- Explain the purpose of the National Standards for Youth Sports

Researchers from the Institute for the Study of Youth Sports, Michigan State University, have described youth sports as athletic endeavors that provide children and youth with a systematic sequence of practices and contests (Seefeldt, Ewing, & Walk, 1991). It has been estimated that as many as 35 million to 40 million youth between 6 and 18 years of age participate in nonschool-sponsored and interscholastic sports. Of these participants, nearly 8 million are participating in interscholastic sports (NFSHSA, 2018). Thus, even though participation rates are known to be overestimated because individuals who participate in more than one activity are counted more than once, these figures show that the number of young people participating in youth sports continues to increase annually.

Researchers have identified several potential benefits that youth sport participants receive, including improvements in academic performance (Eldridge, Palmer, Gillis, et al., 2014), health-related physical fitness (Haapala, Lankhorst, de Groot, et al., 2017), moral development and self-esteem (Malina & Cumming, 2003), development of prosocial values, and general deterrence to negative behaviors such as gang membership, violent behavior (Blon, Bronk, Coakley, et al., 2013), and substance use and abuse (Clark, Camire, Wade, et al., 2015), to name just a few. In this chapter, we examine several factors that influence the development of young people through youth sport participation.

PARTICIPATION

Trends in Participation

As noted earlier, participation in youth sports has continued to increase but mainly at the interscholastic level. Thus, this increased rate of participation is not evident at all age levels and varies by sport. Varying trends and some of the factors influencing these trends in youth sport participation are described below.

Earlier Participation

First, there is a trend toward earlier participation. In the past, growth and development specialists were concerned that children as young as 5 or 6 years of age were participating in team activities such as T-ball and youth football. In 2006, Budhia Singh, a 4-year-old boy from India, set a record for running 40 miles (65 km) in 7 hours and 2 minutes (Wikipedia, 2019). Although authorities recommend children do not begin competing in sports prior to age 8 (Coakley, 1986; Holecko, 2015), children as young as age 3 are currently involved in organized youth sport programs (see Figure 14.1).

The trend toward earlier involvement is, in part, a result of rule changes within selected sports. For example, in T-ball, even the youngest child can perform because the rules allow

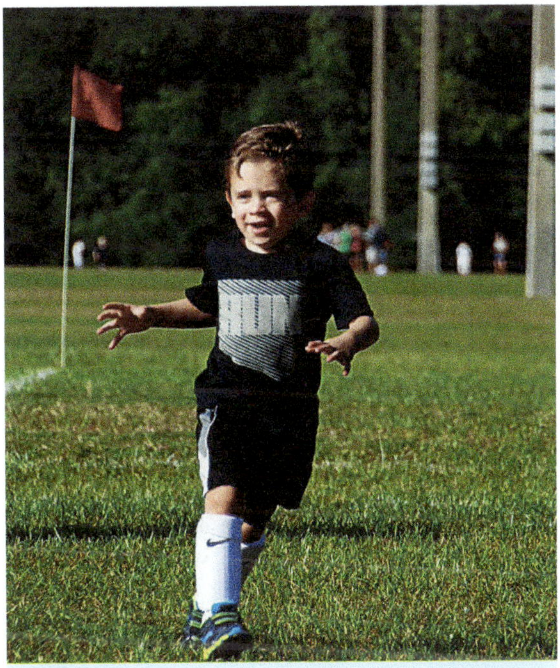

Figure 14.1 Will the trend toward younger sport participation ever end?

Source: Courtesy of Dr. Larry Isaacs.

children to strike a stationary ball. At the same time, defensive performance is no longer required, as rule changes limit the number of players who can bat per inning. Therefore, when the defensive team is unable to get anyone out, the sides at bat change simply because all of the offensive players have had a turn at bat. Irrespective of this earlier participation, the Sports & Fitness Industry Association and the Aspen Institute's "State of Play" report (2018) have noted a drop in youth sport participation among children 6 to 12 years of age. More specifically, in 2008, almost 45 percent of children participated regularly in a team sport. Today that percentage has dropped to 37 percent (Aspen Institute, 2018). This steep drop in participation has been blamed, in part, on poor coaching, increased costs associated with competitive travel teams, and those left behind feel inferior and lose interest in participating.

Female Involvement

A second factor affecting the number of participants in youth sport is an increase in female involvement. In 1971, the year prior to the passing of Title IX, the National Federation of State High School Associations (NFSHSA) identified only 14 interscholastic sports for girls, allowing for only 294,015 participants; by 2018, the number had risen to 41 sports, involving approximately 3.4 million female participants (NFSHSA, 2018). Additionally, some females are now participating in sports that have traditionally been reserved for males. For example, according to a recent survey, 2,237 females now participate in interscholastic 11-player football (NFSHSA, 2018). Table 14.1 reports a longitudinal history of interscholastic sport participation from 1971 through 2018.

Involvement in Nontraditional Sport Activities

A third factor affecting the number of participants in youth sport is that children and young adults in the United States are becoming more involved in what used to be considered nontraditional sport activities. Without doubt, they have been interested in soccer, baseball, football, basketball, and swimming. However, the availability of agency- and community-sponsored programs in such activities as tennis, golf, cycling, bowling, ice hockey, lacrosse, gymnastics, volleyball, track and field, cross-country running, figure skating, downhill and cross-country skiing, and many other sports has opened the door to participation for those youths who are not interested in the more traditional sports.

Participation by Individuals with Disabilities

Finally, there has been a dramatic increase in the number of individuals with disabilities who now actively participate in sports. This increase is directly linked to an increase in agency- and community-sponsored programs that serve people with various degrees of disabilities, including the National Wheelchair Basketball Association; Wheelchair & Ambulatory Sports, USA; US Youth Soccer's TOPSoccer; International Wheelchair Tennis Federation; National Wheelchair Softball Association; United States Quad Rugby Association; and Special Olympics. Additionally, special equipment is now available for individuals with disabilities, further encouraging their participation in sports (see Figure 14.2).

Opportunities for Participation in Sports

Today, children and young adults have many options when it comes to selecting an avenue for youth sport participation. By far, the greatest number of youth sport participants is found in agency-sponsored sports (Little League baseball, Pop Warner football, US Youth Soccer) and in local recreational sport

Table 14.1 Longitudinal history of interscholastic sport participation, 1971 to 2018

Year	Male participants	Female participants	Total
1971/72	3,666,917	294,015	3,960,932
1975/76	4,109,021	1,645,039	5,754,060
1980/81	3,503,124	1,853,789	5,356,913
1985/86	3,344,275	1,807,121	5,151,396
1990/91	3,406,355	1,892,316	5,298,671
1995/96	3,634,052*	2,367,936*	6,001,988*
2000/01	3,921,069	2,784,154	6,705,223
2005/06	4,206,549	2,953,355	7,159,904
2010/11	4,494,406	3,173,549	7,667,955
2013/14	4,527,994	3,267,664	7,795,658
2017/18	4,565,580	3,415,306	7,980,886

Notes: *Total does not include 16,979 participants in coeducational sports.

Any estimate of athletic participation will be inflated because participants are counted more than once if they participate in more than one activity.

Source: NFSHSA (2018). This and other information pertaining to participation may be obtained at www.nfhs.org. Used with permission.

programs. Furthermore, nearly 8 million children and youth now participate in interscholastic sports (NFSHSA, 2018). Table 14.2 lists the 10 most popular interscholastic sports and their numbers of participants. NFSHSA's national survey continues to recognize football as the most popular sport for boys. Nevertheless, the number of young males playing interscholastic football appears to be trending downward. For example, from 2014 to 2018, the number of participants has decreased by over 56,000 (NFSHSA, 2018). This downward trend is most likely, in part, due to news media coverage involving the risk of concussions at all levels of play. This topic will be discussed in greater detail later in the chapter. Outdoor track and field ranks as the most popular interscholastic sport for females.

Reasons for Participating in Sports

Often-cited reasons for participation in youth sports include the following: to improve skills, to have fun, to be with friends, to be part of a team, to experience excitement, to receive awards, to win, and to become more physically fit (Hedstrom & Gould, 2004; Kondric, Sindik, Furjan-Mandic, et al., 2013). Of these reasons, "to have fun" appears to be the predominant reason children and young adults want to be involved in sport (Crane & Temple, 2015). However, the idea of having fun can mean different things to different individuals; what is enjoyable for one may not be enjoyable for another. For this reason, researchers have studied the underlying factors that affect enjoyment of sport.

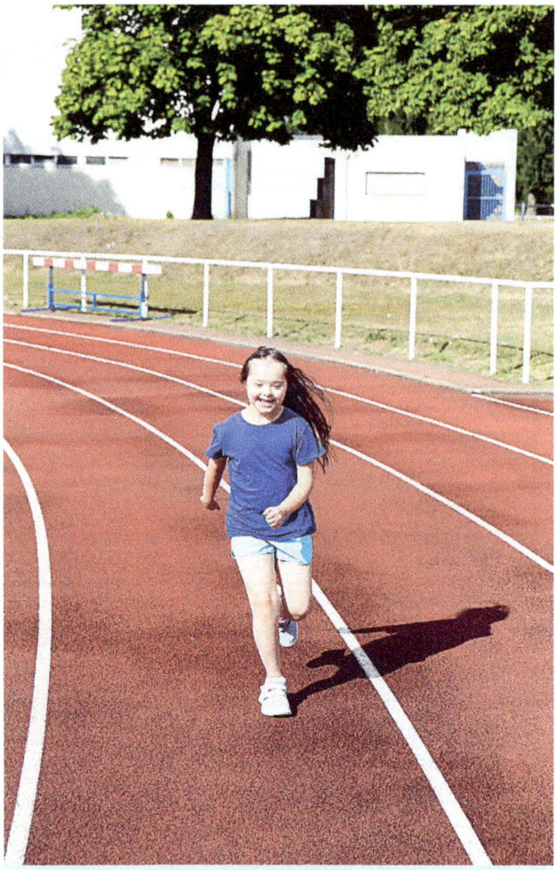

Figure 14.2 An increasing number of children and youths with disabilities now enjoy participation in youth sport activities

Table 14.2 The 10 most popular interscholastic sports for boys and girls

Sport*	Number of participants
Boys	
Football	1,036,842
Outdoor track & field	600,097
Basketball	551,373
Baseball	487,097
Soccer	456,362
Cross-country	270,095
Wrestling	245,564
Tennis	158,151
Golf	144,024
Swimming & diving	138,935
Girls	
Outdoor track & field	488,592
Volleyball	446,583
Basketball	412,407
Soccer	390,482
Fast pitch softball	367,861
Cross-country	223,518
Tennis	190,768
Swimming & diving	175,594
Competitive spirit squads	162,669
Lacrosse	96,904

*Listed from most to least popular. Note that the number of participants is partly determined by the number allowed on a team.

Source: NFSHSA (2018).

Research Findings

In a large-scale study, Wankel and Kreisel (1985) surveyed 822 soccer, baseball, and hockey participants between 7 and 14 years of age (with a 10-item inventory) to determine why they enjoyed sports. Three sport groupings were employed because another purpose was to determine whether reasons for enjoyment differed across sports. Results indicate that the top four enjoyment factors (improving skills, testing abilities against others, excitement of the game, and personal accomplishment—i.e., intrinsic factors) were consistent across all three sport groups. Of moderate importance were the social factors "being on a team" and "being with friends." The extrinsic factors, which included "getting awards" and "pleasing others," were consistently selected as the least important factors for sport enjoyment. Also of interest is the finding that "winning the game" was ranked eighth in the list of 10 factors.

Given these findings, Wankel and Kreisel (1985) offered the following suggestions:

> Emphasis should be on involvement, skill development, and enjoyment of doing the skills. Winning and receiving rewards for playing, aspects that are frequently given considerable emphasis by parents, coaches, and the media, are of secondary importance to the participant's enjoyment and accordingly should not be heavily emphasized. The establishment of rigid schedules and elimination play-offs to declare winners is a questionable practice if the criterion is to provide enjoyment to all participants … Each child should be provided an opportunity to develop his or her skills, be provided with a reasonable challenge, and be afforded an opportunity for personal accomplishment and satisfaction.
>
> (pp. 62–63)

The most comprehensive findings to date on why children and youth participate in sport are from a classic study sponsored by the Athletic Footwear Association (1990). This survey sampled more than 10,000 youths in 11 American cities. Table 14.3 lists the 10 most important reasons children and young adults chose to participate in their favorite sports. Note that they want to participate to have "fun" and that "winning" ranks last. The findings from this study conducted over 30 years ago appear to remain valid. More specifically, when Crane and Temple (2015) analyzed 557 studies, they also concluded that "having fun" was a major reason children and adolescents chose to participate in sport.

Table14.3 The 10 most important reasons I play

	My Best School Sport
1.	To have fun
2.	To improve my skills
3.	To stay in shape
4.	To do something I'm good at
5.	For the excitement of competition
6.	To get exercise
7.	To play as part of a team
8.	For the challenge of competition
9.	To learn new skills
10.	To win

Sample: 2,000 boys and 1,900 girls, grades 7–12, who identified a "best" school sport. Answers above were among 25 responses rated on a 5-point scale.

Source: Athletic Footwear Association (1990). Used with permission.

Competence Motivation Theory

Other researchers have made convincing arguments that participation motivation can be linked to existing theoretical models. One model that is frequently mentioned is Harter's model of perceived competence (Harter, 1988). According to **competence motivation theory**, individuals are motivated to be successful in various achievement areas such as sports (physical), academics (cognitive), or human relationships (social). When performance attempts succeed, the individual experiences a positive effect. This perception of successful competence motivates the individual to continue participation. Similarly, the theory predicts that individuals with low levels of perceived competence will discontinue participation (Weiss & Ferrer-Caja, 2002). Confirming these predictions, Atkins, Johnson, Force, and Petrie (2015) found that a positive motivational climate significantly contributed to sustained sport participation.

Scientific studies designed to test Harter's theory within a sport context have been fairly successful. For example, Roberts, Kleiber, and Duda (1981) found that youth sport participants scored higher in both perceived cognitive and perceived physical competence than did nonparticipants. Feltz and Petlichkoff (1983) reported that current sport participants scored higher on perceived physical competence than did dropouts. However, Ulrich (1987) failed to find among children in grades K-4 a significant relationship between participation in organized sport and perceived physical competence as measured by Harter's Perceived Competence Scale for Children (1982). This contradictory finding may result in part from developmental differences regarding the sources of information that children and young adults use to estimate their physical competence. For example, children aged 8 and 9 tend to use such factors as game outcome and parental feedback. In contrast, youths 10 to 14 years old depend more on social comparisons to peers and evaluations by peers to judge their own physical competence (Horn & Weiss, 1991). Furthermore, it appears that children become more accurate in judging their physical competency as they age and that this increased accuracy may be related to the source of information they use (Horn & Weiss, 1991).

Coaches and teachers should not only be aware of such developmental differences but also be attuned to the value and type of feedback that is most appropriate for their participants. According to Harter's model, if children and youth fail, good social support and positive feedback can increase their perceived competence. Young people should not view mistakes as failures. Instead, parents and coaches should quickly intervene to help them see other reasons why a mistake has occurred. This way, young people will be less likely to view their performance as reflecting a lack of physical ability to accomplish a specific task.

In summary, we can conclude that children and young adults participate in organized sports for a multitude of reasons. Unfortunately, their most often stated reasons for participation (intrinsic reasons) do not always coincide with the program goals established by the adult leadership.

Reasons for Dropping Out of Sports

About 35 percent of the millions of young people who participate in a youth sport will withdraw from the program within any given year. However, contrary to popular belief, most youths do not drop out of a sport because of excessive stress. Instead, empirical evidence suggests that most sport dropouts occur because of interpersonal problems (e.g., disliking the coach) or to pursue other leisure activities (DiFiori, Benjamin, Brenner, et al., 2014). Most often, the other activity is another sport. For example, when they interviewed swimming dropouts, Gould, Feltz, Horn, and Weiss (1982) noted that 80 percent of the youngsters had either reentered or planned to reenter a sport activity. For this reason, sport psychologists recommend caution in interpreting the term *sport dropout*. Obviously, there is a vast difference between young people who withdraw from sports permanently and those who withdraw from one sport activity only to become involved in a different one. In fact, for the youngest participants, frequent withdrawal from sports may signify nothing more than the attempt to sample many different sports before selecting the few that best meet their needs.

As we implied earlier, when sport participation is not fun, there is a greater tendency for young people to drop out (Figure 14.3; see Table 14.4). When children and youth in grades 7 through 12 who had dropped out of a sport were asked what changes would need to be made before they would reenter the sport, both the girls and the boys ranked as most important the need to "make practices more fun" (AFA, 1990). A study involving more than 2,000 girls and boys in grades 3

Table 14.4 The 11 most important reasons children and young adults stopped playing a sport

1.	I lost interest.
2.	I was not having fun.
3.	It took too much time.
4.	Coach was a poor teacher.
5.	There was too much pressure (worry).
6.	I wanted a nonsport activity.
7.	I was tired of it.
8.	I needed more study time.
9.	Coach played favorites.
10.	The sport was boring.
11.	There was an overemphasis on winning.

Sample: 2,700 boys and 3,100 girls who said they had recently stopped playing a school or nonschool sport. Answers above were among 30 responses rated on a 5-point scale.

Source: Athletic Footwear Association (1990). Used with permission.

through 12 confirmed this finding (Sabo & Veliz, 2008). Table 14.5 presents the six most important changes that would need to occur before they would be willing to reenter a sport that they had earlier dropped.

CONTROVERSIES AROUND YOUTH SPORTS

Although involvement in both recreational and competitive athletics contributes significantly to young participants' physical, social, emotional, and cognitive development, sport participation, whether competitive or recreational, is sometimes clouded by controversial issues. This section examines several of the most frequently mentioned issues. For ease of discussion, these controversial issues have been divided into two categories: medical and psychological.

Medical Issues

Potential physical danger is a major criticism of youth sport participation. On average, about 8.6 million sports- and recreational-related injuries are reported each year (Sheu, Chen, & Hedegaard, 2016) and many of these injuries occur within a youth sport setting. In this section, we first examine injury rates of selected sports and then discuss whether the number of injuries can be reduced.

Table 14.5 The six most important changes that would need to occur before children and young adults would be willing to reenter a sport they had previously dropped

"I would play again if. . ."			
Boys		**Girls**	
1.	Practices were more fun.*	1.	Practices were more fun.*
2.	I could play more.	2.	There was no conflict with studies.
3.	Coaches understood players better.*	3.	Coaches understood players better.*
4.	There was no conflict with studies.	4.	There was no conflict with social life.
5.	Coaches were better teachers.*	5.	I could play more.
6.	There was no conflict with social life.	6.	Coaches were better teachers.*

Sample: 2,700 boys, 3,100 girls, grades 7–12, who said they had recently stopped playing a school or nonschool sport. They rated 21 different responses on a 5-point scale.

*Confirmed by Sabo & Veliz (2008).

Source: Athletic Footwear Association (1990). Used with permission.

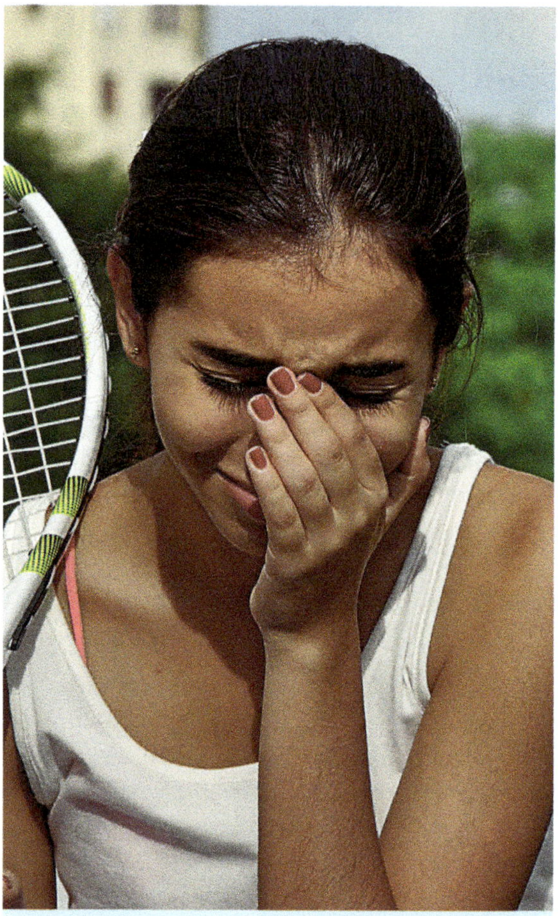

Figure 14.3 When sport participation is not fun, young people will drop out

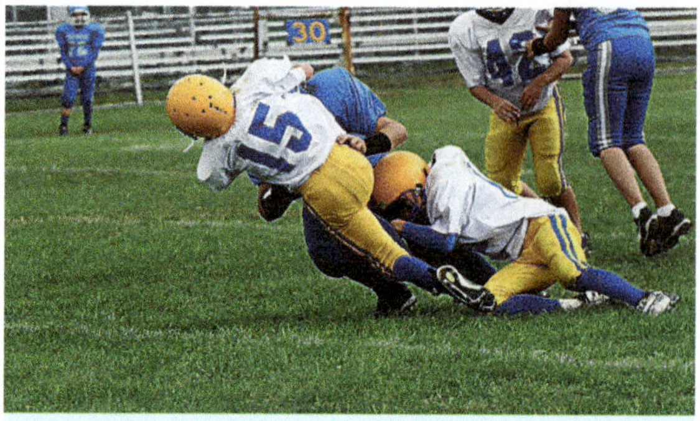

Figure 14.4 Football is classified as a contact/collision sport

Football

Football is classified as a **contact/collision sport** (see Figure 14.4). In general, collision sports have become synonymous with physical injury. Obviously, whenever people are repeatedly running into one another, injuries will occur. But is this true for all ages and levels of play? To provide insight into this question, Stuart, Morrey, Smith, and colleagues (2002) studied the prevalence of injury among 915 youth football players between 9 and 13 years of age. As illustrated in Table 14.6, rates of injury tended to increase as the players matured in age and grade level, a finding that has been confirmed by others (Dompier, Powell, Barron, et al., 2007; Sheu, Chen, & Hedegaard, 2016). Although the highest rate of injury occurred among the players in the oldest age group (eighth-graders), the overall injury rate was only 5.97 percent. This translates to only 8.47 injuries per 1,000 player-games or 0.17 injuries per 1,000 player-plays. More recently, Peterson and colleagues' (2017) review of the literature suggest that youth football injury rates range between 2 to 17.8 injuries per 1000 exposures. When the researchers examined relative prevalence of risk for injury by player position, they determined that 65 percent of injuries occurred to offensive players and 35 percent to defensive players. Among the offensive players, the quarterbacks and the running backs were at greatest risk (30.4 percent). Among the defensive players, the linemen (22.2 percent) and linebackers (10.9 percent) were found to be at greatest risk of injury.

In a large-scale study, Goldberg, Rosenthal, Robertson, and Nicholas (1988) studied the injury experiences of 5,128 boys between 8 and 15 years of age. Only significant injuries were studied (those restricting participation for more than 7 days). Table 14.7 highlights the findings. As in previous small-scale studies, the overall injury rate was rather low (5 percent), with most injuries occurring among older and heavier participants. Unlike injuries common in higher levels of play (college and

Table 14.6 Prevalence of youth football injuries by grade level

Grade	N	% injury prevalence per season	Injuries per 1,000 player-games	Injuries per 1,000 player-plays
4	218	2.73	3.80	0.09
5	211	5.67	7.86	0.16
6	206	6.31	8.74	0.16
7	147	6.00	8.20	0.15
8	133	11.28	15.45	0.33
Overall	915	5.97	8.47	0.17

Source: Stuart et al. (2002).

professional), most significant injuries in youth football involved the upper extremities, particularly the hand and wrist. Because a significant number of major injuries (those restricting participation for more than 21 days) occurred to members of kickoff and punt-return teams, the researchers suggested that youth football administrators consider modifying the sport to eliminate this dangerous aspect of the game. They also recommended that steps be taken to reduce the number of injuries caused by direct impact with the football helmet (18.4 percent).

Concussions, defined as mild traumatic brain injury, have drawn attention from the national media. Concussions were first reported as a major concern among professional football players, and this concern has filtered down to youth who participate in collision sports. For example, Pop Warner football has reported a 9.5 percent decrease in participation and has attributed this decline to concerns over concussions and their potential long-term effects (ESPN, 2013). League officials are currently working to remediate these concerns through enhancing education, teaching appropriate tackling techniques, and studying ways to improve safety equipment. It has been estimated that 3.8 million concussions occur each year during competitive and recreational sport activity, and as many as 50 percent may go unreported (Harmon, Drezner, Gammons, et al., 2013). In its most recent statement, the American Academy of Pediatrics (AAP, 2015) adopted a zero-tolerance stance for illegal, head-first hits. Additionally, in their policy statement on tackle football, a recommendation was made to expand the available of nontackling leagues in an attempt to curtail football injuries. However, a recent study found no significant differences in concussions between tackling and nontackling leagues. In fact, injuries in general were found to occur more frequently in a youth flag football league (Peterson, Kruse, Meester, et al., 2017). Obviously additional research is warranted.

Baseball

Although youth baseball has been a relatively safe activity, two major concerns have surfaced: chest trauma and eye injuries. First and most serious is the potential for sudden death from ventricular fibrillation resulting from nonpenetrating chest trauma. This injury, called **commotio cordis**, is typically encountered when a batter is struck in the chest by a pitched baseball or when the catcher is struck by a foul-tipped baseball. Each year approximately

Table 14.7 Injuries in youth football

Injury rate by weight and age (kg/years)	N	% injury rate	No. of injuries
49.5–67.5/12–15	177	9.6	17
40.5–60.8/11–14	1,160	8.4	97
36–51.8/10–13	1,489	5.8	86
29.3–45/9–12	1,610	2.7	44
22.5–38.3/8–11	692	1.9	13
Overall injury rate	5,128	5.0	257
Most-prone injury sites		**% injury rate**	
Hand/wrist		27.6	
Knee		18.7	
Shoulder/humerus		11.3	
Most common injuries		**% injury rate**	**No. of injuries**
Fractures		35.0	90
Epiphyseal fractures		5.1	13
Sprains		24.5	63
Contusions		16.7	43
Strains		7.0	18
Injury rates by position		**% injury rate**	
Quarterbacks/running backs		30.4	
Defensive linemen		22.2	
Offensive linemen		12.8	
Linebackers		10.9	
Kickoff/punt-return team members		7.4	
Defensive backs		5.8	
Receivers		2.7	
Occurrence of major injuries*		**% injury rate**	
Kickoff/punt-return team members		63.2	
Quarterback/running backs		44.9	
Causes of injuries		**% injury rate**	**No. of injuries**
No unusual occurrence		58.6	150
Helmet		18.4	47
Contact after ball whistled dead		8.6	22
Contact during conditioning drills		8.2	21

*Players restricted for over 21 days.

Source: From Goldberg, Rosenthal, Robertson, & Nicholas (1988). Used with permission via CCC.

SUSTAINING PARTICIPATION

Researchers are interested in studying the sustainability of participation in physical activity as a function of gender, age, and type of athletic activity. With a better understanding of why children and young adults reduce or even stop athletic activity, we can design more effective interventions to improve participation. The need to sustain physical participation is especially important in light of the obesity epidemic in the United States and worldwide and what we know about the health benefits of physical activity. In an attempt to shed light on this subject, Belanger, Gray-Donald, O'Loughlin, and colleagues (2009) undertook a longitudinal investigation of 1,276 youths, who were 12 to 13 years of age at the start of the study. The subjects were assessed every three months over a period of five years. Conclusions were as follows:

- Participation declined in nearly every activity and increased in none. In other words, as young people aged, they became less active in sport.
- Within two years, most youths had discontinued the activities in which they were engaged at the beginning of the study.
- Sustained participation was inversely related to the activity's intensity, for both boys and girls. The more intense the activity, the greater was the dropout rate.
- Activity participation was influenced by the type of athletic activity. Both girls and boys sustained greater rates of participation in individual sports (89 percent girls, 90 percent boys) than in team sports (41 percent girls, 69 percent boys).

10 to 20 new cases are reported (Maron & Estes, 2010). Maron, Gohman, Kyle, and colleagues (2002) examined cases from the U.S. Commotio Cordis Registry and found that most of the victims were boys, with a median age of 14 years.

Among researchers and agencies seeking to eliminate this class of injury, a debate has emerged over the value of using a softer baseball than the standard ball. According to the U.S. Consumer Products Safety Commission (Kyle, 1996), the American Academy of Pediatrics (2001), and the work of Marshall, Mueller, Kirby, and Yang (2003), use of a softer baseball results in fewer and less severe injuries. However, doctors are concerned that the use of a softer baseball may allow a greater portion of the ball to enter the eye's orbit, thus leading to an increase in severe eye injuries. Vinger, Duma, and Crandall (1999) examined baseballs of six different hardnesses and found that the softest of the six intruded significantly into the eye's orbit. The American Academy of Pediatrics suggests that young children may be more susceptible than their older counterparts to sport-related eye injuries because of their athletic immaturity and their slower reaction time. For these and other reasons, the AAP recommends that these young athletes wear protective eyewear when batting. Additionally, children and youths whose corrected visual acuity is less than 20/40, as well as those who have received recent eye trauma, should wear protective eyewear regardless of their playing position (AAP, 2004).

In an attempt to improve youth baseball safety further, researchers are investigating the value of all types of protective equipment, including the softer baseballs just discussed,

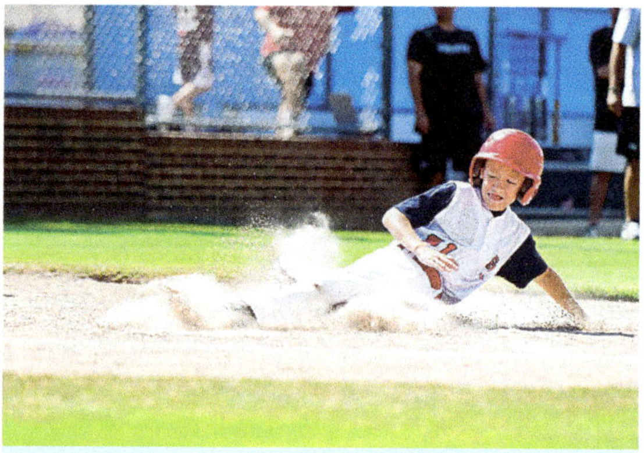

Figure 14.5 Breakaway bases may significantly reduce the number of lower-extremity injuries

chest protectors, batting vests, face masks, and breakaway bases (see Figure 14.5). Regarding chest protectors, researchers, employing an animal model, have now identified a material that has been found to be effective in guarding against commotio cordis (Kymar, Mandleywala, Gannon, et al., 2017). Also under investigation is the influence of aluminum bats on youth baseball injuries. Balls travel faster off an aluminum bat than off a wood bat, thus placing players in the field at greater risk of being hit by a fast-moving ball.

Soccer

Soccer is one of America's fastest-growing sports. In the United States, between 12 and 18 million people participate in soccer. Like American football, soccer is classified as a contact/collision sport. The overall injury rate among professional soccer players is about one injury per season per player. In comparison, injury rates among young soccer players are about 2 per 1,000 participants per year (Leininger, Knox, & Comstock, 2007), and for those youth players older than 12 years of age, the rate is between 4 and 7.6 injuries per 1,000 player hours (Le Gall, Carling, & Reilly, 2008). Nilsson and Roaas's (1978) classic study examined all injuries that occurred during the 1975 and 1977 Norway Cup competitions. During these two tournaments, 25,000 players between 11 and 18 years competed in 2,987 matches. An analysis of the data revealed that girls were twice as likely to be injured as boys, a finding that has been reaffirmed (Koutures & Gregory, 2010). Additionally, Nilsson and Roaas noted that injury rates per 1,000 hours of play were greater in the final rounds of play than during the qualifying rounds. For instance, during qualifying rounds, the rates of injury for boys and girls were 21.5 and 39.5, respectively. However, during the final rounds of play, rates of injury increased to 27.5 for boys and 53.5 for girls, suggesting that fatigue may be a contributing factor. Fortunately, most injuries were minor, and because 9 out of every 10 injured players missed less than 1 day of play, the researchers believed that young soccer players participate in a fairly safe activity. However, concern is increasing over the number of youths who sustain concussions while participating in youth soccer. In one investigation, researchers determined that 47.8 percent of the young adults experienced symptoms of concussion during a single season of soccer play (Delaney, Al-Kashmiri, Drummond, & Correa, 2008). They noted, however, that wearing protective headgear reduced the likelihood of injury during play.

Changes are being made in an attempt to reduce the number of soccer injuries. Because most injuries are caused by person-to-person contact, closer officiating, pregame warnings regarding inappropriate playing tactics (takedowns, hacking, and so forth), and coaching within the spirit of the rules should all be emphasized. In addition, researchers are examining the potential short-term and long-term consequences to youth who repeatedly head the soccer ball (AAP, 2000; see Figure 14.6). For example, one study reports that 49 percent of the 11.5-year-old participants complained of headaches after heading the

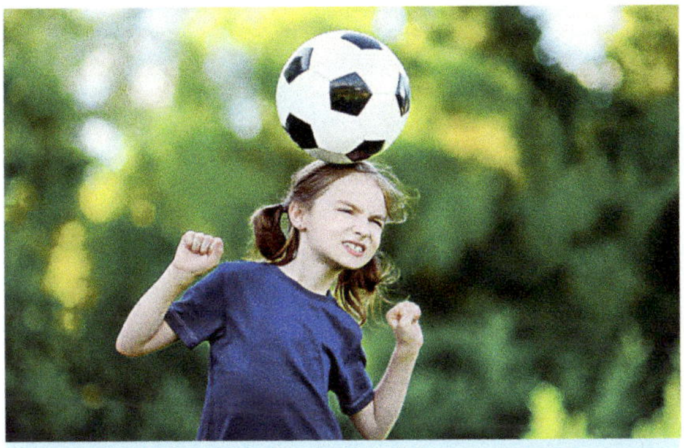

Figure 14.6 Repeated heading may have long-term medical consequences

soccer ball (Janda, Bir, & Cheney, 2002). Research involving adult soccer players indicates that even sub-concussive head impacts, like heading a soccer ball, can have an immediate influence on electrophysiological and cognitive function (Di Virgilio, Hunter, Wilson, et al, 2016). If true for adults, then one can speculate that repeated head trauma to the young developing brain might be even more traumatic. In 2014, a group of concerned parents and young players filed a class action lawsuit against U.S. Soccer and two additional organizations claiming that they were negligent in treating and monitoring head trauma in youth soccer players. In order to settle this litigation, the soccer organizations agreed to develop and implement a new youth soccer concussion policy (Yang & Baugh, 2016). This policy resulted in the following rule changes that went into effect at the beginning of the 2016 youth soccer season: (1) players 10 years of age and under are banned from heading in both games and during practice; and (2) players between 11 and 13 years of age may head during games but cannot perform more than 20 headings per week during practice.

In-Line Skating and Skateboarding

Millions of people participate in skateboarding and/or in-line skating. In fact, in-line roller hockey is quickly replacing ice hockey in many localities. Unfortunately, skateboarding and in-line skating are associated with a high rate of injury. Recent epidemiological data (McKenzie, Fletcher, Nelson, et al., 2016) indicate that on average, 64,572 individuals are treated in emergency departments each year for skateboarding related injuries. It appears that approximately 45 percent of these injuries occurred in children under the age of 15, and boys were involved in the majority of these mishaps. Most injuries requiring hospitalization were diagnosed as either a fracture or dislocation.

Injuries from these activities can be caused by a host of factors. Excessive speed, for example, seems to be a leading culprit, accounting for as much as 35 percent of all in-line skating falls that result in injury (Orenstein, 1996; see Figure 14.7). Normal cruising speeds generally fall between 10 and 17 mph (16 to 27 kph), but speeds in excess of 30 mph (48 kph) are not uncommon (IILSA, 1992). To place these speeds in perspective, consider that young children generally ride a bicycle at 9 mph (14.5 kph) and adults at 13 mph (21 kph; Thompson & Rivara, 1996). In an attempt to improve upon this safety record and to understand better why these mishaps occur, the American Academy of Pediatrics (2002) has made the following determinations:

- Children under 5 years of age should not be allowed to partake in skateboarding activities.
- Close adult supervision is mandatory for children younger than 10 years of age.
- Younger children are more likely to fall because of their higher center of gravity, poor balance, less experience, and slower reaction time.
- Children may overestimate their abilities and underestimate speed, traffic, and other risks.

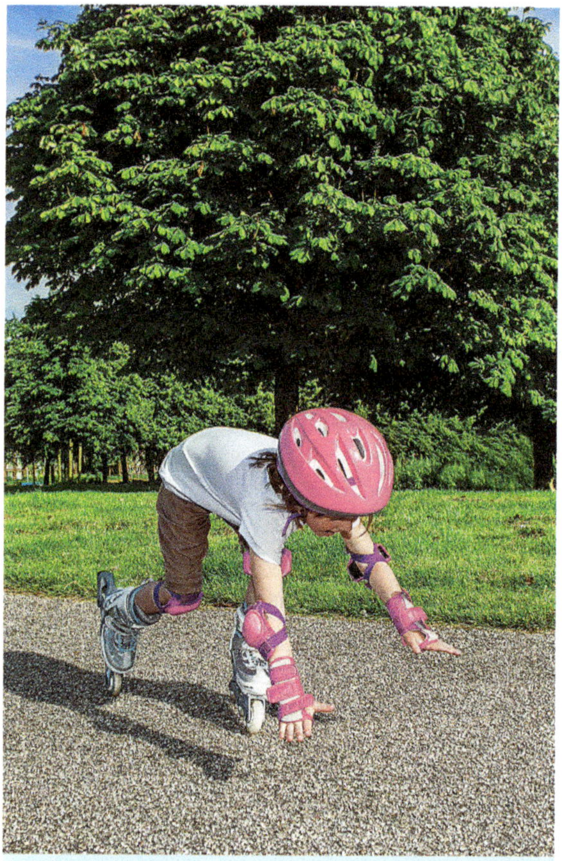

Figure 14.7 Many in-line skating injuries are the result of excessive speed

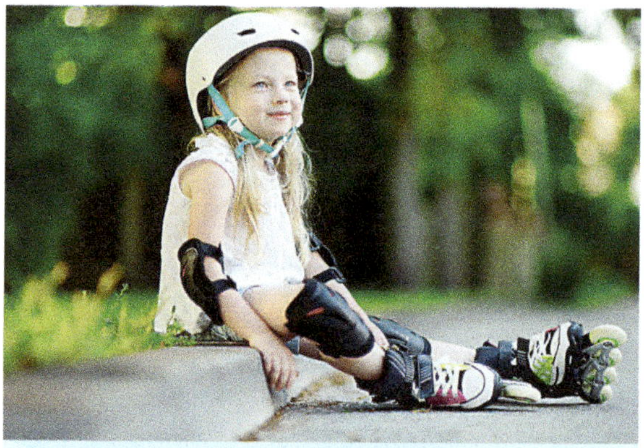

Figure 14.8 Safety equipment significantly reduces in-line skating injuries

- Appropriate safety equipment should be worn at all times (helmet, wrist guards, knee and elbow pads, and so on; see Figure 14.8).

Although researchers have not completely determined why people do not use these safety items, they cite four possible barriers to use: a lack of knowledge as to the importance of wearing protective equipment, discomfort, a perceived unsightly appearance, and cost (Thompson & Rivara, 1996). Individuals who work with in-line skaters and skateboarders should make every attempt to help participants overcome these barriers, because one thing is clear—protective equipment significantly reduces the risk of injury.

Overuse Injuries

Overuse injuries are becoming more prevalent among young athletes in the United States. In fact, it has been estimated that as many as one-third to one-half of youth sport injuries may be caused by overuse (Paterno, Taylor-Haas, Myer, et al., 2013). This should come as no surprise in light of the fact that young athletes are specializing in sports at earlier ages. Specialization generally entails intense, year-round involvement. In fact, it is not uncommon for young athletes to attend sport camps that require them to train 4–6 hours per day. It has been reported that to become a top junior tennis player, the young athlete must practice a minimum of 8–15 hours per week (Wild, 1992). Perhaps even more discouraging are reports that runners as young as 4 years of age are successfully completing marathons (Wikipedia, 2019).

Overuse injuries occur as a result of placing the muscular and skeletal system under repeated stress over long periods. Ewing, Seefeldt, and Brown (1996) note that, "Ironically, there are child labor laws in many countries that forbid stereotype work movements and excessive loading (Roberts, 1995), but these same restrictions do not apply to children's sports" (p. 30). This class of injury should not be taken lightly because, if activity is not curtailed, permanent injury could result. In adults, overuse injuries generally involve bone (stress fractures), tendon (Achilles tendinitis), and fascia (plantar fasciitis). In children and young adults, however, additional prone structures include physes (growth plates), cartilage of the apophyses (a site where the tendon unites with the bone), and articular cartilage. The two most prevalent forms of traction apophysitis are Osgood-Schlatter disease (inflammation of the kneecap ligament at its attachment on the tibia) and Sever's disease (inflammation of the growth plate in the heel). Both diseases are most prevalent in adolescence, when skeletal growth exceeds soft-tissue elongation, thus causing muscle tightness about the prone site. To avoid or reduce the severity of these injuries, young athletes should be encouraged to stretch both before and after physical activity and to discontinue an activity when an overuse injury occurs.

Overuse injuries involving bone can result in stress fractures. These overuse injuries are often the result of an abrupt change in exercise frequency and intensity. Most often the injury site is either the lower extremity or the hip. This type of injury is being seen more frequently and is difficult to diagnose without the use of sophisticated imagery techniques (for example, a CT scan).

"Little League elbow" refers to a class of overuse injuries that result from repeated forces being applied to the medial and lateral structures of the elbow (see Figure 14.9). Most often, the pain occurs on the elbow's medial side. As the name implies, this overuse injury is prevalent in baseball pitchers. In an attempt to protect young athletes from this medical condition, youth sport administrators have changed and modified baseball's rules. Among the most important changes and modifications are the following: T-ball, where the pitcher does not deliver the ball to the batter, is popular among the youngest children; some leagues no longer allow the pitcher to throw a curveball; and most youth leagues now limit the number of pitches per game (see Table 14.8). These pitch count guidelines, referred to as, "Smart Pitch" were established by a joint initiative with Major League Baseball and USA Baseball. Not only do these guidelines establish the maximum number of pitches per game, but also now establishes a required rest period (days off) between games (Major League Baseball, 2019). Table 14.8 presents the Smart Pitch guidelines. A recent national survey supports the need to implement these Smart Pitch guidelines. In this survey (Yang, Mann, Guettler, et al., 2014), youth pitchers between 9 and 18 years of age were required to self-report risk-prone activities. The relationship between these risk-prone activities and reported

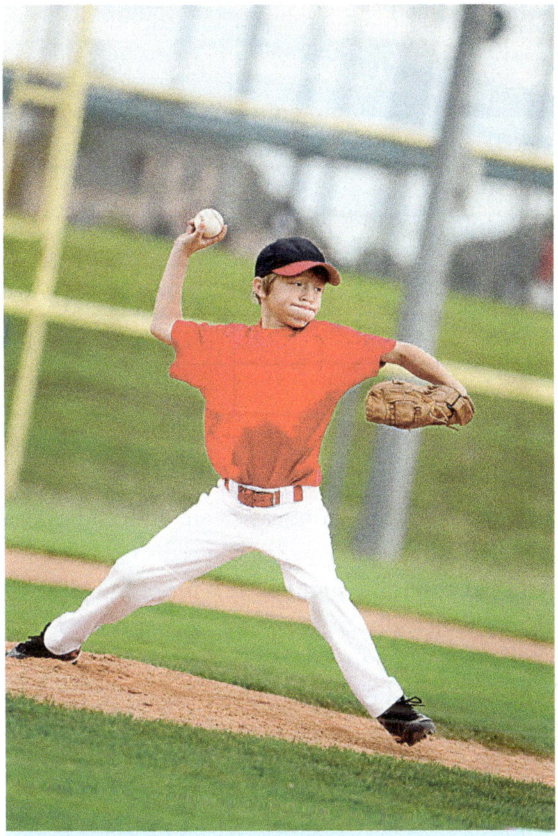

Figure 14.9 Repeated throwing stress can lead to Little League elbow—an overuse injury

Table 14.8 Smart Pitch: Guidelines for youth and adolescent pitchers

Age	Max pitches/gm	0 Days rest	1 Days rest	2 Days rest	3 Days rest	4 Days rest
7–8	50	1–20	21–35	36–50	N/A	N/A
9–10	75	1–20	21–35	36–50	51–65	66+
11–12	85	1–20	21–35	36–50	51–65	66+
13–14	95	1–20	21–35	36–50	51–65	66+
15–16	95	1–30	31–45	46–60	61–75	76+
17–18	105	1–30	31–45	46–60	61–80	81+

Source: Major League Baseball (2019).

shoulder and elbow injuries were assessed. As expected, those involved in the risk-prone activities reported significantly more injuries. More specifically, of the 754 youth pitchers, 43.4 percent pitched on consecutive days, 30.7 percent pitched on multiple teams with overlapping seasons, and 19 percent pitched more than one game on the same day. Additionally, throwing curve balls (70 percent) and pitching with a tired and/or painful arm greatly increased the odds of sustaining an injury.

Little League elbow was once the most frequently treated overuse injury among young athletes, but now physicians are witnessing a significant increase in another overuse injury—runner's knee. This injury is caused by an inappropriate tracking of the kneecap during running.

Because stress injuries are caused by patterns of overuse, young children should be discouraged from specializing in a particular sport during the childhood years. Instead, they should be encouraged to play several sports and even different positions within a selected sport. This way, the child is less likely to overuse a specific body part.

Preventing Youth Sport Injuries

A major challenge for organizers of youth programs is to devise methods and procedures that will curtail the number of injuries among participants. Organizers of youth sport programs need to answer two major questions: (1) are young people's sport injuries avoidable?; and (2) if they are, what steps can be taken to provide a safer and healthier environment?

Experts believe that the number of injuries can be reduced if coaches become more attuned to youngsters' physical and emotional state. Children who are *forced* to participate in sports may experience a higher rate of injury than children who *want* to participate. Furthermore, because many injuries occur late in a game or practice session, coaches should be aware of their players' state of fatigue. The literature also suggests that special precautions should be taken when working with young girls of all ages and with young boys 11–15 years old because these two populations appear to be at the greatest risk for injury.

To answer the question about providing a safe environment, consider the factors that can be addressed to reduce injuries; these are presented in Table 14.9. Pay particular attention to point 10, which notes that organizations are now available to help coaches and parents become better educated in sport safety.

Table 14.9 Factors to be considered in the prevention of injuries

1.	Make sure young athletes have been properly conditioned prior to competing.
2.	Avoid overtraining.
3.	Provide qualified adult supervision.
4.	Change rules to create a safer environment.
5.	Require the use of appropriate safety equipment.
6.	Match competitors according to body size and body weight (consider biological age as opposed to only chronological age or grade level).
7.	Do not allow an injured youth to return to competition until the area of injury has been completely rehabilitated.
8.	Do not allow youths to partake in questionable practices designed to create a competitive edge—that is, rapid weight reduction to qualify for a lower weight class, steroid use, and so forth.
9.	Use coaches who have obtained certification. These coaches tend to have a better understanding of young people's growth and development characteristics and are generally more capable of teaching appropriate skill technique than coaches without certification.
10.	Research the many youth sport organizations and the online courses and certifications in sports safety that they offer—for example, visit the following web address: sports-safety.hss.edu.

Young Athletes' Nutritional Requirements

The young athlete's nutritional requirements are essentially the same as those of any active child. The child's appetite should dictate caloric intake. In general, parents should provide well-balanced meals, being sure to serve appropriate portions. The USDA provides a website for planning and tracking an individual's food intake (see Figure 14.10; visit www.ChooseMyPlate.gov for more information). Unfortunately, problems can arise when parents alter their children's diets in an attempt to give them a competitive edge. For example, because certain sports are organized according to weight, such as wrestling and youth football, children and young adults are sometimes placed on special diets, some even involving periods of fasting, so that these youths can compete in a lower weight class. This practice should be avoided for reasons we will describe.

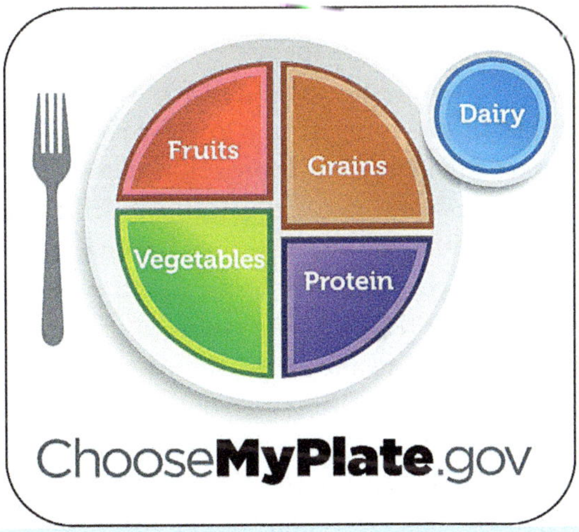

Figure 14.10 MyPlate, the USDA's guide to meal planning
Source: ChooseMyPlate.gov.

Another nutritional concern is the use of dietary supplements, especially vitamins. Generally, the body excretes any excess vitamins that are taken in, but some vitamins are not readily excreted and can accumulate in toxic levels; vitamins A and E, for example, can be harmful when taken in very large doses. Nathan Smith, a well-noted pediatrician, reported five cases of vitamin A poisoning. In one case, the parents of a young tennis player who had experienced vitamin A poisoning repeatedly put the child back on the vitamin (Barnes, 1979), believing that large doses of this vitamin would give the child a competitive advantage. Vitamin supplements are *not* generally necessary when the young athlete is eating balanced meals.

Making Weight and Eating Disorders

In several youth sports, teams are matched for competition on the basis of body weight. The primary intent of using this method is to ensure the safety of those involved and to provide a well-balanced, competitive athletic contest. Despite these positive intentions, adults sometimes employ unacceptable practices to give their child a competitive edge. One such practice is the use of unacceptable means to reduce the athlete's body weight so the youth can compete in a lower weight class. The most widely used approach is depleting the body of its water content; this is achieved by having the youth exercise in a sauna; not letting the young athlete drink water, even to the extent of requiring the youth to spit into a cup instead of swallowing; administering diuretics; and requiring the young person to exercise while wearing a rubber suit. Reducing body weight through rapid dehydration is extremely dangerous and should never be done. Without adequate fluids (water), the body's cells, kidneys, blood, and sweating mechanisms cannot function properly. A 3 percent loss of body fluids can decrease physical performance; a 5 percent loss can cause apparent signs of heat exhaustion; a 7 percent loss can cause hallucinations; a 10 percent loss can lead to heatstroke and circulatory collapse.

The young athlete should not be encouraged to fast. Fasting withholds vital substances that the body needs for proper growth during the formative years. When fasting is carried too far, death can result. A case in point is the story of Christy Henrich. A judge told this young gymnast that if she failed to lose body weight she would never make the Olympic team. At this time, the 15-year-old was only 4 ft 11 in (1.5 m) tall and weighed 90 lb (41 kg). Christy basically stopped eating, and 6 years later she died of multiple organ failure, weighing less than 60 lb (27 kg; Ryan, 1995, as cited in Ewing et al., 1996). In short, coaches must address issues of body weight quite cautiously. When in doubt, they should refer the young athlete to a physician, especially if they suspect an eating disorder.

Psychological Issues: Stress

Critics of youth sports frequently express concern regarding young athletes' ability to handle stressful situations. Limited amounts of stress have been shown to improve motor performance, but critics believe that too much competitive stress can lead to a multitude of negative behavioral, psychological, and even health-related outcomes.

Stress Model in Relation to Sport

Stress is generally viewed as an unpleasant emotional state. Passer's (1982) classic four-stage model precisely illustrates how this unpleasant state is evoked in relation to sport (see Figure 14.11). Passer's four stages are as follows:

- *Situation*. The stress process is evoked whenever individuals are placed in a demanding situation and they view the outcome of the situation as being important.
- *Appraisal*. Individuals appraise the situation in an attempt to determine if they can meet its demands. A young boy may become

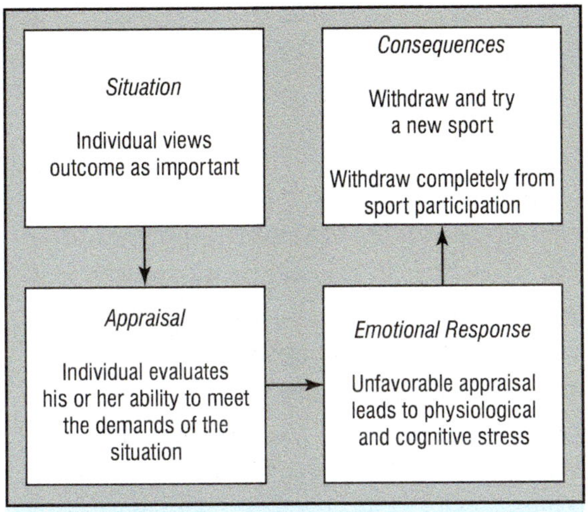

Figure 14.11 Model depicting the development of stress and potential behavioral outcomes

threatened and feel anxious before the start of an athletic contest because he wants to perform well but is not sure that he has the motor skills necessary for success. Thus, the fear of "making a physical game error" can be an intense source of stress among both girls and boys.

- *Emotional response*. Whenever people are threatened, emotional responses become evident. According to Passer, these emotional responses are made up of both physiological components and cognitive-attentional components. For instance, the boy may become so preoccupied with worrying about the outcome of his performance that he does not pay attention to important task-related cues that are necessary for successful performance.
- *Consequences*. This final stage raises the question, What are the outcomes of competitive stress? As mentioned earlier in this chapter, when sport participation loses its appeal, children and young adults frequently either withdraw from the disliked activity to pursue a more enjoyable activity or, in some cases, withdraw completely from sport participation.

Reducing Competitive Stress

Undoubtedly, young people will experience varying degrees of stress from participation in sports. However, steps can be taken to reduce the likelihood that this stress will become excessive.

Increase opportunities for success. One key is to change something about the sport so that success will occur more frequently than failure. For example, in T-ball, the fact that the ball is struck off a stationary batting tee rather than pitched obviously reduces the probability that the young athlete will strike out. In fact, Isaacs (1984) found a strikeout rate of only 4 percent among young T-ball players. Furthermore, according to Isaacs (1981), in basketball, children's shooting performance can be improved by lowering the goal and by using a smaller ball. In short, when children experience a fair amount of success, they develop self-confidence about their ability to meet the demands of the sport, and in turn they feel less threatened when confronted with the demands.

Use skill training. A second way to instill self-confidence and, thus, reduce stress is through skill training. Youth sport personnel, particularly coaches, could spend more practice time teaching motor skills and less time scrimmaging. When scrimmaging is incorporated, the focus should be on reducing performance uncertainty by practicing potential situations that may arise during a competitive contest. Coaches who adhere to these two practices are helping their young players develop self-confidence in their ability not only to meet the physical demands of the sport but also to handle efficiently most situations that may occur during competitive play. Anxiety is reduced whenever the uncertainty surrounding an event is removed or reduced. It is essential that coaches help their players develop an attitude of "I can do it."

STRESS: ANOTHER VIEWPOINT

Proponents of youth sport programs do not argue with the fact that excessive stress is not beneficial. However, they do argue that youth sport participation is by no means the only stressful situation young people encounter in their lives. This view was supported in Simon and Martens's classic work in 1979. These two researchers examined the level of precompetitive **state anxiety** among 468 boys who took part in various youth sport programs and 281 boys who competed in other achievement-oriented activities, including a softball game played in a physical education class, a general school test, group competition within a band, and a band solo competition. As illustrated in Figure 14.12, the researchers found the greatest amount of precompetitive state anxiety among the band solo contestants. Among the 11 sport and nonsport activities examined in the study, state anxiety was greatest in the individual activities. Passer (1982) writes, "This is somewhat ironic because the popular media and youth sport critics typically focus on team sports when discussing or illustrating the stressful nature of athletic competition" (p. 167). In fact, on average, participating in team sports was no more stressful than taking a paper-and-pencil test.

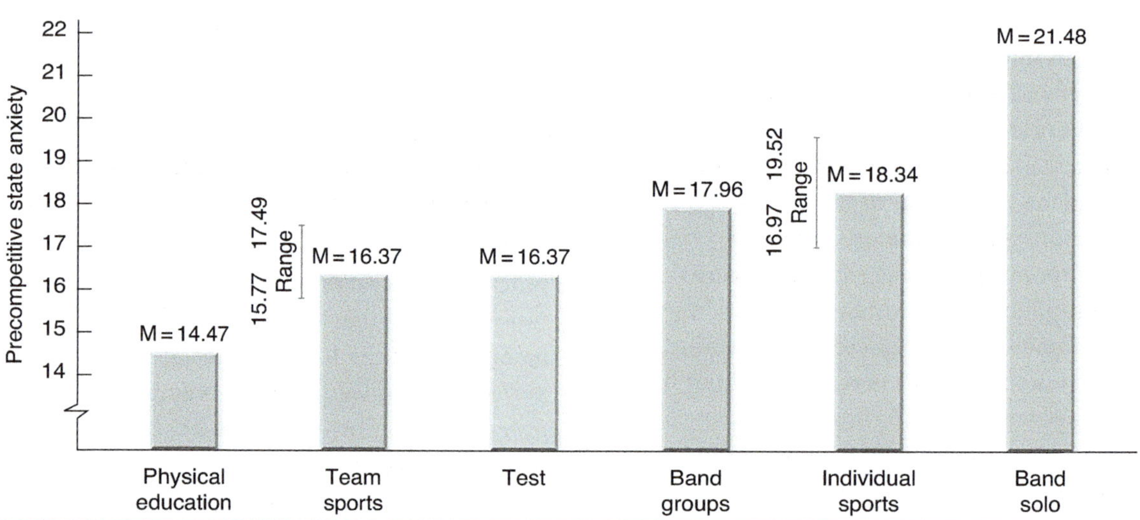

Figure 14.12 Boys' precompetitive state anxiety in 11 sport and nonsport activities. The precompetitive state anxiety scale ranges from 10 to 30. Team sports included football, hockey, baseball, and basketball; individual sports included swimming, gymnastics, and wrestling.

Source: Adapted from Simon and Martens (1979).

De-emphasize contest outcomes. To further reduce competitive stress, coaches should place the outcome of the contest (winning or losing) in perspective. There should not be too much emphasis on winning the game. Recall that the stress process is evoked when the participant views the outcome of the situation as important. To a degree, when there is an increase in the importance of the outcome, an accompanying increase in stress occurs. Thus, other influential people can also help young athletes by not overemphasizing winning. For instance, young children may feel that they have disappointed their parents or their coach if they have not played well. Parents and coaches can reduce stress for these young athletes by making it clear that the outcome of an athletic contest in no way affects their feelings for the children.

Encourage realistic goal setting. Finally, coaches and parents can reduce young athletes' self-imposed stress by helping them set realistic goals. Realistic goals are those that motivate the children to do their personal best and to recognize their own limitations. When realistic goals are established at the beginning of the season, youth sport participants can feel like winners regardless of their team's win/loss record.

YOUTH SPORT COACHING

Without a doubt, a youth sport program is only as good as its adult leaders. With appropriate leadership, the youth sport experience can significantly foster young people's growth and development. In this section, we examine the coaching profession, paying particular attention to volunteer coaches. We also address the controversy regarding the mandatory certification of coaches. Finally, we explore guidelines for effective coaching.

Who's Coaching Our Young People?

Of the approximately 3.5 million coaches in the United States, about 2.5 million are volunteers. Furthermore, as many as 90 percent of these volunteers lack the necessary formal preparation to coach effectively (American Coaching Academy, 2015; Ewing et al., 1996). Researchers from the United States and Canada have attempted to shed light on why so many individuals are motivated to give their valuable time and energy to serve in this voluntary role despite their lack of appropriate training. In one Canadian study, volunteer coaches indicated that the most important reasons for their involvement included personal enjoyment, skill development of players, character development of players, and personal challenge (Hansen & Gauthier, 1988). However, some individuals involved with this study believed that an even stronger motivator was the involvement of the coach's own child in the league. Indeed, 54 percent of the Canadian hockey coaches surveyed had one or two children participating in the league in which they coached. Similar trends have been reported in the United States.

Also of concern is the finding that only about 23 percent of youth sport coaches are female (Solomon & Farrey, 2018). Obviously, we need to find ways to attract more women to coaching (Figure 14.13). There are a number of reasons as to why greater female involvement is important. For example, female coaches

- challenge stereotypical beliefs regarding female sport participation,

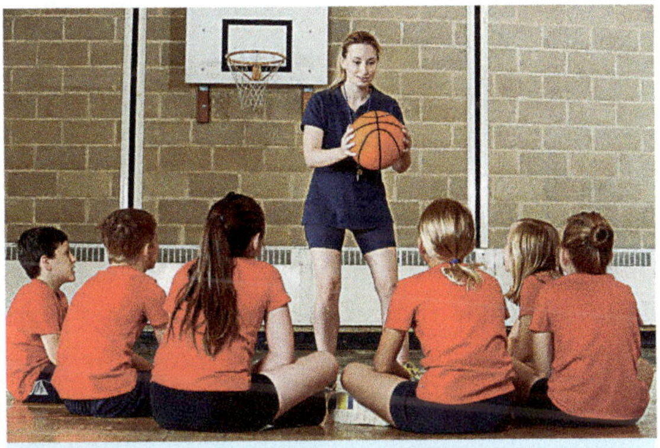

Figure 14.13 There is clearly a need for more involvement of adult women in youth sports

- serve as female role models in leadership positions, and
- provide same-gender role models for girls.

Finally, the question of "who's coaching our kids" arises, in part, because of safety concerns. Parents and youth organizations need to take an active role in screening all potential youth sport coaches, including volunteer coaches, before allowing these individuals to work with young people. Unfortunately, criminals and sex offenders sometimes enter youth sport coaching as a means of preying on children and young adults. Fortunately, organizations now exist that are capable of quickly running criminal background checks on potential youth sport coaches. One such organization is SportsSignup, which offers a background check program called KidsSafePlus. KidsSafePlus is a national screening program for all youth organizations, under which, for a small fee, an organization can obtain instantaneous results for criminal background checks, including a Social Security database search, a Department of Corrections database search, a search of the sex offender registry, and a search of county court records, including a search for pending charges. (To learn more about KidsSafePlus, visit www.sportssignup.com.)

Coaching Certification Programs

A growing number of organizations are providing educational programs for prospective coaches. Graduates of these educational programs have learned how to teach motor skills to children and young adults, organize a practice, physically train young people, prevent and recognize sport injuries, and communicate with and motivate young athletes. Educational information is generally conveyed through video, printed materials, small-group discussions, lectures, and online materials. Several of these organizations are listed in Table 14.10. Through their websites, these organizations offer a wealth of information to individuals desiring to foster the development of children and youth through youth sport.

ARGUMENTS AGAINST MANDATORY COACHING CERTIFICATION

As mentioned earlier, the number of children and young adults participating in both interscholastic and community/agency-sponsored youth sport programs is increasing every year. Unfortunately, this positive trend in participation has its downside. With increased participation comes a need for more sport offerings and, in turn, more coaches. In short, the demand for coaches now exceeds the supply. Those who argue against mandatory coaching certification express concern that making certification mandatory would cause many volunteers to withdraw their service and exacerbate the shortage of coaches. Should this occur, many youth sport programs might have to be eliminated. Others argue that mandatory coaching certification would be expensive; imposing a financial burden that could force some youth sport leagues to fold. Lopiano (1986) argued that this view is short-sighted and analogous to saying that we could reduce the high cost of medical care by eliminating certification of doctors and hospitals.

Table 14.10 Organizations dedicated to the advancement of knowledge through coaching certification

• American Sport Education Program, www.asep.com
• Coaching Association of Canada, www.coach.ca
• Institute for the Study of Youth Sports, edwp.educ.msu.edu/isys
• National Alliance for Youth Sports, www.nays.org
• National Federation of State High School Associations, www.nfhs.org
• North American Youth Sport Institute, www.naysi.com

Guidelines for Effective Coaching

Table 14.11 presents a list of guidelines to enhance the youth sport experience. Not only are these guidelines useful to the coach, but they can also be helpful to the parents of prospective young athletes as they select the best coach to work with their children.

Table 14.11 Guidelines to enhance the youth sport experience

1 Coaches' philosophy of winning:	a. Convey that winning is not everything. b. Do not view losing a game as failing. c. Do not equate winning with success. d. Convey to young people that success is found in striving to do one's best.
2. Coaches' reactions to desirable behaviors:	a. Be generous with positive reinforcement. b. Have realistic expectations of performance. c. Reinforce desired behaviors as quickly as possible. d. Reinforce effort as frequently as performance results.
3. Coaches' reactions to mistakes:	a. Give encouragement. b. Give corrective instruction in a positive manner—but only if you suspect the player is not aware of the corrective information. c. Never punish a young person for making a technical mistake. d. Never administer corrective instruction in a hostile manner.
4. Coaches' reactions to misbehaviors or lack of attention, and coaches' maintenance of discipline:	a. Establish team rules that are clearly understood by all. b. Allow player involvement in the establishment and enforcement of team rules. c. During the game, make sure players understand that all members are part of the team, even those on the bench.
5. Coaches' behaviors:	a. Set a good example as an adult role model. b. Encourage and reinforce both effort and progress. c. Encourage players to be supportive of one another, and reinforce such behaviors. d. Always convey instruction in a positive manner. e. Always be patient and never expect more than a maximum effort from your athletes. f. Be an effective communicator.

Source: Adapted from Smoll and Smith (1984).

PARENTAL EDUCATION: AN ATTEMPT TO CURB VIOLENCE

In addition to the debate over mandatory certification of coaches, there is also debate over proposals to require education of the parents of youth sport participants. These proposals have been made in response to the violent behavior on the part of parents that plagues many youth sport programs. Take, for example, the 34-year-old mother who attacked a 15-year-old soccer referee because she became infuriated during her 11-year-old son's soccer game. Most tragic, an all-time low was reached in August 2000 when a parent beat to death a Massachusetts volunteer coach, in front of the coach's own children, following a youth ice hockey contest for 10-year-olds (Butterfield, 2002).

As a response to these escalating acts of violence, an increasing number of youth sport programs are requiring parental education. One program is the NAYS Parent Orientation & Membership Program (NAYS: National Alliance for Youth Sports, 2019). This program is designed to foster a positive youth sport experience by eradicating parental issues. This is accomplished through video-based training that outlines parental roles and responsibilities. More specifically, parents will receive instruction in: modeling sportsmanship, safety and injury prevention, identifying and preventing steroid abuse, and the importance of maintaining proper behavior, just to name a few.

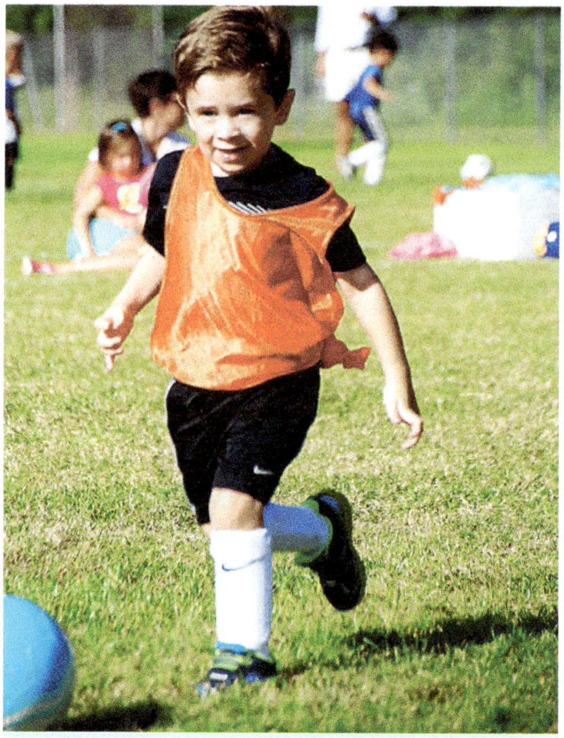

Figure 14.14 All children and young adults should have the right to experience the joy of sports in a safe and healthy environment

Source: Courtesy of Dr. Larry Isaacs.

RIGHTS OF YOUNG ATHLETES

Throughout this chapter we have described and recommended various ways in which the youth sport experience can be enhanced so that all involved may experience the joy of sport to its fullest (Figure 14.14). To this end, we recommend that all youth sport leaders ascribe to and uphold the standards established in the document, National Standards for Youth Sports (NAYS, 2017). **The National Standards for Youth Sports** are intended to provide a framework for the design and execution of youth sport programs. The document is organized around four core components: child centered policies and philosophies, as well as standards for volunteers and parents, and standards for creating a safe playing environment. The document also contains three additional sections that provide information to parents, volunteer coaches, and participants explaining what these standards mean to them (National Alliance for Youth Sports, 2017).

In further attempts to protect young athletes, various organizations have developed position statements regarding recommended practices

Table 14.12 Selected pronouncements of professional organizations regarding youth sports

American Academy of Pediatrics (2015), "Tackling in youth football"	www.pediatrics.org/cgi/doi/10.1542/peds.2015–3282 *Recommendations to improve safety for those playing youth football*
American Academy of Pediatrics (2008), "Strength training by children and adolescents"	http://pediatrics.aappublications.org/content/121/4/835.full *Describes terminology and the risks and benefits of strength training*
American Academy of Pediatrics (2001), "Organized sports for children and preadolescents"	http://pediatrics.aappublications.org/content/107/6/1459.abstract *Lists the safeguards that should accompany children's sports*
American Academy of Pediatrics (2000), "Intensive training and sports specialization in young athletes"	http://pediatrics.aappublications.org/content/106/1/154.full *Reviews the potential risks of high-intensity training and sport specialization in young athletes*
American College of Sports Medicine (2007), "Exercise and fluid replacement"	doi: 10.1249/mss.0b013e31802ca597 *Reviews the effects of dehydration and hydration on human performance*
Major League Baseball (2019), "Guidelines for youth and adolescent pitchers"	www.mlb.com/pitch-smart/pitching-guidelines *Describes the recommended number of pitches allowed per game and amount of rest required between games*
National Strength and Conditioning Association (2009), "Youth resistance training: Position statement"	www.nsca.com/WorkArea/DownloadAsset.aspx?id=1155 *Most comprehensive literature review on youth resistance training*
National Strength and Conditioning Association (2016), "NSCA position statement on long-term athletic development"	www.ncbi.nlm.nih.gov/pubmed/26933920 Describes the 10 pillars of successful long-term athletic development

for young people's athletic endeavors. See Table 14.12 for a list of resources for such practices.

SUMMARY

- The number of young athletes participating in organized youth sport programs continues to grow even though participation in some sports like football appears to be declining. This overall increase in participation is occurring for several reasons. Namely, greater participation at younger ages, greater involvement on the part of girls and young women, greater involvement in nontraditional activities, and greater participation by individuals with disabilities.
- Young people participate in sports for many reasons, but the most often cited reason is "to have fun." Researchers consistently find that children and young adults participate for intrinsic reasons (e.g., fun, to improve skills), not extrinsic reasons (e.g., to win trophies).
- Contrary to popular belief, most youth sport injuries are minor—primarily simple contusions, sprains, and strains. In general, girls tend to be at greater risk of injury than

boys. To reduce the number of youth sport injuries, authorities agree that young people should be encouraged to play many different sports during their formative years. Young athletes who specialize in one activity year-round tend to be at greater risk for stress or overuse injuries. When special precautions are taken, many sport injuries are avoidable.

- The nutritional requirements for a young athlete are the same as for any active young person. Dietary supplements such as vitamins do not give young athletes a competitive edge.
- Some experts believe that competitive stress is the reason why children and young adults discontinue sport participation at increasingly early ages. However, proponents of youth sport programs point out that activities other than sports also produce stress in the lives of young people. Nevertheless, both critics and proponents of youth sport programs agree that steps can be taken to reduce the amount of stress young participants encounter during sport participation. These steps revolve around one central theme: improve the young person's self-confidence concerning her or his ability to meet the demands of the selected sport.
- Most youth sport coaches are in a program because they have a son or daughter involved in the same program. Unfortunately, most of these coaches do not have the appropriate training to foster an optimal youth sport experience. Several organizations provide coaching education for volunteer coaches. Many organizations require certification for youth coaches, as well as criminal background checks before an adult will be allowed to work with children.
- Because of an increase in violence on the part of youth sport participants' parents, many programs require parental education. This training is designed to teach parents about sportsmanship and unacceptable behaviors.
- To enhance the youth sport experience further, the National Alliance for Youth Sports developed the National Standards for Youth Sports with the purpose of providing a framework for the design and execution of youth sport programs.

key concept review

commotio cordis
competence motivation theory
concussion
contact/collision sport
National Standards for Youth Sports
overuse injuries
state anxiety
stress

questions for reflection

1. What are the reasons for increased enrollment in youth sport programs?
2. What (in order) are the 10 most important reasons youths participate in sports?
3. What (in order) are the 11 most important reasons given by young people as to why they drop out of youth sport activities? In addition, what changes would both boys and girls want to see before returning to a sport that they had dropped?
4. What medical issues are associated with each of the following: football, baseball, soccer, and in-line skating/skateboarding? Regarding football, which positions appear to be the most dangerous? What changes could be made to reduce these sport-specific injuries?
5. What are the typical overuse injuries that occur in youth sport participants?

6. What steps can be taken to reduce competitive stress within the youth sport environment?
7. What are the arguments both for and against mandatory coaching certification, as well as for and against mandatory education for parents?
8. Describe the reasons for conducting a criminal and sex offender background check prior to allowing a coach to work with young children. Additionally, identify one organization capable of performing this background check.
9. Can you describe the National Standards for Youth Sports?
10. Can you identify key professional organizations that have published pronouncements regarding youth sports participation?

online resources

Aspen Institute: State of Play: 2018, www.aspeninstitute.org

Coaching Association of Canada, www.coach.ca

In-line Skating Resource Center, www.iisa.org

Institute for the Study of Youth Sports, edwp.educ.msu.edu/isys

National Alliance for Youth Sports, www.nays.org

National Center for Sports Safety, www.sportssafety.org

National Federation of State High School Associations, www.nfhs.org

North American Youth Sport Institute, www.naysi.com

Sports & Fitness Industry Association: www.sfia.org

REFERENCES

American Academy of Pediatrics (2000). Injuries in youth soccer: A subject review (RE9934). *Pediatrics, 105*(3), 659–661.

American Academy of Pediatrics (2001). Risk of injury from baseball and softball in children (RE0032). *Pediatrics, 107*, 782–784.

American Academy of Pediatrics (2002). Skateboard and scooter injuries. *Pediatrics, 109*, 542–543.

American Academy of Pediatrics (2004). Protective eyewear for young athletes. *Pediatrics, 113*, 619–622.

American Academy of Pediatrics (2008). Strength training by children and adolescents. *Pediatrics, 121*, 835–840.

American Academy of Pediatrics (2009). In-line skating injuries in children and adolescents—Reaffirmation of 1998 policy statement. *Pediatrics, 123*, 1421–1422.

American Academy of Pediatrics (2015). Tackling in youth football. *Pediatrics*, 136, e1419–e1430, doi: 10.1542/peds.2015-3282. Retrieved from www.pediatrics.org/cgi/doi/10.1542/peds.2015–3282.

American Coaching Academy (2015). Experts say 90% of youth sports coaches have little to no training, thus putting their athletes at risk. Retrieved from www.prweb.com/releases/sports/coaching/prweb907124.htm.

American Orthopaedic Society for Sports Medicine (2009). Baseball injury prevention. Retrieved from www.orthoinfo.aaos.org/topic.cfm?topic=A00185.

Aspen Institute (2018). *Sport participation and physical activity rates*. Aspen, CO: Author. Retrieved from https://assets.aspeninstitute.org/content/uploads/2018/10/StateofPlay2018_v4WEB_2-final.pdf.

Athletic Footwear Association (1990). *American youth and sports participation*. North Palm Beach, FL: Author.

Atkins, M. R., Johnson, D. M., Force, E. C., & Petrie, T. A. (2015). Peers, parents, and coaches, oh my! The relation of the motivational climate to boys' intention to continue in sport. *Psychology of Sport and Exercise, 16*, 170–180.

Barnes, L. (1979). Preadolescent training: How young is too young? *Physician and Sportsmedicine, 10*, 114–119.

Beets, M. W., & Pitetti, K. H. (2005). Contribution of physical education and sport to health-related fitness in high school students. *Journal of School Health, 75*, 25–30.

Belanger, M., Gray-Donald, K., O'Loughlin, J., Paradis, G., & Hanley, J. (2009). When adolescents drop the ball: Sustainability of physical activity in youth. *American Journal of Preventive Medicine, 37*, 41–49.

Blon, L., Bronk, K., Coakley, J., Lauer, L., & Sawyer, T. (2013). Position statement: Maximizing the benefits of youth sports. *Journal of Physical Education, Recreation & Dance, 84*, 8–13.

Butterfield, F. (2002, Jan. 26). Father in killing at hockey rink is given sentence of 6 to 10 year. *New York Times*. Retrieved from: www.nytimes.com/2002/01/26/us/father-in-kill-ing-at-hockey-rink-is-given-sentence-of-6-to-10-years.html.

Clark, H. J., Camire, M., Wade, T. J., & Cairney, J. (2015). Sport participation and its association with social and psychological factors known to predict substance use and abuse among youth: A scoping review of the literature. *International Review of Sport and Exercise Psychology*, *8*, 224–250.

Coakley, J. (1986). When should children begin competing? A sociological perspective. In M. R. Weiss & D. Gould (Eds.), *Sport for children and youths*. Champaign, IL: Human Kinetics.

Crane, J., & Temple, V. (2015). A systematic review of dropout from organized sport among children and youth. *European Physical Education Review, 21*, 114–118.

Delaney, J. D., Al-Kashmiri, A., Drummond, R., & Correa, F. A. (2008). The effects of protective headgear on head injuries and concussions in adolescent football (soccer) players. *British Journal of Sports Medicine, 42*, 110–115.

DiFiori, J. P., Benjamin, H. J., Brenner, J. S., Gregory, A., Jayanthi, N., Landry, G. L., et al. (2014). Overuse injuries and burnout in youth sports: A position statement from the American Medical Society for Sports Medicine. *British Journal of Sports Medicine*, *48*, 287–288.

Di Virgilio, T. G., Hunter, A., Wilson, L., Stewart, W., Goodall, S., Howatson, G., et al. (2016). Evidence for acute electrophysiological and cognitive changes following routine soccer heading. *EBioMedicine*, *13*, 66–71.

Dompier, T. P., Powell, J. W., Barron, M. J., & Moore, M. T. (2007). Time-loss and non-time-loss injuries in youth football players. *Journal of Athletic Training, 42*, 395–402.

Eldridge, J. A., Palmer, T. B/, Gillis, K., Lloyd, R., Squires, W. G., & Murray, T. D. (2014). Comparison of academic and behavioral performance between athletes and non-athletes. *International Journal of Exercise Science*, *7*, 3–13.

ESPN (2013). Youth football participation drops. *ESPN News Online*. Retrieved from http://espn.go.com/espn/otl/story/_/page/popwarner/pop-warner-youth-football-participation.

Ewing, M. E., Seefeldt, V. D., & Brown, T. P. (1996, March 18). Role of organized sports in the education and health of American children and youth. In A. Poinsett (Ed.), *The role of sports in youth development*. Meeting convened by the Carnegie Corporation of New York.

Feltz, D. L., & Petlichkoff, L. (1983). Perceived competence among interscholastic sport participants and dropouts. *Canadian Journal of Applied Sport Sciences, 8*, 231–235.

Goldberg, B., Rosenthal, P. P., Robertson, L. S., & Nicholas, J. A. (1988). Injuries in youth football. *Pediatrics, 81*, 255–261.

Gould, D., Feltz, D., Horn, T., & Weiss, M.R. (1982). Reasons for discontinuing involvement in competitive youth swimming. *Journal of Sport Behavior*, *5*, 155–165.

Haapala, E. A., Lankhorst, K., de Groot, J., Zwinkels, M., Verschuren, O., Wittink, H., et al. (2017). The associations of cardiorespiratory fitness, adiposity and sports participation with arterial stiffness in youth with chronic diseases or physical disabilities. *European Journal of Preventive Cardiology*, *24*, 1102–1111.

Hansen, H., & Gauthier, R. (1988). Reasons for involvement of Canadian hockey coaches in minor hockey. *Physical Educator, 45*, 147–153.

Harmon, K. G., Drezner, J. A., Gammons, M., Guskiewicz, K. M., Halstead, M., Herring, S. A., et al. (2013). American Medical Society for Sports Medicine position statement: Concussions in sport. *British Journal of Sports Medicine, 47*, 15–26.

Harter, S. (1982). The Perceived Competence Scale for Children. *Child Development, 53*, 87–97.

Harter, S. (1988). Causes, correlates, and the functional role of global self-worth: A life-span perspective. In J. Kolligan & R. Sternberg (Eds.), *Perceptions of competence and incompetence across the life-span*. New Haven, CT: Yale University Press.

Hedstrom, R., & Gould, D. (2004). *Research in youth sports: Critical issues status—White paper summaries of the existing literature*. East Lansing, MI: Institute for the Study of Youth Sports.

Holecko, C. (2015). Is your child old enough for competitive sports? Retrieved from www.familyfitness.about.com/of/kidssports/f/When-Should-Kids-Start-Competitive-Sports.htm.

Horn, T. S., & Weiss, M. R. (1991). A developmental analysis of children's self-ability judgments in the physical domain. *Pediatric Exercise Science, 3*, 310–326.

International In-Line Skating Association (1992). *Guidelines for establishing in-line skate trails in parks and recreational areas*. Minneapolis, MN: Author.

Isaacs, L. D. (1981, December). Factors affecting children's basketball shooting performance: A log-linear analysis. *Carnegie Research Papers*, 29–32.

Isaacs, L. D. (1984). Players' success in T-baseball. *Perceptual and Motor Skills, 59*, 852–854.

Janda, D. H., Bir, C. A., & Cheney, A. L. (2002). An evaluation of the cumulative concussive effect of soccer heading in the youth population. *Injury Control and Safety Promotion, 9*, 25–31.

Jones, M. J., Dunn, J. G. H., Holt, N. L., Sullivan, P. J., & Bloom, G. A. (2011). Exploring the 5C's of positive youth development. *Journal of Sport Behavior, 34*, 250–267.

Kondric, M., Sindik, J., Furjan-Mandic, G., & Schiefler, B. (2013). Participation motivation and student's physical activity among sport students in three countries. *Journal of Sports Science & Medicine*, 12, 10–18.

Koutures, C. G., & Gregory, A. (2010). Clinical report: Injuries in youth soccer. *Pediatrics, 125*, 410–414.

Kyle, S. B. (1996). *Youth baseball protective equipment project: Final report*. Washington, DC: U.S. Consumer Product Safety Commission.

Kymar, K., Mandleywala, S. N., Gannon, M. P., Estes, N. A. M., Weinstock, J., & Link, M. S. (2017). Development of a chest wall protector effective in preventing sudden cardiac death by chest wall impact (Commotio Cordis). *Clinical Journal of Sports Medicine*, 27, 26–30.

Le Gall, F., Carling, C., & Reilly, T. (2008). Injuries in youth elite female soccer players: An 8-season prospective study. *American Journal of Sports Medicine, 36*, 276–284.

Leininger, R. E., Knox, C. L., & Comstock, R. D. (2007). Epidemiology of 1.6 million pediatric soccer related injuries presenting to United States emergency departments from 1990 to 2003. *American Journal of Sports Medicine, 35*, 288–294.

Lloyd, R. S., Cronin, J. B., Faigenbaum, A. D., Kraemer, W. J., Micheli, L. J., Myer, G. D., et al. (2016). National strength and conditioning association position statement on long-term athletic development. *Journal of Strength and Conditioning Research, 30*, 1491–1509.

Lopiano, D. (1986). The certified coach: A central figure. *Journal of Physical Education, Recreation, and Dance, 57*(3), 34–38.

Major League Baseball. (2019). Guidelines for youth and adolescent pitchers. Retrieved from www.mlb.com/pitch-smart/pitching-guidelines.

Malina, R. M., & Cumming, S. P. (2003). Current status and issues in youth sports. In R. M. Malina & M. A. Clark (Eds.), *Youth sports: Perspectives for a new century*. Monterey, CA: Coaches Choice.

Maron, B. J., & Estes, M. (2010). Commotio cordis. *New England Journal of Medicine, 362*, 917–927.

Maron, B. J., Gohman, T. E., Kyle, S. B., Estes, N. A. M., & Link, M. S. (2002). Clinical profile and spectrum of commotio cordis. *Journal of the American Medical Association, 287*, 1142–1146.

Marshall, S. W., Mueller, F. O., Kirby, D. P., & Yang, J. (2003). Evaluation of safety balls and faceguards for prevention of injuries in youth baseball. *Journal of the American Medical Association, 289*, 568–574.

McKenzie, L. B., Fletcher, E., Nelson, N. G., Roberts, K. J., & Klein, E. G. (2016). Epidemiology of skateboarding-related injuries sustained by children and adolescents 5–19 years of age and treated in US emergency departments: 1990 through 2008. *Injury Epidemiology*, 3, 10, doi: 10.1186/s40621-016-0075-6.

National Alliance for Youth Sports (2017). National standards for youth sports. Retrieved from www.nays.org.

National Alliance for Youth Sports (2019). NAYS Parent orientation & membership program. Retrieved from www.nays.org/parents.

National Federation of State High School Association (2018). 2017–2018 high school athletics participation survey. Indianapolis: Author. Retrieved from www.nfhs.org.

Nilsson, S., & Roaas, A. (1978). Soccer injuries in adolescents. *American Journal of Sports Medicine, 6*, 258–361.

Orenstein, J. B. (1996). Injuries and small-wheel skates. *Annals of Emergency Medicine, 27*, 204–209.

Passer, M. W. (1982). Psychological stress in youth sports. In R. A. Magill, M. J. Ash, & F. L. Smoll (Eds.), *Children in sport*. Champaign, IL: Human Kinetics.

Paterno, M. V., Taylor-Haas, J. A., Myer, G. D., & Hewett, T. E. (2013). Prevention of overuse sports injuries in the young athlete. *Orthopedic Clinics of North America, 44*, 553–564.

Peterson, A. R., Kruse, A., J., Meester, S. M., Olson, T. S., Riedle, B. N., Slayman, T. G., et al. (2017). Youth football injuries: A prospective cohort. *The Orthopaedic Journal of Sports Medicine, 5*, doi: 10.1177/2325967116686784.

Roberts, G. C., Kleiber, D. A., & Duda, J. L. (1981). An analysis of motivation in children's sport: The role of perceived competence in participation. *Journal of Sport Psychology, 3*, 206–216.

Roberts, L. (1995). Child labor: A form of modern slavery. In *The way forward: Conference on human rights* (pp. 35–42). Verbier, Switzerland.

Ryan, J. (1995). *Little girls in pretty boxes*. New York: Doubleday.

Sabo, D. & Veliz, P. (2008). *Go out and play: Youth sports in America*. East Meadow, NY: Women's Sports Foundation.

Seefeldt, V., Ewing, M. E., & Walk, S. (1991). Overview of youth sports in the United States. Paper commissioned by the Carnegie Council on Adolescent Development. New York: Carnegie Corporation of New York.

Sheu, Y., Chen, L., & Hedegaard, H. (2016). Sports- and recreation-related injury episodes in the United States, 2011–2014. National Health Statistics Reports, no. 99. Hyattsville, MD: National Center for Health Statistics.

Simon, J., & Martens, R. (1979). Children's anxiety in sport and nonsport evaluative activities. *Journal of Sport Psychology, 1*, 160–169.

Smoll, F. L., & Smith, R. E. (1984). Improving the quality of coach-player interaction. In J. R. Thomas (Ed.), *Motor development during childhood and adolescence*. Minneapolis, MN: Burgess.

Solomon, J. & Farrey, T. (2018). State of play 2018: Trends and developments. The Aspen Institute. Retrieved from www.aspeninstitute.org/blog-posts/10-charts-that-show-progress-challenges-to-fix-youth-sports.

Stuart, M. J., Morrey, M. A., Smith, A. M., Meis, J. K., & Ortiguera, C. J. (2002). Injuries in youth football: A prospective observational cohort analysis among players aged 9 to 13 years. *Mayo Clinic Proceedings, 77*, 317–322.

Thompson, R. S., & Rivara, F. P. (1996). Protective equipment for in-line skaters. *New England Journal of Medicine, 335*, 1680–1682.

Tysvaer, A., & Lochen, E. (1991). Soccer injuries to the brain. *American Journal of Sports Medicine, 19*, 56–60.

Ulrich, B. D. (1987). Perceptions of physical competence, motor competence, and participation in organized sport: Their interrelationships in young children. *Research Quarterly for Exercise and Sport, 58*, 57–67.

Vinger, P. F., Duma, S. M., & Crandall, J. (1999). Baseball hardness as a risk factor for eye injuries. *Archives of Ophthalmology, 117*, 354–358.

Wankel, L. M., & Kreisel, P. S. J. (1985). Factors underlying enjoyment of youth sports: Sport and age group comparisons. *Journal of Sport Psychology, 7*, 51–64.

Weiss, M. R., & Ferrer-Caja, E. (2002). Motivational orientations in youth sports. In T. Horn (Ed.), *Advances in sport psychology*. 2nd ed. Champaign, IL: Human Kinetics.

Wikipedia (2019). Budhia Singh. Retrieved from https://en.wikipedia.org/wilk/Budhia_Singh.

Wild, S. (1992, July–August). Choosing a junior tennis program. *CrossCourt News*, 3.

Yang, J., Mann, B. J., Guettler, J. H., Dugar, J. R., Irrgang, J. J., Fleisig, G. S., & Albright, J. P. (2014). Risk-prone pitching activities and injuries in youth baseball: Findings from a national sample. *The American Journal of Sports Medicine, 42*, 1456–1463.

Yang, Y. T., & Baugh, C. M. (2016). US youth soccer concussion policy: Heading in the right direction. *Pediatrics, 170*, 413–414.

15 MOVEMENT IN ADULTHOOD

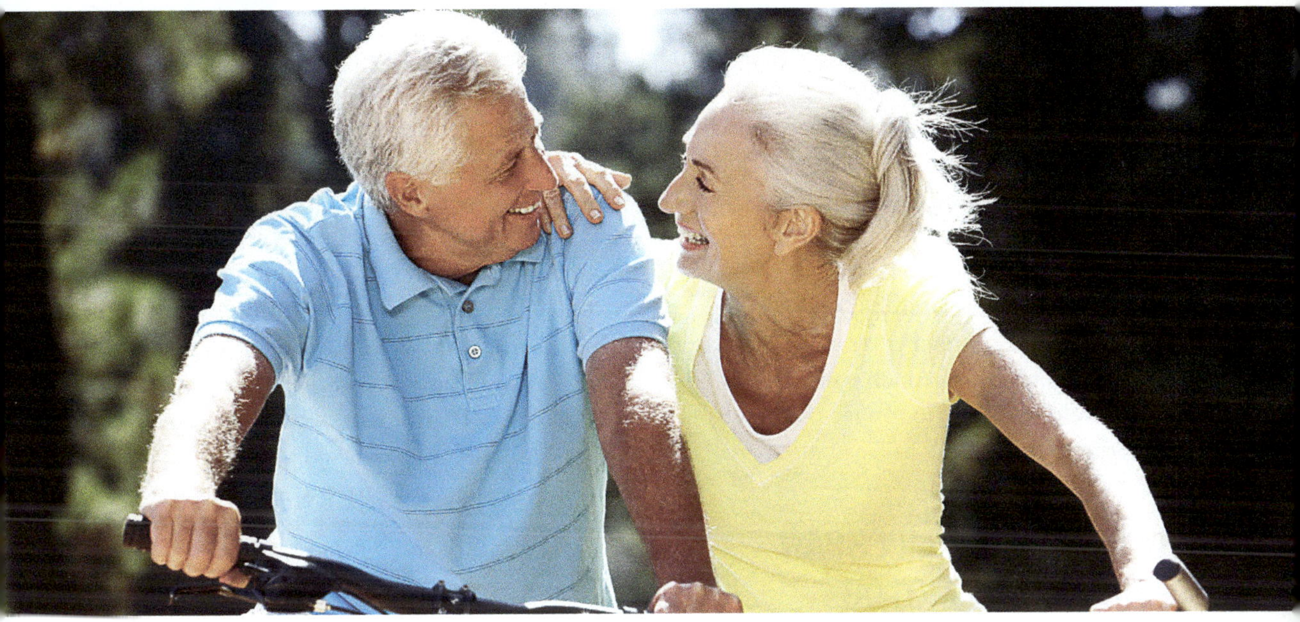

Chapter Objectives

From the information presented in this chapter, you will be able to

- Explain the shift to a lifespan approach in the study of motor development and why it is important
- Explain the important trends in our national and worldwide population related to movement in adults
- Define balance and postural sway and describe the related trends across adulthood
- Describe how walking characteristics change throughout adulthood
- Describe the key issues associated with falls in adulthood and strategies to avoid them
- Explain key issues and factors associated with driving and older adulthood
- Describe activities of daily living in adulthood and what can be done to maintain function with age
- Describe typical changes in movement speed across adulthood
- Define reaction and response time and describe how they relate to aging throughout adulthood
- Explain the national and worldwide trends in physical activity among adults and older adults
- Explain key strategies for maintaining movement ability across adulthood and give key recommendations for quantity and quality of exercise

Recall that motor development is the study of the changes in human motor behavior over the lifespan, the processes that underlie these changes, and the factors that affect them. Although this definition is widely accepted, generally and historically, it has not always been applied. The field of motor development has traditionally emphasized childhood. Adolescence has been examined occasionally; movement in adulthood, seldom. Most motor developmentalists have traditionally maintained an expertise in childhood movement, giving much less attention to the motor changes and related factors of adulthood. For a number of reasons discussed below, that general approach to the study of motor development is no longer the most appropriate.

THE SHIFT TO A LIFESPAN APPROACH TO MOTOR DEVELOPMENT

A lifespan concept of motor development has gained considerable popularity in the academic community over the last quarter century. Taking a lifespan approach to the study of motor development is important because it provides a framework for examining individual changes at all ages throughout life. It also answers important questions as to why certain changing behaviors emerge as we pass from childhood to adolescence to adulthood. Existing research suggests that changes in human movement are similar to what we believe generally happens intellectually: we frequently see performance improve across the childhood years through young adulthood, followed by some plateauing and, later in life, declines in performance. Research has generated results to support this pattern. When they tested fine and gross movement performance across the lifespan, Leversen, Haga, and Sigmundsson (2012) saw improvements in performance from 7- to 9-year-old children to 19- to 25-year-old young adults and declines in performance from young adulthood to 66- to 80-year-old older adults. These findings are typical for studies examining changes in motor development across age and are important general information as they help determine how and where we need to focus efforts to enable people to maintain and improve their movement performance at ages, and in areas, where we now see declines. In short, our interventions can become much more efficient and effective. In addition, though we generally see declines across adulthood with advancing age, considerable research has demonstrated that these declines vary with individuals and can be offset and reversed with carefully designed interventions and wise lifestyle choices. This concept will be discussed in more detail later in the chapter.

This shift to a lifespan study of motor development has been influenced by a number of factors including the increase in the population of older people in the U.S. and throughout the world over the past century. Part of this increase is illustrated in Table 15.1, that depicts the predicted increase of people over 60 years of age from various regions of the world between 2015 and 2030. It ranges from a low of 23 percent in Europe to a high of 71 percent in Latin America and the Caribbean (United Nations Department of Economic and Social Affairs, 2015).

Another way of viewing this phenomenon is presented in Table 15.2 where we can see that, as the number of people over 60, 70, 80, and 90 years of age has increased and is projected to increase, the number of people from birth to 14 years has declined and is projected to decline from 1950 to 2050. Clearly, these are rapid and significant demographic changes that require attention from the developmental community and prompted the National Institute on Aging to state:

Table 15.1 Number (in millions) and distribution of person 60 years or over by region, 2015 and 2030 (rounded to nearest whole number)

Region	60 years or older – 2015	60 years or older – 2030	% change from 2015 to 2030	% of older persons in world – 2015	% of older persons in world – 2030
World	901	1402	56	100	100
Africa	64	105	64	7	8
Asia	508	845	66	56	60
Europe	177	217	23	20	16
North America	75	105	41	8	8
Latin America/Caribbean	71	121	71	8	9
Oceania	7	10	47	1	1

Source: Adapted from World Population Aging, United Nations Department of Economic and Social Affairs (2015).

> [U]nprecedented changes are occurring worldwide as fertility and mortality rates decline in most countries and as populations age. These changes affect individuals, families, governments, and private-sector organizations as they seek to answer questions related to health care, housing, social security, work and retirement, caregiving, and the burden of disease and disability.
>
> (U.S. Department of Health and Human Services, 2017)

By 2030, the number of Americans over 65 years of age will have doubled since the year 2000. The number of Americans over 85 will increase by nearly a million during the decade from 2010 to 2020, so that by 2020 nearly one in five Americans will be over the age of 85. That age group, people 85 years of age and older, are the fastest-growing segment of the population in many countries (USDHHS, National Institute on Aging, 2011).

Worldwide, the number of people over 80 years of age will increase from 14 percent in 2015 to 21 percent in 2050. Those over 60 years of age will increase in number by 56 percent from 2015 to 2030. The number of children from birth to 9 years of age will be exceeded by the number of people over 60 years old by 2030 and one in six people will be over the age of 60 years. Meanwhile, the number of very old, people over the age of 80, is also increasing quickly, especially in developing regions where the rate of increase exceeds that of developed regions. By the year 2050, many regions of the world (i.e., Europe, Latin America and the Caribbean, North America, Oceania) will have a life expectancy of nearly 80 years of age. Throughout the world, women continue to live longer than men with 54 percent of the people over 60 years of age being women. That number increases to 61 percent for those over the age of 80 years (United Nations Department of Economic and Social Affairs, 2015). This dramatic shift in the world's population has occurred, of course, for a number of reasons. Although infectious disease was a major threat early in the last century, major advances have dramatically reduced the incidence of these maladies. The more common causes of death today in the United States are noncommunicable, chronic diseases such as heart disease, diabetes, and cancer. These diseases are often considered "lifestyle" diseases as they are related to unhealthy life choices (e.g., smoking, stress, poor eating habits, physical inactivity).

Table 15.2 Percentages of the world's population by age (in years rounded to the nearest percentage, except for 90+, 2010–2050

Year	0–14	15–24	25–49	50	60+	70+	80+	90+
1950	34	18	32	16	8	3		
1970	38	18	29	16	8	3		
1990	33	19	32	17	9	4	1	0.1
2010	27	18	35	21	11	5	2	0.2
2030	24	15	34	27	16	8	2	0.4
2050	21	14	32	33	21	11	4	0.8

Source: United Nations, Population Division, World population prospects – 2017. population.un.org/wpp/.

Worldwide, the death rates for all chronic diseases rise with increasing age, from approximately 7 million deaths among older adults aged 60 to 69 to 20 million for those 70 and over (World Health Organization, 2005). Another condition whose prevalence increases with age is **frailty**. Approximately 7 percent of people between the ages of 65 and 74 are frail, and that number increases to 18 percent for those aged 75 to 84 and 37 percent for those over 85 years old. Frailty is a "complex health state of increased vulnerability to stressors due to impairments in multiple systems" (Bherer, Erickson, & Liu-Ambrose, 2013, p. 4). Frailty is characterized by increased disability, more falls, more frequent and longer hospitalizations, and an earlier death.

Reducing the incidence of the conditions just described is important to reducing healthcare costs and the human tragedy of the deaths and disabilities these conditions cause. Clearly, the better job we do in keeping our population healthy, active, independent, and socially engaged, the lower our healthcare costs will be and the less misfortune and heartbreak our families will experience. Fortunately, as suggested above, mounting evidence from research shows that well-designed policies and programs can ensure that people live longer and in better health (USDHHS, National Institute on Aging, 2011).

The dramatic increase in the number of older people in the United States and worldwide creates a significant challenge to any number of existing societal infrastructures. More focused attention to this age group should enhance our knowledge of this population, enable the creation of viable programs to assist them in maintaining optimal health and productivity, decrease societal costs, and generally make an important contribution to the health and happiness of all people. The vital and practical application of our knowledge of adulthood will also lead to an improved quality (and perhaps quantity) of life for everyone. Increased knowledge in all areas of development, including motor development, will help us enhance the quality of life for adults of all ages. This chapter addresses issues involving movement in adults. Specifically, we examine balance and postural sway, walking patterns in adulthood, falls and how to avoid them, driving, activities of daily living, movement speed, and maintaining movement ability with increasing age.

BALANCE AND POSTURAL SWAY

One of the most thoroughly investigated characteristics of aging is balance. **Balance**—the ability to control the body's position in space for the purpose of maintaining a static

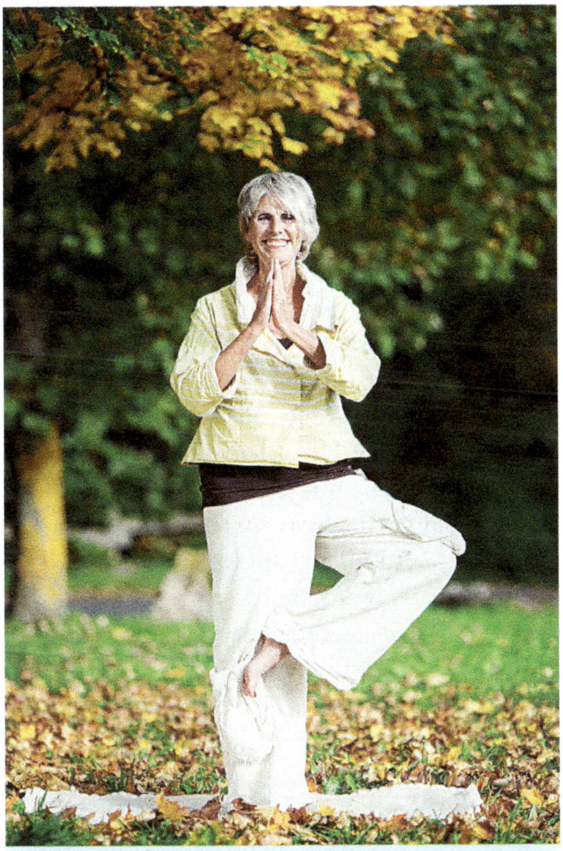

Figure 15.1 Balance in older adulthood is essential for daily function, as well as for most recreational activities

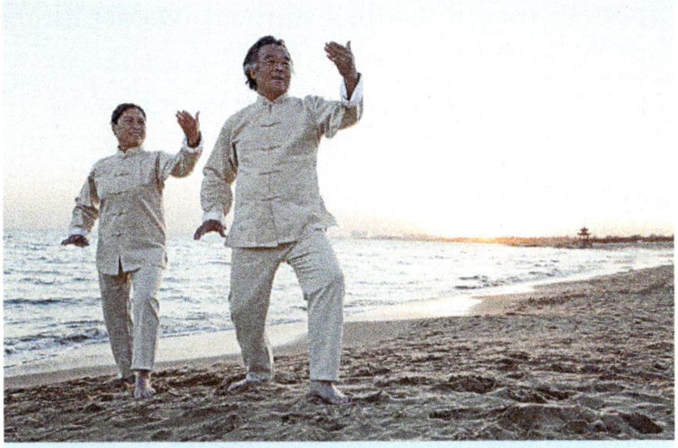

Figure 15.2 Balance is one of our most important daily life skills. Although seemingly simple, it involves a complex integration and synthesis of incoming information, knowledge of our own body's parts in space, and awareness of the surrounding environment.

position or engaging in a dynamic action such as walking—is an important daily-life skill (Figure 15.1). So many goal-directed life and daily tasks require an upright stance, yet standing upright on two feet is an inherently unstable position that is further complicated by the human body's rather high center of body mass. The integrity of one's balance is directly related to risk of falling and is imperative for conducting activities of daily living and maintenance of independent living.

Related Terminology

Static balance occurs when the base of support remains constant and only the center of body mass moves. **Dynamic balance**, in contrast, occurs when the supporting surface and the center of body mass move, as in running (Granacher, Muehlbauer, & Gruber, 2012). A complex process, balance involves the synthesis of incoming sensory information with awareness of the position of the body's parts in space and of the surrounding environment (Figure 15.2). As that information is synthesized, an appropriate movement response is created to control the body's positioning.

Balance is dependent upon, at least, three physiological systems: our senses, our movement ability, and the central processing in our nervous system, which integrates incoming senses and sends the command for the appropriate movement response. Should any one of these systems be impaired, balance can decline. These types of declines are experienced as a result of disease or pathology, or as a part of the typical process of aging. Such a decline is common in old age where as many as 20–50 percent of older adults experience balance issues. Balance is challenged when one's center of mass does not align appropriately with the base of support. Thus, with so much of one's body mass and height residing above a very narrow base of support, human balance has great potential to lose stability. This is further complicated by a large number of destabilizing forces that one typically encounters throughout the day. Loss of balance, and failure to regain it, often result in a fall, a serious consideration for older adults. Thus, we will discuss fall in more detail later in the chapter (Nnodim & Yung, 2015).

Postural sway is a balance-related phenomenon characterized by a nearly imperceptible back-and-forth motion that assists the body in maintaining an upright or standing position. Although one may think of vision as being the most important sense for balance, studies have shown that proprioception is more important than vision for maintaining balance. Postural sway is gradually refined across childhood and adolescence until it becomes well established, fairly early in adulthood (Haddad, Rietdyk, Claxton, & Huber, 2013). The amount of postural sway generally increases linearly once an individual enters adulthood, as deterioration of the postural control mechanisms starts surprisingly early. Declines have been noted as early as 30 years of age in many adults. By 60 years of age, these declines have often become pronounced, resulting in greater amounts of postural sway. Older adults generate more muscle activity, more hip movement, and more overall joint activity than younger adults in their efforts to reduce postural sway. Thus, as aging adults find this muscle and joint activity more and more difficult to maintain, postural sway increases even more.

Balance and Aging

To investigate the effect of increasing task difficulty on balancing, some studies have required participants to perform a second task, or even multiple tasks, while balancing. This requires greater attentional demands as the additional tasks are potential distractors from the requirements of maintaining reduced postural sway. In these studies older adults, when asked to multitask, have exhibited even greater overall displacement than usual, and researchers have concluded that there is an age-related deterioration of the system of postural control. This includes declines in the ability to allocate attention optimally between the postural control requirements and competing tasks. In short, postural sway increases with age, especially in later adulthood and particularly in multi-task situations. To offset these declines, older adults compensate by increasing muscle activity and attempting to make more adjustments at the hip (Granacher et al., 2012).

To investigate further the characteristics of balance performance with age, researchers administered four balance tasks to a large sample of healthy 50- to 64- and 65- to 75-year-old participants (Aslan, Cavlak, Yagci, & Akdag, 2008). The balance tasks included a forward reach that required participants to stand with their feet together and reach forward as far as they could without losing balance. The second, a TUG (Timed Up and Go) test, was a timed test that measured how quickly the subjects could stand from a chair, walk 10 ft (3 m), return, and sit back down. The third, a chair rise, involved standing from a seated position in a chair five times, fully straightening the legs each time. The last test was a timed step in which participants stepped up on a 4-in (10 cm) step five times. Aging was determined to be a clear indicator of balance performance, with the participants exhibiting yearly decreases. At all ages, the males showed significantly more balance than the females. The researchers believed this partially explains the higher incidence of falls among older women compared to older men. Among the younger participants in this study, just under 10 percent had fallen at least once in the last year, while slightly over 25 percent of the older participants had fallen. Those who had fallen performed significantly more poorly on the forward reach test, but no other differences were noted between those who had fallen and those who had not.

These findings were somewhat similar to those generated by a group of French researchers who sought to determine the clinical and biological indicators of balance in older adults (Manckoundia, Buatois, Gueguen, et al., 2008). In an examination of approximately 2,400 participants over the age of 60 years, the researchers performed a number of clinical and balance-related tests. These included blood pressure, body weight, body mass index (BMI), a general health assessment, and a measure of cognitive ability. To demonstrate balance, the participants stood on one leg for a time, rose from a lying position on the floor as quickly as they could, and completed two of the same tasks that were measured in the study by Aslan and colleagues: the TUG test and the chair rise. Consistent with Aslan and colleagues' results, the women were nearly twice as likely to fail on these measures as the men. Being overweight, having low cognitive ability, having a low self-perception of health, and the use of psychotropic drugs were all found to contribute to poor performance on these tasks. The researchers speculated that the declines with age could be related to a decrease in sensory perception, an increase in physical impairments, and poorer vision and vestibular ability. The performance by the female participants was not surprising, as it is consistent with women's increased incidence of falls later in life. The authors posited that the women's poor performance could have resulted from their lack of muscular strength or biomechanical factors related to body weight distribution. Although BMI was directly related to poor performance in both males and females, females' performance declined more significantly than men's with moderate increases in BMI. The researchers believed that a better understanding of these characteristics will aid in diagnosing individuals who may be susceptible to balance problems. This will enable earlier intervention to reduce the likelihood of falls later in life.

Other researchers have examined the effects of various methods to enhance balance or, in some cases, specifically to reduce an individual's deficit in postural control. This is of obvious importance as it relates closely to fall prevention. Granacher, Muehlbauer, Zahner, and colleagues (2011) systematically reviewed the research comparing traditional and more contemporary approaches designed to promote balance and strength. Strength has been shown to be an important underlying correlate to the maintenance of balance across adulthood. According to these researchers, the declines typically seen in postural control with age are a function of a number of factors, which include a decrease in the number and size of muscle fibers and a subsequent reduction in muscle strength and power production, as well as an increasing number of cognitive, visual, vestibular, and proprioceptive impairments.

Granacher and colleagues (2011) also indicated that though balance and strength are closely related, they are independent factors that deserve independent attention and training. Specific research on this topic supports this contention as a combination of balance and strength exercises has been shown to be highly effective in reducing balance deficits while increasing strength. Both balance and strength training, therefore, are important means for fall prevention. Researchers have studied a variety of balance- and strength-related training regimens over the last several decades. Most have been shown to be administratively feasible, safe, and effective in providing benefits for balance, strength, and fall reduction in older adults (Granacher et al., 2011).

WALKING PATTERNS IN ADULTHOOD

As we saw with balance, gait, or walking, patterns change across adulthood (see Figure 15.3), and these changes may be related to declines in balance. Gait changes are relatively

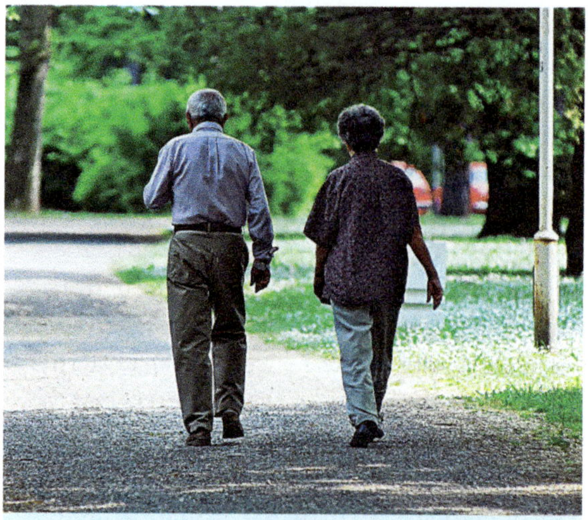

Figure 15.3 Younger and older adult walkers often exhibit different walking characteristics, with older walkers showing less power in the push-off, less hip extension, more variable stride length, and greater hesitancy in walking

subtle across most of adulthood, but they can be pervasive in older adulthood, to the extent that they significantly affect all aspects of an individual's life—physical, psychological, emotional, and social. Declines in qualities of **gait** are most common in individuals who are physically inactive or obese, have reduced strength and balance, or suffer from chronic illness such as diabetes or severe arthritis (Brown & Flood, 2013). Gait speed is of sufficient interest and significance that it has been proposed as a "vital sign" in geriatric assessment, along with blood pressure, respiration, temperature, and pulse (Kuys, Peel, Klein, et al., 2014). A review of the research on gait speed and survival found that gait speed was associated with survival in all studies (Studenski, Perera, Patel, et al., 2011). Thus, it may be a strong indicator of overall health and functional capabilities and, therefore, an important tool in assessing survival potential. This is because gait is a function of many interacting physiological systems, and reduced gait velocity provides an indicator of damage or decline to any one of them. Additionally, slowing gait may initiate a cycle of deconditioning and further, more serious and rapid decline (Studenski et al., 2011).

Gait Changes and Aging

One of the best overall summaries of gait changes with age was provided by Brach and VanSwearingen (2013). They indicated that the characteristics that contribute to "walking problems" (p. 230) with age include:

- forward-flexing trunk posture
- reduced hip extension
- reduced plantar flexion
- reduced power at push-off
- less fluid movement/timing, reducing forward momentum
- more variable stride length and timing
- more hesitancy and greater tendency toward arrhythmic stride.

Brach and VanSwearingen believe that the appearance of any one of these characteristics often interacts with, even contributes to, the occurrence of others. For example, reductions in hip extension decrease the potential energy of the legs, reducing forward momentum and slowing the overall speed of the gait. As we will discuss later, programs to improve gait patterns among older walkers have traditionally focused on improving strength, flexibility, and endurance and can improve underlying impairments, as well as resultant walking characteristics.

In research completed as a part of the Baltimore Longitudinal Study on Aging, Ko and colleagues studied nearly four hundred generally healthy adults ranging in age from 60 to 94 years of age. Their purpose was to determine the relationship between dual task and usual gait patterns in these older adults. Dual task walking is walking while involved in a secondary activity that could potentially take one's attention away from the act of walking. Dual task walking has been associated with progressive declines with age and is considered to be a valuable tool to determine the rate of deterioration in one's walking ability. Thus, it may also be effective in monitoring gait changes while assisting in creating interventions to allay the declines that are common with advancing age.

In this study, participants were asked to walk a 10-meter narrow walkway at their preferred speed. For the dual task activity, they were asked to walk the same runway while reciting the days of the week in reverse order. Participants were considered to have failed the task if they veered off the course while reciting. Those stepping ouside the narrow boundary while walking were considered "failed single motor" and those who passed that test, but ceased or stepped outside the boundary while reciting were considered "failed cognitive." Most participants succeeded on both tests, however, over 20 percent failed on the motor task while just over 10 percent failed on the dual task cognitive test. Participants who were most successful tended to be younger and heavier. Those who failed on the single motor task were slower walkers with a shorter stride, faster cadence, and decreased range of motion at the knee and ankle joints. Those who failed the dual task walking with the cognitive component were found to have a longer double support phase (when both feet are in contact with the floor at the same time). In general, the dual task activity was believed to have created a substantial challenge for many of these older walkers which may be indicative of the increasing attention needed when walking, among older individuals (Ko et al., 2018).

Another study from the Baltimore Longitudinal Study on Aging focused on the specific characteristics associated with the decline in walking speed among older adults. According to the authors, knowing these characteristics and understanding the basic mechanism of slower walking with increasing age can help in the creation of interventions to offset such declines. In this research the 60- to 80-year old participants were tested with follow-up testing done on average within three years. Testing was done in a gait laboratory where characteristics like stride length and width, walking speed, lateral motion, time spent in double support phase, and cadence were determined. Within this sample, nearly one in four participants experienced a notable decline in walking speed at their three-year follow-up. Those with a longer stride and faster cadence were less likely to experience this decline regardless of age. Thus, stride length and cadence, more than the age of the participant, were more closely associated with walking speed declines. These researchers also noted that slower walking had previously been associated with more falls, greater likelihood of being hospitalized, greater chance of intellectual decline, and survival rates at five and ten years from time of testing. Thus, walking speed could be a vital measure for older adults in the medical setting (Jerome et al., 2015).

Boyer, Andriacchi, and Beaupre (2012) studied very active young adult (18–40 years), middle adult (50–64 years), and older adult (65–80 years) walkers. Their purpose was to examine the changes in gait patterns across adulthood to determine if they were as pervasive among a physically active sample of participants. They found that the gait velocity of the older walkers did not vary significantly from that of the other two groups. However, the older walkers achieved their speed by reducing their stride length and increasing their stride speed. Older and middle adult walkers were also found to have a more flat-footed walking style compared to younger walkers as the heel strike was more plantar flexed (i.e., toe-down) upon heel contact. Upon toeing off, the older adults demonstrated less plantar flexion than the younger adults, indicating less range of motion at the ankle joint. The most significant change across the ages was seen in the degree of hip extension, with approximately 20 percent less hip extension demonstrated by the two older groups. The decrease in hip extension has been cited as an important contributor to decreases in walking velocity and increases in falls with age. There was also a progressive decrease in the force of the push-off with age; older groups generated significantly less force than their younger counterparts. In general, these researchers hypothesized that the magnitude of change among these active participants was small compared to what would have been observed in less physically active persons. While it is certainly possible for older adults to maintain a velocity comparable to that of their younger counterparts, changes in gait pattern are still seen, indicating that walking activity may attenuate but not eliminate the effects of aging on movements like walking (Boyer et al., 2012).

In an examination of gait and physical activity, Van Emmerik, Jones, Busa, and Baird (2013) reiterated that gait speed generally declines with age. The decrease in speed is frequently associated with shorter strides and increased time in the double support phase. A shortened stride length is associated with reduced motion of the pelvis and decreased plantar flexion when pushing off. Compared to young adults, healthy older adults also tend to generate less acceleration during push-off and are delayed in shifting their weight to the advancing forward leg. These may be subtle, even subconscious compensating movements to ensure stability during walking. Despite these changes in gait, Van Emmerik and his team maintain that an active life-style is integral to maintaining a healthy gait as people age. Physical activity has been shown to reduce the likelihood, or delay the onset, of gait-related disabilities and to slow the declines in gait patterns. In some cases the effects of physical activity have restored function and even enhanced mobility and the independence that comes with maintenance of a healthy walking pattern.

FALLS

Falling can be a serious problem, especially for older adults. Annually in the United States, more than 30 percent of people over 65 years of age experience a fall, and people over the age of 85 years are more than four times as likely to fall as people 65 to 74 years of age. Falling has become the leading cause of injury among those over 65 and the leading cause of death resulting from injury, with the risk of serious harm from falling increasing with age. In a systematic review and meta-analysis on walking patterns, researchers found that fear of falling was significantly related to a cautious gait. The cautious gait was characterized by increased variability, which the researchers determined by measuring the rhythm of the gait (the time required for each stride; Ayoubi, Launay, Annweiler, & Beauchet, 2015). Table 15.3 lists a number of important facts regarding falls, their incidence and severity. Fortunately, a number of

Table 15.3 Facts and figures about falls and falling from the Centers for Disease Control (2017)

Twenty-five percent of people over 65 years fall each year
Even one fall doubles the chance of falling again
800,000 patients per year are hospitalized because of falling (usually a hip or head injury)
Nearly a third of a million people are hospitalized annually for hip fractures
Ninety-five percent of hip fractures are fall induced
Falls are the biggest cause of traumatic brain injuries
Falls lead to fear of falling, reduced activity, reduced strength, and more falls

precautionary measures can reduce the incidence of falling, thus protecting an individual's mobility and ability to maintain independent living (Centers for Disease Control, 2017). Those measures will be discussed later in the chapter.

Causes of Falls

Table 15.4 lists some of the many factors that contribute to the increased incidence of falls among people over 65. The causes of falls are clustered into two general categories: **intrinsic** and **extrinsic causes.** Intrinsic causes are directly related to the inherent physiology or cognitive ability of the individual. Extrinsic causes are linked to the environmental situation surrounding the fall (Ambrose, Paul, & Hausdorff, 2013).

Intrinsic Causes

An intrinsic cause of falling that has become increasingly significant over the last few decades is obesity. Nearly 35 percent of older adults in the United States are obese, and the number of older adults who are obese is expected nearly to double over the next 40 years. An individual's degree of obesity appears to be directly related to his or her difficulty in walking and, therefore, his or her potential for falling. Though difficulty walking is rarely considered as serious or life-threatening as many chronic diseases (e.g., cancer, diabetes), it is directly related to a person's mortality (Himes & Reynolds, 2012).

In addition, the relative risk of a fall from slipping is nearly four times greater for people who are obese than for those who are not,

Table 15.4 Contributors to falls among older adults

Intrinsic causes		Extrinsic causes
Balance problems		Alcohol use
Declining flexibility		Improper clothing or attire
Disease		Darkness
Cardiovascular	Arthritis	Environmental obstacles
Parkinson's	Maladies of the feet	Irregular walking surfaces
Dementia	Hypothyroidism	Slippery surfaces
Cerebral vascular	Osteoporosis	Uneven stairs
Dizziness		Cracked sidewalks
Fainting		Medication
Fatigue		Rushing
Reduced joint mobility		
Declining strength and endurance		
Increased (i.e., slower) reaction time		
Visual impairment		
General difficulty in walking (e.g., reduced step height)		
Obesity		

when exposed to the same magnitude of postural disturbance. A number of factors may be at work here. For example, avoiding a fall often requires a rapid postural compensation or a compensatory step to regain balance. This may be more challenging for people who are obese simply because the mechanics of their condition interfere with the quick movement needed to compensate successfully. Also, given that obesity is often associated with reduced muscular strength and power, adults who are obese and older may be unable to generate sufficient strength and power to compensate successfully during a fall. Thus, fall prevention interventions should focus on increasing lower body strength (Madigan, Rosenblatt, & Grabiner, 2014) in addition to decreasing adiposity.

Extrinsic Causes

Conditions in the environment can also contribute to an increased incidence of falls. Examples of extrinsic causes include chairs or toilets that are too low, an absence of handrails, uneven step heights, slippery surfaces, and inappropriate footwear. Loose rugs and poor lighting can also be problematic, especially for older people with vision impairments or reduced capacity to perceive contrast. Home intervention strategies have been shown to be effective in reducing the incidence of falls, though they are only one approach of the many needed to overcome a problem that is becoming more pervasive (Ambrose et al., 2013).

Another prominent extrinsic cause of falls is the use of medications, especially those that impair balance. For example, psychotropic medications, which are often used for depression, can cause such side effects as drowsiness and confusion. Such medications may nearly double older adults' chance of falling (Ambrose et al., 2013). Compounding the problem, these individuals may be overmedicated, a condition referred to as **polypharmacy**. This can result in a negative interaction among drugs, which in turn can cause dizziness or difficulty in balance. Kelly, Pickett, Yiannakoulias, and associates (2003) examined the relationship between falls causing injury (requiring emergency room treatment) and the use of medication. Participants were adults 66 years of age and older living in a community of older adults. The researchers used local hospital databases to determine fall incidence and linked that information with medication use for 30 days prior to the fall. They found the fall rate to be 31.6 per 1,000 persons per year. The researchers determined that the use of certain types of medications (e.g., narcotic painkillers, antidepressants, anticonvulsants) was related to the chance of suffering an injurious fall.

Similar research was conducted on Brazilian women 60 years of age and older. All of the subjects were living in a regular community setting, and all completed a questionnaire regarding their history of falls over the previous 12 months and any medications they had taken. The participants were clustered into those who had no falls, those who had fallen one or more times, and those who had fallen two or more times. Of the 634 women who participated, 23.3 percent reported one fall in the previous year. Slightly less, 14 percent, reported two or more falls. Less than 10 percent of the women had taken no medications during the year. Over 50 percent had been taking between 1 and 4 medications, over 34 percent had been taking 5 to 10 medications, and slightly less than 4 percent had been taking 11 medications or more. Those taking medications were more likely to have fallen. Specifically, the women taking diuretics were found to be 1.6 times as likely to have fallen as those taking no medication. Similarly, those taking beta blockers were twice as likely to have fallen as those who were not using these medications (Rozenfeld, Camacho, & Veras, 2003).

Consequences of Falling

Unfortunately, many older adults who fall never regain functional walking, and the potential for serious injury from falling increases as individuals age. Furthermore, just under 90 percent of deaths from falling occur among people over the age of 75 years. Men are nearly 50 percent more likely to die from a fall than women, though women are nearly 70 percent more likely than men to fall nonfatally and are more likely to incur a fracture from their fall (Centers for Disease Control, 2016). A fifth of the older adults who fall suffer injuries such as hip fracture or head trauma, with falls being the most common cause of broken bones for this age group.

One of the most feared consequences of falling is a fractured hip. More than 90 percent of hip fractures in older adults are caused by falls. Estimates suggest that as many as half a million hip fractures per year will occur by the year 2040. Tragically, 20 percent of hip fracture victims will die within a year of the fracture. For those who survive and who had been living alone prior to the injury, nearly 25 percent will require dependent care, in addition to continued medical care and physical therapy, for a minimum of a year during their recuperation. Over 75 percent of patients with hip fractures are women, and for both men and women the incidence of this injury increases exponentially with age, with those over 85 years of age experiencing 10 to 15 times more fractures than those who are 60 to 65 years old.

Because falls can be so serious, a fall quadruples the likelihood of a person over the age of 75 years seeking long-term care in a rehabilitation or assisted living facility. Falling can diminish the individual's self-efficacy and confidence, leading to a reduction in overall activity level that can further diminish the person's fitness level, overall mobility, and ability to maintain independence. Fear of falling can also lead to avoidance of physical activity. In other words, a negative cycle—the exercise-aging cycle discussed in Chapter 3—ensues. With reduced activity, physiological parameters begin to decline. This initiates a downward cycle of further decreases in activity, increases in disease, and eventually death.

Kumar and associates (2016) indicate that fear of falling is strongly related to self-efficacy (i.e., one's belief in own abilities), balance confidence, and general concern about falling. Just over 30 percent of older people who have not fallen, according to these authors, report a fear of falling. Among those who have fallen, that number increases to well over 60 percent. These numbers are significant as this kind of fear can lead to reduced physical activity, fewer social interactions, and an overall reduction in life quality. It also increases the liklihood that one may fall again. In previous research a number of interventions were found to be effective in reducing this type of fear. Those interventions that were multi-pronged (e.g., included both physical activity and behavioral approaches) were most successful. They included behavioral activities to reduce negative perceptions about falls and activities to eliminate avoidance behaviors in addition to physical activities specifically designed to reduce falling (e.g., balance and strength training). To examine this phenomenon more precisely, Kumar's research team conducted a systematic review and meta-analysis on this topic. This included over thirty studies from several countries including the United States and Australia. Examples of interventions in these studies included programs to enhance balance, strength, flexibility, and gait technique lasting less than 12 weeks to over 26. The meta-analysis indicated that, immediately following the intervention, there was typically an overall small to moderate reduction in fear of falling. Over the longer term, approximately 6 months later, the effect was found to be small and not statistically significant. These findings led the researchers to conclude that these kinds of interventions are probably useful to a small degree over the short term. Though these findings were less encouraging, Kumar and associates noted that, based on previous research, these kinds of interventions, though not as promising in reducing fear, are effective in reducing the number of falls in elderly people (Kumar et al., 2016). Fortunately, as we will see, regular physical activity, careful monitoring of medications, periodic eye exams, and scrutiny of potential fall hazards in the home can dramatically reduce the risk of falling.

Strategies to Avoid Falls

Unquestionably, the number of falls among older adults can be reduced. The Centers for Disease Control cite a number of factors as common causes of falling. These include too little lower body strength, too little Vitamin D, walking and balance issues, various medications including some over-the-counter medications, poor vision and unsuitable footwear, foot pain, broken or uneven stairs, and clutter that can cause trips. Most falls, they say, are caused by more than one factor. Fortunately, the risk of falling can be reduced a number of ways. Table 15.5 indicates a number of these recommendations from the Centers for Disease Control (2017).

Table 15.5 Centers for Disease Control's precautions to avoid falling

• Be medically evaluated; see a doctor
• Review your medications
• Do strength and balance exercises
• Have your eyes checked
• Make your home safer:
• Keep it well lit
• Install grab bars near toilets, showers, and baths
• Eliminate sources of trips (e.g., extension cords, rumpled rugs, clutter)
• Install railings on stairs

Source: Adapted from Centers for Disease Control – Important facts about falls (2017).

Perhaps most importantly, the Centers for Disease Control (2017) recommends regular exercise to enhance or maintain strength and balance. A physical fitness program can offset declines in these areas, as well as enhance such characteristics as balance and reaction time. A more physically fit older adult is less likely to become ill and experience the need for medications that could cause falls. Exercises specifically designed to increase strength, reduce excess body weight, and improve balance can reduce the likelihood of falls.

In a meta-analysis on the effect of fall prevention programs, an exercise program designed to prevent falls was found to be an effective approach to fall reduction (El-Khoury, Cassou, Charles, & Dargent-Molina, 2013). This research statistically summarized the findings of several studies on this topic and determined that fall prevention exercise programs decreased the number of falls experienced by people over the age of 60 years and also reduced the number of injuries sustained from falling. Importantly, the effect was most notable for the most serious injuries, with the estimated reduction in potential falls ranging from 37 percent for generally injurious falls to 43 percent for "severe injury falls," to 61 percent for the most serious category, "falls resulting in fractures" (p. 11). All of the exercise programs found to be effective in fall reduction included some form of balance training. Most of the effective programs, however, involved a number of components, such as muscle strength, endurance, and flexibility training. The researchers posited that these programs reduce falls by improving important related characteristics such as reaction time, general physical condition, and even cognitive function. Faster reactions, the researchers stated, reduce the likelihood of a fall, and increased muscle mass may reduce the impact and therefore, the potential for injury upon falling. According to the research team, these findings should encourage medical professionals to recommend fall prevention programs to their patients and encourage policy-makers to provide funding for such programs.

In a similar systematic review and meta-analysis of studies conducted on fall prevention, Sherrington, Whitney, Lord, and colleagues (2008) sought to determine what kinds of fall prevention programs are available for older people, with special interest in determining which types of exercise programs lead to better outcomes. Citing the fact that a third of all individuals over the age of 65 years experience at least one fall per year, contributing to over half of the hospitalizations related to injuries, these authors called the need for better fall intervention programs an "urgent global health challenge" (p. 2234). Sherrington and colleagues further noted that falls do not occur randomly in this age group, but instead are quite predictable based on the presence of risk factors, such as reductions in muscle strength and balance, gait impediments, reduced visual ability, and intake of certain prescription medications. Exercise-based fall prevention programs have been effective in overcoming some of these risk factors, but questions still exist as to which types of exercise programs are most effective in reducing the number of falls among older adults. Results from this research reconfirmed that exercise programs are effective in reducing fall rates. Specifically, a 17 percent reduction in falls was found in this review of 44 studies examining the efficacy of exercise in fall prevention. Three factors were found to be of particular importance in fall reduction: balance training, the amount of exercise undertaken, and, interestingly, reduced levels of walking. Overall program length was found to be a significant factor, with longer program participation leading to greater fall prevention. These researchers hypothesized that the minimum criterion for an effective fall prevention program would equate to a 25-week-long program that met twice per week (Sherrington et al., 2008).

Perhaps the most interesting finding from this study was that programs that did not include walking as an exercise medium yielded better outcomes related to fall prevention. This result may be attributable to the fact that walking itself increases the risk of falling. A second possible explanation is that an individual's time spent walking replaces time involved in other activities that may be more conducive to reducing falls. Despite this finding, the authors emphasized that walking programs provide valuable overall health benefits (such as weight reduction, blood pressure reduction, and overall improvement in fitness). Nevertheless, if fall prevention is the main objective of the program, this research determined that walking may not be an ideal exercise medium (Sherrington et al., 2008).

In a more recent and specific study on exercises to enhance balance in the eldery, Hamed, Bohm, Mersman, and Arampatzis (2017) compared the effectiveness of various exercise interventions. This research was considered necessary as older individuals generally demonstrate a declining ability to respond to rapidly occurring instability to regain their balance and avoid falling. Thus, falls become more common and are a leading cause of injury and death throughout the world and an economic weight on society. Both age-related declines in the ability to correct and maintain posture and reductions in muscle strength are thought to be contributory factors. Thus, just under fifty participants ranging in age from 63 to 80 years of age were placed in one of three conditions: a muscle-strengthening group, a perturbation group, and a control group. The muscle-strengthening group routinely completed leg and trunk exercises while they completed stability-related exercises on an unstable platform. Both groups trained twice a week for 14 weeks. The third group did no exercises as they were simply for control purposes. Strength, balance, and the ability to recover from instability were tested before and after training. The researchers concluded that both interventions were effective for balance recovery compared to the control group. The muscle-strengthening group and the perturbation group both improved in plantar flexion strength, but only the strengthening group improved in knee extension strength. Nevertheless, only the perturbation group improved significantly in their standing balance ability. Thus, the perturbation group was concluded to be the most effective for dynamic stability in older individuals as it can potentially improve strength, and sensory processing to adjust for rapid and sudden changes in one's base of support. Thus, it could also be effective in reducing the number of falls in the elderly (Hamed et al., 2017).

DRIVING IN OLDER ADULTHOOD

One of the most serious aspects of aging is the decline in driving ability that older adults experience (see Figure 15.4). Although young drivers (under 25 years old) receive more citations, are more likely to have their driving privileges suspended, and are more likely to be involved in an accident than any other age group, the number of serious accidents rises after the age of 75. More fatal crashes are experienced by drivers of this age group than all other age groups. The increase in fatalities is likely attributable in part to the increased frailty among this older age group, in that these individuals may find it difficult to recover from injuries sustained in a crash. Also, driving skills may be reduced among older drivers, for example, they may fixate more on their driving route as opposed to scanning for driving risks. Older drivers have been shown to respond more slowly when a decision must be made, perceive visual contrast more poorly, and have decreased ability to detect road hazards (Yeung & Wong, 2015). In addition, older drivers are particularly more likely to be involved in accidents that involve an intersection turn across opposing traffic, merging into moving traffic, or changing lanes.

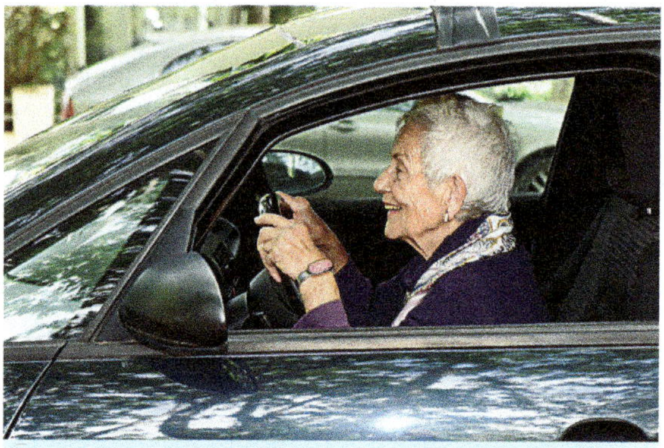

Figure 15.4 The incidence of serious driving accidents increases notably after the age of 75 years. Many factors affect this phenomenon, with some of the most significant being reduced vision, slowing of reaction time, and, for some, reductions in cognitive ability. Many diseases, such as arthritis, can also impair an individual's driving ability.

Nevertheless, enabling older drivers to continue to drive is critical to assuring their continued independence and maintaining the quality of their health and life in general. Therefore, simply depriving older people of driving privileges may not be the simple solution that it seems. A worthy goal would be to enhance the safety of roads and highways while reducing the impact on life quality, safety, and even the financial stability of older drivers. Research by Adriana and colleagues considered this predicament when undertaking their research on executive function and driving ability of older drivers. Driving, they say, is an extremely complicated task that requires visual, intellectual, and movement abilities that may be deleteriously affected with age. These changes may be contributors to increased risk for accidents created by older drivers. Intellectual decline often seen with aging has frequently been cited as a major contributor to decrements in driving safety for older drivers, so these researchers sought to determine the relationship between executive function (group of mental processes for goal-directed activity) and driving performance. Well over a hundred drivers in France, ranging in age from 20 to 82 years of age completed a lengthy on-road driving test in addition to several tests of executive function. One aspect of executive function, inhibition (mentally restraining a behavior or desire), was found to decline with age and driving performance was found to be impaired, in part, by this declining ability. Thus, this research team concluded that declines in inhibition, at any age, would affect driving performance, but that these types of deficiencies are most common with older drivers. Thus, intervention designed to enhance driving among older drivers, especially as it relates to improving inhibition are indicated and may be one way to enable older drivers to continue to drive and drive more safely (Adriana, Moessinger, Charles, & Postal, 2019).

The plight of the older driver is compelling. For example, in the United States alone, there were 35 million drivers in 2011 who were 65 years old or older, making up 16 percent of all American drivers. With our population aging rapidly, that number is expected to increase to 40 million by the year 2020 (National Highway Traffic Safety Adminstration, 2013). As discussed, the simple solution may seem to be prohibiting driving past a certain age, although such a policy would entail a number of sacrifices. For example, public transportation, as well as families and other individuals, would have to assume a greater burden in transporting older adults. In addition, the cessation of driving for older adults has been associated with increases in depression and in feelings of isolation and loneliness, and a decreased overall quality of life (Boot, Stothart, & Charness, 2014). As noted, the loss of driving ability has tremendous implications for an individual's opportunities to be mobile, stay engaged with society, and maintain dignity. Driving offers access to friends, family, jobs, shopping, education, culture, and religion, as well as considerable personal choice. Losing the ability to drive can be considered a major life crisis.

Factors Related to Declines in Driving Ability

Declines in vision, hearing, speed of processing, and the ability to take in relevant environmental information efficiently are all thought to contribute to the incidence of serious accidents among older adults (Boot et al., 2014).

Vision and hearing. Vision, of course, is critical to safe driving. People begin to lose their ability to focus efficiently in their forties as a result of the natural thickening of the lens. This affects the ability to process driving-related information accurately as vision shifts from far to near (e.g., from down the road to the instrument panel). By the age of 65, an individual's eyes may have difficulty adapting to changing light conditions, making night driving particularly challenging, and reductions in depth perception can affect a person's ability to anticipate merging and lane changes. Eye diseases become more common in later adulthood (e.g., macular degeneration, cataracts, glaucoma) and can make driving less comfortable, more difficult, and more dangerous. Similar declines are often exhibited with hearing; these declines are particularly common in men after the age of 60 years. Declines in hearing are especially significant when accompanied by declines in vision (Boot et al., 2014).

Processing and response time. Declines in processing and response speed (discussed in more detail later in the chapter) also contribute to declines in driving ability with age. Older adults may take up to twice as long to process perceptual or cognitive information as younger adults. Thus, related movement responses, such as the application of brakes, can be delayed.

Chronic conditions. This population is also more likely to experience any number of chronic conditions (e.g., heart disease, cancer, diabetes, dementia) whose symptoms, or the medications taken to allay these symptoms, may affect driving. Older adult drivers who have diabetes or dementia are 1.5 and 3 times, respectively, as likely to have an accident that is their fault (Boot et al., 2014).

Physical fitness. A lack of physical fitness has also been associated with an increase in crashes, perhaps because decreased cognitive abilities, attention, and psychomotor speed frequently accompany declining fitness. The increased incidence of accidents may also relate to factors such as decreased neck, shoulder, and trunk flexibility; greater stress; a greater tendency to fatigue; and reduced overall alertness, which are also associated with reduced fitness (Alosco, Penn, Spitznagel, et al., 2015). Research examining the effects of short-term home and community-based fitness programs on older drivers' safety has indicated that increased fitness can stabilize driving performance and reduce driving errors (Golisz, 2014).

Obesity. Obesity has also been studied for its impact on driving as we age. This condition is a particular concern for truck drivers: according to studies, between 40 percent and 50 percent of truck drivers are obese, perhaps as a result of the sedentary nature of the work, its impact on sleep and eating patterns, and drivers' lack of regular exercise. Commonly associated with obesity is obstructive sleep apnea, a condition that is nearly universal among individuals with a BMI of 40 or more. This condition increases the chance of a driving accident by nearly four times, and drivers with sleep apnea routinely perform more poorly on driving simulation tests than control groups without apnea (Kay & McLaughlin, 2014).

Consequences of Age-Related Driving Changes

The typical, though not fixed, series of events that is associated with age-related driving changes is depicted in the **Mobility Consequences Model** (see Figure 15.5). The progression often begins with the older adult experiencing physical and/or mental changes, such as reduced vision or reaction time. These changes lead to a reduction in driving skill, an increase in the number of actual accidents while driving, and, inevitably, reduced driving. Reduced driving, in turn, hampers general mobility, which can dramatically impact the person's quality of life. This process usually takes place over the course of many years, gradually narrowing the person's scope of activities. Though this series of events often occurs, it is not universal, as many drivers do not experience the functional declines described in this section until they reach very advanced ages. Thus, they can continue to drive safely until they are quite old (Burkhart, Berger, Creedon, & McGavock, 1998).

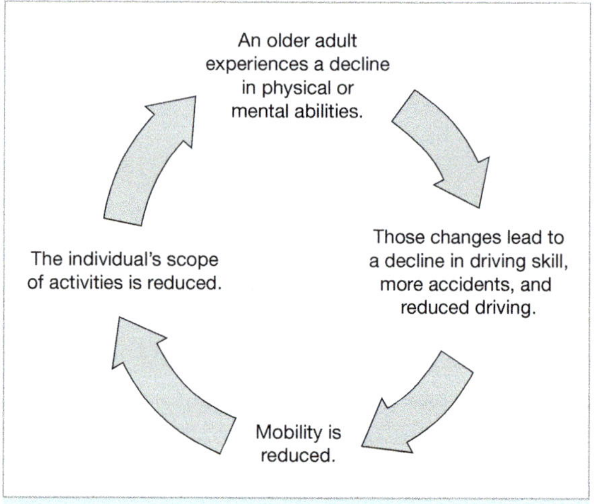

Figure 15.5 The Mobility Consequences Model
Source: Adapted from Burkhart et al. (1998).

Adapting to Age-Related Changes in Driving Ability

Andrews and Westerman (2012) note that one of the ways older adults can adapt to declines in driving skill is through "**strategic compensation**" (p. 661). That is, they can take unique compensatory steps to improve the safety of their driving. For example, they can be more selective as to when and where they drive, and choose driving conditions that are suited to their capabilities. This might include avoiding highspeed routes, rush-hour driving, and night driving. They can also adopt strategies such as driving more slowly, allowing more space between their car and the vehicle in front of them, waiting for bigger gaps between cars when merging into traffic, and not driving when they are rushed or feeling stressed.

For individuals who lose the ability or confidence to drive, alternatives must be made available. The severity of the Mobility Consequences Model is lessened when alternatives exist. Obviously, mass transit can provide some assistance. Some experts have recommended support groups where older drivers who have made a successful transition to no driving assist others and share ideas. Unquestionably, education and counseling are other effective options. Of course, changing societal attitudes and eliminating the stigma of losing the privilege of driving might also help to reduce the impact on older adults. Perhaps the most successful interventions in this area would be those that provide alternative forms of transportation along with efforts to maintain and restore the dignity, independence, and security of older adults who have lost the ability to drive. More research in this area is imperative.

ACTIVITIES OF DAILY LIVING

One of the most serious aspects of aging can be the loss of ability to perform **activities of daily living (ADLs)** or **instrumental activities of daily living (IADLs)**. ADLs are self-care activities that include eating, rising from a chair, getting in and out of bed, brushing teeth, dressing, and bathing (see Figure 15.6). IADLs include activities that are less fundamental for function but necessary to maintain independent living, such as cooking, shopping, doing laundry, walking, taking medications, and handling personal finances. Both ADLs and IADLs are measures of functional status. Inability to perform them successfully indicates that an individual is losing the ability for self-care and independence and represents a significant disability (Dunlop, Song, Arnston, et al., 2015).

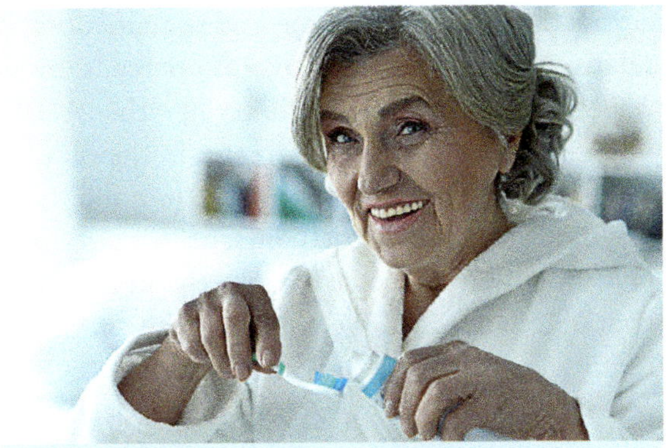

Figure 15.6 Brushing your teeth is an example of an activity of daily living (ADL), a self care activity

Prevalence of Related Disability

A 2011 study sought to determine the percentage of people aged 65 years and older who reported some degree of disability related to ADLs and IADLs. The study also determined how this percentage changed across the decade from 1998 to 2008. The average age of the participants was just over 74 years with slightly over half of the respondents being women. Interestingly, despite purported increases in chronic disease across this same time period, the percentage of persons reporting difficulty with ADLs remained relatively constant at just under 20 percent. The percentage of those reporting IADL disability was slightly higher across this same time frame and remained relatively constant at just over 25 percent. In 2008, the incidence of disability in either ADL or IADL was significantly greater in the oldest age group, the over 85-year-olds, than the 65- to 69-year-old participants, at just over 50 percent and 17 percent respectively. In 2008, overall, 7 percent of the older women surveyed reported greater disability than the men, a statistically significant figure. The researchers concluded that although disability in the older population continues to be substantial, it is not increasing in incidence (Hung, Ross, Boockvar, & Siu, 2011).

Factors Affecting Functionality

Factors associated with an individual's ability to maintain functionality have also been studied. In a large-scale study of more than 4,000 participants over the age of 65 years, the researchers administered a questionnaire and physical fitness test to determine the factors that most strongly related to ADLs. Of the factors studied, experiencing pain generated one of the strongest relationships, though cognitive function, vision and hearing problems, and a high BMI were also strongly related to poorer performance on ADLs (Komatsu, Nezu, Tomioka, et al., 2013).

Sedentary Behavior

A large-scale study, conducted with more than 2,000 subjects 60 years of age and older, focused on the relationship between sedentary behavior and ADLs. One purpose of the study was to explore the relationship between the magnitude of a person's sedentary activity and the person's degree of disability in ADLs. Although a sedentary lifestyle has long been known to be related to increased mortality, evidence indicates that a sedentary lifestyle may be a separate factor from physical activity level in its effects on health (e.g., heart disease, diabetes, mortality in general), obesity level, ADLs, and overall quality of life. In this research, being older, being female, having a lower level of education, and having a lower income were all found to be associated with disability on ADLs (Dunlop et al., 2015).

The likelihood of having an ADL-related disability increased by more than 50 percent for each hour per day of sedentary time. Importantly, this finding appeared to be independent of an individual's involvement in moderate to vigorous activity, indicating that sedentary behavior is a significant and independent risk factor for ADL disability. The risk associated with sedentary behavior, according to the researchers, appeared to be especially significant for people who were over the age of 70 years and for African Americans. This study also found that ADL disability was more strongly related to the negative effects of sedentary behavior than to the positive effects of moderate to vigorous physical activity. Given that an average older adult in the United States spends nearly 70 percent of her or his waking time being sedentary, this is a particularly important finding. Sedentary behavior, therefore, is risky and potentially costly to society, and a strong rationale now exists for developing policy-level strategies for education regarding the perils of sedentary living (Dunlop et al., 2015).

Physical Activity

Physical activity, however, is also clearly a variable that affects an individual's ability to perform ADLs and IADLs. In a systematic review and meta-analysis of the effect of various kinds of physical activity on ADLs, Roberts, Phillips, Cooper, Gray, and Allen (2017) noted that aging is typically associated with deterioration in a number of physiological systems that impact one's ability to perform daily functions. Inability to perform routine activities like grooming, eating, moving from place to place, go grocery shopping, and cleaning one's house certainly reduce the overall quality of living. Thus, strategies to overcome these deficits are warranted. One such strategy is to increase the level of physical activity to enhance strength, endurance, and flexibility and, therefore, functionality. To assess the efficacy of such interventions, this research team systematically analyzed nearly fifty studies involving participants 60 years of age and older and the benefits of physical activity programs on their ability to perform activities of daily living. They performed this research in light of increasing numbers of similar large-scale studies indicating that physical activity does positively affect the ability of an older adult to perform their daily activities in addition to improving strength, balance, movement ability, intellect, and fall reduction. Specific results of this study indicated that the greatest impact on ADL performance came from physical activity programs that employed moderate levels of physical activity in addition to stressing intellectual, physical, and social skill. This led the researchers to conclude that physical activity programs, when appropriately designed, can positively affect performance of ADLs among the elderly population. In addition, this information is valuable in creating and implementing intervention programs for older adults who are, or could be, struggling in their daily functionality (Roberts et al., 2017).

MOVEMENT SPEED IN ADULTHOOD

Although human beings display significant individual differences in the way their movement changes with age, norms have been observed for the speed of various adult movements. As discussed earlier, walking speed generally decreases with age, particularly in late adulthood. The speed of many other kinds of movements, such as running, also appears to be affected.

Physiological Functional Capacity and Speed of Performance

The capacity to undertake the physical tasks of daily life with success and with a given level of ease is known as **physiological functional capacity** (**PFC**; Tanaka & Seals, 2003, p. 2152). PFC typically declines with age throughout adulthood. In extreme cases, declines in PFC can lead to a dramatic drop in functional capacity. This can particularly have an impact on persons in physically demanding occupations and can even result in an inability to perform the activities of daily living. It is difficult to predict when PFC declines will begin, because many factors affect its onset. A few examples of such factors are changing levels of physical activity and their effects on muscular strength, flexibility, cardiovascular endurance, and even body composition; the increased incidence of disease; changing societal expectations; and reduced motivation to perform with age.

One approach that researchers have taken to examining this phenomenon has been to study and compare young and older adult athletes and changes in their performance levels across time. Research in this area has determined that endurance running performance decreases with age, though it is generally well maintained in elite runners through approximately 35 years of age (see Figure 15.7). From 35 to 50 or 60 years of age, additional, modest decreases are noted. Thereafter, running declines become more significant and are influenced by an increase in orthopedic injuries, often associated with running. Researchers in this area have noted that these declines tend to be three times greater in females than in males. The most significant gender differences are seen after 60 years of age. Tanaka and Seals (2003) have speculated that these gender differences may have a strong biological basis, but they are also very likely to be linked to differing societal

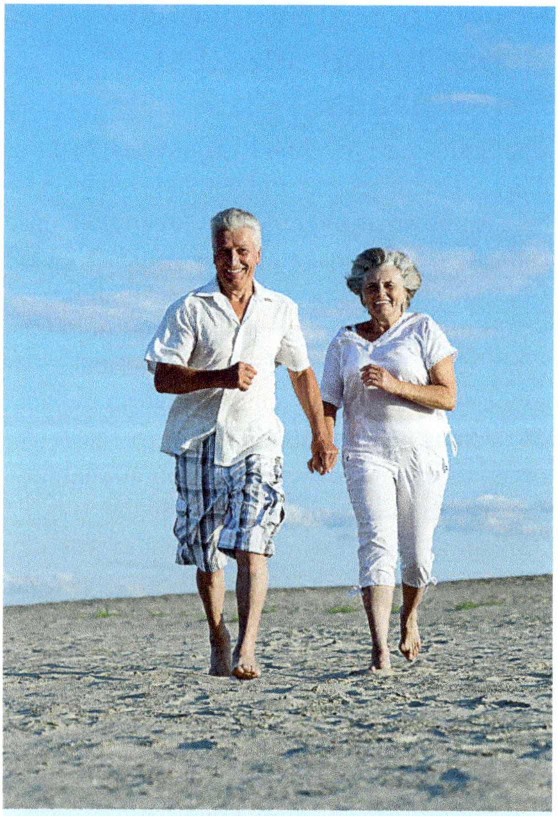

Figure 15.7 Running speed for short distances normally declines considerably with age, but the relative running speed for longer distances is often well preserved

expectations for men and women, especially at advanced ages.

Tanaka and Seals (2003) also examined age-related swimming performance. These authors believe that analyses of swimming performance were more accurate indicators of age-related declines in physiological functional capacity, because swimming is a non-weight-bearing activity. Thus, swimming would be less affected by factors such as the skeletal and orthopedic maladies commonly found in runners. In addition, unlike with running, similar numbers of older men and women swim. This enables researchers examining PFC to accommodate with more accuracy the effects of sociological factors differentially affecting men and women. Tanaka and Seals found that Masters swimmers often achieve their best swimming performances as late as 40 to 50 years of age. Nevertheless, swimming performance generally declines with age in both women and men, with performance declining a third less than in running. In addition, the point at which declines become "exponential" occurs much later in swimming (approximately 70 years of age) versus running (approximately 60 years of age). Clearly, according to Tanaka and Seals, the decline in PFC is age-associated but is also strongly influenced by the task in question. Gender also appeared to influence performance in swimming, as the declines in women occurred faster than in men, especially over shorter distances. Significant gender differences in the rate of decline were not found in the longer-distance events. Tanaka and Seals indicated that this could be attributable to the fact that physiological factors linked to success in sprinting events (such as strength and power) decline faster in women than do the physiological factors linked to endurance events (such as maximal cardiovascular capacity). Interestingly, this relationship between gender, performance, and distance was not found in other sports, such as running, where gender-related declines in women were greater than those in men regardless of distance (Tanaka & Seals, 2003).

The overall acceleration in declines in performance at approximately 60 to 70 years of age was of particular interest to these researchers. Research findings have consistently shown a decline in performance with age—even in research on choice of walking speeds, which slow very little up to the age of 60 and then drop significantly thereafter. A similar pattern has been observed in weight lifting, with consistent declines until 60 years of age and accelerated declines thereafter. Initial interpretations of these phenomena point to dramatic physiological declines that increase at this age. However, "biobehavioral" adaptations may also partially explain the drops. Perhaps older athletes simply decline in their interest in or motivation to engage in physical activity, leading researchers to consider sociocultural factors such as reduced expectations for older athletes—and, therefore, athletes' reduced expectations for themselves—at that time of life. A more complete understanding of these factors is important for developing strategies to improve health, functional capacity, and the ability to maintain independent living among older members of society (Tanaka & Seals, 2003).

Reaction, Response, and Movement Times

Related Terminology

In addition to speed of performance, motor development professionals are also interested in other forms of movement speed. Aging is associated with slower **reaction times**. Two of the most common types of reaction time are simple and choice reaction time. **Simple reaction time** is how quickly we respond to a stimulus. More specifically, it is the elapsed time from the occurrence of some sort of stimulus (e.g., a flashing light or a buzzer) to the initiation of the related response (e.g., pressing a button). **Choice reaction time** is slightly more complex. In choice reaction time, any one of several stimuli may appear, and the response may differ based on which stimulus appears. For example, one of several different-colored lights may appear, and the button to be pushed depends on which colored light appears. This is a very laboratory-based example, but various forms of reaction time are important in daily life. For example, when driving in heavy traffic, one may have to brake or accelerate (make a choice) depending on what one or more other cars do. As an example of simple reaction time, hitting the brakes quickly when driving is an important response to the stimulus of a car suddenly swerving out of control in front of you. Reaction time has been studied extensively, and psychologists often use it as an indicator of the status of the central nervous system and, therefore, of cognitive function.

Reaction time is different from movement time. **Movement** time is the period of time from the beginning of a movement until its completion. The movement could be very short and simple, such as pressing a button, or longer and more complex, such as running a 50-meter sprint or even a complete marathon (Schmidt & Lee, 2014).

Reaction, Response Time, and Aging

The correlation between aging and slowing is high, and the gap in timing between older and younger performers widens as the complexity of the task increases. Choice reaction time, being more complex than simple reaction time, is an example. Verhaegen (2014), in a meta-analysis on age and movement speed, observes that we begin life relatively slowly as children; gradually increase in movement speed across childhood, adolescence, and early adulthood; and then gradually slow thereafter. Hence, processing speed is both age-sensitive (p. 5) and curvilinear. Verhaegen claims that processing time increases by 1.5 milliseconds with each additional year of adulthood. On average, he claims, a 70-year-old exhibits speed that is similar to an 8-year-old's.

Though declines with age are evident in both simple and choice reaction time, researchers have noted that the decline for simple reaction time is less evident than that of choice reaction time. In simple reaction time, only a mild decline in performance has been observed across adulthood, until the age of 50 years. In choice reaction time, the decline is evident across most of adulthood. In an extensive study of nearly 8,000 participants aged 30 through over 80, the participants were stratified to represent the entire population of Finland, where the research was conducted. As expected, the results showed a consistent and statistically significant decline across adulthood in movement times and in the time it took for the subjects to make decisions regarding movements. The declines in performance started early in adulthood and became more prominent with age. Even the 40- to 49-year-olds showed significant degrees of slowing when compared to the 30- to 39-year-olds. The magnitude of slowing was also found to increase after the age of 70. The difference between the young and old participants was 90 percent for simple reaction time and 140 percent for choice reaction time. The time it took to make a decision prior to responding was 40 percent longer in the oldest participants than in their youngest counterparts. This difference increased to 65 percent for choice reaction time. The difference between the youngest and the oldest participants varied depending on the performance measure. Another finding, which has been replicated repeatedly in previous research, is that movement times were shorter for men than women across all age groups (Era, Sainio, Koskinen, et al., 2011).

The results of this research are typical of other studies conducted over the years and would be expected for almost all forms of movement. One particularly important finding of this research was that some of the older adults generated results similar to those of much younger people. Somehow, these people appeared to have overcome the decline in speed generally seen. The researchers theorized that the physical activity level of these individuals may have offset the slowing, or they may have been extremely fast as younger adults, making their declines less evident (Era et al., 2011).

In another large-scale study, this one examining the effects of age and education on reaction time, Tun and Lachman (2008) examined more than 3,600 participants ranging in age from 32 to 85 years of age. Participants were tested following a brief hearing assessment and an interview. All tests were conducted over the telephone and were shown to be satisfactorily reliable compared to face-to-face testing of reaction time. As in most previous investigations of this kind, reaction times were found to slow as the complexity of the task increased. More complicated tasks were also found to have a greater negative effect on the reaction time of older participants. Interestingly, education level was found to have a positive effect on performance, especially for the more complex tasks. Participants with more education performed as well as those with less education who were up to 10 years younger. To some extent these findings parallel research that indicates that education level has a positive effect on intellectual function with age and reduces the risk of dementia in old age. However, this effect did not hold for the 75- to 85-year-old participants, the oldest age group in this research. For these older adults, the authors posited that "biological declines predominate" (p. 1421).

The phenomenon in which people maintain speed for relatively simple movements longer than for more complex movements has been partially explained by the **last-in-first-out hypothesis**. This hypothesis suggests that the neural and muscular capability to perform simple movement acts, such as reflexive movements or other integrated movements, is developed early in life and is relatively resistant to decline with aging. However, more coordinated, goal-oriented, or complicated movements are developed later in life and begin to decline in people as young as 30 (Spirduso, Francis, & MacRae, 2005).

Though slowing is a common and expected age-related phenomenon, exceptions exist. One is **saccadic movements**, the micro-adjustments that the eyes make in order to work together as they scan a line of words on a written page or sweep across a horizontal or vertical landscape. These movements are believed to be the fastest produced by the human body, and they can be produced both voluntarily and reflexively. Pratt,

Dodd, and Welsh (2006) examined saccadic movements in younger and older adults with average ages of approximately 19 and 66 years, respectively. Generally these researchers determined that the saccadic system appears to be relatively "impervious" (p. 373) to the kinds of slowing seen in other human movements in adulthood. Even among generally sedentary individuals, very high levels of saccadic movement are continually produced. The systems that produce saccadic movement may simply maintain a higher level of fitness compared with those muscular systems that show greater rates of decline with age.

As evidenced by saccadic movements, the continued use of various bodily systems may prevent or reduce declines that people may otherwise experience. Bherer and colleagues (2013) examined this very issue as it relates to the effects of physical activity and exercise on various brain functions and cognition. In psychology, as mentioned earlier, reaction time is often employed as a measure of central nervous system integrity and, therefore, cognitive function. This relationship strengthens as the complexity of the speed task increases. According to Bherer and associates, lifestyle factors affect the rate of slowing in reaction time. To offset reductions in speed, they recommend maintaining strong social ties, seeking intellectually stimulating leisure activities, and, most important, maintaining a physically active lifestyle. As we know, physical activity is strongly linked to reduced incidence of chronic diseases and even provides some degree of protection from dementia.

The typical reduction in the speed of mental processing is associated with anatomical changes in the brain. Specifically, researchers have observed a loss of the brain's white matter in most aging adults. The overall volume of the brain also decreases. This is especially notable after the age of 50 years, when decreases of 0.35 percent per year have been observed. For younger adults, the annual loss is approximately one-third of this rate. Reductions in size are seen in specific brain structures, including the hippocampus, which is believed to be instrumental in memory. Physical activity, however, has been shown to offset many of these declines to some extent. Cognitive function, for example, is strongly related to an individual's level of cardiorespiratory fitness: studies have shown that people who are active demonstrate less decline, especially those who are vigorously active. In fact, some studies have demonstrated that physical activity (e.g., aerobic exercise) often generates improved cognition. Studies have also found that other forms of exercise, such as resistance and balance training, can improve cognition in certain areas. Clearly, cardiorespiratory and resistance training should be strong considerations for any adult who seeks to maintain and possibly even improve cognition with increasing age (Bherer et al., 2013).

To add specific support to this conclusion, Renaud, Maquestiaux, and Joncas (2010) studied the effects of a 3-month aerobic training program on reaction time performance. These researchers provided further support for the idea that aging generally leads to cognitive declines. Cognitive declines affect an individual's level of control over attention, which affects the ability to prepare for optimal performance on response speed tasks. Not surprisingly, like cognition in general, attentional control can decline with age. To study the effects of enhanced physical activity on reaction time measures, thought to be indicators of attentional control and preparation, these researchers examined a group of 60- to 80-year-old sedentary persons. Some served as the treatment group and exercised for an hour, 3 times per week for 3 months, and others served as the control group and did not exercise. Sedentary, in this study, was defined as exercising fewer than two times per week. In the end, the treatment group improved in cardiorespiratory fitness by 25 percent on a Rockport 1-mile (1.6 km) test and demonstrated improvement on the reaction time tasks, especially on the choice reaction time tasks. These researchers concluded that enhanced cardiorespiratory fitness positively affected the brain, especially those areas most closely associated with attention, preparation, and speed of response. In addition, they concluded that this type of exercise would yield greater improvement in more complex tasks (e.g., choice versus simple reaction time). Given the low relative cost and the general accessibility of exercise programs for most older adults, these programs are a viable means of intervention to reduce certain common declines with age.

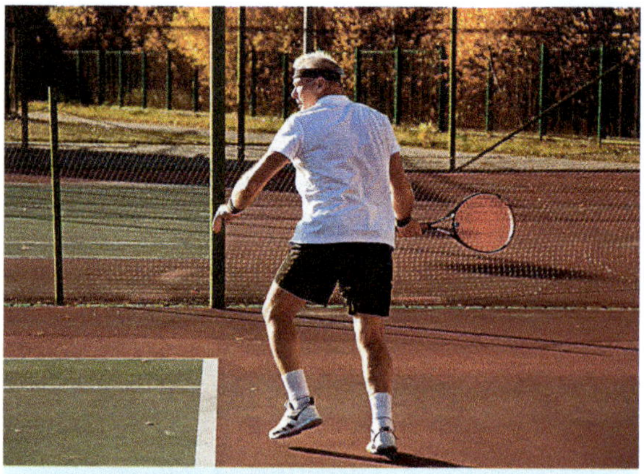

Figure 15.8 As many active older adults know, pacing is often an effective way to compensate for declines in speed, strength, and endurance

MAINTAINING MOVEMENT ABILITY

Most adults show decline in movement ability as they age. However, this decline, although inevitable for many people, does not have to begin as early or be as abrupt or severe as it is for some adults. Clearly, by maintaining a physically active life, individuals can delay, postpone, or in some cases reverse regression or decline in movement ability. Certain compensatory strategies, as well as exercise and general physical activity, can be highly effective in allaying the typical declines seen with increasing age.

Compensation for Movement Decline

There are many ways older adults can compensate for such phenomena as reduced speed, strength, and endurance and maintain high levels of performance. For example, in longer activities where fatigue might be a factor, older adults can learn to conserve energy by pacing their effort: doling out energy cautiously and avoiding unnecessary expenditures of effort. Many performers, such as distance runners, cyclists, and swimmers, consciously practice pacing, and in some older adults a certain amount of pacing occurs subconsciously as they moderate their performance through a constant concern for preserving their energy (see Figure 15.8).

Older adults may also practice other subconscious or automatic compensatory tendencies. For example, they may apply more effort than would a younger person. However, this mode of compensation does not work for extended periods because fatigue occurs more readily than it does with pacing. Some older adults may compensate for movement deficits by short- and long-term anticipation of movement. Short-term anticipation occurs, for example, when a racquetball player focuses on an opponent's movement so as to gain insight into proper positioning on the court. Examples of long-term anticipation are practice and securing sufficient rest in preparation for an upcoming movement activity, and these might increase the success of performance in the activity.

Older adults are often willing to sacrifice speed for accuracy in movement activities and occasionally may use this tactic as a form of compensation. This tactic also may be a result of the older person's more cautious approach to movement (Schmidt & Lee, 2014). The **speed/accuracy trade-off** is particularly common and useful among skilled adults. For example, in a game of tennis, an older adult might overcome reduced mobility or forehand velocity on the court through strategic and accurate ball placement back to the opponent. However, this form of compensation, although useful in many situations, cannot fully overcome movement deficits because the additional time the older adult gains may be insufficient to overcome the speed and accuracy of a younger opponent.

Finally, older performers may be able to compensate somewhat by maintaining high criteria or expectations concerning their own performance rather than expecting low performance. This tactic has been found particularly effective in certain memory tasks, as well as in tests involving sensory discrimination. No doubt, setting high expectations for one's own performance often helps an individual overcome some portion of the movement deficits that result from aging.

Physical Activity

Individuals can maintain and even improve their movement ability well into late adulthood by avoiding a sedentary lifestyle and participating in physical activity or exercise programs. Although any number of factors (social involvement, leisure-time cognitive activity, and so forth) can contribute to delaying many of the characteristics associated with aging, physical activity provides the most protection. Physical activity is the general term for engagement in energy-expending bodily movements that activate skeletal muscles. Exercise is a specific subset of physical activity that is "planned, structured, and purposive to improve specific physical skills or physical fitness" (Bherer et al., 2013).

For many of the reasons mentioned above, we have seen a cascade of research on the importance of physical activity for people of all ages, including adults and older adults. In a 2015 review of this research, Macera, Cavanaugh, and Bellettiere indicated that the most common chronic diseases in the United States are arthritis, cardiovascular disease, diabetes, chronic obstructive pulmonary disease, cancer, depression, and cognitive impairment. Physical activity has been shown to have a positive, ameliorating effect on all of these conditions while reducing the pain or physical limitations that often accompany these maladies and increasing age in general. For example, an additional 1,000 walking steps per day were found to reduce the functional limitations of osteoarthritis by over 15 percent. In general, modest decreases in physical inactivity resulted in "profound effects in attenuating the risk of future disability" (p. 4).

Similar results were generated by Guo, Shi, Yu, and Qiu (2016) in a systematic review of benefits derived for older adults from traditional Chinese sports and physical activities. In this review of studies specifically focused on Chinese people over the age of 50 years, this research team selected nearly a hundred studies for examination. Though a number of traditional Chinese sports were included, the main focus tended to be on the effects of Tai Ji Quan (Tai Chi), a slow, deliberate, and ancient form of exercise that included meditation and breathing exercises. Benefits from Tai Ji Quan included enhanced balance, hand grip, limb strength, and joint proprioception. In addition, oxygen uptake and several measures of lung function were enhanced as well as a number of measures of intellectual and psychological health. Practitioners were also found to have reduced incidence of several chronic diseases. Of particular interest, participation in Tai Ji Quan was found to reduce the incidence of metabolic syndrome with as little as one hour of participation per week. In general, Guo and colleagues concluded that strong evidence suggests that many of these traditional Chinese sports and physical activities, especially Tai Ji Quan, are promising interventions to enhance many aspects of health in older Chinese (Guo, Shi, Yu, & Qiu, 2016).

Being physically active even appears to have an ameliorating effect for older adults who are frail. One would think that physical activity would be contraindicated for these individuals; however, when introduced progressively, it may be one of the most important approaches to overcoming this condition. Research has shown that physical activity can offset the incidence of frailty and even reverse related characteristics, such as reductions in functional capabilities and losses of muscle mass and strength (Bherer et al., 2013).

Adult Physical Activity and Performance Patterns

Knowledge of the physical activity and performance trends across adulthood is essential to the eventual creation of strategies to avoid or slow the decline in functional ability often seen with increasing age. Toward this end Hall and associates (2017) studied physical activity and performance starting at age 18 and included participants into their early nineties. Physical activity was measured several ways including daily steps, overall time involved in moderate to vigorus physical activity, overall time spent in sedentary activity, and by using accelerometry to literally measure quantitiy of movement. Measures of performance included walking speed, balance tests, lower body strength testing, and a 6-minute walk to determine cardiovascular endurance.

Males performed better than females across all ages though performance declined at a similar rate for both genders across all decades of adulthood. However, more physically active participants experienced smaller declines in performance. More specifically, notable declines were seen as early as the forties in lower leg strength and balance. Gait speed and endurance slowed notably in the fifties. Of interest, the power of the association between physical activity and performance increased with age indicating the importance of maintaining a physically active lifestyle in older age. The strongest association was found for the 80- to 90-year-olds, but similar associations were found at younger ages as well. For example, significant correlations were found in the 40- to 50-year-olds between physical activity, leg strength, and aerobic endurance. Performance and activity level differences between age groups increased in magnitude with increasing age. Thus, the greatest declines in performance and activity were seen in the older age groups. This is to be expected as the older age groups were most likely to experience sedentary to light activity, a high rate of physical inactivity, and only moderate amounts of moderate to vigorous physical activity. However, a high rate of sedentary behavior was determined for all age groups, lending credibility to the authors' conclusion that strategies to enhance physical activity and performance should be initiated relatively early in adulthood (Hall et al., 2017).

As discussed in Chapter 3, *Healthy People 2020* (USDHHS, 2010) indicates that only 20 percent of adults in the United States achieve recommended levels of physical activity. Attainment of advanced education, greater income, a history of physical activity participation, ease of access to exercise or fitness facilities, and living in a safe neighborhood all increase the likelihood that an individual will engage in physical activity. Older people with low incomes, less time, poor motivation, disabilities, or even perceived poor health are less likely to achieve the recommended amounts of physical activity. Fortunately, some positive trends appear to be emerging, as from 1997 to 2012

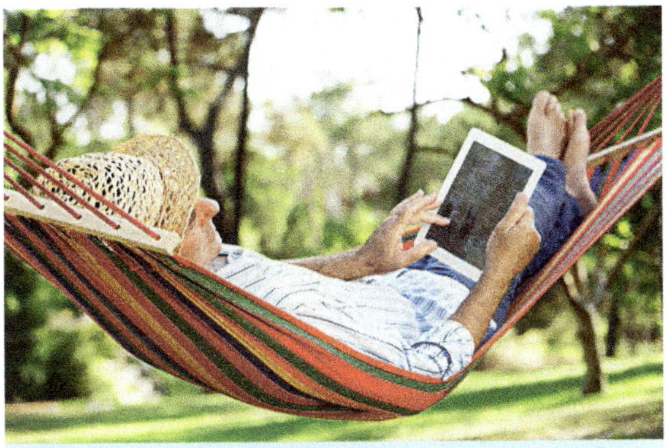

Figure 15.9 The incidence of sedentarism in the United States has decreased over time with the most sedentary people becoming moderately active. Nevertheless, we continue to see worldwide declines in physical activity, and projections indicate that physical inactivity will become even more common in years to come.

the number of adults (i.e., those over 18 years) who experienced no leisure-time activity decreased by over 25 percent. Nevertheless, nearly one in three adults still did not participate in any leisure-time physical activity (see Figure 15.9). This proportion increased with age: approximately 23 percent of young adults, nearly 32 percent of middle adults, and over half of people 75 years of age participated in no leisure-time physical activity. The numbers tended to be slightly higher for females than males across adulthood.

To get a sense of adult physical activity patterns worldwide, Ng and Popkin (2012) gathered information from some of the most populous countries in the world: the United States, the United Kingdom, Brazil, China, and India. Based on the information they collected, these researchers determined a physical activity pattern for each country and projected trends for the future. Their general conclusion was that physical activity is declining "rapidly" (p. 666) across the globe. Of the countries studied, this trend was most notable in China and Brazil, where the greatest overall declines in physical activity occurred. The declines seemed to be related to physical activity decreases at home and at work, an expected finding given that both countries have experienced increases in home technology and shifts away from manual forms of work (e.g., agriculture) to more mechanized labor in manufacturing. Predictions regarding physical activity levels were considered "bleak" (p. 666), with activity levels among Americans and Britons projected to decline and the Chinese and Brazilian people projected to experience even steeper declines. The researchers concluded that India is experiencing a smaller decrease nationwide, but a societal dichotomy exists, where a major decline is occurring among wealthier Indians while many other Indians continue to engage in occupational physical labor. In addition, the significant declines in the United States, the United Kingdom, Brazil, and China are thought to be strongly related to the dramatic increase in technology, especially technology related to the media (TV, Internet, cable access, and so forth). To date, technology has had less impact in India, according to these researchers.

The research also showed clear differences in physical activity patterns in the United States, the United Kingdom, and China between women and men. Declines appear to be greater among women, who have typically assumed responsibility for child and household care while sometimes maintaining an outside occupation, as well. Yet, for women in the United States, domestic physical activity was believed to have fallen by a third during the 30-year period ending in 1995. The authors also noted that in the United States the amount of activity allotted to preparing food has dropped by nearly 75 percent with the increasing availability of processed foods (Ng & Popkin, 2012).

To study more specifically the decline in physical activity with age, another research team examined the rate of decline with increasing age. The researchers measured the total daily activity of more than 500 older adults by using portable activity monitors. The average age of the participants was just over 80 years. Daily activity was found to be negatively correlated with age; that is, as age increased, activity level declined. The researchers determined that the rate of decline increased by approximately 3 percent for each additional year of age. The rate of decline for a 91-year-old would be nearly twice that of a 71-year-old. The researchers posited that this acceleration in the decline in physical activity in older people resulted from the aggregation of impairments in physiological abilities that enable physical activity in younger persons. Interestingly, more highly educated participants seemed to experience slower rates of decline. Nevertheless, the general increasing rate of decline in physical activity with age among older adults is a serious societal issue and an important public health challenge, especially given the dramatic rise in the number of older Americans (Buchman, Wilson, Yu, et al., 2014).

Adult Physical Activity Recommendations

Given that physical activity is so important for people of all ages, and especially for adults and older adults, the United States Department of Health and Human Services released the second edition of the *Physical Activity Guidelines for Americans* (2018). This document clearly states the importance of regular physical activity at all ages and notes that it is "essential" for healthy aging (see Figure 15.10). Specific recommendations for adults include doing a minimum of 150–300 minutes of activity per week at moderate intensity and 75–150 minutes of vigorous aerobic activity. Muscle-strengthening activities are advised on at least two days per week. Doing more than the recommended amounts of activity generally leads to additional benefits. Older adults are also advised to supplement these recommendations with balance training. More generally, the guidelines stipulate that less sitting and more moving are in the best interest of nearly everyone and even the least active segment of the population will benefit from minor increases in moderate to vigorous activity levels. The guidelines further indicate that improvements in health and wellness often begin immediately following physical activity with research indicating that nearly everyone (i.e., both genders, all races, all ages, people with disabilities or cronic conditions, etc.) will benefit. They state that the research on the positive outcomes associated with physical actitivity are well established. For those who have not previously exercised, the guidelines advise starting slowly and working up to increasingly greater intensity of exercise though any amount of physical activity is better than doing none. For older adults, the guidelines state that accruing better health through physical activity may be easier than once believed. Even one bout of moderate-to-vigorous physical activity can enhance sleep, relaxation, improve thought processes, lower blood pressure, and improve insulin sensitivity over the short term immediately after the exercise. In addition, whereas previous evidence suggested that aerobic activity required accumulated bouts of a minimum duration (e.g., 10 minutes), the new guidelines indicate that a predetermined duration is not essential to benefit health. Even small bouts of activity (e.g., walking up stairs, or walking across a parking lot) all contribute to daily physical activity and can be health-enhancing.

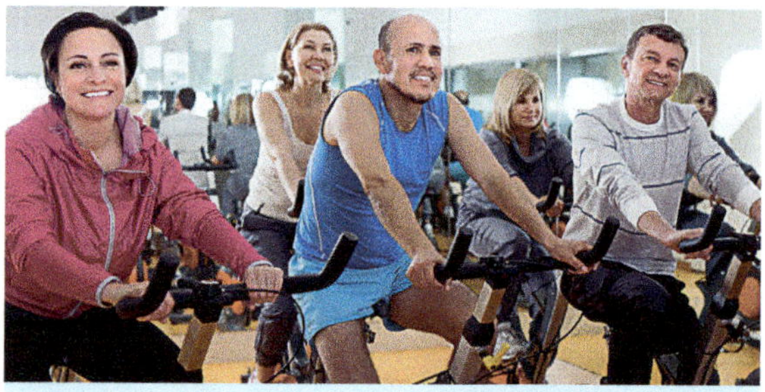

Figure 15.10 Exercise programs in mid- and older adulthood can be beneficial in a variety of ways

Older adults who are physically active can more easily execute their activities of daily living, have reduced chance of falling, and are less prone to injury (Piercy et al., 2018). A more comprehensive list of benefits derived from physical activity are listed in Table 15.6.

Table 15.6 Health benefits derived from physical activity for adults and older people

Benefits from Physical Activity for Adults and Older Adults
Lower risk
• all-cause mortality
• cardiovascular disease mortality
• cardiovascular disease (e.g., heart disease, stroke)
• hypertension
• type 2 diabetes
• adverse blood lipid profile
• anxiety
• depression
• weight gain
• falling
• fall related injuries
• cancer of the bladder, breast, colon, endometrium, oesophagus, kidney, lung and stomach
• dementia
Improved
• cognition
• quality of life
• sleep
• bone health
• physical function

Source: U.S. Department of Health and Human Services (2018).

Factors Affecting Involvement in Physical Activity

With the benefits of physical activity and exercise being well established, one might expect more people to engage in an active lifestyle. As we seek ways to increase people's activity levels, examining their perceptions about physical activity may be beneficial. Franco, Tong, Howard, and colleagues (2015) studied people from around the world and their perspectives on physical activity. Interestingly, these researchers concluded that many older adults are still unaware of the beneficial effects of exercise; some even believe it can be harmful. In general, these researchers found that the major barriers to engaging in physical activity included:

- lacking adequate social support
- having physical limitations
- having a history or habit of being inactive
- having other priorities
- lacking convenient access to facilities
- simply not caring enough.

The authors also indicated that some of the adults they studied perceived themselves to be too frail to be active and considered their aged condition to be inevitable. Clearly, enhanced education would be a partial solution to some of these barriers. In addition, Franco's team concluded that more social interaction should enhance the desirability of physical activity, especially when it includes people of a similar age and background.

Finally, in an article entitled "The Secrets of Highly Active Older Adults," Franke, Tong, Ashe, and colleagues (2013) sought to determine the factors that enable certain individuals to remain relatively active at older ages (see Figure 15.11). By use of intensive, qualitative interviews with community-dwelling older adults, all of whom were 65 years of age or older, the researchers were able to probe the factors that promoted involvement in physical activity. They also employed accelerometers to determine the participants' daily activity levels.

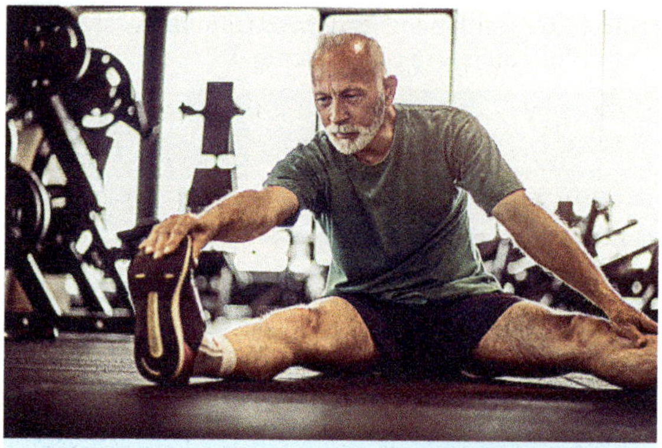

Figure 15.11 By maintaining an active, exercising lifestyle, most adults can postpone or avoid many forms of movement decline. In fact, improvements in motor performance can frequently be achieved throughout the lifespan.

The research team identified three general factors that were most important in enabling physically active lifestyles. They were:

1. *Resourcefulness*. Those people who had a greater sense of self-help, self-efficacy, self-control, and adaptability, even under adverse conditions, were more likely to exhibit a physically active lifestyle. Participants with these characteristics also gave themselves higher scores on health and independence.
2. *Maintaining social networks*. Having friends and family nearby and being connected to them, as well as being involved in regular social activities—especially those that promote physical activity—enhanced participants' ability to stay active. Related factors included the quality of the participants' living situation, their connections to people around them, and their general sense of belonging.
3. *Living where the surrounding built and natural environment included physical structures that were conducive to being active*. Examples included everything from sidewalks to the scenery in the surrounding area to access to recreational areas and facilities that would promote physical activity. In general, "movement friendly" (p. 405) environments were important to staying active.

In general, the highly active older adults in this study lived alone, had better coping skills than their less active counterparts, and continued their physically active lifestyle even when presented with significant personal challenges (Franke, et al., 2013).

Knowing and understanding the factors that influence continued activity, even for older adults, are integral to establishing health policies, designing and implementing programs, and generally developing innovative and evidence-based strategies to keep the growing number of older adults in our society physically active. The highly active older adults in this study are a testament to the fact that older people can remain physically active.

SUMMARY

- Traditionally, the study of adult development has been overshadowed by the study of children and adolescents. However, because of changing population trends and rapidly increasing numbers of individuals approaching middle and late adulthood, many developmentalists now focus their attention on the adult years. The number of people over 65 years of age is expected to triple from 2010 to 2050, so understanding changes in movement across adulthood is becoming increasingly important. Taking a lifespan approach to the study of development will yield insights that will help people maintain and improve function as they age.
- Balance is a complex skill that is integral to many daily tasks. As we age, balance often requires greater conscious awareness. Increases in postural sway and losses in balance-related functions lead to increasing numbers of falls among older adults.

Training programs, especially those that emphasize both balance and strength training, have been found to be effective in reducing the declines in balance that individuals commonly experience with increasing age.

- Walking patterns across adulthood have been studied extensively. Though changes across most of adulthood are subtle, they become more pervasive in older age and can significantly affect daily function. Gait speed and length often decline with age and are considered to be an important "vital sign" of overall health and functionality. Research comparing older adults who had fallen to those who had not found that those who had fallen took shorter strides, demonstrated a greater stride frequency, had greater lateral sway, and generally exhibited less consistent walking patterns than their counterparts who had not fallen. In general, research indicates that a physically active lifestyle can help a person preserve and even enhance gait characteristics in older adulthood.
- Falls cause more deaths among older adults than any other type of accidents; each year, nearly a third of older adults experience a fall. Many factors, particularly a lack of physical activity and declining physical parameters, contribute to these falls. Falls can be devastating, as they hinder an individual's self-efficacy, reduce confidence and activity, and lead to a decline in overall mobility and fitness. Fortunately, several strategies can help people avoid falling. These include exercise programs to enhance strength, balance, and flexibility; careful screening and control of medication; and thorough analysis of the home environment to reduce factors that contribute to falling. The increase in obesity levels in the United States has also contributed to fall rates. Adults who are obese are at greater risk of falling because of such factors as slower compensatory movements to avoid the fall and the decreased muscle mass and strength that often accompany obesity.
- Driving is one of the most important skills for older adults. As older adults age, the number of accidents in which they are involved and their anxiety about driving increase while their driving frequency decreases. With the population of older adults growing so rapidly, the number of traffic accidents among older drivers could triple within the next 30 years. The Mobility Consequences Model depicts a progression common among older drivers: Mental and/or physical changes lead to a loss of driving skill, which increases accidents. Eventually, driving frequency is reduced, affecting the individual's quality of life by narrowing the scope of activities. For older adults, finding safe and viable transportation alternatives is imperative. Older drivers can strategically compensate while driving to decrease the likelihood of an accident. By driving at safer times on safer routes, adapting strategies such as allowing more space between cars before merging, and not driving while rushed, older adults can reduce their risk of driving accidents.
- The ability to perform activities of daily living and instrumental activities of daily living is also found to decline in later life. ADLs include self-care activities such as brushing one's teeth and eating, whereas IADLs are less fundamental to function; they include activities such as cooking and cleaning. A decline in both categories indicates a significant loss of function and independence. Nearly half of people over 85 years report difficulty with one or more ADLs or IADLs. A sedentary lifestyle has been found to contribute greatly to declines in these abilities. Physical activity programs, especially those involving progressive resistance, balance, and functional training, are viable ways to overcome declines in the ability to perform ADLs and IADLs.

- In research on physiological functional capacity (the ability to succeed in physical tasks of daily life), the performance of older athletes has been compared to that of younger athletes. Running performance decreases with age beginning at about 35 years. Injuries may be a factor in this decline. Females seem to decline more quickly than males. Smaller declines have been found in swimming performance, perhaps because swimming is not a weight-bearing activity. Many Masters swimmers achieve their best times at 40 to 50 years of age; however, among both runners and swimmers, an acceleration of decline was found to occur beginning around 60 to 70 years of age.
- Declines in movement ability are extremely common among aging people, but these declines can be postponed or even, in some cases, avoided. Several strategies may compensate for age and help older adults maintain movement ability. Examples include pacing oneself carefully, applying extra effort, anticipating upcoming activity, setting high expectations for performance rather than accepting low performance, and making a speed/accuracy tradeoff. More important, regular practice and exercise are extremely effective in helping individuals maintain and even improve their movement ability in adulthood.
- Reaction time is a specific measure of how quickly a person responds to a stimulus. Simple reaction time involves one stimulus and one type of response. Choice reaction time often involves several different stimuli, requiring different responses. Both forms of reaction time are important in daily activities, such as driving or reacting to avoid a fall. Both decline with age, though simple reaction time appears to begin to slow around age 50, whereas declines in the more complex choice reaction time begin much earlier in adulthood. The saccadic movements of the eyes appear to maintain their speed throughout life, perhaps as a result of constant use of these movements, even among sedentary people. Exercise programs, especially programs emphasizing cardiorespiratory fitness, have been effective in enhancing brain function, which appears to be fundamental to our speed of reaction.
- Physical activity has clearly been found to be beneficial in attenuating many of the declines in movement ability seen across adulthood, even among older adults who are frail. Physical activity reduces the potential for frailty and has even been shown in some cases to reverse the characteristics of frailty. Unfortunately, only 20 percent of adults in the United States achieve the recommended levels of physical activity. Only around a third participate in leisure-time physical activity in middle adulthood, and that proportion decreases further through older adulthood. Trends of decreasing levels of physical activity have been seen worldwide; contributory factors include technology and increased viewing of media. This lack of activity presents a significant public health challenge in the United States and throughout the world. As a response, the United States Department of Health and Human Services has published *Physical Activity Guidelines for Americans* encouraging people of all ages to exercise. This document makes specific recommendations for the quantity and quality of exercise and the ways in which it is beneficial for health and wellness.
- Many people are still unaware of the benefits of exercise as we age. Some even believe that exercise is harmful for older people. Research on highly active older people, however, has shown that resourcefulness, having a positive and encouraging social network, and living near a built and natural environment conducive to physical activity can enhance a person's physical activity levels and assist in maintaining quality of life.

key concept review

activities of daily living (ADLs)
balance
choice reaction time
dynamic balance
extrinsic causes
frailty
gait
instrumental activities of daily living (IADLs)
intrinsic causes
last-in-first-out hypothesis
Mobility Consequences Model
movement time
physiological functioning capacity (PFC)
polypharmacy
postural sway
reaction time
saccadic movements
simple reaction time
speed/accuracy trade-off
static balance
strategic compensation

questions for reflection

1. Discuss trends in population growth in the United States and the world. What implications do these trends hold for the future?
2. How does balance performance change over the lifespan?
3. What methods have been found to be effective in improving balance in older adults?
4. What are the important findings comparing gait patterns in early versus late adulthood?
5. What causes can be linked to the increasing number of falls seen in older adults?
6. What can be done to decrease falls among adults and older adults?
7. Describe the Mobility Consequences Model and what it has to say about driving and physical activity as we age.
8. Which factors might contribute to declines in running speed with age?
9. What is the difference between reaction time and movement time? Define each.
10. What are the trends in reaction time with age and the factors that affect them?
11. What do we mean by the term *speed/accuracy trade-off?* Can you provide two examples of this phenomenon?
12. What is unique about saccadic movements and what implications does this have for other types of human movement?
13. What are some national and worldwide trends in physical activity patterns with regard to age?
14. What is the relationship between aging and physical activity? List several reasons why people should stay physically active as they age.
15. What specific recommendations regarding quality and quantity of exercise would you make for an adult looking to start an exercise program?
16. What are some factors that influence physical activity levels among active older adults?

online resources

Administration on Aging, acl.gov/about-acl/administration-aging
American College of Sports Medicine, Updated Physical Activity Guidelines, www.acsm.org/read-research/newsroom/news-releases/news-detail/2018/11/12/updated-physical-activity-guidelines-now-available
American Senior Fitness association, www.seniorfitness.net
Centers for Disease Control, Falls www.cdc.gov/homeandrecreationalsafety/falls/adultfalls.html
Healthy People 2020 and 2030, www.healthypeople.gov

National Council on Aging, www.ncoa.org
National Highway Traffic Safety, Enhancing Safety for Aging Road Users www.nhtsa.gov/events/enhancing-safety-aging-road-users
National Institute on Aging, www.nia.nih.gov
National Institute for Occupational Safety and Health, Falls in the Workplace www.cdc.gov/niosh/topics/falls/
National Physical Activity Guidelines, https://health.gov/paguidelines/about/
U.S. Census Bureau, www.census.gov
U.S. Department of Health and Human Services, www.hhs.gov
U.S. Department of Labor, Occupational Safety and Health Administration, Fall Prevention Campaign, www.osha.gov/stopfalls/

REFERENCES

Adriana, J., Moessinger, M., Charles, A., & Postal, C. (2019). Exploring the contribution of executive functions to on-road driving performance during aging: A latent variable analysis. *Accident Analysis & Prevention*, doi.org/10.1016/j.aap.2019.02.010.

Alosco, M. L., Penn, M. S., Spitznagel, M. B., Cleveland, M. J., Ott, B. R., & Gunstad, J. (2015). Reduced physical fitness in patients with heart failure as a possible risk factor for impaired driving performance. *The American Journal of Occupational Therapy*, doi: 10.5014?ajot.2015.013573.

Ambrose, A. F., Paul, G., & Hausdorff, J. M. (2013). Risk factors for falls among older adults: A review of the literature. *Maturitas, 75*, 51–61.

Andrews, E. C., & Westerman, S. J. (2012). Age differences in simulated driving performance: Compensatory processes. *Accident Analysis and Prevention*, *45*, 660–668.

Aslan, U. B., Cavlak, U., Yagci, N., & Akdag, B. (2008). Balance performance, aging, and falling: A comparative study based on a Turkish sample. *Archives of Gerontology and Geriatrics*, *46*, 283–292.

Ayoubi, F., Launay, C. P., Annweiler, C., & Beauchet, O. (2015). Fear of falling and gait variability in older adults: A systematic review and meta-analysis. *Journal of the American Medical Directors Association*, *16*, 14–19.

Bherer, L., Erickson, K. I., & Liu-Ambrose, T. (2013). A review of the effects of physical activity and exercise on cognitive and brain functions in older adults. *Journal of Aging Research*, doi.org/10.1155/2013/657508.

Boot, W. R., Stothart, C., & Charness, N. (2014). Improving safety of aging road users: A mini-review. *Gerontology*, doi: 10.1159/000354212.

Boyer, K. A., Andriacchi, T. P., & Beaupre, G. S. (2012). The role of physical activity in changes in walking mechanics with age. *Gait & Posture*, *36*, 149–153.

Brach, J. S., & VanSwearingen, J. M. (2013). Interventions to improve walking in older adults. *Current Translational Geriatrics and Gerontology Reports*, *2*, 230–238.

Brown, C. J., & Flood, K. L. (2013). Mobility limitation in the older patient: A clinical review. *Journal of the American Medical Association*, *310*, 1168–1177.

Buchman, A. S., Wilson, R. S., Yu, L., James, B. D., Boyle, P. A., & Bennett, D. A. (2014). Total daily activity declines more rapidly with increasing age in older adults. *Archives of Gerontology and Geriatrics*, *58*, 74–79.

Burkhart, J. E., Berger, A. M., Creedon, M., & McGavock, A. T. (1998). Mobility and independence: Changes and challenges for older drivers. Administration on Aging, Retrieved from www.aoa.gov/research/drivers.html.

Centers for Disease Control (2016). Hip fractures among older adults. Retrieved from www.cdc.gov/homeandrecreationalsafety/falls/adulthipfx.html.

Centers for Disease Control and Prevention (2017). Important facts about falls. Retrieved from www.cdc.gov/homeandrecreationalsafety/falls/adultfalls.html.

Dunlop, D. D., Song, J., Arnston, E., Semanik, P., Lee, J., Chang, R. W., & Hootman, J. M. (2015). Sedentary time in U.S. older adults associated with disability in activities of daily living independent of physical activity. *Journal of*

Physical Activity and Health, *12*, doi: 10.1123/jpah.2013–0311.

El-Khoury, F., Cassou, B., Charles, M., & Dargent-Molina (2013). The effect of fall prevention exercise programmes on fall induced injuries in community dwelling older adults: Systematic review and meta-analysis of randomized controlled trials. *BMJ*, *347*, doi: 10.1136/bmj.f6234.

Era, P., Sainio, P., Koskinen, S., Ohlgren, J., & Harkanen, T. (2011). Psychomotor speed in a random sample of 7979 subjects aged 30 years and over. *Aging Clinical and Experimental Research*, *23*, 135–144.

Franco, M. R., Tong, A., Howard, K., Sherrington, C., Ferreira, P. H., Pinto, R. Z., & Ferreira, M. L. (2015). Older people's perspectives on participation in physical activity: A systematic review and thematic synthesis of qualitative literature. *British Journal of Sports Medicine*, doi: 10.1136/bjsports-2014–094015.

Franke, T., Tong, C., Ashe, M. C., McKay, H., Sims-Gould, J., & The Walk the Talk Team (2013). The secrets of highly active older adults. *Journal of Aging Studies*, *27*, 398–409.

Golisz, K. (2014). Occupational therapy interventions to improve driving performance in older adults: A systematic review. *The American Journal of Occupational Therapy*, *68*, 662–669.

Granacher, U., Muehlbauer, T., & Gruber, M. (2012). A qualitative review of balance and strength performance in healthy older adults: Impact for testing and training. *Journal of Aging Research*, doi: 10:1155/2012/708905.

Granacher, U., Muehlbauer, T., Zahner, L., Gollhofer, A., & Kressig, R. (2011). Comparison of traditional and recent approaches in the promotion of balance and strength in older persons. *Sports Medicine*, *41*, 377–400.

Guo, Y., Shi, H., Yu, D., & Qiu, P. (2016). Health benefits of traditional Chinese sports and physical activity for older adults: A systematic review of evidence. *Journal of Sport and Health Science*, doi.org/10.1016/j.jshs.2016.07.002.

Haddad, J. M., Rietdyk, S., Claxton, L. J., & Huber, J. (2013). Task-dependent postural control throughout the lifespan. *Exercise and Sport Sciences Reviews*, *41*, 123–132.

Hall, K.S., Cohen, H.J., Pieper, C.F., Fillenbaum, G.G., Kraus, W.E., Huffman, K.M., et al. (2017). Physical performance across the adult life span: Correlates with age and physical activity. *The Journals of Gerontology*, doi-org.libaccess.sjlibrary.org/10.1093/gerona/glw120.

Hamed, A., Bohm, S., Mersmann, F., & Arampatzis, A., (2017). Exercises of dynamic stability under unstable conditions increase muscle strength and balance ability in the elderly. *Scandinavian Journal of Medicine & Science in Sports*, doi: 10.1111/sms.13019.

Himes, C. L., & Reynolds, S. L. (2012). Effect of obesity on falls, injury, and disability. *Journal of the American Geriatric Society*, *60*, 124–129.

Hung, W. H., Ross, J. S., Boockvar, K. S., & Siu, A. L. (2011). Recent trends in chronic disease, impairment and disability among older adults in the United States. *BMC Geriatrics*. Retrieved from www.biomedcentral.com/1471–2318/11/47.

Jerome, G. J., Ko, S., Kauffman, D., Studenski, S. A., Ferrucci, L., & Simonsick, E. M. (2015). Gait characteristics associated with walking speed decline in older adults: Results from the Baltimore Longitudinal Study of Aging. *Archives of Gerontology and Geriatrics*, doi.org/10.1016/j.archger.2015.01.007.

Kay, G. C., & McLaughlin, D. (2014). Relationship between obesity and driving. *Current Obesity Reports*, *3*, 336–340.

Kelly, K. D., Pickett, W., Yiannakoulias, N., Rowe, B. H., Schop-flocher, D. P., Svenson, L., et al. (2003). Medication use and falls in community-dwelling older persons. *Age and Ageing*, *32*(5), 503–509.

Ko, S., Jerome, J. G., Simonsick, E. M., Studenski, S., Hausdorff, J. M., & Ferrucci, L. (2018). Differential associations between dual-task walking abilities and usual gait patterns in healthy older adults: Results from the Baltimore Longitudinal Study of Aging. *Gait & Posture*, doi.org/10.1016/j.gaitpost.2018.04.039.

Komatsu, M., Nezu, S., Tomioka, K., Hazaki, K., Harano, A., Morikawa, M., et al. (2013). Factors associated with activities of daily living (ADL) in independently living elderly person in a community: A baseline examination of a large scale cohort study, Fujiwara-kyo study. *Europe PubMed Central*, doi: 10.1265/jjh.68.22.

Kumar, A., Delbaer, K., Zijlstra, G. A. R., Carpenter, H., Iliffe, S., Masud, T., et al. (2016). Exercise for reducing fear of falling in older people living in the community. *Cochrane Systematic Review and Meta-Analysis. Age and Ageing*, doi: 10.1093/ageing/afw036.

Kuys, S. S., Peel, N. M., Klein, K., Slater, A., & Hubbard, R. E. (2014). Gait speed in ambulant older people in long term care: A systematic review and meta-analysis. *Journal of the American Medical Directors Association, 15*, 194–200.

Leversen, J. S. R., Haga, M., & Sigmundsson, H. (2012). From children to adults: Motor performance across the life-span. *PLOS One*, doi: 10.1371/journal.pone.0038830.

Macera, C. A., Cavanaugh, A., & Bellettiere, J. (2015). State of the art: Physical activity and older adults. *American Journal of Lifestyle Medicine*. doi: 10.1177/1559827615571897.

Madigan, M., Rosenblatt, N. J., & Grabiner, M. D. (2014). Obesity as a contributing factor to falls by older adults. *Current Obesity Reports, 3*, 348–354.

Manckoundia, P., Buatois, S., Gueguen, R., Perret-Guillaume, C., Laurain, M., Pfitzenmeyer, P., et al. (2008). Clinical determinants of failure in balance tests in elderly subjects. *Archives of Gerontology and Geriatrics, 47*, 217–228.

National Highway Traffic Safety Administration, National Center for Statistics and Analysis (2013). Traffic safety facts: 2011 data—Older population (Publication No. DOT HS 811 745). Retrieved from www-nrd.nhtsa.dot.gov/Pubs/811745.pdf.

Ng, S. W., & Popkin, B. M. (2012). Time use and physical activity: A shift away from movement across the globe. *Obesity Reviews, 13*, 659–680.

Nnodim, J.O., & Yung, R.L. (2015). Balance and its clinical assessment in older adults: A review. *Journal of Geriatrics and Medical Gerontology*, doi: 10.23937/2469-5858/1510003.

Piercy, K. L., Troiano, R. P., Ballard, R. M., Carlson, S. A., Fulton, J. E., Galuska, G., et al. (2018) Special Communication: The Physical Activity Guidelines for Americans. *JAMA*, doi:10.1001/jama.2018.14854.

Pratt, J., Dodd, M., & Welsh, T. (2006). Growing older does not always mean moving slower: Examining aging and the saccadic motor system. *Journal of Motor Behavior, 38*, 373–382.

Renaud, M., Maquestiaux, F., & Joncas, S. (2010). The effect of three months of aerobic training on response preparation in older adults. *Frontiers in Aging, 2*, doi: 10.3389/fnagi. 2010.00148.

Roberts, C. E., Phillips, L. H., Cooper, C. L., Gray, S. & Allan, J. L. (2017). Effect of different types of physical activity on activities of daily living in older adults: Systematic review and meta-analysis. *Journal of Aging and Physical Activity*, doi.org/10.1123/japa.2016-0201.

Rozenfeld, S., Camacho, L. A., & Veras, P. (2003). Medication as a risk factor for falls in older Brazilian women. *Revista Panamericana de Salud Publica, 13*(6), 369–375.

Schmidt, R. A., & Lee, T. D. (2014). *Motor learning and performance*. 5th ed. Champaign, IL: Human Kinetics.

Sherrington, C., Whitney, J. C., Lord, S. R., Herbert, R. D., Cumming, R. G., & Close, J. C. T. (2008). Effective exercise for the prevention of falls: A systematic review and meta-analysis. *Journal of the American Geriatrics Society, 56*, 2234–2243.

Spirduso, W., Francis, K. L., & MacRae, P. G. (2005). *Physical dimensions of aging*. 2nd ed. Champaign, IL: Human Kinetics.

Studenski, S., Perera, S., Patel, K., Rosano, C., Faulkner, K., Inzitari, M., et al. (2011). Gait speed and survival in older adults. *Journal of the American Medical Association, 305*, 50–58.

Tanaka, H., & Seals, D. R. (2003). Invited review: Dynamic exercise performance in Masters athletes: Insight into the effects of primary human aging on physiological functional capacity. *Journal of Applied Physiology, 95*, 2152–2162.

Tun, P. A., & Lachman, M. E. (2008). Age difference in reaction time and attention in a national telephone sample of adults: Education, sex, and task complexity matter. *Developmental Psychology, 44*, 1421–1429.

United Nations Department of Economic and Social Affairs (2015). *World population ageing – 2015*. New York: United Nations.

United Nations, Population Division, *World population prospects – 2017*. www.population.un.org/wpp/.

U.S. Department of Health and Human Services (2010). *Healthy People 2020*. Retrieved from www.healthypeople.gov/2020/topics-objectives/topic/physical-activity.

U.S. Department of Health and Human Services (2018). *Physical Activity Guidelines for Americans*, 2nd ed. Washington, DC: U.S. Department of Health and Human Services.

U. S. Department of Health and Human Services, National Institute on Aging (2011). *Global health and aging*, NIH publication no. 11–7737. Retrieved from www.nia.nih.gov/research/pub-lication/global-health-and-aging/preface.

U.S. Department of Health and Human Services, National Institute on Aging (2017). *Global aging*. Retrieved from www.nia.nih.gov/research/dbsr/global-aging (accessed March 31 2019).

Van Emmerik, R. E. A., Jones, S. L., Busa, M. A., & Baird, J. L. (2013). A systems perspective on postural gait stability: Implications for physical activity in aging and disease. *Kinesiology Review*, 2, 17–28.

Verhaegen, P. (2014). *The elements of cognitive change: Metaanalysis of age-related differences in processing speed and their consequence*. New York: Oxford University Press.

World Health Organization (2005). Preventing chronic diseases: A vital investment. Retrieved from www.who.int/chp/chronic_disease_ report/contents/part2.pdf.

Yeung, J. S., & Wong, Y. D. (2015). Effects of driver age and experience in abrupt-onset hazards. *Accident Analysis and Prevention*, *78*, 110–117.

PART V

Assessing Motor Development

16 ASSESSMENT

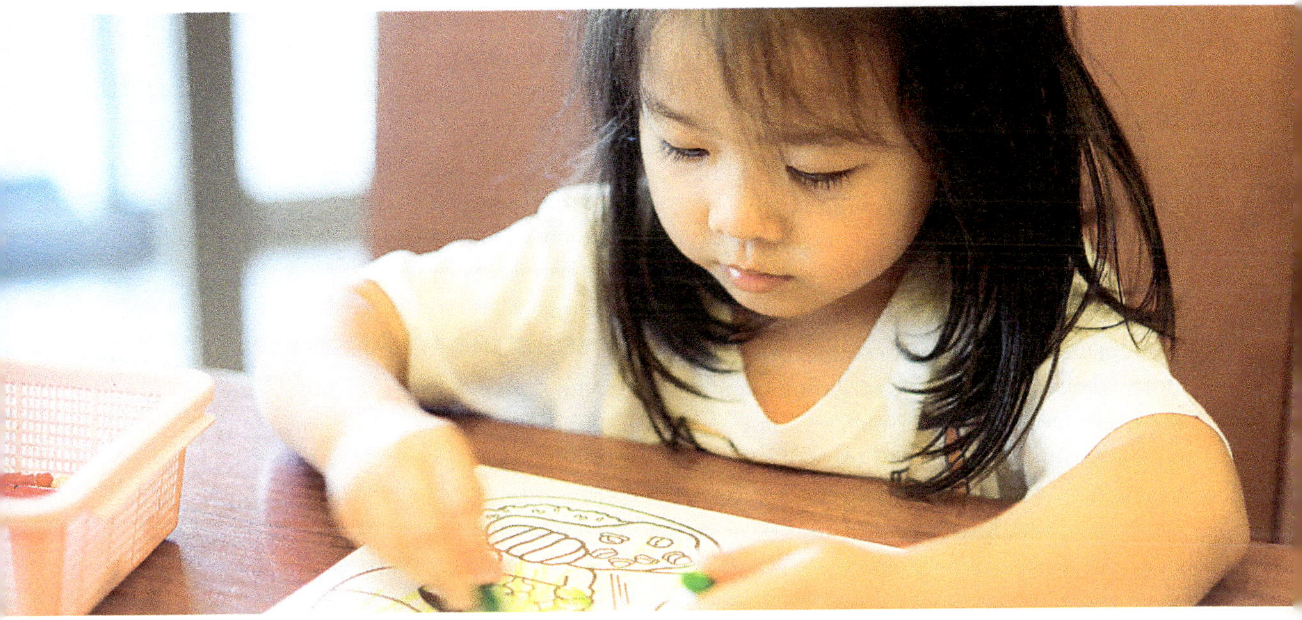

Chapter Objectives

From the information presented in this chapter, you will be able to

- Describe how to select and administer an appropriate assessment instrument and interpret and share assessment results
- Describe the advantages and disadvantages of both norm-referenced and criterion-referenced assessment instruments
- Provide a comparative example of a product-oriented versus a process-oriented assessment
- Describe these norm-referenced assessment instruments: Bayley-4, Bruininks-Oseretsky Test of Motor Proficiency-2, and the Test of Gross Motor Development-3
- Describe these process-oriented assessment instruments: SIGMA, Developmental Sequence of Motor Skills—Component Approach, and Developmental Sequence of Motor Skills Inventory—Total Body Approach
- Describe three popular assessment instruments used in assessing individuals with disabilities
- Identify several aids that can help you acquire valid assessment data
- Describe test batteries specifically designed to assess the health-related physical fitness of both children and adults
- Describe the instruments for assessing the physical and functional fitness of older adults

Throughout your study of human motor development you have encountered many research studies. In most of these studies, the motor development researcher had to administer some type of assessment in order to gather the data needed to answer the study's questions. Collecting data is an important component in other professions, as well. For example, physical education teachers should assess their students' motor behaviors prior to and following instructional units. Physical therapists assess their patients to uncover deficiencies or delays in motor development prior to and following the implementation of a corrective program. In short, whenever teaching or training occurs, it is important to assess performance and/or developmental level prior to formal instruction or movement skill remediation.

All too often, however, this important step is not performed. Why does this problem exist? It is often claimed that tests are too difficult, too time-consuming, and too expensive to administer, but many valid assessment instruments are available that professionals in school and non-school settings can feasibly administer. We believe the primary culprit is lack of training—many professionals simply do not fully understand the role of assessment and do not know how to select and administer tests. This chapter has been designed to help overcome this deficiency. It describes why you should assess, what should be assessed, how to prepare participants for assessment, and how to select the best assessment instrument for a particular situation. In addition, we describe and review several popular assessment instruments.

GUIDELINES FOR ASSESSMENT

The assessment process should not be approached haphazardly; it should be planned systematically. The following are important questions to consider before beginning an assessment:

1. Why do you want to make an assessment?
2. What variables do you plan to assess?
3. Which tests purport to assess the important variables that you have identified?
4. How will you prepare yourself for collecting the data?
5. Do you have the statistical skills to interpret the assessment data?
6. How, and with whom, will you share the assessment results?

Reasons to Assess

Many professionals assess performance as a simple matter of course, probably because when they were in school their instructor periodically assessed their performance or stressed the importance of assessment. However, assessment of performance should be carried out with a specific purpose in mind, such as one of the following:

1. *Screening*: Screening is a process whereby people are assessed to determine whether they should be referred for further testing or whether they need a special intervention or program of instruction. For example, school personnel may want to screen students at the beginning of a school year to identify children who have special needs, exercise specialists screen clients before prescribing an exercise training program, and clinicians screen patients before beginning an intervention.
2. *Program content*: Assessment results are helpful during the planning of the content of a program. An assessment of participants' incoming ability allows the professional to write program or treatment objectives that challenge the participants.
3. *Evaluating progress*: Assessment can also be used to determine how well participants are proceeding toward the objectives.

4. *Program evaluation*: A performance assessment will reveal whether a specific program of instruction is fostering motor skill or physical fitness development.
5. *Classification*: Through assessment, it is possible to place participants in homogeneous or heterogeneous groups. For example, when a coach is preparing rosters for teams that will compete against one another, she will attempt to create teams with similar overall skill levels.

Variables to Assess

Once you have determined why you need to make an assessment, you will want to determine which variables to assess. The selection of variables should be based on your objectives for the program or treatment. Instructional units that are tied to specific course objectives generally indicate which variables need to be assessed; for example, in a gymnastics unit, you may want to assess balance and upper-body strength. In short, assess those variables that reflect your objectives for an individual or group of individuals.

Selecting the Best Test

To select the best test, review all available tests that purport to assess the variables of interest. Popular measurement textbooks contain descriptions of available tests (Burton & Miller, 1998; Lacy & Williams, 2018; Morrow, Mood, Disch, & Kang, 2016), as does the classic *Mental Measurements Yearbook* (Carlson, Geisinger, & Jonson, 2017). Additionally, professional organizations, such as the ACSM and APTA, frequently introduce and critique popular instruments, and these organizations can be additional sources for instruments. (See "Online Resources" at the end of the chapter.)

After consulting these references, you should be able to identify several tests that assess the variables in which you are interested. Now you must decide which test instrument best meets your needs. To make this decision, consider each of the following questions:

1. Is the test statistically valid, reliable, and objective?
2. If the test is norm-referenced, are the norms established for a population similar to the one you plan to assess?
3. Is the test instrument feasible to administer?

Characteristics of Ideal Tests

Acceptable test instruments should be valid, reliable, and objective. A *valid* test measures what it claims to measure. One type of validity frequently used in motor development and physical education is content validity. An instrument with **content validity** contains tasks that measure specific content of interest. This type of validity is often determined by a panel of experts through logic. For example, experts have determined that the 50-yard dash is a valid indicator of running speed because it measures how fast a person runs. Other types of validity are statistically determined, and a detailed discussion of them is beyond the scope of this text.

Consistency of results is another important characteristic of a good test. A test is *reliable* if participants' scores do not significantly vary from day to day, assuming that they have not received additional instruction or training. Thus, **test reliability** indicates the test score's freedom from error.

The third characteristic of an ideal test is **objectivity** (sometimes called **inter-rater reliability**), which is the degree of accuracy to which a test is scored. Content validity is frequently determined subjectively, but both reliability and objectivity are determined statistically. To make these statistical determinations, we computed a **correlation coefficient** for two sets of scores. For example, to determine objectivity, a set of ratings compiled by one scorer is correlated with scores obtained by a second scorer to determine if the two sets of scores are consistent. A correlation coefficient of 0.80 or 0.90 is generally deemed acceptable.

Population-Specific Nature of Norms

Norms describe how large groups of people score in regard to selected variables. Because one large group can differ from another large group in regard to a variable of interest, norms are population-specific. An example is norms for height. Because Americans are generally taller than Japanese people, the normative values for each population would be different, and it would be inappropriate to use values established for one population when evaluating data from another. The same holds true regarding tests of motor proficiency and tests of physical fitness.

Therefore, if you decide to use a norm-referenced test, make certain that the norms were established on a population similar to the one you intend to assess.

Test Feasibility

You may find several tests that meet all of the selection criteria, so the next step is to determine which of these tests is most feasible to administer. Consider the following points:

1. Which test can be administered in the least amount of time?
2. Do you have to administer the test individually, or can it be administered to groups?
3. Do you have the training and expertise to administer the test? Some tests require extensive training.
4. Do you have all of the supplies and equipment needed for test administration? Some tests must be purchased as part of a test kit that may cost several hundred dollars.
5. Do you have the training and expertise to interpret the test results?

Besides referring to the publications mentioned earlier in this section, consult the test manual that accompanies most tests. Generally, the manual describes in detail how the test was developed and how it should be administered.

Preparing Participants for Assessment

Without a doubt, requiring people to perform strange motor tasks, in unfamiliar surroundings, in front of strangers, while sometimes using strange-looking equipment can produce a great deal of test anxiety among the participants. However, several steps can help reduce the uneasy feeling. Before conducting an assessment, consider the test environment and the participants' physical and psychological needs.

Test Environment

The area where the assessment is to be administered should be as comfortable as possible, and its temperature and lighting should be ideal. The testing area should be free of unnecessary furniture or other obstacles and free from distractions, such as high noise levels. Above all, the area should be free of potential hazards.

Meeting Physical Needs

Consider the participants' physical needs. For example, participants who are thirsty or those who must use the restroom will be distracted from the assessment. Establish a procedure whereby, before assessment begins, you ask whether any participants need to be excused.

Meeting Psychological Needs

The following procedures help reduce test anxiety:

1. When participants arrive, do not rush into the assessment. Engage them in informal conversation for a few minutes. Introduce yourself and encourage the participants to

talk about themselves. Ask a question such as, "What are some of your favorite activities?" Informal conversation about the participants relaxes them by making them focus their attention on themselves instead of the assessment.

2. Tell the participants what they will be doing during the assessment. In other words, reveal the unexpected.
3. When talking with the participants, avoid using the word *test*, which makes many people nervous.
4. If equipment is to be used during the assessment, give participants an opportunity to explore it before the assessment begins. For example, before requiring participants to catch a ball, let them informally play with the ball, so they can experience for themselves that the ball is soft and will not harm them. This procedure would also be helpful when working with older adults who may have reduced vision and slower reaction times.

Administrator Preparation and Data Collection

After selecting an assessment instrument and preparing your participants for assessment, there is one additional step in preparation—you must now be certain that you are adequately prepared to administer the assessment. To help prepare yourself, ask the following questions:

- Do I have the necessary equipment to administer the assessment?
- If administering a standardized assessment, can I accurately deliver the standardized directions to the participants?
- Do I have an appropriate score sheet, with extra pencils on hand?
- Am I adequately prepared to administer the assessment without constantly referring to the test manual?

In short, you must think through and even pilot (test run) the procedures prior to administering the assessment.

If the assessment requires you to observe and then rate developmental movement performance, do you possess valid observational skills? In other words, do you have a complete understanding of the developmental milestones being assessed? Are you able to recognize deviations from the norm? Finally, of utmost importance, have you thought through observational vantage points for each skill being assessed? For example, say that you are planning to observe an individual's stage of development for the fundamental locomotor skill of running. As the participant performs, from what angle will you be observing? Will the runner be coming directly toward you or running away from you, or will you be observing the runner from a side view? Obviously, the answer depends on which component of the skill is being evaluated. If you are assessing the relationship of the heel to the buttock, then a side view would be most appropriate. However, if you are observing the runner to determine whether the hands are crossing the body's midline, then requiring the runner to run directly toward you would be most appropriate. In other words, you should plot observational vantage points for each skill being assessed, prior to assessment.

Interpreting the Assessment Data

The most frequently asked question following data collection is, "How well did the participant perform in accordance with accepted criteria or norms?" To answer this question, you will need to have at least an introductory understanding of two measurement concepts: measures of central tendency and measures of variability.

Measures of central tendency include the mean, the median, and the mode. The *mean* is simply the arithmetic average. To calculate it, add all the raw scores and divide by the number of individuals who took part in the assessment. The *median* is the 50th percentile, the exact midpoint of a distribution of scores. The *mode*, the crudest measure of central tendency, is the score that appears most frequently within the distribution.

Measures of variability describe the spread of the scores. The most frequently used measure of variability is the **standard deviation,** which measures the degree to which the scores vary about the mean of the distribution. The concept of standard deviation can be best illustrated by its relationship to the normal bell-shaped curve, shown in Figure 16.1. This curve is a theoretical model based on laws of chance, describing the phenomenon observed when large groups of individuals are tested. The area under the curve represents performance occurrences. Notice that the curve consists of three positive and three negative standard deviation (σ) units. The area within +1σ and –1σ of the mean contains 68.26 percent of a normally distributed population. Within +2σ and –2σ of the mean we will find 95.4 percent of the population. Finally, 99.7 percent of the population will fall somewhere between +3σ and –3σ.

When analyzing assessment data, you will be interested in determining whether the raw score of interest falls above or below the mean and how far the score deviates from the mean score. When real data are involved, σ units are transformed into actual scores. Here is an example to illustrate the point. Suppose Billy's mother is interested in how her son performed on a test measuring abdominal strength/endurance (sit-up test). Billy was able to perform 35 sit-ups. How does Billy's performance rank among his classmates or among students in a standardized population? To answer this question, you need to know the mean and standard deviation of the distribution of scores, which includes Billy's score. Let's say that the mean of the distribution of sit-up scores is 45 and the standard deviation is 10. With this

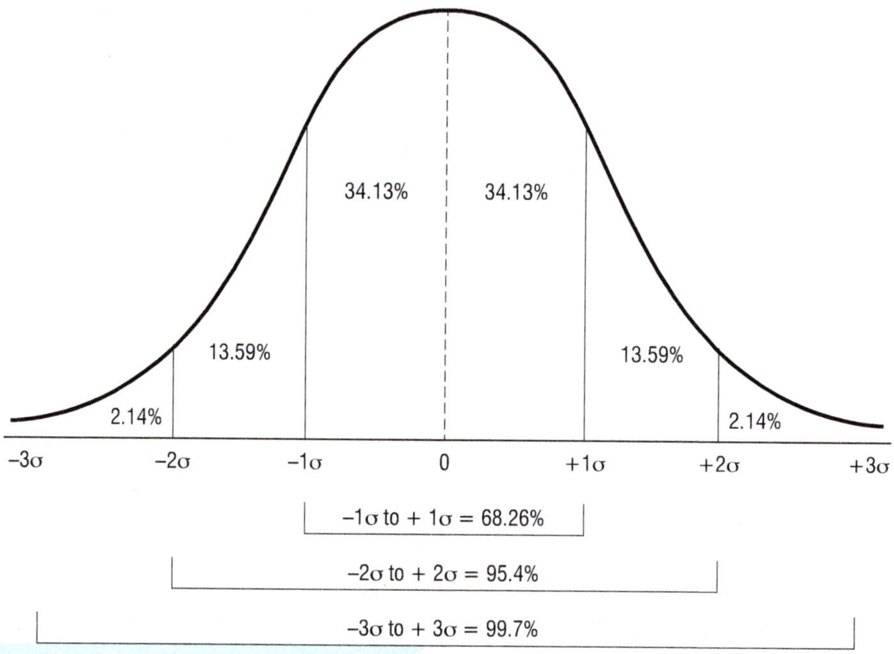

Figure 16.1 The normal bell-shaped curve

information, we can now say that Billy's score is below the average score. Not only is his score below average, but also it is -1σ below the mean. Therefore, we can say that about 84 percent of the individuals within this distribution performed better than Billy; conversely, Billy performed better than 16 percent of the individuals within this distribution.

Informal Assessment

We generally think of assessment as being a very detailed, formal process. This formal process generally occurs in any situation in which individuals are aware that they are being observed and evaluated. Unfortunately, many individuals become anxious and "tighten up" in these formal settings. As a result, a true performance score is probably not being obtained. For this reason, you may choose to engage regularly in informal assessment. When assessment is performed in an informal manner, the individual is not generally aware that an observation is being made.

For young children, Linder (1996, 2008a, 2008b) has described a type of informal assessment known as transdisciplinary **play-based assessment**. This type of informal assessment often involves either unstructured or structured motor play. The play-based assessment is accomplished by allowing the child free play within an approved area, in the presence of an adult facilitator. At first, the facilitator simply plays along and models the child's play behavior. However, later on, the facilitator will coax the child into exhibiting new movement tasks that the child did not spontaneously initiate. During this time, an evaluation is being conducted, but the child is not aware of it. In fact, video recording the play session is recommended. An administration guide is available which provides comprehensive instructions on conducting these play sessions. The guide also includes reproducible forms and information designed to link assessment to intervention (Linder, 2008c).

Sharing Assessment Results

Once you have analyzed and interpreted the results of your assessment, you will want to share the information with the appropriate people. Depending on the circumstances, these people can include the subjects, appropriate family members (e.g., caregivers, spouses, children), and relevant professionals (e.g., physical therapists, physicians, or a host of others). Individual face-to-face communication is best. Realistically, however, individual conferences are not always possible when large groups of people are involved. Whether you convey assessment results individually or through written communication, the goal of the communication is the same: an explanation of why you assessed, what you assessed, and what the assessment revealed. Remember that those involved are going to be interested in knowing what they can do to improve the participant's motor or fitness abilities, so be prepared to offer program suggestions.

TYPES OF ASSESSMENT INSTRUMENTS

After realistically considering the questions mentioned earlier, you will be in a position to choose the type of test that will best meet your needs. This section examines the advantages and disadvantages of several assessment tools.

Norm-Referenced (NR) Instruments

Norm-referenced (NR) assessment instruments are basically **quantitative evaluations** designed to compare a person's skills and abilities with those of others from similar age, gender, and socioeconomic groups. Because the normative scales are derived from statistical procedures, these types of instruments are sometimes referred to as **psychometric.** Currently popular NR tests are the Bayley Scales of Infant and Toddler Development-4 (Bayley & Aylward, 2019), Bruininks-Oseretsky Test of Motor Proficiency-2 (Bruininks & Bruininks, 2005), and the Test of Gross Motor Development-3 (Ulrich, 2019).

Advantages

Norm-referenced tests are popular because most (but not all) are easy to administer. The administrator needs minimal training to administer the test, and the scoring procedures generally are simple. The assessment score provides information as to where a person stands in relation to peers.

Disadvantages

Because NR scales provide information concerning a person's "average" functioning, they are not precise and cannot pinpoint the cause of skill or developmental deficits. They simply supply information as to where a given person stands in comparison to people with similar characteristics. Scores obtained from NR tests offer little insight into programming considerations.

Criterion-Referenced (CR) Instruments

Criterion-referenced (CR) assessment instruments evaluate the "quality" of a person's performance. Because human development proceeds along a predictable sequence of milestones, it is possible to determine where a person's performance lies on this continuum. One major difference between NR and CR assessments is that with CR assessments, we can compare people "against themselves" over time as they meet criteria along the continuum. In contrast, NR assessments compare people to a standardized population at a given point in time. With CR tests, the administrator's primary interest, for example, is not how far a person can throw a ball but rather the technique (form) the person uses when projecting the ball. Similarly, a therapist would be interested in evaluating a client's walking technique as opposed to walking speed, and this can be done with a CR test. Motor development professionals frequently refer to this type of assessment as "process oriented," which is discussed later in this chapter.

Advantages

Results from CR assessment instruments lend more insight into programming considerations than do results from NR tests. The CR test also provides for true developmental assessment—that is, comparing individuals' own performances as they develop along a continuum from immature to mature performance styles.

Disadvantages

CR tests can be more complicated to administer than NR tests, hence, much more training may be needed. Frequently, the administrator must learn many functional definitions for intraskill components, and confusion about them often causes scoring difficulties.

Product-Oriented Assessment

Motor development researchers in the first half of the twentieth century relied heavily on the use of **product-oriented assessments.** When employing this approach, the administrator is more interested in performance outcomes—for instance, how far or how fast a person can throw a ball—than the technique used to perform the task. The form or technique is generally of little interest to the product-oriented assessment administrator. Without a doubt, the simplest product-oriented assessment is the pass/fail system. Consider, for example, that you wish to assess the catching ability of a 20-year-old female college student. In a pass/fail system, you would assess the student's performance by determining the number of thrown balls that she retains versus the number of balls she drops. To score, you might award 1 point for each retained ball and 0 points for each dropped ball.

Thus, product-oriented assessments are similar to NR assessments because both measure quantitative performance outcomes. They differ in that with NR assessments, normative data have been established for the quantitative measures. The advantages and disadvantages of product-oriented assessments are similar to those of NR assessments.

Process-Oriented Assessment

Unlike product-oriented assessment, which is concerned only with the outcome of performance, **process-oriented assessment**, as the term implies, is concerned with the process or technique used to accomplish the task. For example, not how far did the college student throw the ball (product-oriented), but instead, what technique did she use to throw the ball (process-oriented). Did she take a step in the direction of the intended throw? If so, was the step taken with the leg opposite the throwing arm? Researchers have constructed developmental sequences describing various stages of maturity for a number of fundamental locomotor skills and fundamental object-control skills. However, as we have mentioned in previous chapters, the process-oriented assessment can take one of two forms, based on different philosophies: the component approach, developed primarily by Roberton and Halverson (1984), or the total body approach, developed by researchers from Michigan State University (Haubenstricker, 1990). Both approaches are described in detail later in the chapter.

SELECTED NORM-REFERENCED INSTRUMENTS

This section briefly describes three popular norm-referenced assessment instruments, namely, the Bayley Scales of Infant and Toddler Development-4, the Bruininks-Oseretsky Test of Motor Proficiency-2, and the Test of Gross Motor Development-3.

Bayley Scales of Infant and Toddler Development-4

The fourth edition of the Bayley Scales of Infant and Toddler Development (Bayley-4) was released in 2019 (Bayley & Aylward, 2019). This early childhood assessment instrument, which was first published in 1969, has now been in use for over 50 years. This assessment instrument consists of a battery of five subtests designed to identify delays in young children between 16 days and 42 months of age. The five domains assessed include: cognitive, language, social-emotional, adaptive behavior, and motor. New to the fourth edition, the motor response items are now presented in a separate Motor Response booklet. Of particular interest to readers of this textbook is this motor subtest. This subtest assesses degree of body control, large muscle coordination, fine motor manipulation skills involving use of the hands and fingers, dynamic movement, dynamic praxis, postural imitation, and stereognosis (perceiving and understanding the form and nature of objects by the sense of touch). Additionally, the child's caregiver is engaged in order to support responses where appropriate. Depending upon the child's age, the assessment can be administered in about 30–90 minutes. Also new to the fourth edition are updated norms based on data collected between 2017 and 2019. Updated reliability and validity studies are also included. Scoring can be accomplished manually or through a web-based application.

Because the Bayley-4 is classified as a "level B" product, it can be purchased only by individuals who have a Master's degree in psychology or related field; or practice in an allied health field; or have the qualifications to interpret clinical assessments, in accordance with the 2014 Standards for Education and Psychological testing (American Psychological Association, 2014).

Bruininks-Oseretsky Test of Motor Proficiency-2

The Bruininks-Oseretsky Test of Motor Proficiency-2 (BOTMP-2) is a norm-referenced **test battery** of eight subtests made up of 53 items (see Table 16.1). A short form, comprised of 14 items from the complete battery, can be used as a quick screening device. The battery provides both a comprehensive index of motor proficiency and individual measures of fine and gross motor skills for individuals of 4–21 years of age. The complete battery can be administered in 45–60 minutes; the short form takes approximately 15–20 minutes.

Table 16.1 Subtests for the Bruininks-Oseretsky Test of Motor Proficiency-2

Subtest	# of items	Selected sample tasks
Fine Motor Precision	7	Cutting out a circle, connecting dots
Fine Motor Integration	8	Copying a star, copying a square
Manual Dexterity	5	Stringing blocks, sorting cards
Bilateral Coordination	7	Tapping foot and finger, doing jumping jacks
Balance	9	Walking on a line, one-leg balance on beam
Running Speed & Agility	5	Shuttle run, one-legged side hop
Upper-Limb Coordination	7	Throwing a ball at a target, catching a ball
Strength	5	Standing long jump, sit-ups

Source: Bruininks and Bruininks (2005).

Test of Gross Motor Development-3

The Test of Gross Motor Development-3 (TGMD-3) represents a major revision to this assessment instrument, which was first released in 1985 (Ulrich, 2019). The primary purpose of this norm-referenced instrument is to identify children between the ages of 3.0 years and 10.11 years of age who may be lagging significantly behind their peers in the development of gross motor skills. Additionally, the instrument can also be used to aid in the planning of a gross motor development instructional program; to assess individual progress in gross motor development; to evaluate the success of a gross motor developmental program; and is frequently employed in research involving the study of gross motor development.

The test assesses 13 motor skills, which are divided into two subtests: locomotor skills and ball skills. Locomotor skills measured are running, galloping, hopping, skipping, the horizontal jump, and sliding; ball skills include two-hand strike of a stationary ball, one-hand forehand strike of a self-bounced ball, one-hand stationary dribble, two-hand catch, kick a stationary ball, overhand throw, and an underhand throw.

Clinicians appreciate the scoring system, which allows the test to be individually administered in approximately 15–20 minutes. The TGMD-3 score sheet lists performance criteria that are associated with a mature pattern of performance for each of the locomotor and ball skills being assessed. If the child exhibits the performance criteria, a score of 1 is recorded. For each performance criterion not exhibited, a score of 0 is given.

see Figure 16.2. A manual supplied with the test kit provides tools for calculating subtest performance, as well as composite performance (see Figure 16.3). The test manual is well written and easy to understand.

One study found that 88 percent of physical education students and 96 percent of physical education teachers could correctly classify a special education student's level of motor development following only three 50-minute training sessions with the Test of Gross Motor Development (Suomi & Suomi, 1997). This finding supports Ulrich's (1984) earlier statement that the Test of Gross Motor Development can be used with minimal training to assess accurately the motor performance of children both with and without disabilities, including those with mild to moderate intellectual disabilities.

SELECTED PROCESS-ORIENTED ASSESSMENT INSTRUMENTS

This section describes three process-oriented assessment instruments: the Ohio State University Scale of Intra-Gross Motor Assessment (SIGMA), the Developmental Sequence of Motor Skills—Component Approach, and the Developmental Sequence of Motor Skills Inventory—Total Body Approach.

SIGMA

The Ohio State University Scale of Intra-Gross Motor Assessment (SIGMA) (Loovis & Ersing, 1979) is a criterion-referenced assessment tool designed to evaluate the motor behavior of typical preschool and elementary school children, as well as young children with intellectual disabilities. Each of the 11 fundamental motor skills examined (walking, stair climbing, running, throwing, catching, jumping, hopping, skipping, striking, kicking, and ladder climbing) is presented in four developmental levels. The authors state that SIGMA is unique among tests in that it can be administered in formal testing situations or in an informal free-play setting. Test administration is simplified through the use of a skill format sheet. Each sheet provides five sources of information to help the administrator: (1) equipment needed to administer the test; (2) directions about the test conditions; (3) criterion test performance; (4) references from which more information about the skill can be obtained; and (5) summative terms/phrases that best describe the child's performance.

One unique aspect of the SIGMA is its accompanying program, the Performance Base Curriculum (PBC). The PBC is essentially an instructional program that states objectives and activities for each developmental level within each skill. The PBC is directly related

Section 6. Record of Item Performance

Locomotor Subtest

Skill	Materials	Directions	Performance Criteria	Trial 1	Trial 2	Score
1. Run	60 feet (18.3 meters) of clear space to run, and two cones or markers	Place two cones 50 feet (15.2 meters) apart. Make sure there is at least 8–10 feet (2.4–3.1 meters) of space beyond the cone for a safe stopping distance. Tell the child to run fast from one cone to the other cone when you say, "Go." Repeat a second trial.	1. Arms move in opposition to legs with elbows bent			
			2. Brief period where both feet are off the surface			
			3. Narrow foot placement landing on heel or toes (not flat-footed)			
			4. Non-support leg bent about 90 degrees so foot is close to buttocks			
					Skill Score	

Figure 16.2 Sample excerpt from the TGMD-3 score sheet

Source: Copyright © Pro-Ed. Used by permission.

Test of Gross Motor Development–Third Edition

TGMD-3

Examiner Record Form

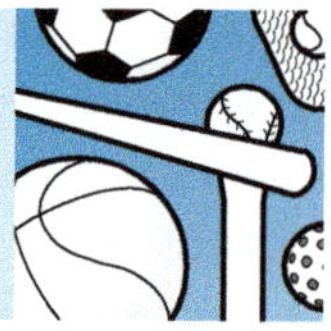

Ages 3-0 to 10-11

Dale A. Ulrich

Section 1. Identifying Information

Name ______				Female ☐ Male ☐
	Year	Month	Day	School ______
Date Tested	______	______	______	Preferred Hand: Right ☐ Left ☐ Not Established ☐
Date of Birth	______	______	______	Preferred Foot: Right ☐ Left ☐ Not Established ☐
Age*	______	______	______	Examiner's Name ______
				Examiner's Title ______

*When accessing the normative tables, use years and months. Do not round up.

Section 2. Subtest Performance

Subtest	Raw Score	Age Equivalent	%ile Rank	Scaled Score	___% Confidence Interval	Descriptive Term	Difference Between Scaled Scores
Locomotor	___	___	___	☐	___ to ___	______	☐
				+			
Ball Skills	___	___	___	☐	___ to ___	______	☐ Not important
				=			☐ Statistical 3 or above
		Sum of Scaled Scores		☐			☐ Clinical 6 or above

Section 3. Composite Performance

	Sum of Scaled Scores	%ile Rank	Gross Motor Index	___% Confidence Interval	Descriptive Term
Gross Motor	☐	___	☐	___ to ___	______

Section 4. Descriptive Terms

Scaled Score	1–3	4–5	6–7	8–12	13–14	15–16	17–20
Descriptive Term	Impaired or Delayed	Borderline Impaired or Delayed	Below Average	Average	Above Average	Superior	Gifted or Very Advanced
Index Score	<70	70–79	80–89	90–109	110–119	120–129	>129

Section 5. Administration and Scoring Guidelines

- Directions for all test items require you to first give the child a good demonstration of the skill, which includes all of the performance criteria. Next, give the child a practice trial, followed by two trials that you score. If you are unsure of whether the child performed a performance criterion correctly, administer another trial, look at only that performance criterion, and score it.
- Score each performance criterion as:
  - 1 = performs correctly
  - 0 = does not perform correctly
- **Performance criteria scores** are calculated by summing the scores on Trial 1 and Trial 2 for each performance criterion.
- **Skill Scores** are calculated by summing all of the performance criteria scores for each skill.
- The **Locomotor Total Raw Score** is calculated by summing the 6 Locomotor Skill Scores.
- The **Ball Skills Total Raw Score** is calculated by summing the 7 Ball Skills Scores.

1 2 3 4 5 6 7 8 9 10 28 27 26 25 24 23 22 21 20 19

14807

Additional copies of this form (#14807) may be purchased from PRO-ED, 8700 Shoal Creek Blvd., Austin, TX 78757-6897 800/897-3202, Fax 800/397-7633, www.proedinc.com

Figure 16.3 Examiner Record Form from the TGMD-3

Source: Copyright © Pro-Ed. Used by permission.

to the SIGMA, providing a critical link between assessment and program intervention.

Developmental Sequence of Motor Skills: Component Approach

Within the discipline of motor development, the most widely discussed process-oriented assessments are those Roberton and Halverson (1984) have described. Their technique is based on the idea that because development occurs at different times for different body components, assessment of motor behavior should involve a segmental or component approach. This component approach requires the identification of developmental characteristics of body parts in the performance of a selected task. Refer to Table 13.3, which illustrates the hypothesized developmental sequence for two-handed catching. Note that the emphasis in this type of assessment is how each body component reacts to the oncoming projectile. In addition, refer to Chapters 12 and 13, which present in detail the component approach for assessing running, jumping, hopping, skipping, throwing, catching, and punting.

Roberton and Halverson, both noted for their use of process-oriented assessment, have pointed out a few major drawbacks of the component approach. Specifically, they believe that a comprehensive understanding of the developmental steps and a prolonged period of study and practice of the technique are required for a proper assessment using the component approach. In an attempt to minimize these drawbacks, Stephen Langendorfer has constructed a series of forms designed to facilitate the efficient use of the component approach to assess some of the fundamental motor skills. Each of his forms lists the component being observed, observation criteria upon which a decision is made as to developmental level (decision rules), and names for each developmental level. Figure 16.4 presents the Developmental Sequence Decision Rule form for the fundamental motor skill of overarm throw for force. The form gives specific directions for its use. Appendix C.1 contains this and additional Decision Rule checklists for assessing a sampling of fundamental motor skills using the component approach.

Developmental Sequence of Motor Skills Inventory: Total Body Approach

Instead of the component analysis that Roberton and colleagues favored, some professionals prefer a more global analysis based on the configuration of the total body during performance of a task. This assessment technique has evolved from identification of developmental sequences for selected skills. Each developmental sequence consists of three to five stages, stated in terms of observable behaviors. The assessment administrator's task is to observe children performing the skills and then to classify them according to their level of development. To date, developmental sequences have been studied for running, hopping, skipping, galloping, long jumping, throwing, catching, striking, kicking, and punting. Table 16.2 highlights the characteristics of stages in the development of the fundamental motor skill of running. See Appendix C.2 for a usable assessment, which includes the characteristics of stages for each of the fundamental motor skills. These developmental sequences are the result of data collected at the Michigan State University Motor Performance Study. Most of these skills were presented in detail in Chapters 12 and 13.

ASSESSING INDIVIDUALS WITH DISABILITIES

Comparative studies of populations support the contention that although individuals with selected special needs perform behind their peers without disabilities, children in both groups may follow similar patterns of development. Unfortunately, many assessment instruments, both norm- and criterion-referenced, are geared toward the population without disabilities and so they cannot be appropriately used with special populations. For instance, a child with spina bifida who uses a wheelchair may have typical motor ability in the upper extremities, but because the child does not use the legs while throwing a ball, normative performance data comparisons are inappropriate.

Special populations pose other potential concerns regarding the use of assessment instruments geared to populations without disabilities. Frequently, the developmental starting points for children with special needs are so low that their scores are not included in the assessment materials. Clearly, there is a need for the development of more valid test instruments to assess the motor development of children with disabling conditions. However, some do exist. In the following sections, we present two popular assessment instruments frequently used by professionals who work with individuals with special needs.

DEVELOPMENTAL SEQUENCE DECISION RULE CHECKLIST—OVERARM THROW FOR FORCE (© 2007, S. J. Langendorfer)

Observer ____________ Performer Observed ____________ Media ____________

Observing the **Overarm Throw for Force** using movement component developmental sequences: For each observation question, circle **Y** for YES; **N** for NO (see additional instructions at bottom)

COMPONENT OBSERVED	OBSERVATION CRITERIA/DECISION RULE (circle best choice)	Y	N	DEVELOPMENTAL LEVEL NAME	EVALUATIVE COMMENTS
Preparatory Arm Backswing	Does the arm move away form the throw direction?	Y	N	1. No backswing	
	If Yes, is action a large circular motion with partially extended elbow?	Y	N	2. Shoulder/elbow flexion	
	If Yes, is direction of the arm movement beyond the width of the shoulders?	Y	N	3. Upward circle	
	If Yes, at the point of farthest backswing are the throwing wrist and forearm pronated so the ball faces backwards?	Y	N	4. Lateral swing, supinated action	
	If Yes, then prep. backswing is most advanced level: #5, *lateral swing, pronated action*			5. Lateral swing, pronated action	
Step/Leg Action	Does at least one foot move forward?	Y	N	1. No step	
	If Yes, is step with foot opposite to throw arm?	Y	N	2. Homolateral step	
	If Yes, is opposite step ≥ 50% of standing height?	Y	N	3. Contralateral step	
	If Yes, step action is the most advanced level: #4, *long (≥ 50% height), contralateral step*			4. Long, contralateral step	
Trunk Action	Does any part of trunk/pelvis turn or rotate back?	Y	N	1. No trunk rotation	
	If Yes, do hips begin forward turn while shoulders are still turning backward or held back?	Y	N	2. Block rotation	
	If Yes, trunk action is the most advanced level: #3: *differentiated, pelvic-lead rotation*			3. Differentiated, pelvis-lead rotation	
Humerus Action	Is the humerus at a 90° angle from the trunk?	Y	N	1. Humerus oblique	
	If Yes, is humerus aligned 180° at front facing?	Y	N	2. Humerus aligned, but independent	
	If Yes, humerus action is the most advanced level: #3, *humerus lag*			3. Humerus lag	
Forearm Action	Does hand with the ball appear to stop or move downward during the forward propulsive motion?	Y	N	1. No forearm lag	
	If Yes, is deepest "lag"of ball at front facing?	Y	N	2. Forearm lag	
	If Yes, forearm action is the most advanced level: #3, *delayed, forearm lag*			3. Delayed forearm lag	

Please note that an answer of NO (N) to any question assesses a performer's developmental level for that component at the level on that adjacent line in the 5th column (Developmental level name). When you answer YES (Y), then use the next question to evaluate that component further, until you *either* answer NO (N) *or* reach the last question in that component.

References

Haywood, K., & Getchell, N. (2009). Chapter 8, Development of ballistic skills (pp. 143–167). *Life Span Motor Development* (5th ed.). Champaign, IL: Human Kinetics.

Haywood, K. M., Roberton, M. A., & Getchell, N. (2012). Chapter 7 – Development of ballistic skills (pp. 153–176). *Advanced Analysis of Motor Development*. Champaign, IL: Human Kinetics.

Roberton, M. A., & Halverson, L. E. (1984). Developing children—*Their changing movement* (pp. 102–121). Philadelphia, PA: Lea & Febiger.

Figure 16.4 Developmental Sequence Decision Rule form for the fundamental motor skill of overarm throw for force

Table 16.2 Sample excerpt from the Summary of Fundamental Motor Skill Stage Characteristics—MSU Motor Performance Study: Total Body Approach

Fundamental motor skills	Stage 1	Stage 2	Stage 3	Stage 4	Stage 5
Run	Arms—high guard	Arms—middle guard	Arms—low guard	Heel-toe contact (toe-heel when sprinting)	
	Flat-footed contact	Vertical component still great	Arm opposition—elbows nearly extended	Arm-leg opposition	
	Short stride	Legs near full extension	Heel-toe contact	High heel recovery	
	Wide stride, shoulder width			Elbow flexion	

Source: Haubenstricker (1990). Used with permission from Dr. John Haubenstricker.

Peabody Developmental Motor Scales-2

The Peabody Developmental Motor Scales-2 (PDMS-2) is one of the most frequently used assessment instruments to measure motor skill development in young children between birth and 5 years of age (Folio & Fewell, 2000). The PDMS-2 is specifically designed to assess both qualitative and quantitative aspects of motor development, for both gross motor and fine motor skills. Additionally, the assessment kit includes a Motor Activity Program for use in planning individualized interventions. Professional therapists, psychologists, and diagnosticians consider the PDMS-2 to be one of the most reliable test instruments for children with special needs. The performance norms provided in the test manual are based on a nationally representative age-stratified sample of 2,003 children from 46 states. The assessment can be administered in approximately 45–60 minutes. Six subtests make up the PDMS-2:

1. *Reflexes*: An examination of eight reflexes in young children who are 11 months of age or younger.
2. *Stationary*: An evaluation designed to measure the child's ability to maintain balance or equilibrium.
3. *Locomotion*: An evaluation of the child's ability to move; includes tasks in crawling, walking, running, and similar actions.
4. *Object Manipulation*: Administered to children older than 11 months of age; an evaluation of the child's ability to manipulate a ball. This subtest involves activities such as throwing, catching, and kicking a ball.
5. *Grasping*: A measurement of the child's ability to use the small muscles of the hand to grasp and control objects.
6. *Visual-Motor Integration*: A measurement of eye-hand coordination, plus an evaluation of the child's visual perception. Examples of subtests include building with blocks and copying designs.

The test kit can be purchased online from Western Psychological Services (WPS) at www.wpspublish.com/store/p/2900/peabody-developmental-motor-scales-second-edition-pdms-2.

AIDS IN ASSESSING MOTOR SKILLS

As mentioned, one disadvantage of many tests is the need for the test administrator to learn many functional definitions describing the criterion behavior associated with each developmental level of a given skill. Checklists or reminder sheets that list key descriptive terms for each developmental level can jog the administrator's memory (see Figure 16.2). Regardless of a person's expertise with the developmental stages of selected tasks, it is still an excellent idea to have such a checklist at hand to ensure consistent scoring.

Video recording individual performances is another way to assess motor skills. Certain motor skills must be executed at high rates of speed, so even an experienced administrator may have difficulty denoting exactly what took place within each body segment during the performance of the task. Watching a slow-motion video affords a more precise analysis of most motor skills. However, one motor skill that does not lend itself to video analysis is the overarm throw for force, because the video device's framing rate is usually not fast enough to freeze the ballistic movement of the throwing arm. As a result, the throwing arm is likely to be blurred.

Another advantage of video recording is that it decreases the number of times a participant must perform a task to allow the administrator to evaluate the developmental level of each body segment. In a given test session, for example, a very young child or an older adult may become fatigued if required to perform a certain task many times. With video recording, the participant must perform only a few trials. The administrator can play back the recording as often as necessary to evaluate each body segment.

Brigance Diagnostic Inventory of Early Development-III

The Brigance Diagnostic Inventory of Early Development-III (BDIED-III; Brigance, 2014) is a criterion-referenced test with norms. The BDIED divides behaviors into 11 domains, illustrated in Table 16.3. Of the 11 domains, the first four are generally considered the most relevant for professionals working in the discipline of motor behavior (perambulatory motor skills and behaviors, gross motor skills and behaviors, fine motor skills and behaviors, and self-help skills). This multidomain test is designed for use with individuals between birth and 7 years of age. The test is easy to administer, and interpretation of the results is aided by the identification of developmental age levels for each skill sequence. These developmental age levels indicate roughly when a certain behavior

Table 16.3 Brigance Diagnostic Inventory of Early Development: Assessment categories

• Preambulatory motor skills and behaviors
• Gross motor skills and behaviors
• Fine motor skills and behaviors
• Self-help skills
• Prespeech behaviors
• Speech and language skills
• General knowledge and comprehension
• Readiness skills
• Basic reading skills
• Writing skills
• Math skills

typically starts to be exhibited and when that same behavior is typically mastered. Because of the wide range of skills assessed and the flexible testing format, the BDIED is very useful for assessing young individuals with severely disabling conditions (Bagnato, Neisworth, & Pretti-Frontczak, 2010).

ASSESSING PHYSICAL FITNESS

To this point, we have focused our attention on the assessment of motor skills. There is, however, a rapidly growing body of knowledge regarding the assessment of health-related physical fitness. In the sections that follow, we describe several of the most frequently used physical fitness test batteries: the FITNESSGRAM®, the Presidential Youth Fitness Program, and the Brockport Physical Fitness Test.

The FITNESSGRAM® and ACTIVITYGRAM®

Developed by the Cooper Institute for Aerobics Research, the FITNESSGRAM® and ACTIVITYGRAM® have rapidly become the world's most widely used instruments for the assessment of health-related physical fitness for students 5 to 18 years of age. This instrument is currently used worldwide in over 20,000 schools involving 10 million students (Cooper Institute, 2019).

The FITNESSGRAM® is a criterion-referenced instrument in the form of web-based software that assesses aerobic capacity, body composition, muscular strength, muscular endurance, and flexibility. Table 16.4 outlines the tests used to assess each of these components. The FITNESSGRAM® is more than a physical fitness assessment instrument, however; it is a comprehensive educational, reporting, and promotional tool. Once test data are entered into the software, reports can be generated. One such report is the cornerstone FITNESSGRAM® Student Report (see Figure 16.5). This report presents performance scores along with recommendations to the student for activities that can help the student achieve a Healthy Fitness Zone (HFZ) score (students are assigned their own login and can view their test results using a customizable dashboard). HFZ scores identify levels of physical activity that are associated with good overall health. HFZs are established by a panel of experts and are based on best practices and the best current research available.

The FITNESSGRAM® software includes the ACTIVITYGRAM®, a behaviorally based physical activity assessment tool. Students are required to record their physical activity each 30 minutes over a 3-day period (2 school days and 1 non-school day). See Figure 16.6.

Table 16.4 FITNESSGRAM test items

Aerobic capacity (select one):
The PACER* (a 20-meter progressive, multistage shuttle run set to music)
1-mile run
Walk test (ages 13 and older)
Body composition (select one):
Skinfold measurement* (triceps and calf skinfold)
Body mass index (weight in kilograms divided by height in meters squared)
Bioelectric impedance analyzer
Muscular strength and muscular endurance
Abdominal strength: Curl-up test* Trunk-extension strength and flexibility:
Trunk lift*
Upper-body strength (select one):
90° push-up*
Flex-arm hang
Modified pull-up
Flexibility (select one):
Back-saver sit-and-reach
Shoulder stretch

*Recommended test item.

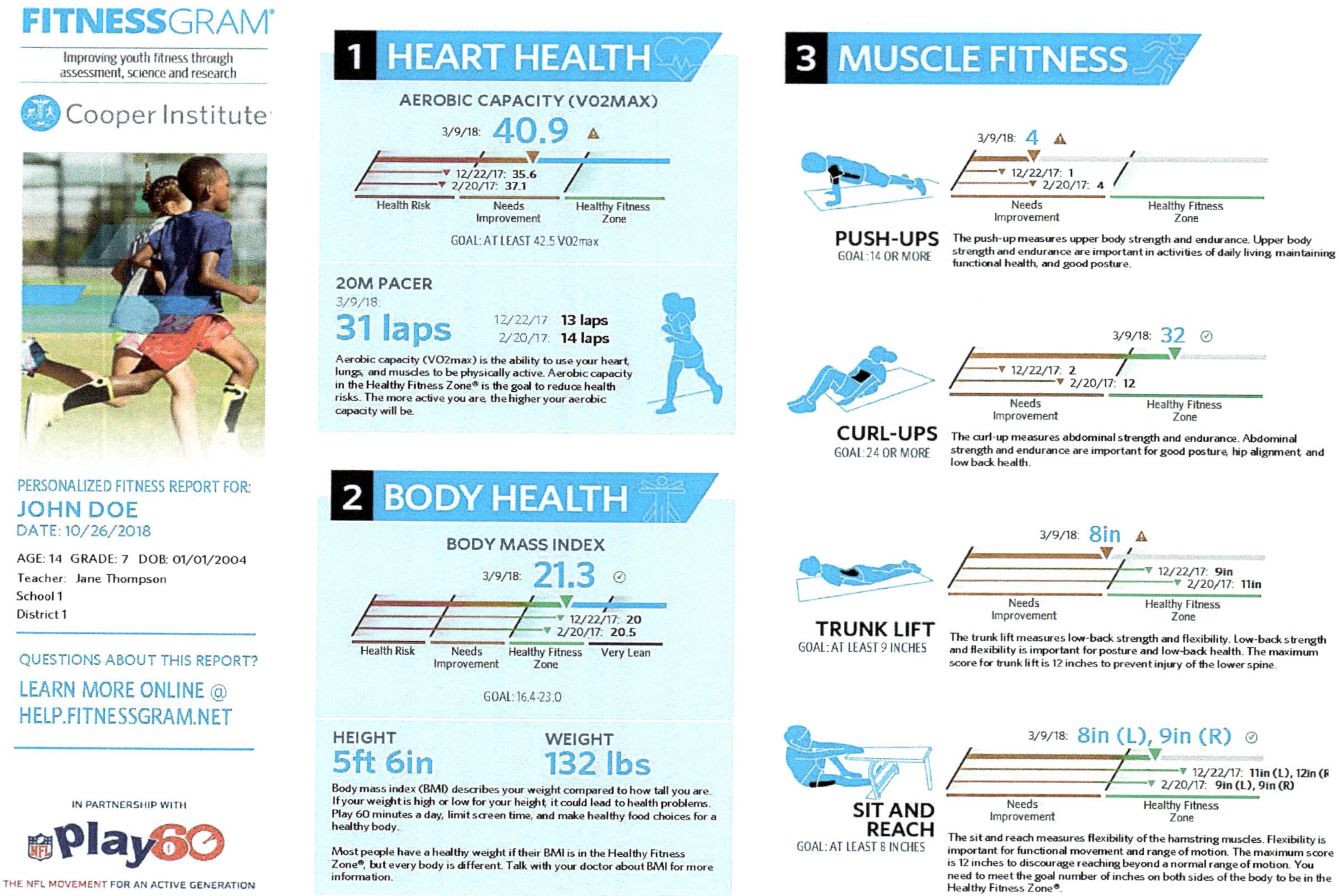

Figure 16.5 FITNESSGRAM® student report

Source: Copyright © 2018 by The Cooper Institute. Reprinted with permission of The Cooper Institute, Dallas, TX.

The ACTIVITYGRAM® allows students and their caregivers to determine whether the activity goal of participating in moderate or vigorous activity for 60 minutes on most days of the week is being met.

Also available with FITNESSGRAM® is NUTRIGRAM®, a log of dietary activity to allow assessments of nutritional knowledge and eating habits. The FITNESSGRAM® Kit, including the FITNESSGRAM® Administration Manual (Cooper Institute, 2017) is available from Human Kinetics Publishers (www.us.humankinetics.com).

Presidential Youth Fitness Program

Launched in 2012, the Presidential Youth Fitness Program (PYFP) replaced the longstanding, norm-referenced President's Challenge Physical Fitness Test (Presidential Youth Fitness Program, 2013). The newer program bases its physical fitness awards on the FITNESSGRAM®'s health-related fitness assessment. To receive the Presidential Youth Fitness Award, a participant must achieve a Healthy Fitness Zone score in each of the five test events (aerobic capacity, muscular strength, muscular endurance, flexibility, and body composition). For children with disabilities who are unable to perform select FITNESSGRAM® tests, the PYFP encourages physical educators to use the Brockport Physical Fitness Test, described in the next section.

The PYFP was established through a joint partnership between the President's Council on Fitness, Sports, & Nutrition, the Centers for Disease Control and Prevention, the National Foundation on Fitness, Sports & Nutrition, SHAPE America, and the Cooper Institute. This partnership is important because the PYFP is much more than a physical fitness assessment. For example, the PYFP also includes programs to foster professional development for physical educators. Additionally, a non-federal partner, the General Mills Foundation, established grants to support the implementation of the program.

Two recent evaluations of this program highlight the program's success. Namely, the PYFP was found to be effective in fostering fitness education, fitness assessment, and measuring student progress within the physical education setting. It was also noted that those students who participated in PYFP increased their aerobic capacity significantly more than control subjects. Administratively, however, identified barriers to PYFP implementation revolved around challenges associated with using the FITNESSGRAM® software, as well as the lack of time being devoted to physical education in schools (Presidential Youth Fitness Program, 2016, 2018).

The Brockport Physical Fitness Test

The Brockport Physical Fitness Test (Winnick & Short, 2014) was specifically designed to assess the health-related fitness of youths with physical or intellectual disabilities. Compatible with the FITNESSGRAM®, the Brockport test is criterion-referenced; thus, scores are compared to carefully developed standards rather than to national averages for youths without disabilities. Criterion-referenced standards are provided for such disabilities as visual impairments, spinal cord injuries, cerebral palsy, and congenital anomalies or amputations. The test consists of 27 health-related fitness tests, and instructors can select individual items to create a test for a particular individual or group. As mentioned earlier, the Presidential Youth Fitness Program has adopted this test as its assessment program for children with disabilities.

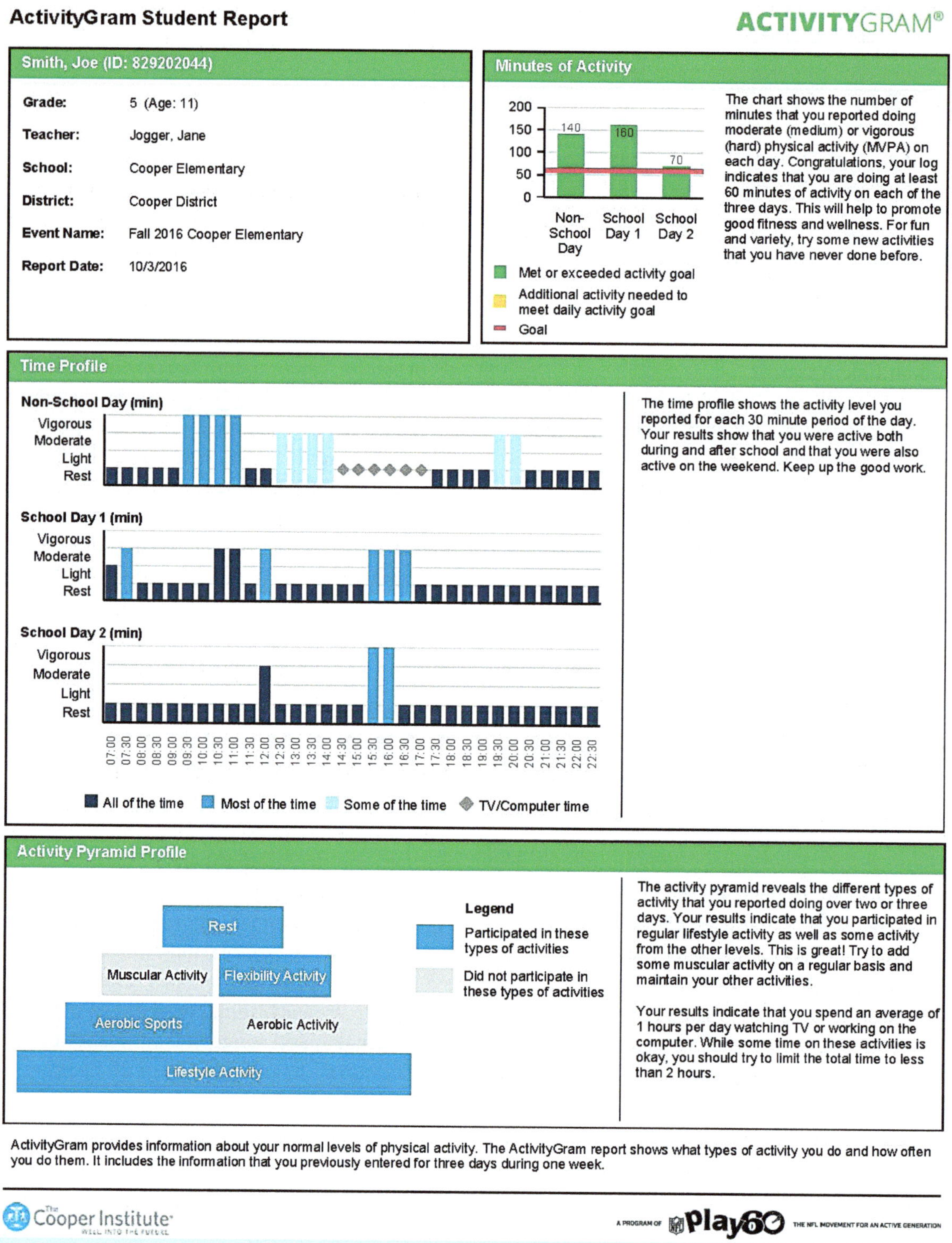

ActivityGram Student Report ACTIVITYGRAM®

Smith, Joe (ID: 829202044)

Grade: 5 (Age: 11)
Teacher: Jogger, Jane
School: Cooper Elementary
District: Cooper District
Event Name: Fall 2016 Cooper Elementary
Report Date: 10/3/2016

Minutes of Activity

The chart shows the number of minutes that you reported doing moderate (medium) or vigorous (hard) physical activity (MVPA) on each day. Congratulations, your log indicates that you are doing at least 60 minutes of activity on each of the three days. This will help to promote good fitness and wellness. For fun and variety, try some new activities that you have never done before.

Time Profile

The time profile shows the activity level you reported for each 30 minute period of the day. Your results show that you were active both during and after school and that you were also active on the weekend. Keep up the good work.

Activity Pyramid Profile

The activity pyramid reveals the different types of activity that you reported doing over two or three days. Your results indicate that you participated in regular lifestyle activity as well as some activity from the other levels. This is great! Try to add some muscular activity on a regular basis and maintain your other activities.

Your results indicate that you spend an average of 1 hours per day watching TV or working on the computer. While some time on these activities is okay, you should try to limit the total time to less than 2 hours.

ActivityGram provides information about your normal levels of physical activity. The ActivityGram report shows what types of activity you do and how often you do them. It includes the information that you previously entered for three days during one week.

The Cooper Institute · A program of Play60

Figure 16.6 ACTIVITYGRAM® student report

Source: Copyright © 2018 by The Cooper Institute. Reprinted with permission of The Cooper Institute, Dallas, TX.

ASSESSING FUNCTIONAL AND PHYSICAL FITNESS OF OLDER ADULTS

In this section we describe two instruments that assess older adults' ability to maintain activities of daily living skills, which are essential to preserve a high quality of life. We will describe the Senior Fitness Test and the Short Physical Performance Battery.

The Senior Fitness Test

The Senior Fitness Test (Rikli & Jones, 2013) consists of a battery of six test items designed to evaluate the physical and **functional fitness** of older adults. This easy-to-administer test has been scientifically validated. Performance norms are available, which were established by testing more than 7,000 men and women from the United States between the ages of 60 and 94. Additionally, these norms have also been shown to be appropriate for use in an elderly Norwegian population (Langhammer & Stanghelle, 2011). Thus, it is suggested that the use of the Senior Fitness Test norms may be appropriate for individuals living in similar countries (Langhammer & Stanghelle, 2015). Listed below is a brief description of the six tests that comprise this fitness assessment:

1. *Chair Stand*: Serves as a measure of functional lower-body strength. Requires the participant to place the arms across the chest and then to stand up and sit down as many times as possible in 30 seconds.
2. *Arm Curl*: Serves as a measure of functional upper-body strength. Requires the participant to perform a bicep curl as many times as possible in 30 seconds. Women use a 5-pound (2.3 kg) weight and men use an 8-pound (3.6 kg) weight.
3. *2-Minute Step Test*: Serves as a measure of physical stamina. Requires the participant to step (march in place) for a period of 2 minutes. The number of full cycle steps completed is recorded. Step height is calculated as a height located midway between the kneecap and the iliac crest (hip bone).
4. *Chair Sit-and-Reach*: Serves as a measure of lower-body and hamstring flexibility. While sitting on the front of a chair, the participant extends one leg straight and then bends forward at the hip as if attempting to touch the toes. This position is held for 2 seconds, and a measurement is taken according to the procedure described in the test manual.
5. *Up and Go*: Serves as a measure of walking speed, agility, and balance. The individual is timed as he or she rises from a chair, walks forward and around a marker, and returns to a seated position.
6. *Back Scratch Test*: Serves as a measure of upper-body flexibility. The participant points one elbow toward the sky with the hand behind the head, places the other arm behind the back, and attempts to touch the fingers. The administrator uses a ruler to measure the distance between the fingertips.

According to health professionals, the test is easy to administer, and both educational and motivating for participants to increase their physical activity (Jong, Peters, Gawler, et al., 2018). Appendix C.3 contains the scorecard for the test. Complete instructions, along with published norms, are available by purchasing the *Senior Fitness Test Manual*, 2nd edition, at www.us.humankinetics.com

Short Physical Performance Battery

Unlike the Senior Fitness Test, which assesses both upper- and lower-body functioning, the Short Physical Performance Battery (SPPB; Figure 16.7; Gurainik, Simonsick, Ferrucci, et al., 1994) focuses entirely on the functioning of the lower extremities. The SPPB is used to assess the current level of lower-extremity

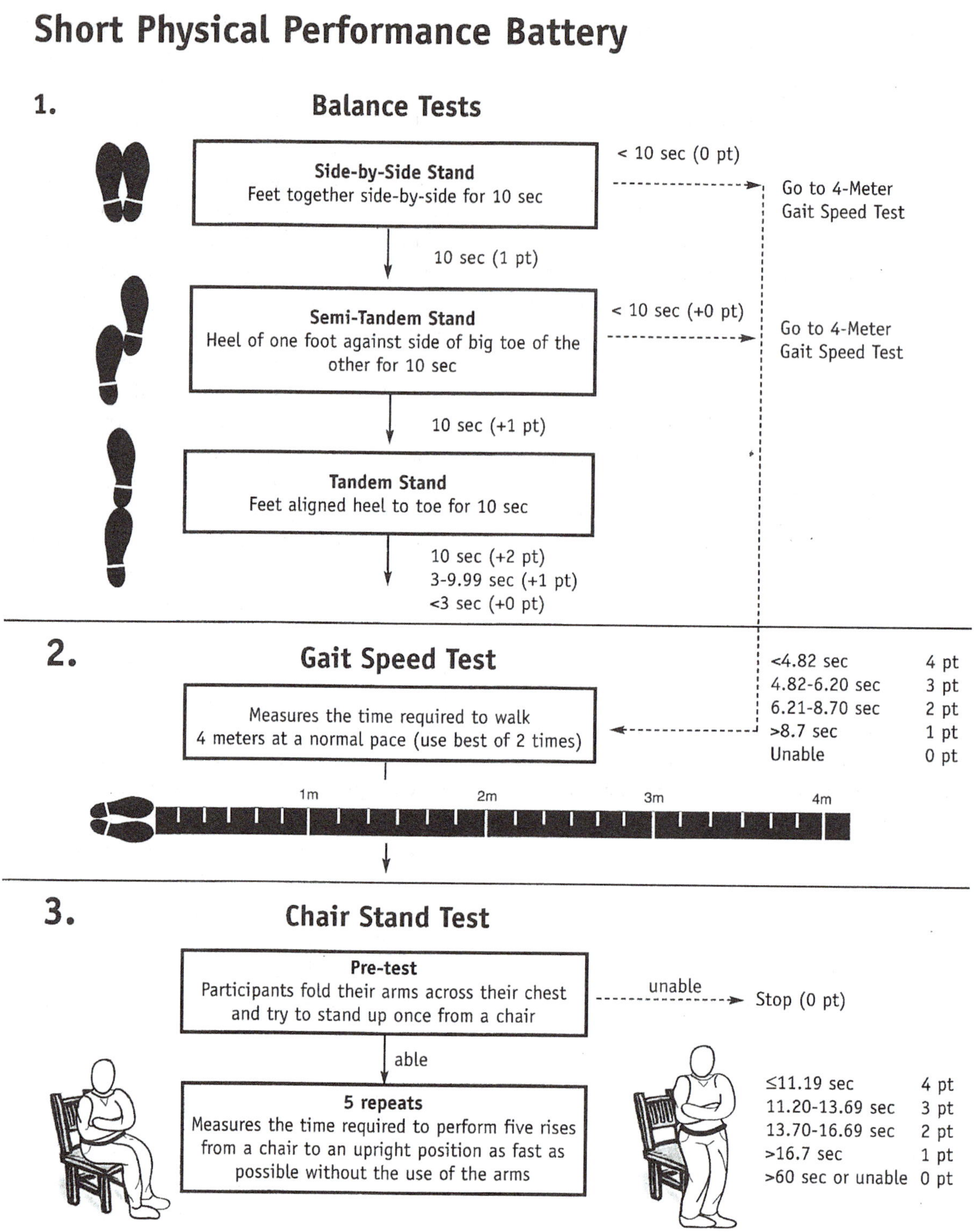

Figure 16.7 The Short Physical Performance Battery

Source: National Institute on Aging.

functioning, and it has also been proven to be a useful tool for predicting the future onset of disability (Cress, Gondo, Davey, et al., 2010). More specifically, lower SPPB scores have been associated with an increased risk of falls (Veronese, Bolzetta, Toffanello, et al., 2014) and predictive of a poor outcome following a hospital stay (Volpato, Cavalieri, Sioulis, et al., 2011). This latter point is important since the identification of future disability could permit the disability to be prevented or reduced through early intervention. Additionally, the SPPB can accurately measure mobility limitations in individuals diagnosed with COPD (Bernabeu-Mora, Medina-Mirapeix, Liamazares-Herran, et al., 2015).

The SPPB is not a complicated assessment instrument. In fact, it can be administered in as little as 10 minutes and consists of only the following three items:

1. a 4-meter (4.4-yard) walk to measure walking speed and gait;
2. a series of four standing static balances with the feet placed in different positions;
3. a measure of the ability to get in and out of a chair.

Each of these areas of assessment is vital for independent living during older adulthood.

See Appendix C.4 for a score sheet for the SPPB. The SPPB assessment package, containing complete administration instructions, can be obtained through the National Institute on Aging (www.grc.nia.nih.gov/branches/leps/sppb/index.htm).

SUMMARY

- Psychomotor assessment should be systematically—not haphazardly—approached and based on a plan that links assessment with curricular programming.
- It is important to select an appropriate test instrument. The instrument should be valid, reliable, objective, and feasible to administer and interpret. However, the most important characteristic is test validity. If the test fails to assess what it purports to assess, the instrument is of no value.
- Norm-referenced test instruments are popular because most (but not all) are easy to administer, and they usually require minimal training of the administrator. This type of assessment provides information about a person's average functioning. In contrast, criterion-referenced assessment instruments evaluate the quality of an individual's performance or set a level for mastery.
- Norm-referenced assessment instruments include the Bayley Scales of Infant and Toddler Development-4, the Bruininks-Oseretsky Test of Motor Proficiency-2, and the Test of Gross Motor Development-3.
- Popular process-oriented assessment instruments include the Ohio State University Scale of Intra-Gross Motor Assessment (SIGMA), the Developmental Sequence of Motor Skills—Component Approach, and the Developmental Sequence of Motor Skills Inventory—Total Body Approach.
- When assessing persons with disabilities, it is important to use an assessment instrument geared to populations with disabilities rather than an instrument intended for use with typically developing participants. At present, there is a need for more assessment instruments to be validated with populations with disabilities.
- Another area of interest to motor behavior specialists is the assessment of physical fitness. Popular fitness test batteries for children and adolescents include the FITNESSGRAM® and ACTIVITYGRAM®, the Presidential Youth Fitness Program, and the Brockport Physical Fitness Test.
- To assess functional and physical fitness in older adults, two popular instruments are the Senior Fitness Test and the Short Physical Performance Battery.

key concept review

content validity
correlation coefficient
criterion-referenced (CR) assessment instruments
functional fitness
interrater reliability
norm-referenced (NR) assessment instruments
objectivity
play-based assessment
process-oriented assessment
product-oriented assessment
psychometric
quantitative evaluations
standard deviation
test battery
test reliability

questions for reflection

1. What are the six guidelines for systematically preparing to perform an assessment? Explain each.
2. Can you discuss five reasons for assessing student performance?
3. Why are norms population-specific?
4. What are three areas that must be addressed when preparing students for assessment?
5. When students are assessed, they are often nervous. What steps can be taken to reduce test anxiety?
6. Can you define validity, reliability, and objectivity? Explain each and give two practical examples of each.
7. Can you draw and label the "bell-shaped" curve? Include in your illustration the standard deviations and the percentages of area under the curve associated with each standard deviation unit.
8. What are norm-referenced assessment instruments? Can you identify the advantages and disadvantages associated with this type of assessment instrument?
9. What are criterion-referenced assessment instruments? Can you identify the advantages and disadvantages associated with this type of assessment instrument?
10. What is the difference between product-oriented assessment instruments and process-oriented assessment instruments? What are the advantages and disadvantages of each?
11. Can you describe in detail the Test of Gross Motor Development-3?
12. How does using checklists, an observation plan, and video recording aid in conducting an assessment?
13. What popular instruments are used to assess health-related physical fitness?
14. What popular instruments are used to assess functional and physical fitness in older adults?

online resources

American College of Sports Medicine, www.acsm.org
American Physical Therapy Association, www.apta.org
Cooper Institute, www.cooperinstitute.org
FITNESSGRAM®/ACTIVITYGRAM®, www.fitnessgram.net
Human Kinetics Publishers, www.us.humankinetics.com
National Center on Health, Physical Activity and Disability, www.nchpad.org
National Institute on Aging, www.nia.nih.gov
Presidential Council on Sports, Fitness & Nutrition, www.hhs.gov/fitness/index.html
Presidential Youth Fitness Program, www.pyfp.org

REFERENCES

American Psychological Association. (2014). *Standards for educational and psychological testing*. Washington, DC: American Psychological Association.

Bagnato, S. J., Neisworth, J. T., & Pretti-Frontczak. K. (2010). *Linking authentic assessment & early childhood intervention: Best measures for best practices*, 2nd ed. Baltimore, MD: Paul H. Brookes.

Bayley, N. (2005). *Bayley scales of infant and toddler development*, 3rd ed. San Antonio, TX: Psychological Corporation.

Bayley, N., & Aylward, G. P. (2019). *Bayley scales of infant and toddler development*, 4th ed. San Antonio, TX: Psychological Corporation.

Bernabeu-Mora, R., Medina-Mirapeix, F., Liamazares-Herran, E., Garcia-Guillamon, G., Gimerez-Gimerez, L. M., & Sanchez-Nieto, J. M. (2015). The short physical performance battery is a discriminative tool for identifying patients with COPD at risk of disability. *International Journal of Chronic Obstructive Pulmonary Disease, 10*, 2619–2626.

Brigance, A. H. (2014). *Brigance inventory of early development-III*. North Billerica, MA: Curriculum Associates, Inc.

Bruininks, R. H., & Bruininks, B. D. (2005). *Bruininks-Oseretsky test of motor proficiency*, 2nd ed. San Antonio, TX: Pearson Assessments.

Burton, A. W., & Miller, D. E. (1998). *Movement skill assessment*. Champaign, IL: Human Kinetics.

Carlson, J. F., Geisinger, K. F., & Jonson, J. L. (2017). *The twentieth mental measurements yearbook*. Lincoln, NE: Institute of Mental Measurements.

Cooper Institute (2017). *FITNESSGRAM administration manual*, 5th ed. Dallas: The Cooper Institute.

Cooper Institute (2019). Why FITNESSGRAM? Dallas: The Cooper Institute. www.cooperinstitute.org/fitnessgram/why.

Cress, M. E., Gondo, Y., Davey, A., Anderson, S., Kim, S., & Poon, L. W. (2010). Assessing physical performance in centenarians: Norms and an extended scale from the Georgia centenarian study. *Gerontology and Geriatrics Research*, http://dx.doi.org/10.1155/2010/310610.

Folio, R., & Fewell, R. R. (2000). *Peabody developmental motor scale*, 2nd ed. Los Angeles: Western Psychological Services.

Gurainik, J. M., Simonsick, E. M., Ferrucci, L., Glynn, R. J., Berkman, L. F., Blazer, D. G., et al. (1994). A short physical performance battery assessing lower extremity function: Association with self-reported disability and prediction of mortality and nursing home admission. *Journal of Gerontology, 49*, M85–94.

Haubenstricker, J. (1990). Summary of fundamental motor skill stage characteristics: Motor performance study—MSU. Unpublished materials, Michigan State University, East Lansing, MI.

Jong, L. D., Peters, A. D., Gawler, S., Chalmers, N., Henderson, C., Hooper, J., et al. (2018). The appeal of the Functional Fitness MOT to older adults and health professionals in an outpatient setting: A mixed-method feasibility study. *Clinical Interventions in Aging, 13*, 1815–1829.

Lacy, A. C. & Williams, S. M. (2018). *Measurement and evaluation in physical education and exercise science*, 8th ed. London: Taylor & Francis.

Langhammer, B., & Stanghelle, J. K. (2011). Functional fitness in elderly Norwegians measured with the senior fitness test. *Advances in Physiotherapy, 13*, 137–144.

Langhammer, B., & Stanghelle, J. K. (2015). The senior fitness test. *Journal of Physiotherapy, 61*, 163.

Linder, T. W. (1996). *Observing Kassandra: A transdisciplinary play-based assessment of a child with severe disabilities* (videotape). Baltimore, MD: Paul H. Brookes.

Linder, T. W. (2008a). *Transdisciplinary play-based assessment*, 2nd ed. Baltimore, MD: Paul H. Brookes.

Linder, T. W. (2008b). *Transdisciplinary play-based intervention*, 2nd ed. Baltimore, MD: Paul H. Brookes.

Linder, T. W. (2008c). *Administration guide for TPBA2 & TPBA2*. Baltimore, MD: Paul H. Brookes.

Loovis, E. M., & Ersing, W. F. (1979). *Assessing and programming gross motor development for children*, 2nd ed. Loudonville, OH: Mohican Textbook Publishing.

Morrow, J., Mood, D., Disch, J., & Kang, M. (2016). *Measurement and evaluation in human performance*, 5th ed. Champaign, IL: Human Kinetics.

Plowman, S. A., & Meredith, M. D. (Eds.) (2013). *FITNESSGRAM/ACTIVITYGRAM reference guide*, 4th ed. Dallas: The Cooper Institute.

Presidential Youth Fitness Program (2013). *Presidential youth fitness program physical educator resource guide* (Internet Resource). Silver Spring, MD: National Foundational on Fitness, Sports and Nutrition.

Presidential Youth Fitness Program (2016). Presidential youth fitness program evaluation report: 2013–2016. Retrieved from https://pyfp.org/doc/PYFP_Process_Evaluation_Report_2013_2016_cleared.pdf.

Presidential Youth Fitness Program (2018). Presidential youth fitness program summary evaluation report. Retrieved from https://pyfp.org/doc/icf_pyfp_summary_evaluation_report_11_30_18_final.pdf.

Rikli, R. E., & Jones, C. J. (2013). *Senior fitness test manual*, 2nd ed. Champaign, IL: Human Kinetics.

Roberton, M. A., & Halverson, L. E. (1984). *Developing children—their changing movement.* Philadelphia, PA: Lea & Febiger.

Suomi, R., & Suomi, J. (1997). Effectiveness of a training program with physical education students and experienced physical education teachers in scoring the test of gross motor development. *Perceptual and Motor Skills, 84*, 771–778.

Ulrich, D. A. (1984). The reliability of classification decisions made with the objectives based motor skill assessment instrument. *Adapted Physical Activity Quarterly, 1*, 52–60.

Ulrich, D. A. (2019). *Test of Gross Motor Development-3*. Austin, TX: Pro-Ed.

Veronese, N., Bolzetta, F., Toffanello, E. D., Zambon, G., Rui, M. D., Perissinotto, E., et al. (2014). Association between short physical performance battery and falls in older people: The Progetto Veneto Anziani study. *Rejuvenation Research*, *17*, doi.org/10.1089/rej.2013.1491.

Volpato, S., Cavalieri, M., Sioulis, F., Guerra, G., Maraldi, C., Zuliani, G., et al. (2011). Predictive value of the short physical performance battery following hospitalization in older patients. *The Journal of Gerontology, 66A*, 89–96.

Winnick, J. P. & Short, F. X. (2014). *Brockport Physical Fitness Test manual*, 2nd ed. Champaign, IL: Human Kinetics.

APPENDICES CONTENTS

APPENDIX A
Growth Charts: National Center for Health Statistics

APPENDIX B
Mean Changes in Height, Weight, and BMI Across the Lifespan

APPENDIX C
Sample Assessment Tools

APPENDIX A GROWTH CHARTS: NATIONAL CENTER FOR HEALTH STATISTICS

APPENDIX A.1 BOYS: BIRTH TO 36 MONTHS. LENGTH-FOR-AGE AND WEIGHT-FOR-AGE PERCENTILES. CDC GROWTH CHARTS: UNITED STATES

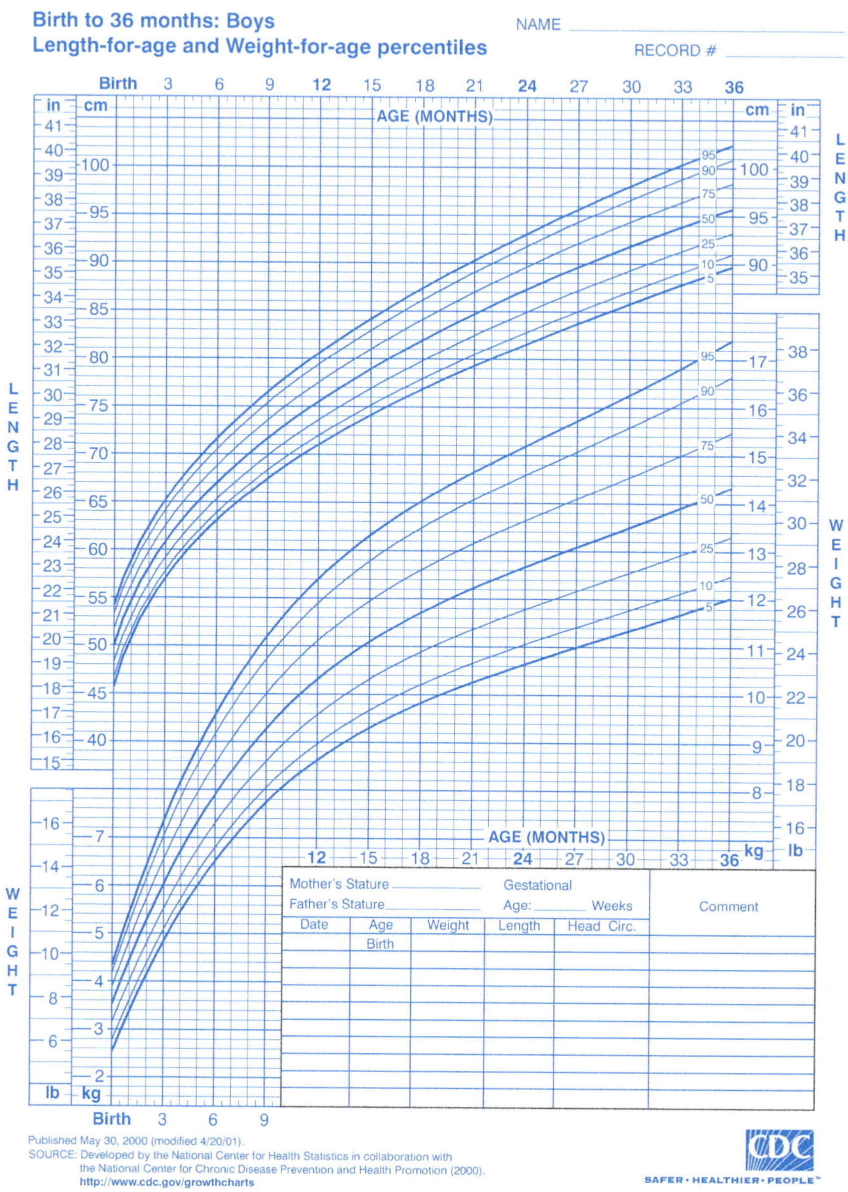

Source: Developed by the National Center for Health Statistics in collaboration with the National Center for Chronic Disease Prevention and Health Promotion (2000), www.cdc.gov/growthcharts.

APPENDIX A.2 BOYS: BIRTH TO 36 MONTHS. HEAD CIRCUMFERENCE-FOR-AGE AND WEIGHT-FOR-LENGTH PERCENTILES. CDC GROWTH CHARTS: UNITED STATES

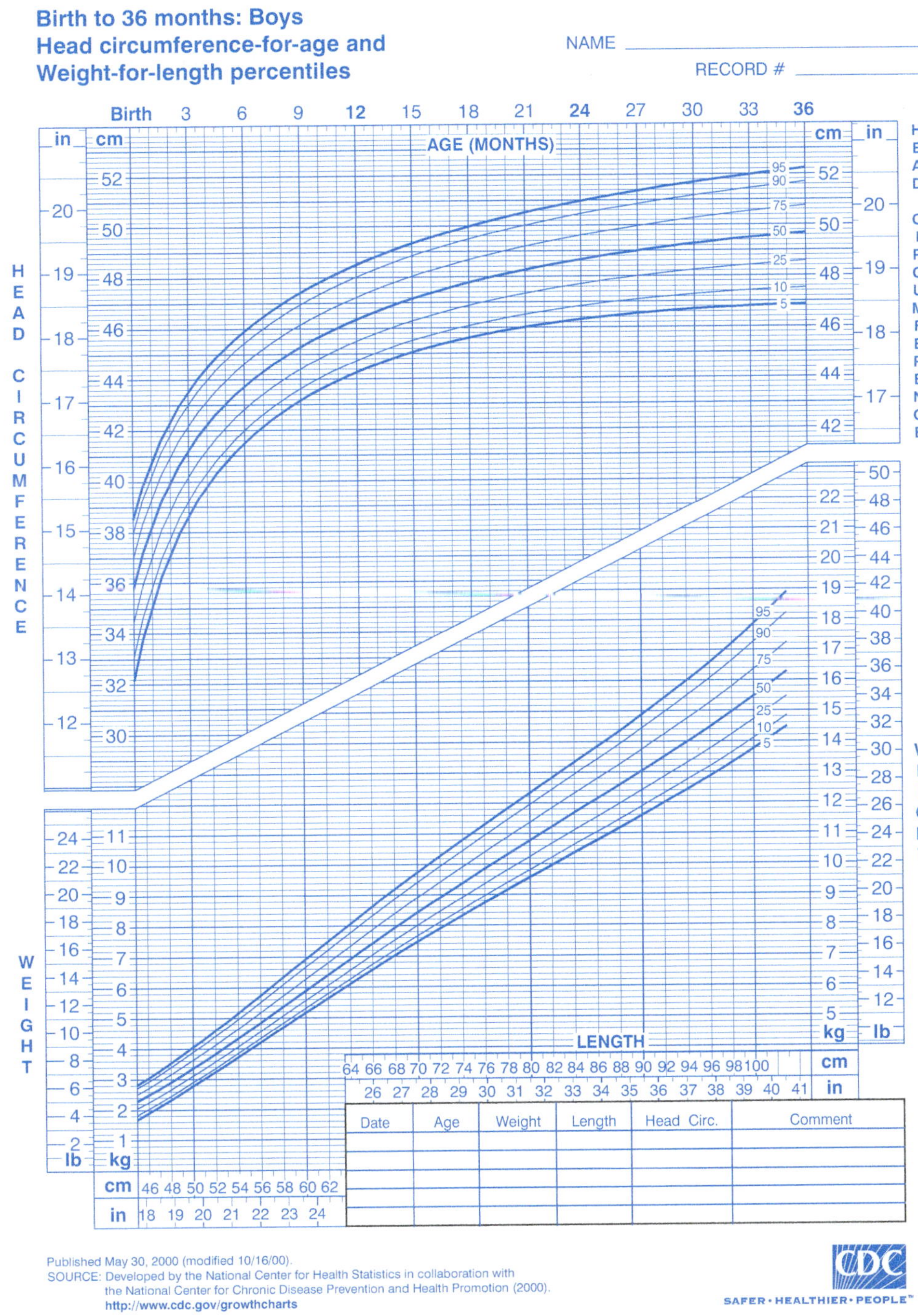

Source: Developed by the National Center for Health Statistics in collaboration with the National Center for Chronic Disease Prevention and Health Promotion (2000), www.cdc.gov/growthcharts.

APPENDIX A.3 GIRLS: BIRTH TO 36 MONTHS. LENGTH-FOR-AGE AND WEIGHT-FOR-AGE PERCENTILES. CDC GROWTH CHARTS: UNITED STATES

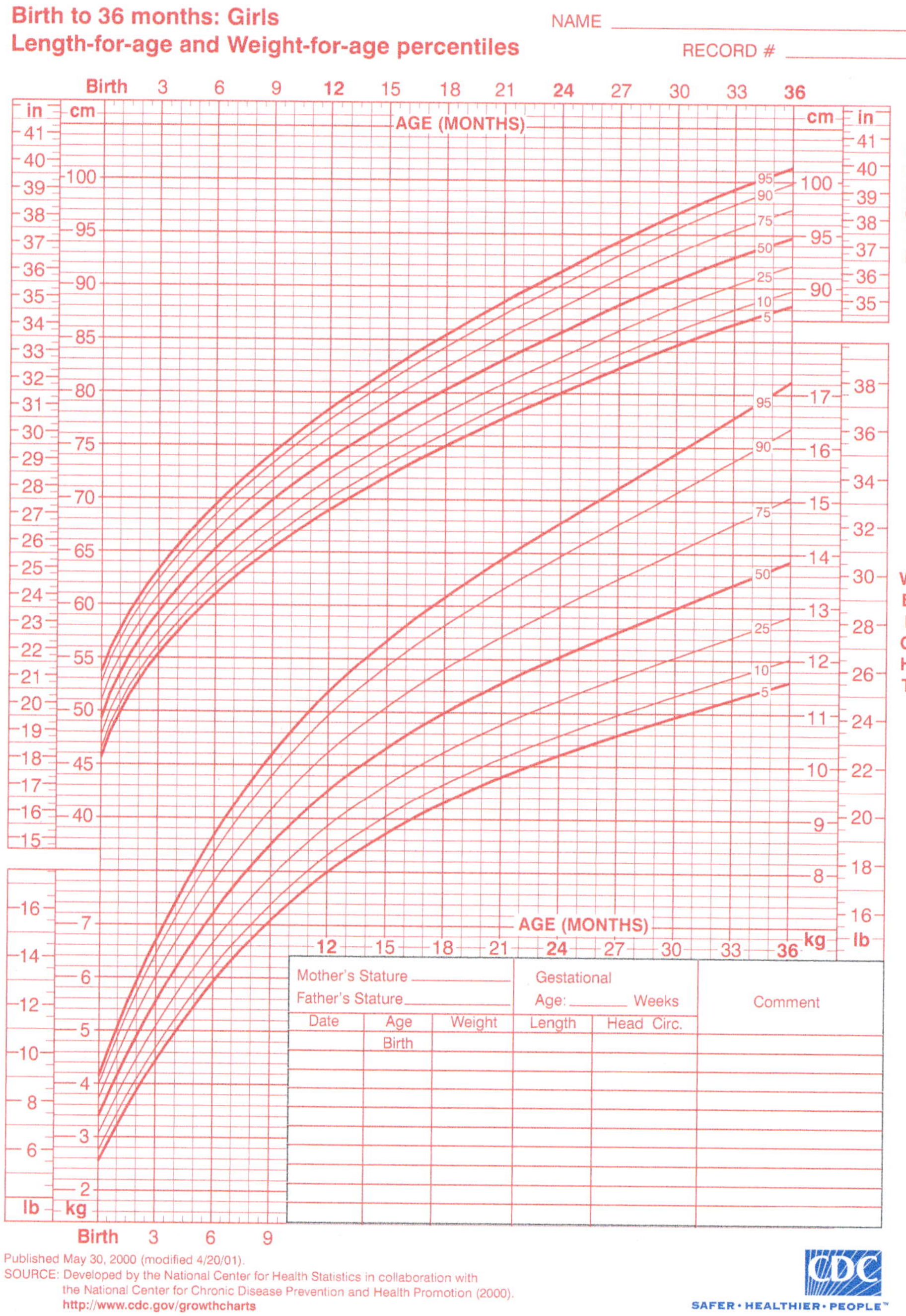

Source: Developed by the National Center for Health Statistics in collaboration with the National Center for Chronic Disease Prevention and Health Promotion (2000), www.cdc.gov/growthcharts.

APPENDIX A.4 GIRLS: BIRTH TO 36 MONTHS. HEAD CIRCUMFERENCE-FOR-AGE AND WEIGHT-FOR-LENGTH PERCENTILES. CDC GROWTH CHARTS: UNITED STATES

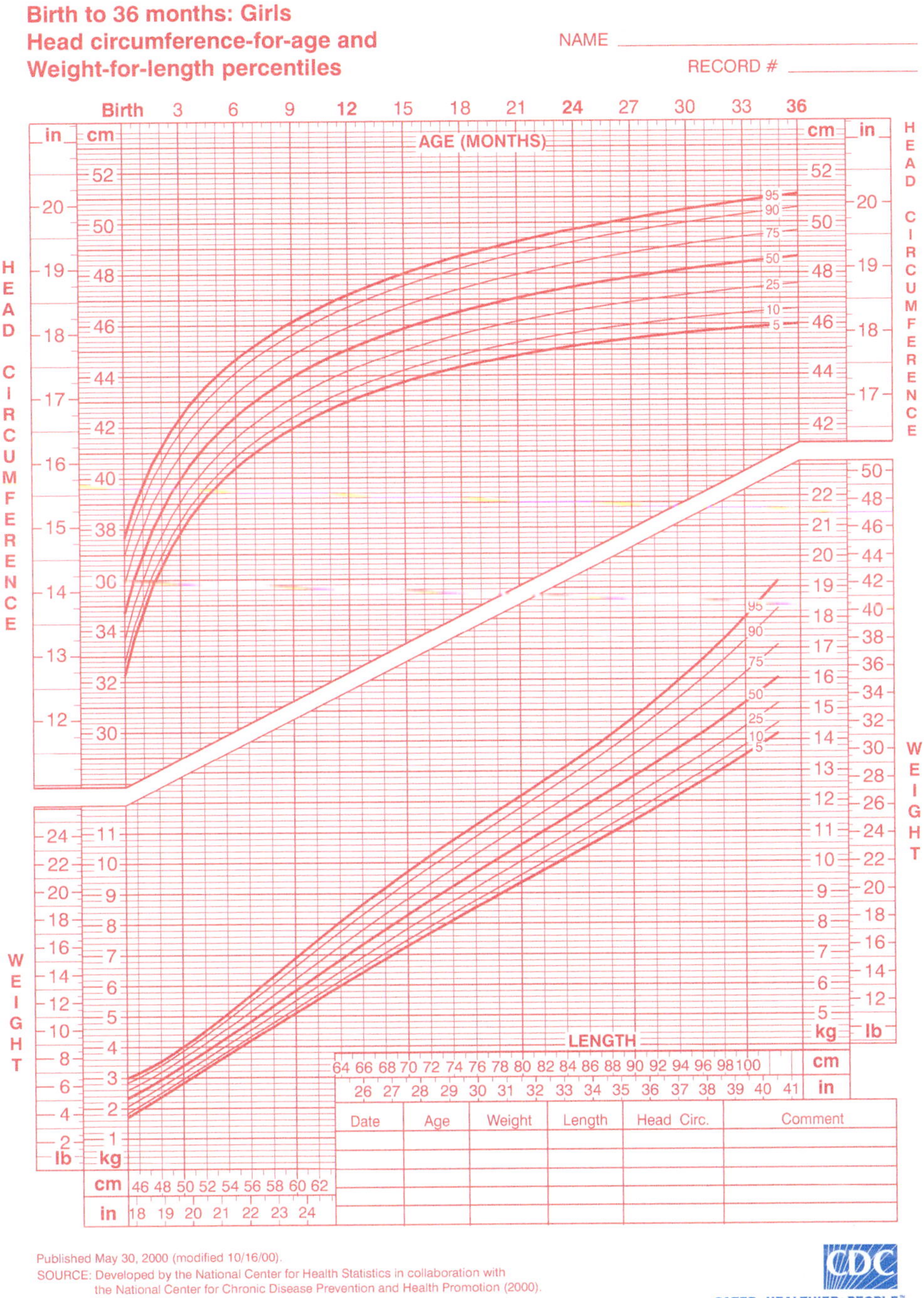

Source: Developed by the National Center for Health Statistics in collaboration with the National Center for Chronic Disease Prevention and Health Promotion (2000), www.cdc.gov/growthcharts.

APPENDIX A.5 BOYS: 2 TO 20 YEARS. STATURE-FOR-AGE AND WEIGHT-FOR-AGE PERCENTILES. CDC GROWTH CHARTS: UNITED STATES

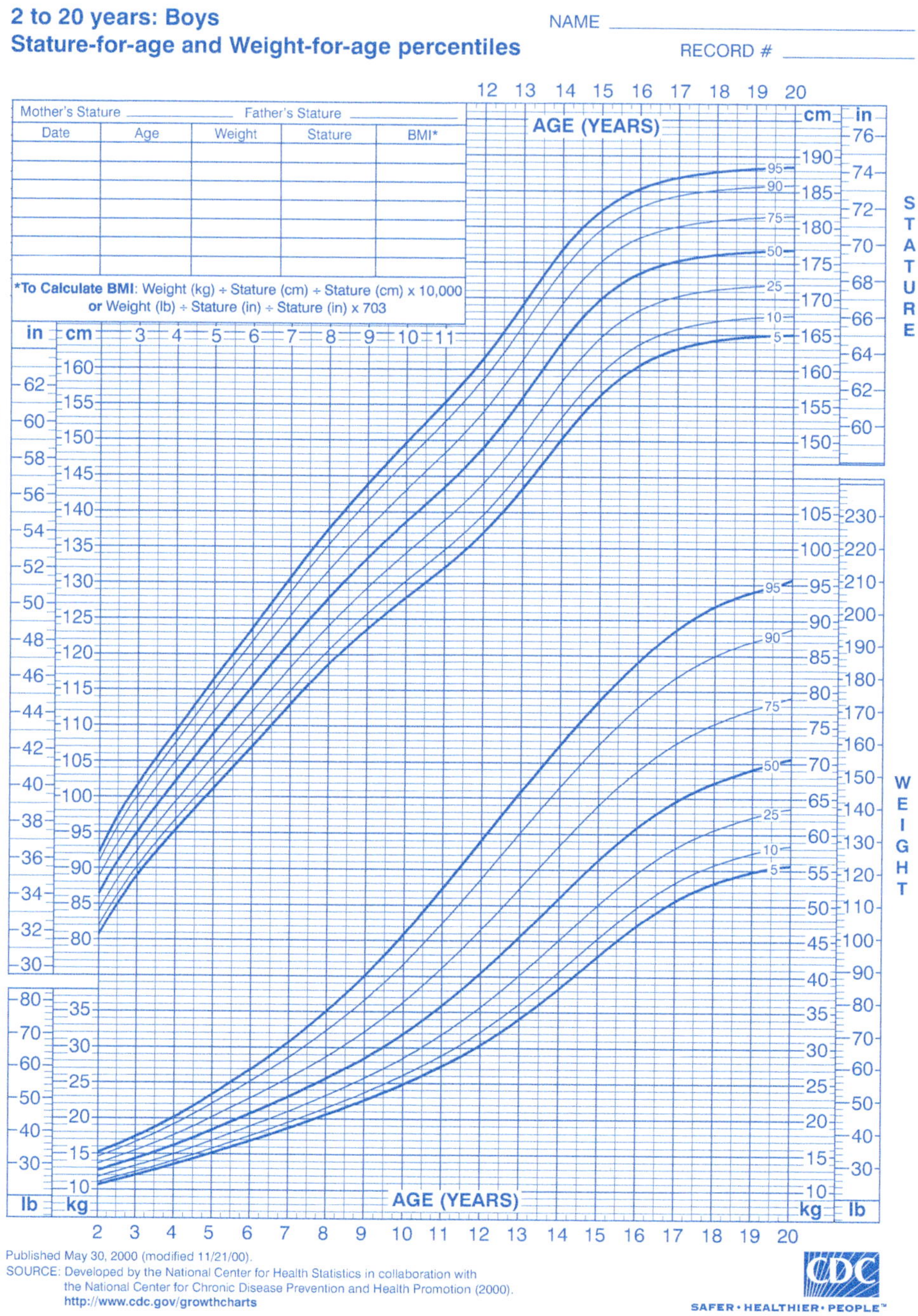

Source: Developed by the National Center for Health Statistics in collaboration with the National Center for Chronic Disease Prevention and Health Promotion (2000), www.cdc.gov/growthcharts.

APPENDIX A.6 BOYS: 2 TO 20 YEARS. BODY MASS INDEX-FOR-AGE PERCENTILES. CDC GROWTH CHARTS: UNITED STATES

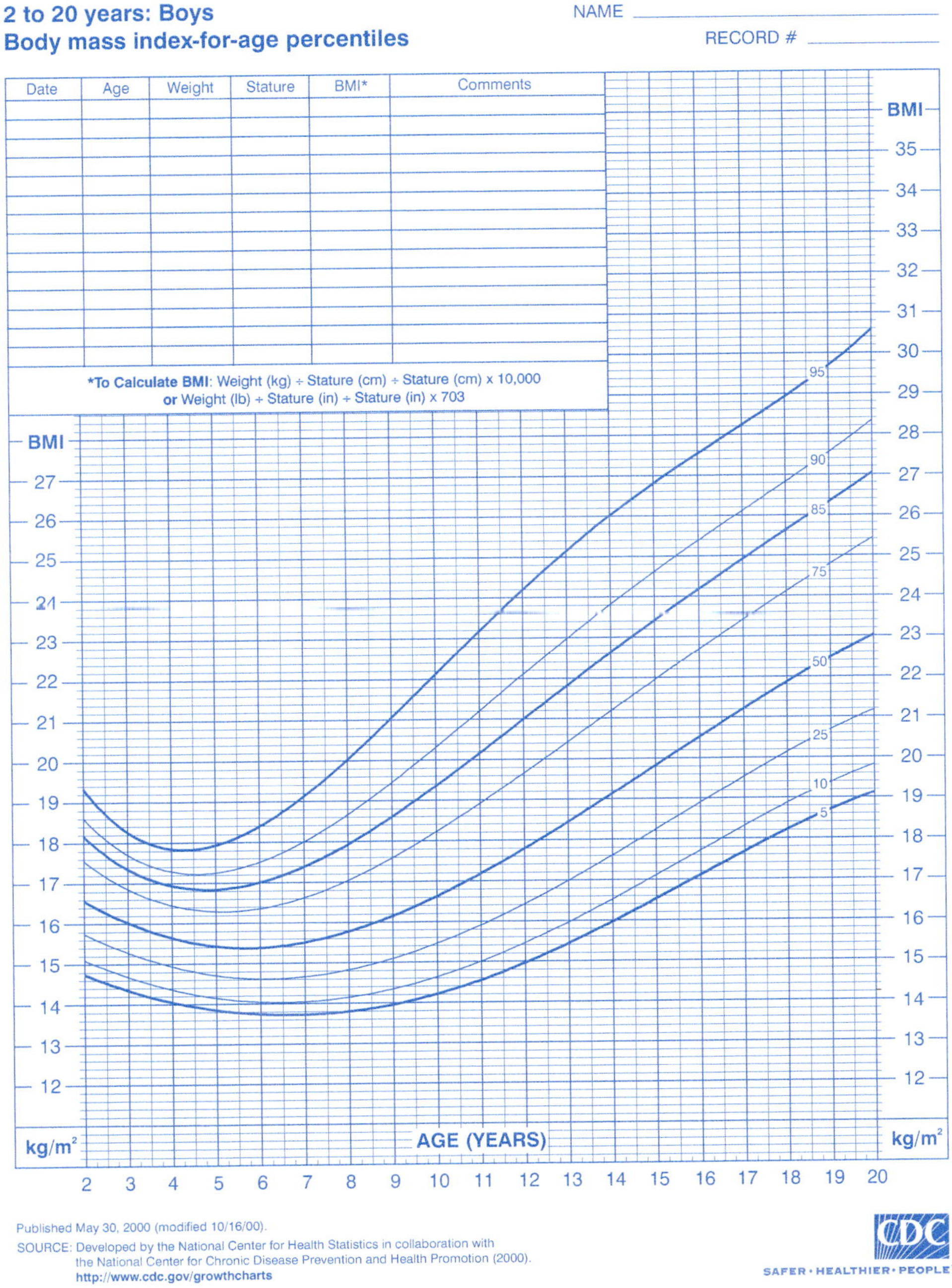

Source: Developed by the National Center for Health Statistics in collaboration with the National Center for Chronic Disease Prevention and Health Promotion (2000), www.cdc.gov/growthcharts.

APPENDIX A.7 GIRLS: 2 TO 20 YEARS. STATURE-FOR-AGE AND WEIGHT-FOR-AGE PERCENTILES. CDC GROWTH CHARTS: UNITED STATES

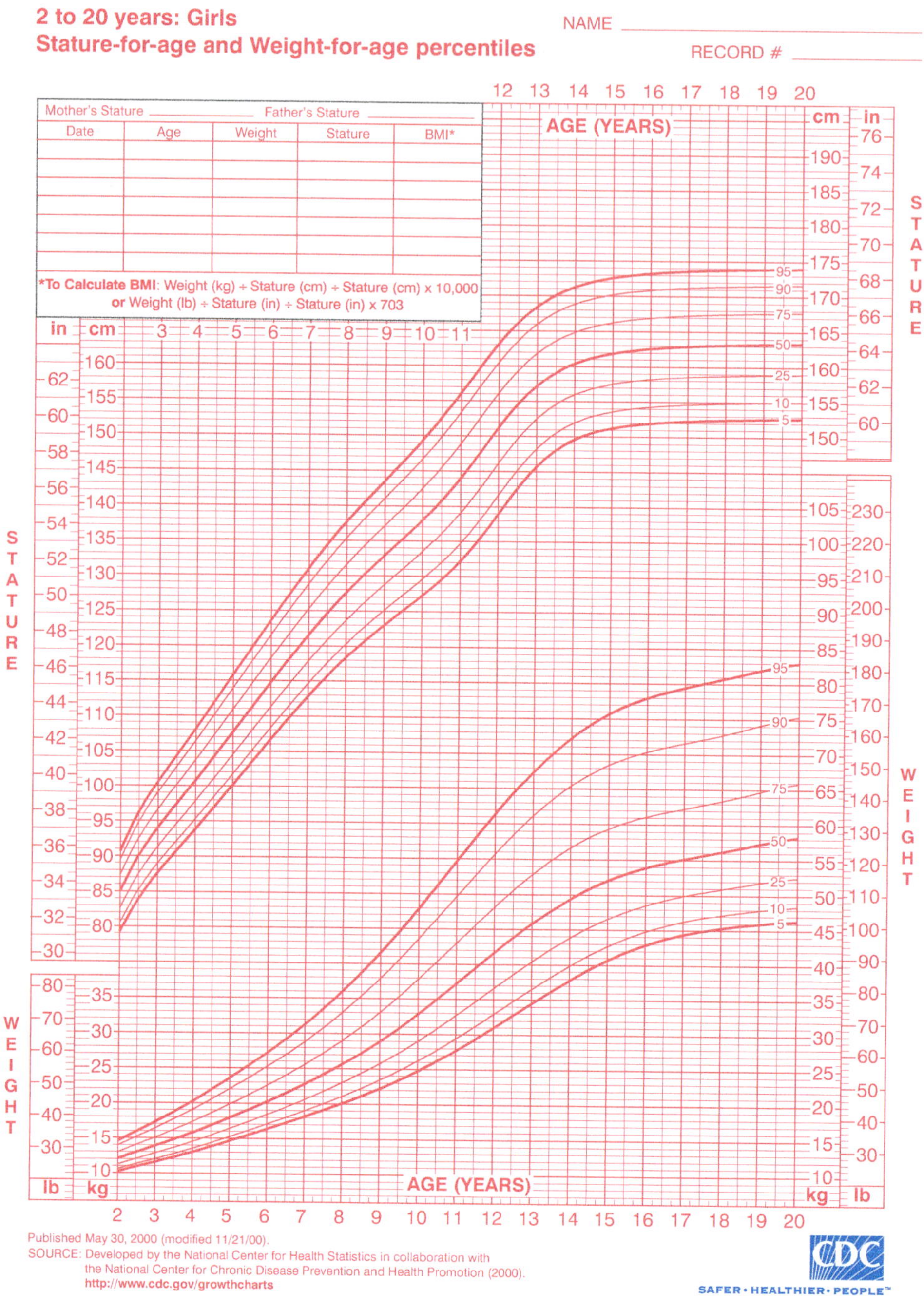

Source: Developed by the National Center for Health Statistics in collaboration with the National Center for Chronic Disease Prevention and Health Promotion (2000), www.cdc.gov/growthcharts.

APPENDIX A.8 GIRLS: 2 TO 20 YEARS. BODY MASS INDEX-FOR-AGE PERCENTILES. CDC GROWTH CHARTS: UNITED STATES

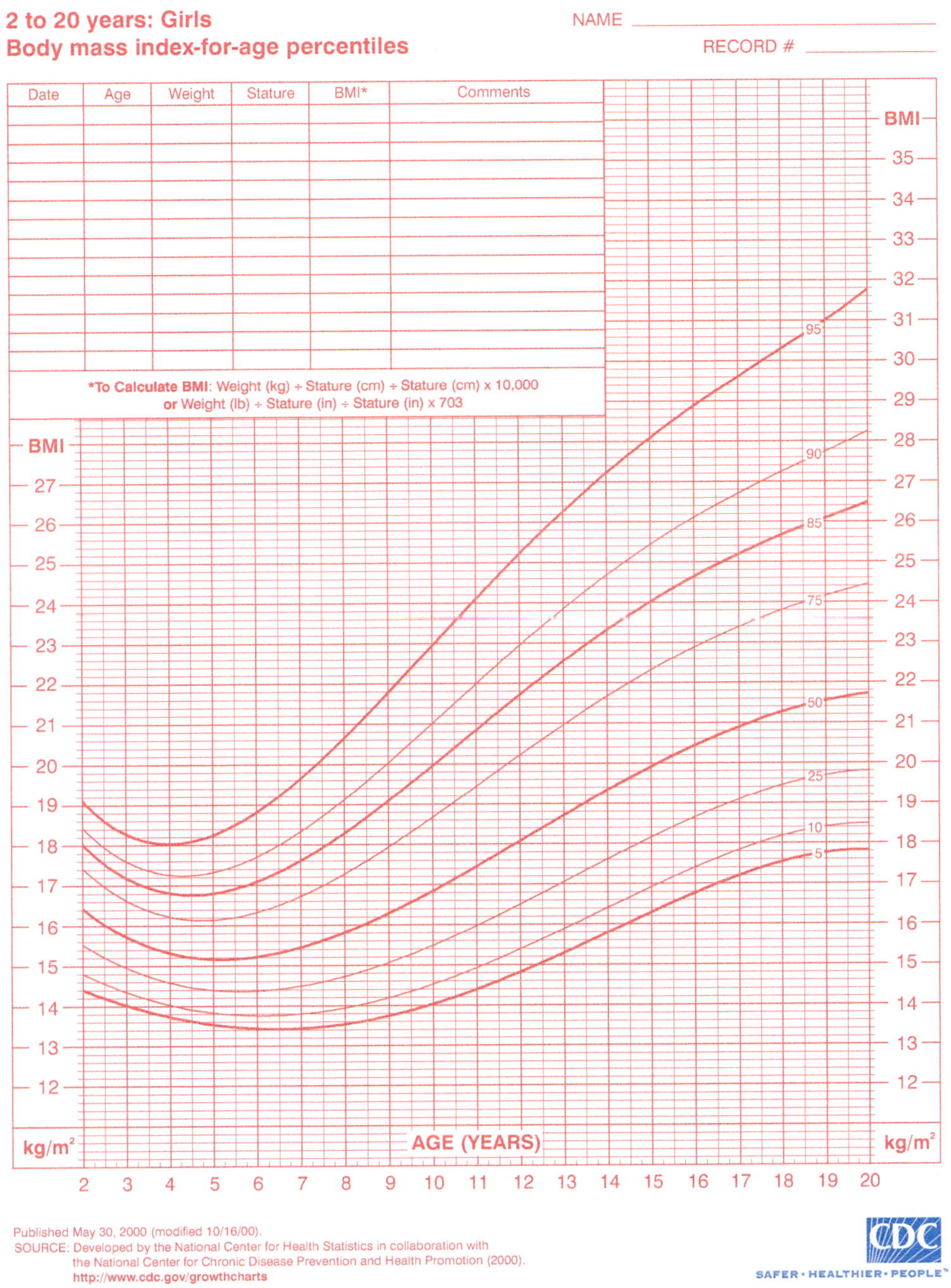

Source: Developed by the National Center for Health Statistics in collaboration with the National Center for Chronic Disease Prevention and Health Promotion (2000), www.cdc.gov/growthcharts.

APPENDIX A.9 BOYS: WEIGHT-FOR-STATURE PERCENTILES. CDC GROWTH CHARTS: UNITED STATES

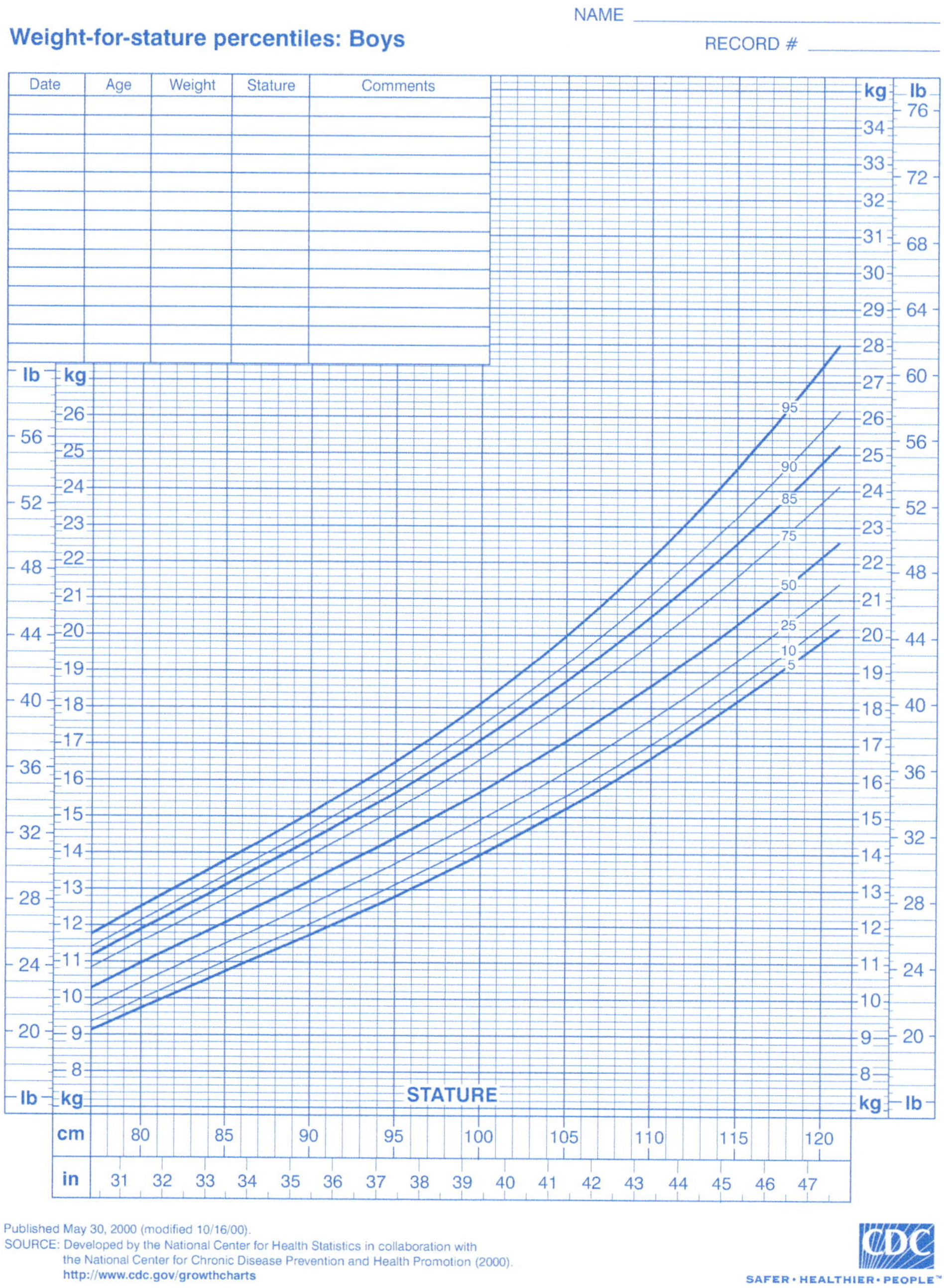

Source: Developed by the National Center for Health Statistics in collaboration with the National Center for Chronic Disease Prevention and Health Promotion (2000), www.cdc.gov/growthcharts.

APPENDIX A.10 GIRLS: WEIGHT-FOR-STATURE PERCENTILES. CDC GROWTH CHARTS: UNITED STATES

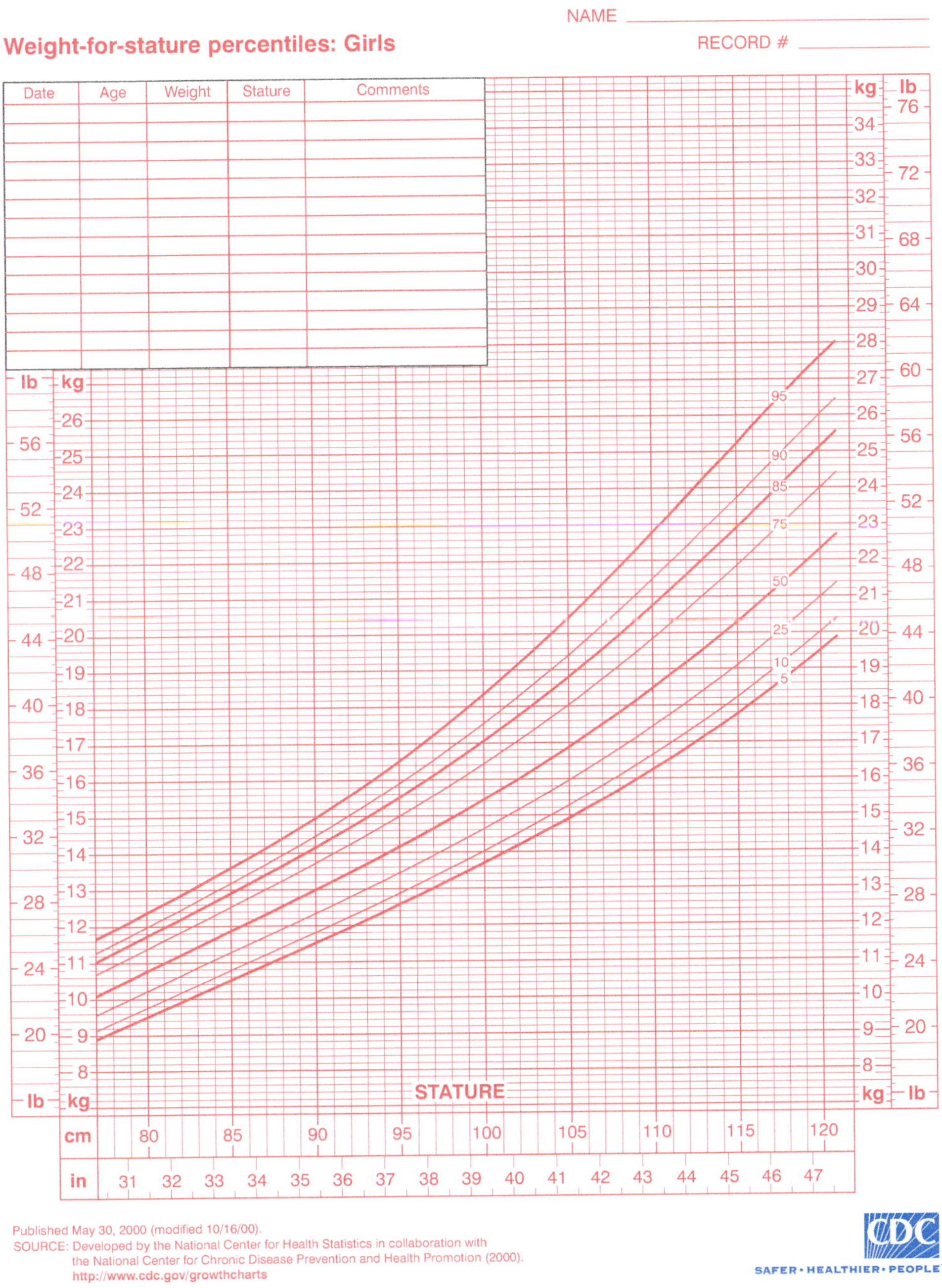

Source: Developed by the National Center for Health Statistics in collaboration with the National Center for Chronic Disease Prevention and Health Promotion (2000), www.cdc.gov/growthcharts.

APPENDIX B MEAN CHANGES IN HEIGHT, WEIGHT, AND BMI ACROSS THE LIFESPAN

APPENDIX B.1 MEAN HEIGHT* (INCHES) FOR PERSONS 2 TO 80+ YEARS OF AGE

AGE (YEARS)	MALE	FEMALE
2	36.3	35.4
3	39.0	38.6
4	42.0	41.7
5	44.8	44.2
6	47.2	46.7
7	49.8	49.0
8	51.9	51.8
9	53.7	54.2
10	56.3	56.8
11	59.2	59.3
12	61.4	61.5
13	64.3	62.4
14	66.7	63.1
15	68.3	64.4
16	68.5	63.9
17	68.9	64.0
18	69.1	63.6
19	69.4	64.2
20–29	69.4	64.1
30–39	69.5	64.3
40–49	69.4	64.1
50–59	69.3	63.7

AGE (YEARS)	MALE	FEMALE
60–69	69.0	63.2
70–79	68.1	62.7
80 yrs and over	67.6	61.3

*Based on NHANES 2011–2014.

Source: Fryar, Gu, Ogden, & Flegal (2016).

Reference

Fryar, C. D., Gu, Q., Ogden, C. L., & Flegal, K. M. (2016). Anthropometric reference data for children and adults: United States, 2011–2014. National Center for Health Statistics. *Vital Health Statistics* 3(39).

APPENDIX B.2 MEAN WEIGHT* (POUNDS) FOR PERSONS 2 TO 80+ YEARS OF AGE

AGE (YEARS)	MALE	FEMALE
2	31.3	29.3
3	35.3	34.5
4	40.8	40.3
5	46.6	45.0
6	52.8	52.4
7	61.9	58.7
8	69.4	69.9
9	74.4	82.7
10	88.7	90.9
11	107.0	104.5
12	111.6	122.9
13	133.9	122.4
14	145.2	131.4
15	157.3	141.7
16	164.1	143.3
17	165.5	148.5
18	179.4	148.2
19	174.0	150.9
20–29	186.8	161.8
30–39	198.8	172.9
40–49	201.7	173.1
50–59	199.5	174.4
60–69	199.7	168.8
70–79	189.3	165.8
80 yrs and older	174.6	141.9

*Based on NHANES 2011–2014.

Source: Fryar, Gu, Ogden, & Flegal, (2016).

Reference

Fryar, C. D. Gu, Q., Ogden, C. L., & Flegal, K. M. (2016). Anthropometric reference data for children and adults: United States, 2011–2014. National Center for Health Statistics. *Vital Health Statistics* 3(39).

APPENDIX B.3 MEAN BODY MASS INDEX FOR PERSONS 2 TO 80+ YEARS OF AGE*

AGE (YEARS)	MALE	FEMALE
2	16.8	16.6
3	16.3	16.3
4	16.2	16.2
5	16.3	16.1
6	16.5	16.7
7	17.4	17.0
8	17.9	18.1
9	18.0	19.6
10	19.5	19.5
11	21.2	20.7
12	20.6	22.6
13	22.6	22.0
14	22.8	23.2
15	23.6	24.6
16	24.5	24.6
17	24.5	25.4
18	26.3	25.7
19	25.4	25.8
20–29	27.2	27.6
30–39	28.9	29.4
40–49	29.4	29.6
50–59	29.1	30.2
60–69	29.4	29.7
70–79	28.6	29.6
80 yrs and over	26.7	26.6

*Pregnant women excluded. Based on NHANES 2011–2014.

Source: Fryar, Gu, Ogden, & Flegal, (2016).

Reference

Fryar, C. D., Gu, Q., Ogden, C. L., & Flegal, K. M. (2016). Anthropometric reference data for children and adults: United States, 2011–2014. National Center for Health Statistics. *Vital Health Statistics* 3(39).

APPENDIX C SAMPLE ASSESSMENT TOOLS

APPENDIX C.1 A DEVELOPMENTAL SEQUENCE OF MOTOR SKILLS—COMPONENT APPROACH

DEVELOPMENTAL SEQUENCE DECISION RULE CHECKLIST-OVERARM THROW FOR FORCE (© 2007, S. J. Langendorfer)

Observer ______________________ Performer Observed ____________________ Media ___________________

Observing the Overarm Throw for Force using movement component developmental sequences: For each observation question, circle **Y** for YES; **N** for NO (see additional instructions at bottom)

COMPONENT OBSERVED	OBSERVATION CRITERIA/ DECISION RULE (circle best choice)	Y	N	DEVELOPMENTAL LEVEL NAME	EVALUATIVE COMMENTS
Preparatory Arm Backswing	Does the arm move away from the throw direction? If Yes, is action a large circular motion with partially extended elbow? If Yes, is direction of the arm movement beyond the width of the shoulders? If Yes, at the point of farthest backswing are the throwing wrist and forearm pronated so the ball faces backwards? If Yes, then prep. backswing is most advanced level: #5, *lateral swing, pronated action*	Y Y Y Y	N N N N	1. No backswing 2. Shoulder/elbow flexion 3. Upward circle 4. Lateral swing, supinated action 5. Lateral swing, pronated action	
Step/Leg Action	Does at least one foot move forward? If Yes, is step with foot opposite to throw arm? If Yes, is opposite step > 50% of standing height? If Yes, step action is the most advanced level: #4, *long (≥ 50% height), contralateral step*	Y Y Y	N N N	1. No step 2. Homolateral step 3. Contralateral step 4. Long, contralateral step	

COMPONENT OBSERVED	OBSERVATION CRITERIA/ DECISION RULE (circle best choice)	Y	N	DEVELOPMENTAL LEVEL NAME	EVALUATIVE COMMENTS
Trunk Action	Does any part of trunk/pelvis turn or rotate back?	Y	N	1. No trunk rotation 2. Block rotation 3. Differentiated, pelvis-lead rotation	
	If Yes, do hips begin forward turn while shoulders are still turning backward or held back?	Y	N		
	If Yes, trunk action is the most advanced level: #3: *differentiated, pelvic-lead rotation*				
Humerus Action	Is the humerus at a 90° angle from the trunk?	Y	N	1. Humerus oblique 2. Humerus aligned, but independent 3. Humerus lag	
	If Yes, is humerus aligned 180° at front facing?	Y	N		
	If Yes, humerus action is the most advanced level: #3, *humerus lag*				
Forearm Action	Does hand with the ball appear to stop or move downward during the forward propulsive motion?	Y	N	1. No forearm lag 2. Forearm lag 3. Delayed forearm lag	
	If Yes, is deepest "lag" of ball at front facing?	Y	N		
	If Yes, forearm action is the most advanced level: #3, *delayed, forearm lag*				

Please note that an answer of NO (N) to any question assesses a performer's developmental level for that component at the level on the adjacent line in the 5th column (Developmental level name). When you answer YES (Y), then use the next question to evaluate that component further, until you *either* answer NO (N) *or* reach the last question in that component.

References

Haywood, K., & Getchell, N. (2009). Chapter 8, Development of ballistic skills (pp. 143–167). *Life span motor development* (5th ed.). Champaign, IL: Human Kinetics.

Haywood, K. M., Roberton, M. A., & Getchell, N. (2012). Chapter 7 - Development of ballistic skills (pp. 153–176). *Advanced analysis of motor development*. Champaign, IL: Human Kinetics.

Roberton, M. A., & Halverson, L. E. (1984). *Developing children: Their changing movement* (pp. 102–121). Philadelphia, PA: Lea & Febiger.

APPENDIX C.1 B DEVELOPMENTAL SEQUENCE OF MOTOR SKILLS—COMPONENT APPROACH

DEVELOPMENTAL SEQUENCE DECISION RULE CHECKLIST—ONE-HAND SIDEARM STRIKING

Observer ____________________ Performer Observed ____________________ Media ____________________

Observing the One-Hand Sidearm Striking using movement component developmental sequences: For each observation question, circle **Y** for YES; **N** for NO (see additional instructions at bottom)

COMPONENT OBSERVED	OBSERVATION CRITERIA/ DECISION RULE (circle best choice)	Y	N	DEVELOPMENTAL LEVEL NAME	EVALUATIVE COMMENTS
Preparatory Backswing Action	Does arm/implement move away from ball direction in anticipation?	Y	N	1. No backswing 2. Upward 3. Sideward 4. Cocked back	
	If Yes, does arm/implement mainly move downward or sideways and not upward over the shoulder?	Y	N		
	If Yes, does the arm/implement reach behind the body?	Y	N		
	If Yes, prep. backswing is most advanced level:				
Step/Leg Action	Does one foot make a step/ weight shift toward ball?	Y	N	1. No step 2. Back foot step 3. Partial/long step 4. Balanced contralateral step	
	If Yes, does foot closest to ball step forward (or rear foot step backward)?	Y	N		
	If Yes, is front foot step less than 1/4 body hgt?	Y	N		
	If Yes, step action is the most advanced level: *#4, balanced front foot step*				
Trunk Action	Does any part of trunk/pelvis turn/rotate backward?	Y	N	1. No rotation 2. Block rotation 3. Differentiated, pelvis-lead rotation	
	If Yes, do hips begin forward turn while shoulders are still turning backward or held back?	Y	N		
	If Yes, trunk action is the most advanced level: *#3, differentiated, pelvic-lead rotation*				

COMPONENT OBSERVED	OBSERVATION CRITERIA/ DECISION RULE (circle best choice)	Y	N	DEVELOPMENTAL LEVEL NAME	EVALUATIVE COMMENTS
Implement Lag Action	Does the implement lag momentarily during forward propulsion motion?	Y	N	1. No implement lag 2. Implement lag 3. Delayed lag	
	If Yes, is implement lag delayed until trunk front facing?	Y	N		
	If Yes, implement action is most advanced level: #3, delayed implement lag				

Please note that an answer of NO (N) to any question assesses a performer's developmental level for that component at the level on the adjacent line in the 5th column. When you answer YES (Y), then use the next question to evaluate that component further, until you *either* answer NO (N) *or* reach the last question in that component.

References

Langendorfer, S. J. (1987). Prelongitudinal screening of overarm striking development performed under two environmental conditions. In J. E. Clark & J. H. Humphrey (Eds.), *Advances in motor development research*, Volume I (pp. 17–47). New York: AMS Press.

Roberton, M. A., & Halverson, L. E. (1984). *Developing children: Their changing movement* (pp. 115–123). Philadelphia, PA: Lea & Febiger.

Used with permission of Dr. Stephen Langendorfer.

APPENDIX C.1 C DEVELOPMENTAL SEQUENCE OF MOTOR SKILLS—COMPONENT APPROACH

HYPOTHESIZED DEVELOPMENTAL SEQUENCE DECISION RULE CHECKLIST-FORCEFUL KICKING (Adapted from categories originally hypothesized by Michelle Lisy © 2002 and Mally, et al., 2011)

Observer ____________________ Performer Observed ____________________ Media ____________________

Observing **Forceful Kicking** using movement component developmental sequences: For each observation question, circle **Y** for YES; **N** for NO (see additional instructions at bottom)

COMPONENT OBSERVED	OBSERVATION CRITERIA/ DECISION RULE (circle best choice)	Y	N	DEVELOPMENTAL LEVEL NAME	EVALUATIVE COMMENTS
Approach Phase— Leg Action	Does either foot make a forward, lateral, or backward stepping action before the ball is kicked? If no,	Y	N	1. No step 2. Step after kick 3. Contralateral step 4. Contralateral leap 5. Contralateral extended leap	
	If yes, does the support foot (i.e., opposite kicking foot) take a forward step? If no,	Y	N		
	If yes, is the final support foot action a *leap* (i.e., flight phase)? If no,	Y	N		
	If yes, are the thighs spread >90° at the frame just before support foot contact? If no,	Y	N		
	If yes, then most advanced approach leg action level: #5, *contralateral extended leap*				
Follow-through Phase— Arm Action	During and after ball contact, are one or both arms held below the shoulders? If no,	Y	N	1. High guard, winging 2. Bilateral, middle guard 3. Asymmetric opposition 4. Bilateral opposition	
	If yes, after ball contact, does arm opposite kicking leg move in opposition to kicking leg? If no,	Y	N		
	If yes, after ball contact, do *both* arms move in opposition to legs? If no,	Y	N		
	If yes, then most advanced approach phase arm action level: #4, *bilateral opposition*				

COMPONENT OBSERVED	OBSERVATION CRITERIA/ DECISION RULE (circle best choice)	Y	N	DEVELOPMENTAL LEVEL NAME	EVALUATIVE COMMENTS
Follow-through Phase—Leg Action	After ball contact, does the kicking leg take a forward step? If no,	Y	N	1. No follow-through 2. Follow-through	
	If yes, do both feet leave the ground at some time after ball contact? If no,	Y	N	3. Hop/jump flight, support leg lands first	
	If yes, does the foot of the kicking leg land first? If no,	Y	N	4. Leap flight, kick leg lands first	
	If yes, then most advanced follow-through phase leg action level: #4, *leap flight, kicking leg lands first*				

Please note that an answer of NO (N) to any question assesses a performer's developmental level for that component at the level on the adjacent line in the 5th column. When you answer YES (Y), then use the next question to evaluate that component further, until you *either* answer NO (N) *or* reach the last question in that component.

References

Lisy, M. (2002). Testing developmental sequences for the forceful kick. Unpublished Masters research project, Bowling Green State University, Bowling Green, OH.

Mally, K. K., Battista, R. A., & Roberton, M. A. (2011). Distance as a control parameter for place kicking. *Journal of Human Sport & Exercise*, 6(1), 122–134.

Used with permission of Dr. Stephen Langendorfer.

APPENDIX C.1 D DEVELOPMENTAL SEQUENCE OF MOTOR SKILLS—COMPONENT APPROACH

DEVELOPMENTAL SEQUENCE DECISION RULE CHECKLIST-STANDING LONG JUMP
(Adapted from Clark & Phillips, 1985; Haywood & Getchell, 2005)

Observer ____________________ Performer Observed ________________ Media ________________

Observing the **Standing Long Jump** using movement component developmental sequences: For each observation question, circle **Y** for YES; **N** for NO (see additional instructions at bottom)

COMPONENT OBSERVED	OBSERVATION CRITERIA/ DECISION RULE (circle best choice)	Y	N	DEVELOPMENTAL LEVEL NAME	EVALUATIVE COMMENTS
Arm action	Do the arms swing forward at any time during jump?	Y	N	1. No arm action 2. Arms swing forward 3. Arms extend, then partially flex 4. Arms extend, then fully flex	
	If yes, do the arms swing backward before moving forward?	Y	N		
	If yes, do the arms swing forward in the sagittal plane and reach a point of full (180°) shoulder flexion and full (180°) elbow extension?	Y	N		
	If yes, then most advanced level: #4, *arms extend, then full flex*				
Leg action	Does the takeoff occur with two feet simultaneously?	Y	N	1. One-foot takeoff 2. Knee extension first 3. Simultaneous extension 4. Heels up first	
	If yes, do the knees and hips both extend simultaneously?	Y	N		
	If yes, do the heels rise off the ground *before* the knees extend?	Y	N		
	If yes, then the most advanced level: #4, *heels up first*				

Please note that an answer of NO (N) to any question assesses a performer's developmental level for that component at the level on the adjacent line in the 5th column. When you answer YES (Y), then use the next question to evaluate that component further, until you *either* answer NO (N) *or* reach the last question in that component.

References

Clark, J. E., & Phillips, S. J. (1985). A developmental sequence of the standing long jump. In J. Clark & J. Humphrey (Eds.), *Motor development*: Vol. 1. *Current selected research* (pp. 73–85). Princeton, NJ: Princeton Book.

Haywood, K. M. & Getchell, N. (2005). *Life span motor development* (4th ed.). Champaign, IL: Human Kinetics.

Used with permission of Dr. Stephen Langendorfer.

APPENDIX C.2 A DEVELOPMENTAL SEQUENCE OF MOTOR SKILLS INVENTORY-TOTAL BODY APPROACH

Student Name:	Date:
RUN	
Stage 1 ☐ Arms in high guard—shoulder high ☐ Short stride (shoulder width) ☐ Flat-footed contact with surface ☐ Little knee flexion ☐ Feet remain near surface	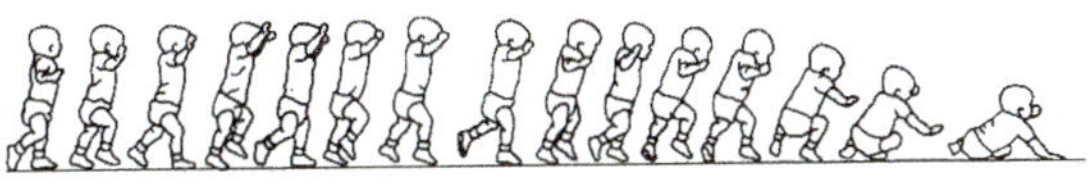
Stage 2 ☐ Arms in middle guard—waist high ☐ Stride longer than in stage 1; approaches midsagittal line ☐ Usually flat-footed contact with surface ☐ Greater knee flexion than in stage 1 ☐ Swing leg flexed with anterior-posterior movement	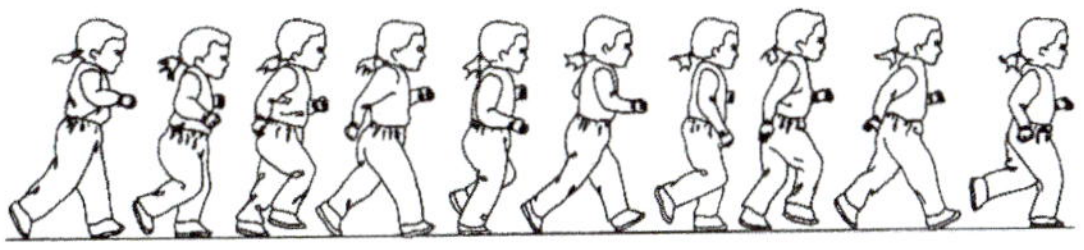
Stage 3 ☐ Arms—low guard ☐ Arm opposition—elbows nearly extended ☐ Heel-toe contact	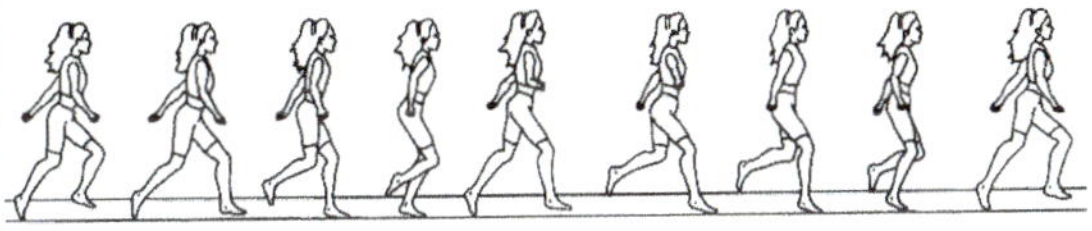
Stage 4 ☐ Heel-toe foot contact with surface at slow speeds ☐ Foot contact on metatarsal arch when sprinting ☐ Arm action in direct opposition to leg action ☐ Swing leg flexes, nearly contacts buttocks during recovery phase	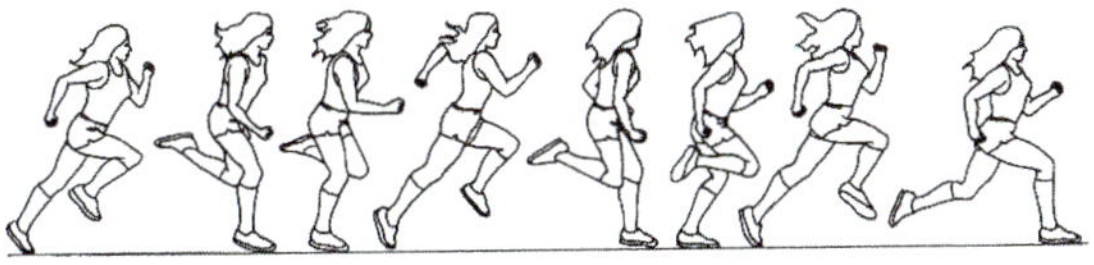
Student's Stage:	Comments:

Based on the following sources: Fountain et al. (1981); Seefeldt and Haubenstricker (1982); Seefeldt, Reuschlein, and Vogel (1972).

References

Fountain, C., Ulrich, B., Haubenstricker, J., & Seefeldt, V. (1981). Relationship of developmental stage and running velocity in children 2.5 to 5 years of age. Paper presented at the Midwest District convention of the American Alliance for Health, Physical Education, Recreation, and Dance, Chicago.

Seefeldt, V., & Haubenstricker, J. (1982). Patterns, phases, or stages: An analytical model for the study of developmental movement. In J. A. S. Kelso & J. E. Clark (Eds.), *The development of movement control and coordination*. New York: Wiley.

Seefeldt, V., Reuschlein, P., & Vogel, P. (1972). Sequencing motor skills within the physical education curriculum. Paper presented at the American Association for Health, Physical Education, and Recreation, Houston, TX.

Compiled by Dr. Larry Isaacs. All material used with permission of Dr. John Haubenstricker.

APPENDIX C.2 B DEVELOPMENTAL SEQUENCE OF MOTOR SKILLS INVENTORY – TOTAL BODY APPROACH

Student Name: Date:

STANDING LONG JUMP

Stage 1

- ☐ Vertical force greater than horizontal force (more upward than forward movement)
- ☐ Angle of takeoff is above 45°
- ☐ Arms move backward acting as a brake as legs extend forward

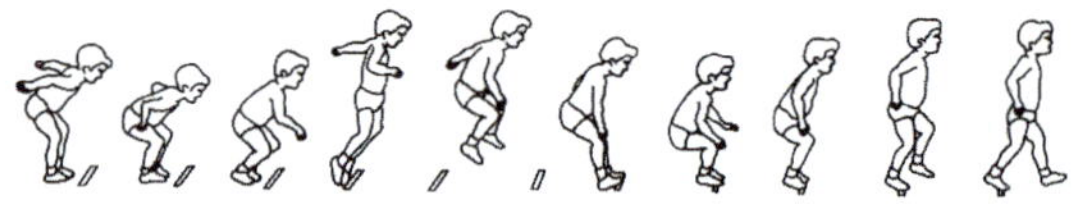

Stage 2

- ☐ During preparatory phase arms move in anterior-posterior direction
- ☐ In-flight arms move sideward (chicken wing)
- ☐ Knee and hip flexion is greater than that exhibited in stage 1
- ☐ Angle of takeoff still above 45°
- ☐ Landing made with center of gravity above base of support
- ☐ At landing thighs are perpendicular to surface

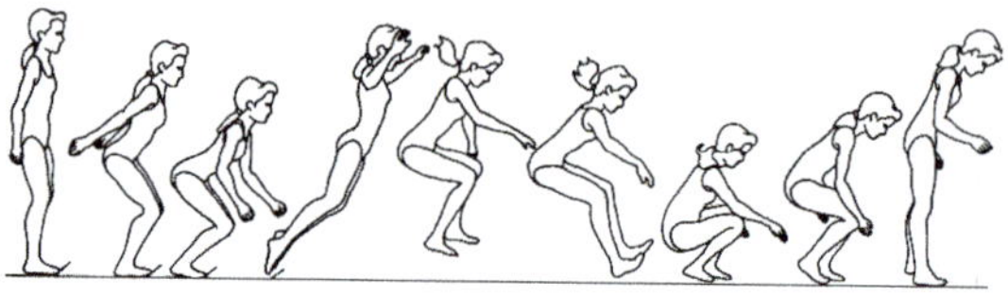

Stage 3

- ☐ Arms move forward then backward during prep phase
- ☐ Knees and hips flex fully prior to takeoff
- ☐ At takeoff arms extend forward but do not exceed head height
- ☐ Possible full knee extension at takeoff
- ☐ Angle of takeoff remains above 45°
- ☐ At landing thigh remains less than parallel to landing surface
- ☐ At landing center of gravity is near base of support

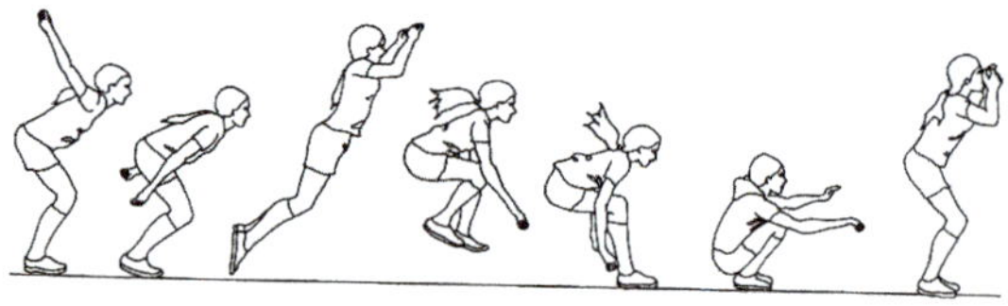

Stage 4

- ☐ At takeoff, arms vigorously extended forward and upward, above head level
- ☐ At takeoff, hip and knees fully extended
- ☐ Angle of takeoff is 45° or less
- ☐ In preparation for landing, arms brought downward and legs thrust forward, thighs parallel to surface
- ☐ At landing, center of gravity far behind base of support at foot contact, knees flex, arms thrust forward to maintain momentum

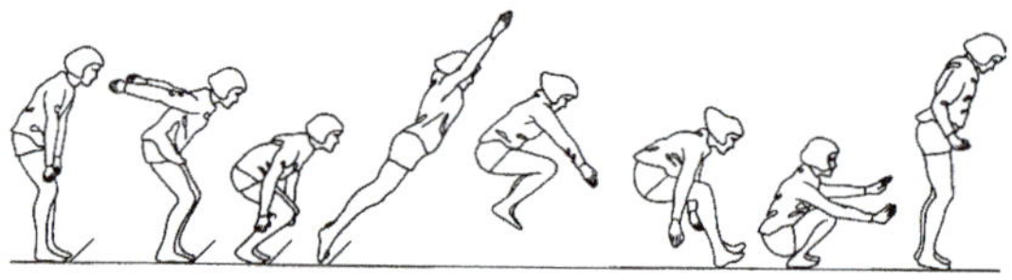

Student's Stage: Comments:

Based on the following sources: Haubenstricker, Seefeldt, and Branta (1983); Seefeldt and Haubenstricker (1982); Seefeldt, Reuschlein, and Vogel (1972).

References

Haubenstricker, J., Seefeldt, V., & Branta, C. (1983). Preliminary validation of a developmental sequence for the standing long jump. Paper presented at the annual convention of the American Alliance for Health, Physical Education, Recreation, and Dance, Minneapolis.

Seefeldt, V., & Haubenstricker, J. (1982). Patterns, phases, or stages: An analytical model for the study of developmental movement. In J. A. S. Kelso & J. E. Clark (Eds.), *The development of movement control and coordination*. New York: Wiley.

Seefeldt, V., Reuschlein, P., & Vogel, P. (1972). Sequencing motor skills within the physical education curriculum. Paper presented at the American Association for Health, Physical Education, and Recreation, Houston, TX.

Compiled by Dr. Larry Isaacs. All material used with permission of Dr. John Haubenstricker.

APPENDIX C.2 C DEVELOPMENTAL SEQUENCE OF MOTOR SKILLS INVENTORY – TOTAL BODY APPROACH

Student Name: Date:

HOP

Stage 1

- ☐ Nonsupport knee flexed at 90° or less, thigh parallel to surface
- ☐ Nonsupport foot in front of body
- ☐ Body upright with arms flexed at elbows
- ☐ Hands held near shoulders, slightly to side
- ☐ Limited force production, little height or distance achieved in a single hop

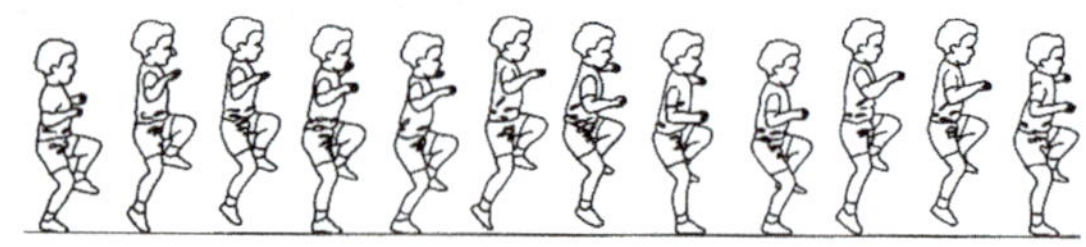

Stage 2

- ☐ Nonsupport knee fully flexed so foot is near buttocks
- ☐ Thigh of nonsupport leg nearly parallel to surface
- ☐ Truck slightly flexed at hip, causing slight forward lean
- ☐ Considerable height achieved by flexing and extending support leg
- ☐ Arms participate vigorously in force production, moving up and down bilaterally
- ☐ Thigh of nonsupport leg aids force production by flexing at hip joint
- ☐ Flexion at hips and support knees absorbs force of landing
- ☐ Can generally perform two to four hops before losing balance

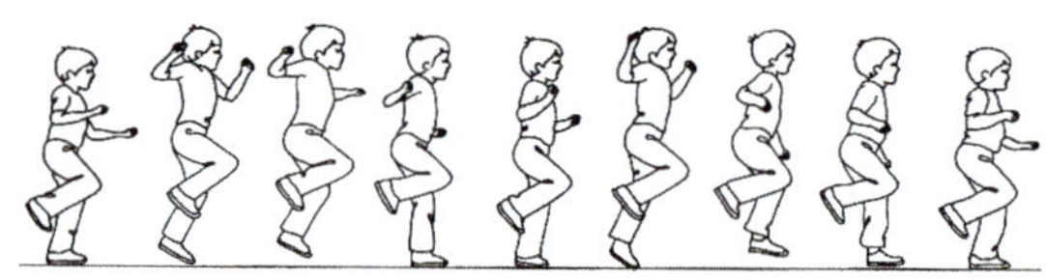

Stage 3

- ☐ Nonsupport thigh vertical with knee flexed at 90° or less
- ☐ Greater forward body lean than in stages 1 and 2, hips further in front of support leg at takeoff
- ☐ Greater distance achieved in relation to height of hop
- ☐ Arms moved upward during the force production phase

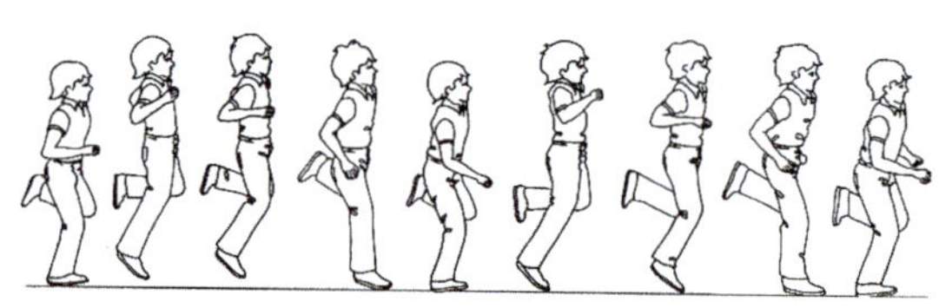

Stage 4

- ☐ Nonsupport knee flexed 90° or less
- ☐ Nonsupport leg swings forward and backward like pendulum to aid force production
- ☐ Arms positioned close to sides of body, elbows flexed at 90°
- ☐ As nonsupport leg increases force production, force production of arms diminishes

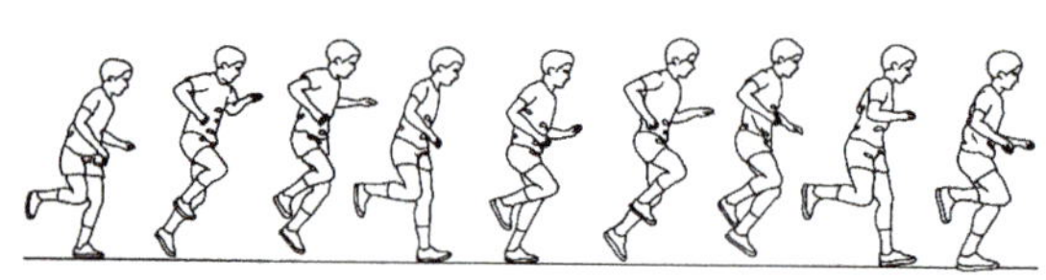

Student's Stage: Comments:

Based on the following sources: Haubenstricker, Henn, and Seefeldt (1975); Haubenstricker et al. (1989); Seefeldt and Haubenstricker (1974, 1982).

References

Haubenstricker, J., Henn, J., & Seefeldt, V. (1975). Developmental sequence of hopping. Rev. ed. Unpublished materials, Michigan State University, East Lansing, MI.

Haubenstricker, J., Branta, C., Seefeldt, V., Brakora, L., & Kiger, J. (1989). Prelongitudinal screening of a developmental sequence for hopping. Paper presented at the annual convention of the American Alliance for Health, Physical Education, Recreation, and Dance, Boston.

Seefeldt, V., & Haubenstricker, J. (1974). Developmental sequence of hopping. Unpublished materials, Michigan State University, East Lansing, MI.

Seefeldt, V., & Haubenstricker, J. (1982). Patterns, phases, or stages: An analytical model for the study of developmental movement. In J. A. S. Kelso & J. E. Clark (Eds.), *The development of movement control and coordination*. New York: Wiley.

Compiled by Dr. Larry Isaacs. All material used with permission of Dr. John Haubenstricker.

APPENDIX C.2 D DEVELOPMENTAL SEQUENCE OF MOTOR SKILLS INVENTORY – TOTAL BODY APPROACH

Student Name:	Date:
GALLOP	
Stage 1 ☐ Pattern resembles a rhythmically uneven run, can revert to traditional running pattern ☐ Relatively fast tempo with inconsistent rhythm ☐ Trail leg crosses in front of lead leg during airborne phase and remains in front at contact ☐ Trail leg flexed at $<45^{\circ}$ during airborne phase; both feet generally contact floor in a heel-toe pattern, although either may strike surface flat-footed	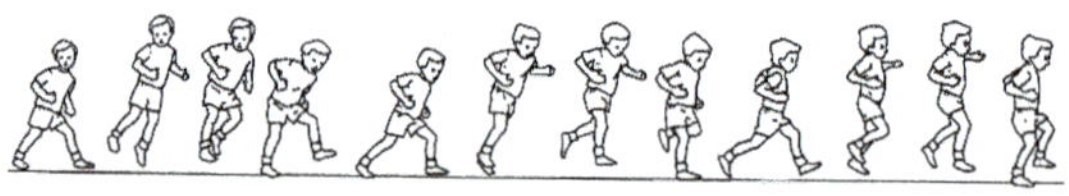
Stage 2 ☐ Pattern slow-to-moderate tempo; rhythm can appear choppy ☐ Trail leg in front of, adjacent to, or behind lead leg during airborne phase; at contact always adjacent to or behind lead leg ☐ Trail leg extended during airborne phase, often causing trail foot to turn out and lead leg to flex at $<45^{\circ}$ ☐ Feet usually contact floor in a heel-toe/heel-toe or toe/toe combination; transfer of weight appears stiff and exaggerated ☐ Vertical component often exaggerated as trunk extends to lift body up	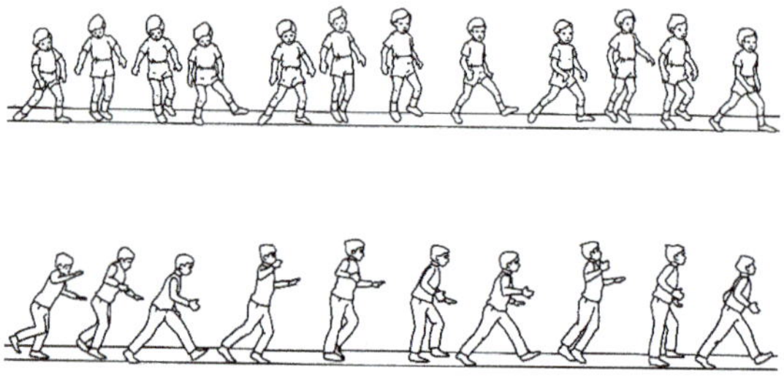
Stage 3 ☐ Pattern smooth, rhythmical, executed at moderate tempo ☐ Trail leg may cross in front of or move adjacent to lead leg during airborne phase; placed adjacent to or behind lead leg at contact ☐ Both lead and trail legs flexed at $<45^{\circ}$, feet close to surface during airborne phase ☐ Lead foot meets surface with heel-toe pattern; transfer of weight to ball of trail foot	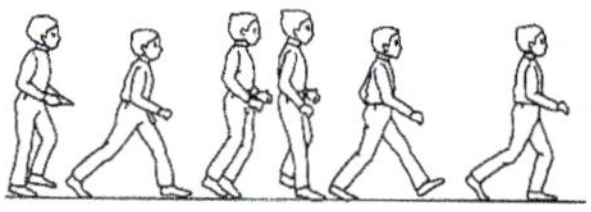
Student's Stage:	Comments:

Based on the following source: Sapp (1980).

Reference

Sapp, M. (1980). The development of galloping in young children: A preliminary study. Unpublished master's project, Michigan State University, East Lansing, MI.

Compiled by Dr. Larry Isaacs. All material used with permission of Dr. John Haubenstricker.

APPENDIX C.2 E DEVELOPMENTAL SEQUENCE OF MOTOR SKILLS INVENTORY – TOTAL BODY APPROACH

Student Name: ______________________ Date: ______________________

SKIP

Stage 1 □ Deliberate step-hop pattern employed with occasional double hop □ Little effective use of the arms to provide momentum □ Exaggerated step or leap present during transfer of weight from limb to limb □ Total action appears to be segmented	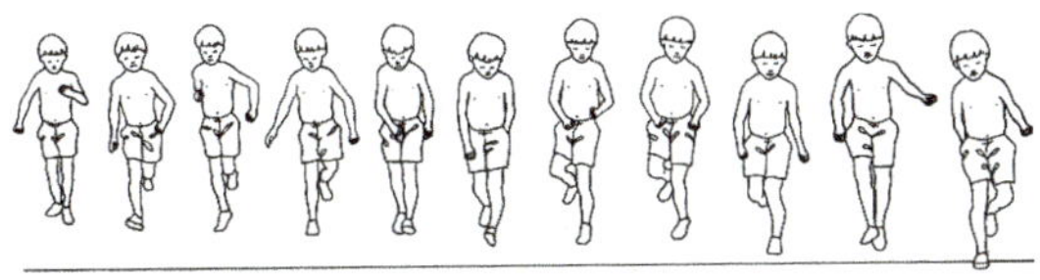
Stage 2 □ Rhythmical transfer of weight during step phase □ Increased use of arms in providing forward and upward momentum □ Vertical component exaggerated while executing the hop	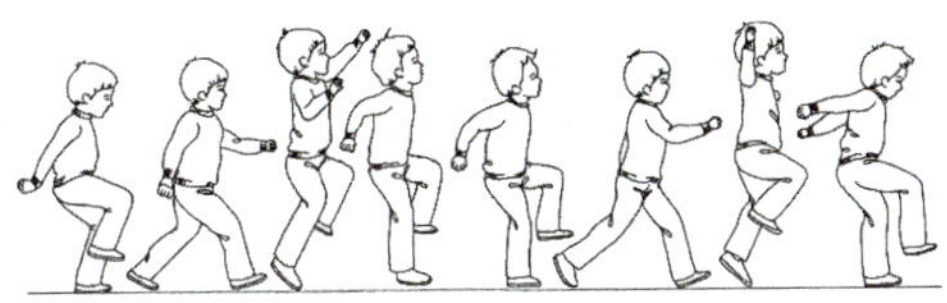
Stage 3 □ Rhythmical transfer of weight during all phases □ Reduced arm action during the transfer of weight phase □ Foot of supporting limb carried near the surface during the hopping phase	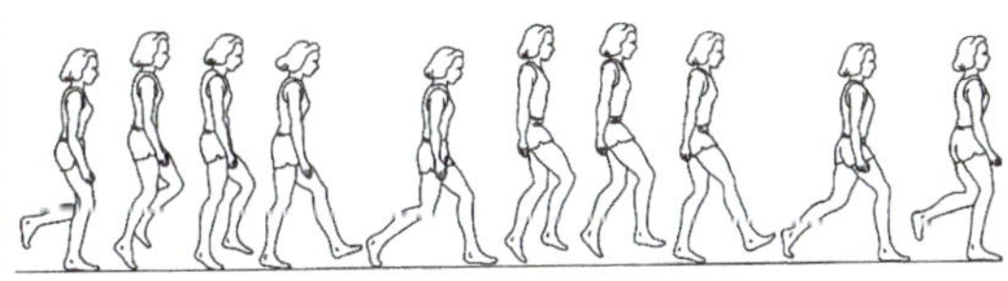
Student's Stage:	Comments:

Based on the following sources: Sapp (1980); Seefeldt and Haubenstricker (1974, 1982).

References

Sapp, M. (1980). The development of galloping in young children: A preliminary study. Unpublished master's project, Michigan State University, East Lansing, MI.

Seefeldt, V., & Haubenstricker, J. (1974). Developmental sequence of hopping. Unpublished materials, Michigan State University, East Lansing, MI.

Seefeldt, V., & Haubenstricker, J. (1982). Patterns, phases, or stages: An analytical model for the study of developmental movement. In J. A. S. Kelso & J. E. Clark (Eds.), *The development of movement control and coordination*. New York: Wiley.

Compiled by Dr. Larry Isaacs. All material used with permission of Dr. John Haubenstricker.

APPENDIX C.2 F DEVELOPMENTAL SEQUENCE OF MOTOR SKILLS INVENTORY – TOTAL BODY APPROACH

Student Name: Date:

THROW

Stage 1 ☐ Throwing motion essentially posterior-anterior in direction ☐ Feet usually stationary during throw ☐ Little to no trunk rotation ☐ Ball projection force usually comes from hip flexion, shoulder protraction, and elbow extension	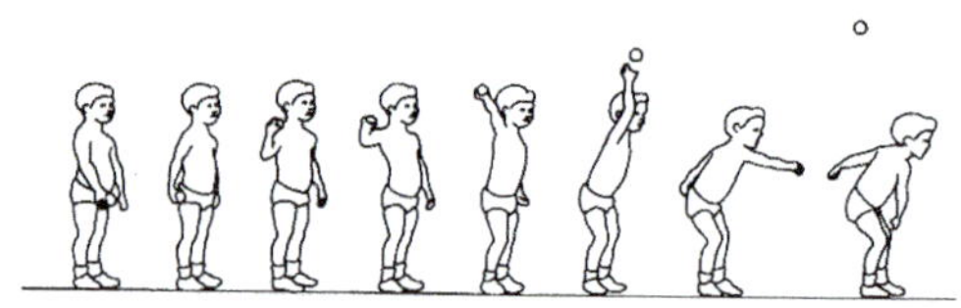
Stage 2 ☐ Most distinctive feature: Rotation of body about imaginary vertical axis with hips, spine, and shoulders rotating as one unit ☐ Forward step with ipsilateral or contralateral pattern ☐ Arm brought forward in transverse plane (resembling "sling" rather than throw)	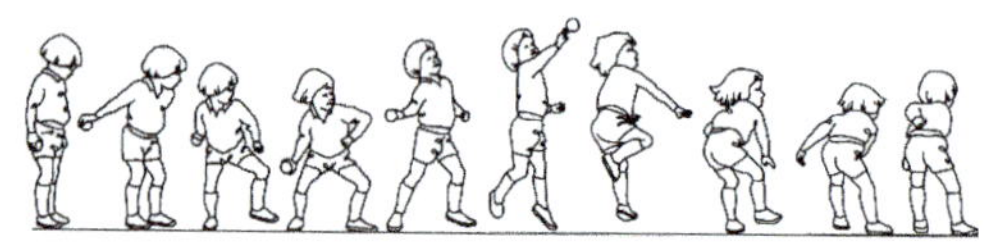
Stage 3 ☐ Most distinctive feature: Ipsilateral arm-leg action ☐ Arm moves above shoulder by vertical and posterior motion at time of step ☐ Little or no rotation of spine and hips in preparation for throw ☐ Follow-through phase includes flexion at hip joint, some trunk rotation toward side opposite throwing arm	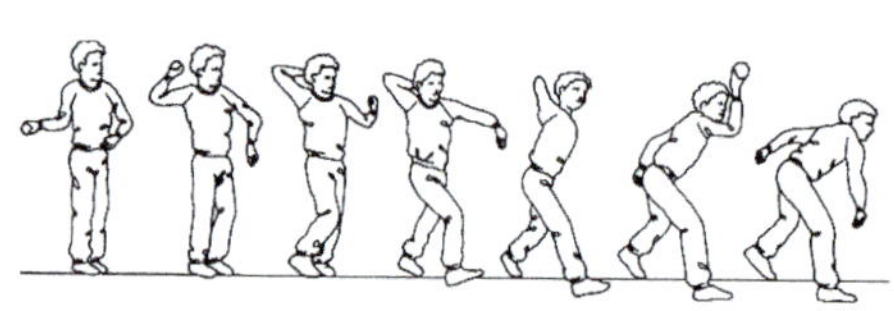
Stage 4 ☐ Forward step taken with leg opposite throwing arm (contralateral) ☐ During contralateral step, throwing arm moved in vertical and posterior direction ☐ During wind-up phase, little to no rotation of hips and spine (resembles look of stages 1 and 3) ☐ During force production phase, contralateral step results in wide base of support and greater stability	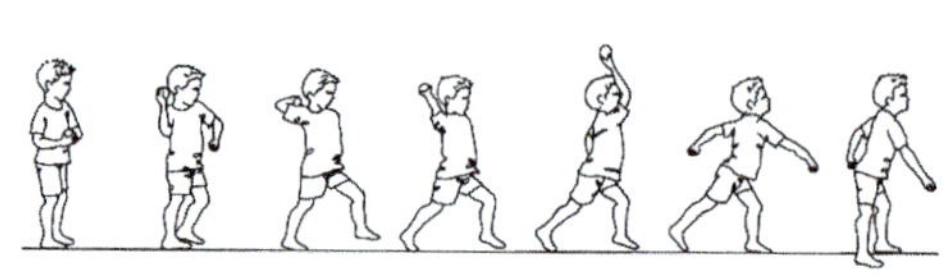
Stage 5 ☐ During wind-up phase, throwing hand moves downward then backward as contralateral hand moves forward ☐ Hips and spine rotate ☐ Contralateral leg strikes surface as hips, spine, and shoulder begin sequential derotation ☐ Contralateral leg begins extension at knee providing equal and opposite reaction to throwing arm	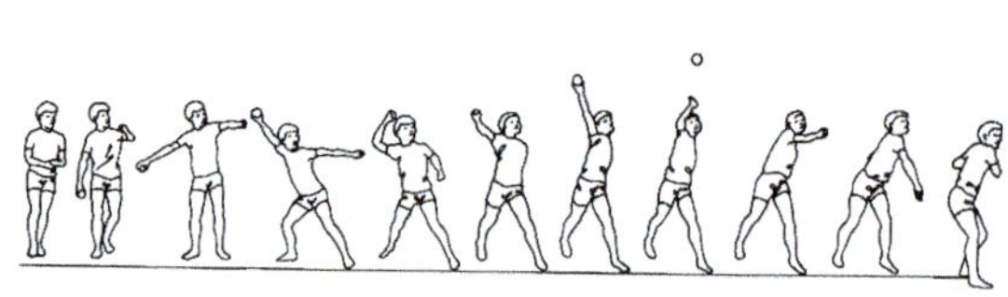

Student Name:	Date:
THROW	
☐ Arm opposite throwing limb moves forcefully toward body to assist in equal and opposite reaction	
Student's Stage:	Comments:

Based on the following sources: Haubenstricker, Branta, and Seefeldt (1983); Seefeldt and Haubenstricker (1976, 1982); Seefeldt, Reuschlein, and Vogel (1972).

References

Haubenstricker, J., Branta, C. & Seefeldt, V. (1983). Preliminary validation of a developmental sequence for throwing and catching. Paper presented at the annual convention of the North American Society for the Psychology of Sport and Physical Activity, East Lansing, MI.

Seefeldt, V., & Haubenstricker, J. (1976). Developmental sequence of throwing. Rev. ed. Unpublished manuscript. Michigan State University, East Lansing, MI.

Seefeldt, V., & Haubenstricker, J. (1982). Patterns, phases, or stages: An analytical model for the study of developmental movement. In J. A. S. Kelso & J. E. Clark (Eds.), *The development of movement control and coordination*. New York: Wiley.

Seefeldt, V., Reuschlein, P., & Vogel, P. (1972). Sequencing motor skills within the physical education curriculum. Paper presented at the American Association for Health, Physical Education, and Recreation, Houston, TX.

Compiled by Dr. Larry Isaacs. All material used with permission of Dr. John Haubenstricker.

APPENDIX C.2 G DEVELOPMENTAL SEQUENCE OF MOTOR SKILLS INVENTORY – TOTAL BODY APPROACH

Student Name:	Date:
CATCH	
Stage 1 ☐ Arms presented in front of body, elbows extended, palms facing upward or inward ☐ As ball contacts hands or arms, elbows flexed and arms and hands attempt to secure ball by holding it against chest	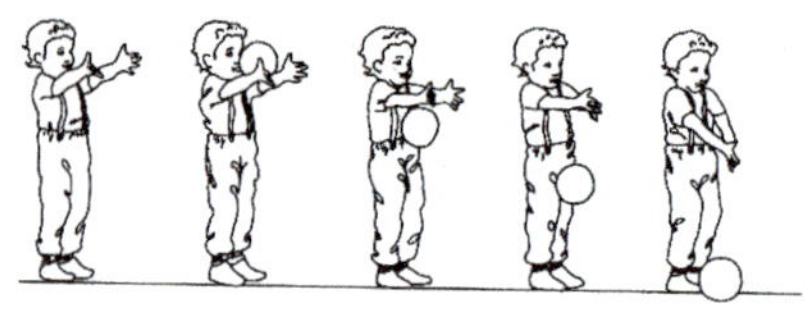
Stage 2 ☐ Arms in front of body, elbows extended or slightly flexed ☐ As ball approaches, arms begin encircling motion that culminates by securing ball against chest ☐ Arm action initiated prior to all-arm contact	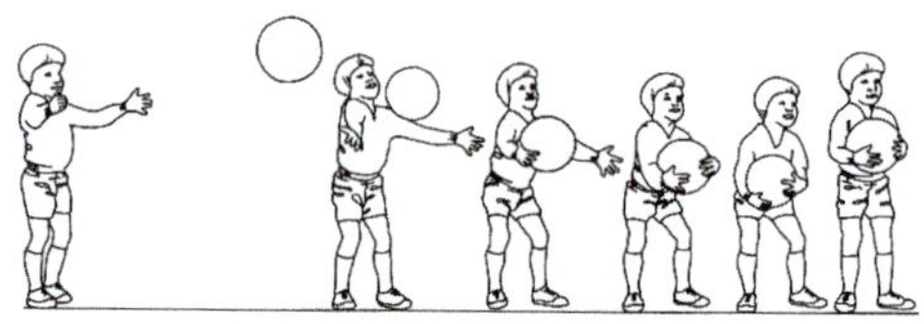
Stage 3 ☐ Arms slightly flexed, extended at shoulder ☐ Substage 1: Uses chest as first contact with ball, attempts to hold ball against chest with hands and arms ☐ Substage 2: Attempts to catch ball with hands. Upon failure, ball is maneuvered to chest, controlled by hands and arms	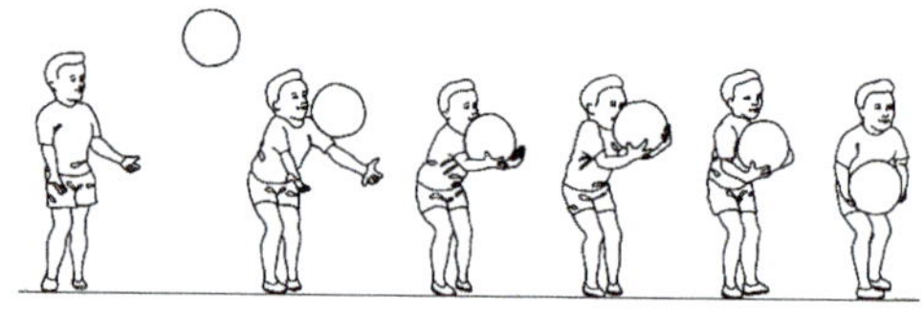
Stage 4 ☐ Preparation is made to receive ball by flexing elbows and presenting arms ahead of frontal plane ☐ Elbows may be kept by sides and flexed simultaneously as they move to meet ball ☐ Catch is made with hands only	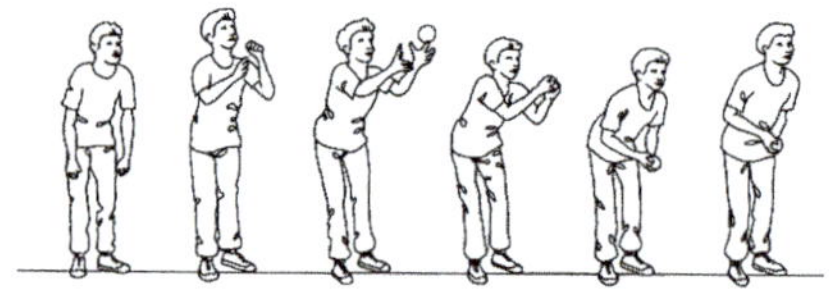
Stage 5 ☐ Same upper segmental actions as described in stage 4 ☐ In stage 5 performer changes base of support to receive ball	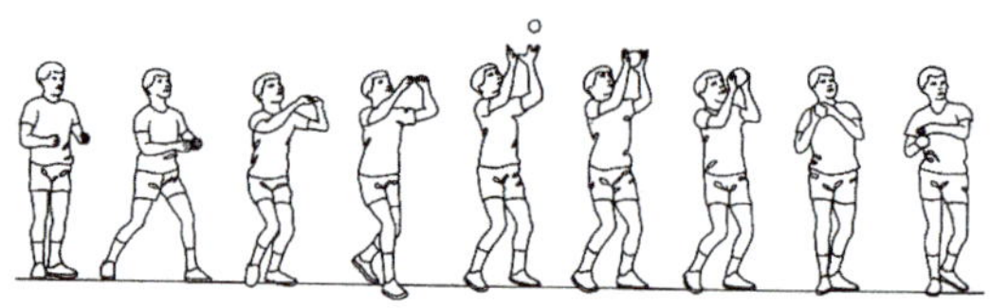
Student's Stage:	Comments:

Based on the following sources: Haubenstricker, Branta, and Seefeldt (1983); Seefeldt (1972); Seefeldt and Haubenstricker (1982).

References

Haubenstricker, J., Branta, C. & Seefeldt, V. (1983). Preliminary validation of a developmental sequence for throwing and catching. Paper presented at the annual convention of the North American Society for the Psychology of Sport and Physical Activity, East Lansing, MI.

Seefeldt, V. (1972) Developmental sequence of catching skill. Paper presented at the annual convention of American Association for Health, Physical Education and Recreation, and Houston, TX.

Seefeldt, V., & Haubenstricker, J. (1982). Patterns, phases, or stages: An analytical model for the study of developmental movement. In J. A. S. Kelso & J. E. Clark (Eds.), *The development of movement control and coordination*. New York: Wiley.

Compiled by Dr. Larry Isaacs. All material used with permission of Dr. John Haubenstricker.

APPENDIX C.2 H DEVELOPMENTAL SEQUENCE OF MOTOR SKILLS INVENTORY – TOTAL BODY APPROACH

Student Name:	Date:
STRIKE	
Stage 1 ☐ Motion primarily posterior-anterior in direction ☐ Movement begins with hip extension, slight spinal extension, and shoulder retraction on striking side of body ☐ Elbows fully flexed ☐ Feet remain stationary	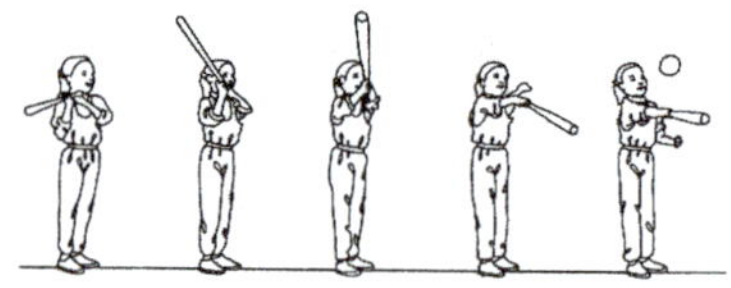
Stage 2 ☐ Primary pattern is unitary rotation of hip-spinal linkage about imaginary vertical axis ☐ Forward movement of bat in transverse plane ☐ Feet remain stationary or either foot may receive weight as body moves toward approaching ball	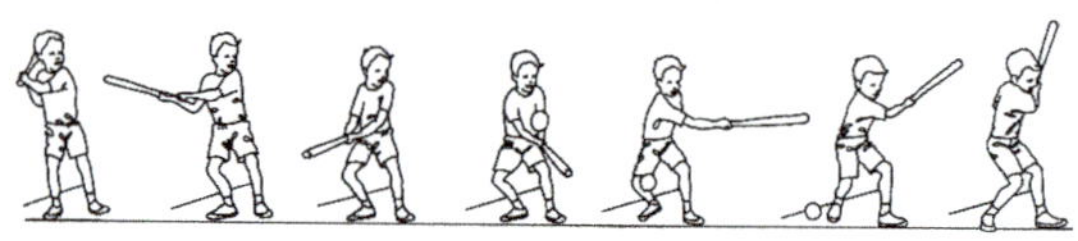
Stage 3 ☐ Shift of weight to front, supporting foot occurs in ipsilateral* pattern ☐ Trunk rotation-derotation decreased markedly in comparison with stage 2 ☐ Movement of bat in oblique-vertical plane	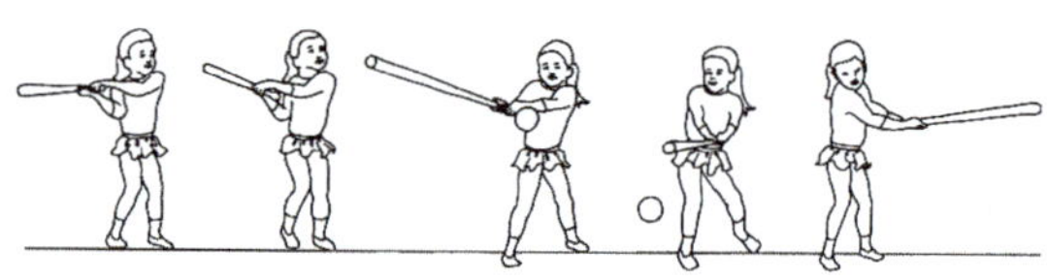
Stage 4 ☐ Transfer of weight in rotation-derotation in contralateral pattern ☐ Transfer of weight made with bat still moving backward ☐ At initiation of forward movement bat is kept near body ☐ Supination-pronation of hands do not occur until arms and hands are well-forward and ready to extend bat to meet ball ☐ At bat-ball contact weight is on forward foot	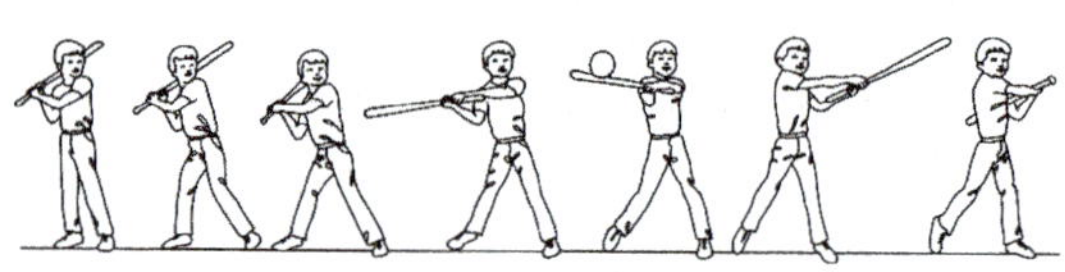
Student's Stage:	Comments:

*Same as both *unilateral* and *homolateral—stepping* forward with the foot that is on the same side of the body as the throwing arm. Based on the following source: Seefeldt and Haubenstricker (1982).

Reference

Seefeldt, V., & Haubenstricker, J. (1982). Patterns, phases, or stages: An analytical model for the study of developmental movement. In J. A. S. Kelso & J. E. Clark (Eds.), *The development of movement control and coordination*. New York: Wiley.

Compiled by Dr. Larry Isaacs. All material used with permission of Dr. John Haubenstricker.

APPENDIX C.2 I DEVELOPMENTAL SEQUENCE OF MOTOR SKILLS INVENTORY – TOTAL BODY APPROACH

Student Name: Date:

KICK

Stage 1

- ☐ Preparatory phase: Usually stationary, positioned near ball
- ☐ If performer moves, steps are short and concerned with spatial relationships, not taken to improve momentum
- ☐ Force production phase: Thigh of kicking leg moves forward with knee flexed, nearly parallel to surface at time of foot-ball contact
- ☐ Knee joint extension occurs after contact resulting in push, not strike
- ☐ Upper extremity action usually bilateral
- ☐ Follow-through phase: Knee of kicking leg extends until approaching 180°
- ☐ If trunk inclined forward at contact, forward step taken to regain balance
- ☐ If trunk inclined backward at contact, kicking leg will move backward after ball contact to regain balance

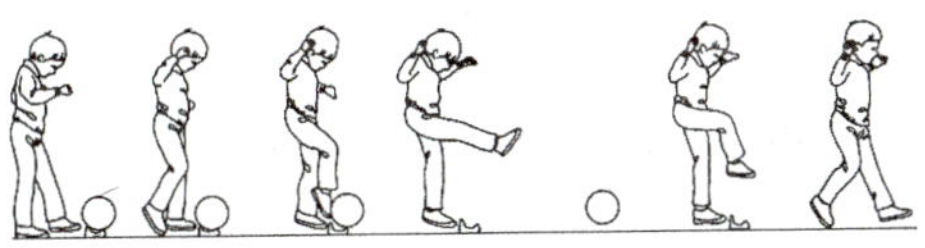

Stage 2

- ☐ Preparatory phase: Performer is stationary
- ☐ Initial action involves hyperextension at hips and flexion at knee
- ☐ Force production phase: Kicking leg moves forward with knee joint in flexed position
- ☐ Knee joint extension begins just prior to foot-ball contact
- ☐ Arm-leg opposition occurs during kick
- ☐ Follow-through phase: Knee extension continues after foot-ball contact but force of kick not usually sufficient to move body forward. Instead, performer usually steps sideward or backward

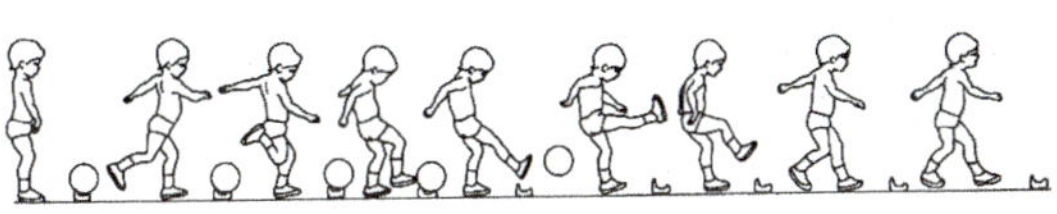

Stage 3

- ☐ Preparatory phase: One or more deliberate steps to approach ball
- ☐ Support leg placed near ball, slightly to side
- ☐ Force production phase: Kicking foot stays near surface, less knee flexion than stage 2
- ☐ Trunk remains nearly upright preventing max force production
- ☐ Knee extension begins prior to foot-ball contact
- ☐ Arm-leg opposition evident
- ☐ Follow-through phase: Force of kick may carry performer past point of foot-ball contact

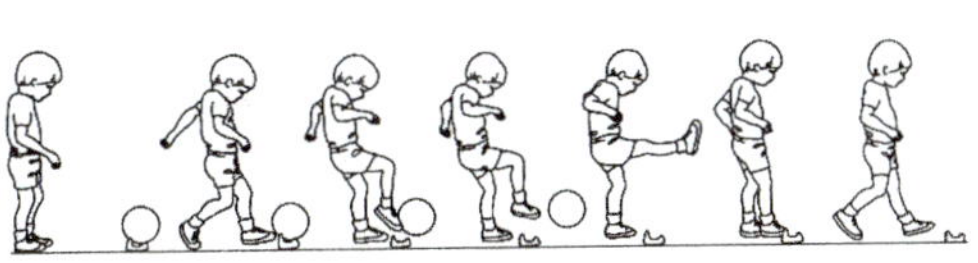

Student Name:	Date:
KICK	
Stage 4 ☐ Preparatory phase: Approach involves one or more steps, final "step" is a leap onto support leg ☐ Force production phase: Shoulders retracted and trunk inclined backward as support leg makes contact with surface ☐ Movement of thigh nearly stops as knee joint begins rapid extension forward ☐ Arm-leg opposition present as in stage 3	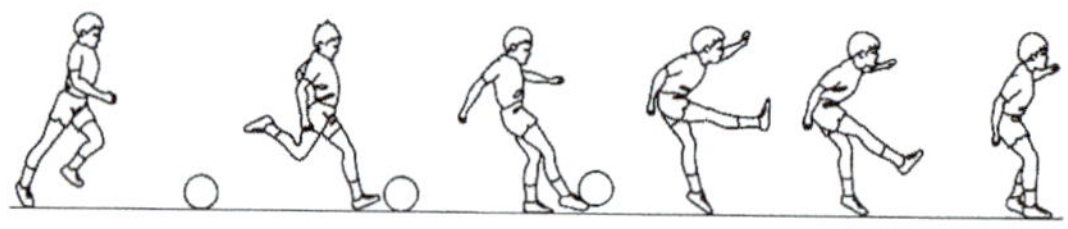
Student's Stage:	Comments:

Based on the following sources: Haubenstricker et al. (1981); Seefeldt (1972); Seefeldt and Haubenstricker (1975, 1982).

References

Haubenstricker, J., Seefeldt, V., Fountain, C., & Sapp, M. (1981). Preliminary validation of a developmental sequence for kicking. Paper presented at the Midwest District convention of the American Alliance for Health, Physical Education, Recreation, and Dance, Chicago.

Seefeldt, V. (1972). Developmental sequence of kicking. Unpublished materials. Michigan State University, East Lansing, MI.

Seefeldt, V., & Haubenstricker, J. (1975). Developmental sequence of kicking. Rev. ed. Unpublished materials. Michigan State University, East Lansing, MI.

Seefeldt, V., & Haubenstricker, J. (1982). Patterns, phases, or stages: An analytical model for the study of developmental movement. In J. A. S. Kelso & J. E. Clark (Eds.), *The development of movement control and coordination*. New York: Wiley.

Compiled by Dr. Larry Isaacs. All material used with permission of Dr. John Haubenstricker.

APPENDIX C.2 J DEVELOPMENTAL SEQUENCE OF MOTOR SKILLS INVENTORY – TOTAL BODY APPROACH

Student Name: Date:

PUNT

Stage 1

- ☐ Performer is stationary
- ☐ Ball held with both hands at waist height or higher
- ☐ Ball may be manipulated:
    - ☐ Held with both hands as foot is lifted forward and upward with hip and knee flexion
    - ☐ Ball may be tossed up and forward into air. Punter must move body forward into punting position
    - ☐ Performer may bounce ball and attempt to punt upon rebound
    - ☐ Flexion at hip and knee of punting leg places these segments in front of the midfrontal plane

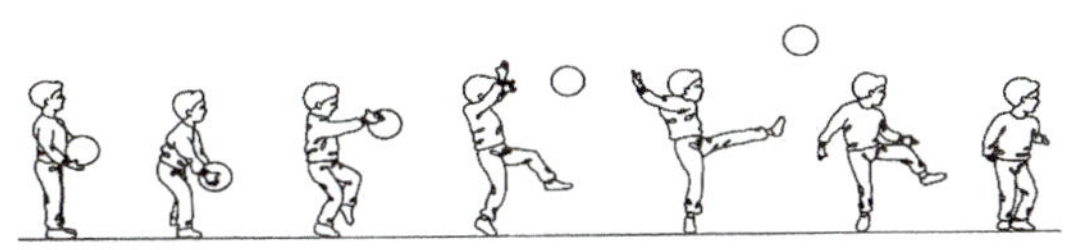

Stage 2

- ☐ Preparatory phase: Performer is stationary
- ☐ Ball held in both hands
- ☐ Ball may be dropped or tossed forward or upward
- ☐ Nonsupport leg flexed at knee, thigh perpendicular to surface or behind midfrontal plane
- ☐ As punting leg moves forward, momentum may carry performer forward for a step; generally force is upward

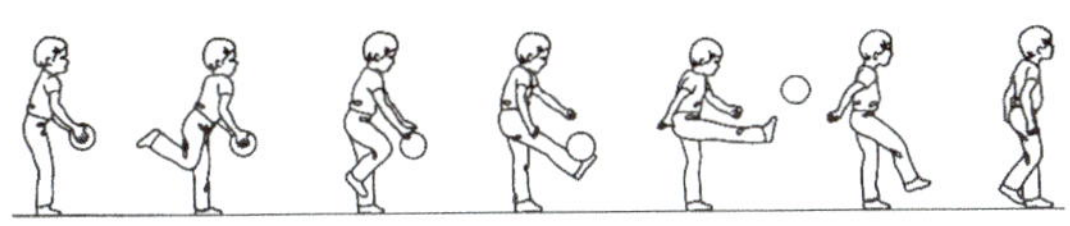

Stage 3

- ☐ Moves forward deliberately one or two steps in preparation for punt
- ☐ Ball released in forward and downward direction
- ☐ Knee flexed at 90° or less; thigh farther behind midfrontal plane than in stage 2
- ☐ Follow-through of striking leg generally carries punt ahead of point where ball was contacted

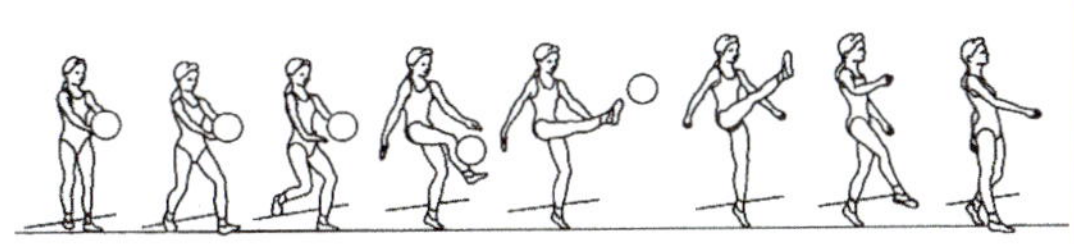

Stage 4

- ☐ Approach rapid, usually comprising one or more steps
- ☐ Leap performed just prior to contacting ball
- ☐ Ball released in forward and downward direction
- ☐ Ball contacted at or below knee height
- ☐ After the punt, momentum of swinging leg carries performer off the surface in upward and forward direction

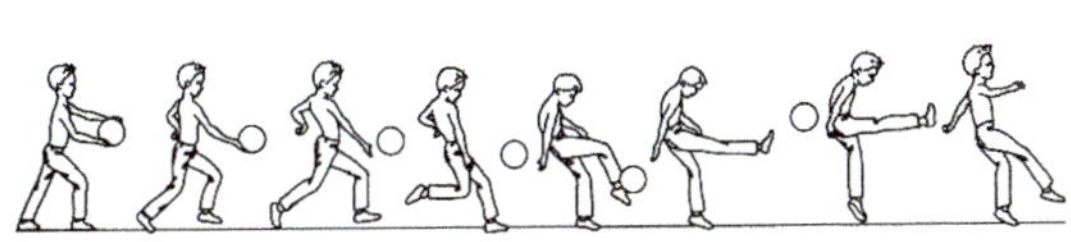

Student's Stage:

Comments:

Based on the following source: Seefeldt and Haubenstricker (1975).

Reference

Seefeldt, V., & Haubenstricker, J. (1975). Developmental sequence of punting. Rev. ed. Unpublished materials. Michigan State University, East Lansing, MI.

Compiled by Dr. Larry Isaacs. All material used with permission of Dr. John Haubenstricker.

APPENDIX C.3 SENIOR FITNESS TEST SCORECARD

SCORECARD: SENIOR FITNESS TEST

Name: ______________________________ Date: ____________________

☐ Male ☐ Female Age:__________ Ht:__________ Wt:__________

TEST ITEM	TRIAL 1	TRIAL 2	COMMENTS
1. Chair stand test (# in 30 sec)	______	______	____________ ____________
2. Arm curl test (# in 30 sec)	______	______	____________ ____________
3. 2-minute step test (# of steps) or 6-minute walk test (# of yds)	______	______	____________ ____________
4. Chair sit-and-reach test (nearest 1/2 in.: +/–)	______	______	____________ ____________
5. Back scratch test (nearest 1/2 in.: +/–)	______	______	____________ ____________
6. 8-ft up-and-go test (nearest 1/10 sec)	______	______	____________ ____________

Source: Rikli & Jones (2013).

Reference

Rikli, R. E., & Jones, C. J. (2013). *Senior fitness test manual.* 2nd ed. Champaign, IL: Human Kinetics, p. 57.

APPENDIX C.4 SHORT PHYSICAL PERFORMANCE BATTERY PROTOCOL AND SCORE SHEET

Study ID Date Tester Initials

All of the tests should be performed in the same order as they are presented in this protocol. Instructions to the participants are shown in bold italic and should be given exactly as they are written in this script.

1. BALANCE TESTS

The participant must be able to stand unassisted without the use of a cane or walker. You may help the participant to get up.

Now let's begin the evaluation. I would now like you to try to move your body in different movements. I will first describe and show each movement to you. Then I'd like you to try to do it. If you cannot do a particular movement, or if you feel it would be unsafe to try to do it, tell me and we'll move on to the next one. Let me emphasize that I do not want you to try to do any exercise that you feel might be unsafe.

Do you have any questions before we begin?

A. Side-by-Side Stand

1. ***Now I will show you the first movement.***
2. (Demonstrate) ***I want you to try to stand with your feet together, side-by-side, for about 10 seconds.***
3. ***You may use your arms, bend your knees, or move your body to maintain your balance, but try not to move your feet. Try to hold this position until I tell you to stop.***
4. Stand next to the participant to help him/her into the side-by-side position.
5. Supply just enough support to the participant's arm to prevent loss of balance.
6. When the participant has his/her feet together, ask ***"Are you ready?"***
7. Then let go and begin timing as you say, ***"Ready, begin."***
8. Stop the stopwatch and say ***"Stop"*** after 10 seconds or when the participant steps out of position or grabs your arm.
9. If participant is unable to hold the position for 10 seconds, record result and go to the gait speed test.

B. Semi-Tandem Stand

1. ***Now I will show you the second movement.***
2. (Demonstrate) ***Now I want you to try to stand with the side of the heel of one foot touching the big toe of the other foot for about 10 seconds. You may put either foot in front, whichever is more comfortable for you.***
3. ***You may use your arms, bend your knees, or move your body to maintain your balance, but try not to move your feet. Try to hold this position until I tell you to stop.***
4. Stand next to the participant to help him/her into the semi-tandem position.
5. Supply just enough support to the participant's arm to prevent loss of balance.
6. When the participant has his/her feet together, ask ***"Are you ready?"***
7. Then let go and begin timing as you say ***"Ready, begin."***

Source: Gurainik, Simonsick, Ferrucci, et al., 1994; available: www.grc.nia.nih.gov/branches/leps/sppb/index.htm. Additional information and instructions are available here: www.youtube.com/watch?v=XgiuciJXPm4.

Study ID ____ Date ____ Tester Initials ____

8. Stop the stopwatch and say ***"Stop"*** after 10 seconds or when the participant steps out of position or grabs your arm.
9. If participant is unable to hold the position for 10 seconds, record result and go to the gait speed test.

C. Tandem Stand

1. ***Now I will show you the third movement.***
2. (Demonstrate) ***Now I want you to try to stand with the heel of one foot in front of and touching the toes of the other foot for about 10 seconds. You may put either foot in front, whichever is more comfortable for you.***
3. ***You may use your arms, bend your knees, or move your body to maintain your balance, but try not to move your feet. Try to hold this position until I tell you to stop.***
4. Stand next to the participant to help him/her into the tandem position.
5. Supply just enough support to the participant's arm to prevent loss of balance.
6. When the participant has his/her feet together, ask ***"Are you ready?"***
7. Then let go and begin timing as you say, ***"Ready, begin."***
8. Stop the stopwatch and say ***"Stop"*** after 10 seconds or when the participant steps out of position or grabs your arm.

If participant did not attempt test or failed, circle why:

Tried but unable	1
Participant could not hold position unassisted	2
Not attempted, you felt unsafe	3
Not attempted, participant felt unsafe	4
Participant unable to understand instructions	5
Other (specify) ________	6
Participant refused	7

SCORING:

A. Side-by-Side-Stand

Held for 10 sec	☐ 1 point
Not held for 10 sec	☐ 0 points
Not attempted	☐ 0 points

If 0 points, end Balance Tests

Number of seconds held if less than 10 sec:____: __ __ sec

B. Semi-Tandem Stand

Held for 10 sec	☐ 1 point
Not held for 10 sec	☐ 0 points
Not attempted	☐ 0 points *(circle reason above)*

If 0 points, end Balance Tests

Number of seconds held if less than 10 sec:____: __ __ sec

C. Tandem Stand

Held for 10 sec	☐ 2 points
Held for 3 to 9.99 sec	☐ 1 point
Held for < than 3 sec	☐ 0 points
Not attempted	☐ 0 points *(circle reason above)*

Number of seconds held if less than 10 sec: ____: __ __ sec

D. Total Balance Tests score ____________ (sum points)

Comments:

____

____

____

____

Study ID Date Tester Initials

2. GAIT SPEED TEST

Now I am going to observe how you normally walk. If you use a cane or other walking aid and you feel you need it to walk a short distance, then you may use it.

A. First Gait Speed Test

1. ***This is our walking course. I want you to walk to the other end of the course at your usual speed, just as if you were walking down the street to go to the store.***
2. Demonstrate the walk for the participant.
3. ***Walk all the way past the other end of the tape before you stop. I will walk with you. Do you feel this would be safe?***
4. Have the participant stand with both feet touching the starting line.
5. ***When I want you to start, I will say: "Ready, begin."*** When the participant acknowledges this instruction say: ***"Ready, begin."***
6. Press the start/stop button to start the stopwatch as the participant begins walking.
7. Walk behind and to the side of the participant.
8. Stop timing when one of the participant's feet is completely across the end line.

B. Second Gait Speed Test

1. ***Now I want you to repeat the walk. Remember to walk at your usual pace, and go all the way past the other end of the course.***
2. Have the participant stand with both feet touching the starting line.
3. ***When I want you to start, I will say: "Ready, begin."*** When the participant acknowledges this instruction say: ***"Ready, begin."***
4. Press the start/stop button to start the stopwatch as the participant begins walking.
5. Walk behind and to the side of the participant.
6. Stop timing when one of the participant's feet is completely across the end line.

Gait Speed Test Scoring:

Length of walk test course: Four meters ☐ Three meters ☐

A. Time for First Gait Speed Test (sec)

1. Time for 3 or 4 meters _____ _____. _____ _____ sec
2. If participant did not attempt test or failed, circle why:

Tried but unable	1
Participant could not walk unassisted	2
Not attempted, you felt unsafe	3
Not attempted, participant felt unsafe	4
Participant unable to understand instructions	5
Other (Specify) ______________________	6
Participant refused	7

Complete score sheet and go to chair stand test

3. Aids for first walk: None ☐ Cane ☐ Other ☐

Study ID Date Tester Initials

Comments:

B. **Time for Second Gait Speed Test (sec)**

1. Time for 3 or 4 meters ___ ___. ___ ___ sec
2. If participant did not attempt test or failed, circle why:

Tried but unable	1
Participant could not walk unassisted	2
Not attempted, you felt unsafe	3
Not attempted, participant felt unsafe	4
Participant unable to understand instructions	5
Other (Specify) ____________________	6
Participant refused	7

3. Aids for second walk: None ☐ Cane ☐ Other ☐

What is the time for the faster of the two walks ☐

Record the shorter of the two times ___ ___. ___ ___ sec

[If only 1 walk done, record that time] ___ ___. ___ ___ sec

If the participant was unable to do the walk: 0 points

For 4-Meter Walk:

If time is more than 8.70 sec:	☐ 1 point
If time is 6.21 to 8.70 sec:	☐ 2 points
If time is 4.82 to 6.20 sec:	☐ 3 points
If time is less than 4.82 sec:	☐ 4 points

For 3-Meter Walk:

If time is more than 6.52 sec:	☐ 1 point
If time is 4.66 to 6.52 sec:	☐ 2 points
If time is 3.62 to 4.65 sec:	☐ 3 points
If time is less than 3.62 sec:	☐ 4 points

3. CHAIR STAND TEST

Single Chair Stand

1. ***Let's do the last movement test. Do you think it would be safe for you to try to stand up from a chair without using your arms?***
2. ***The next test measures the strength in your legs.***
3. (Demonstrate and explain the procedure.) ***First, fold your arms across your chest and sit so that your feet are on the floor; then stand up keeping your arms folded across your chest.***
4. ***Please stand up keeping your arms folded across your chest.*** (Record result).
5. If participant cannot rise without using arms, say ***"Okay, try to stand up using your arms."*** This is the end of their test. Record result and go to the scoring page.

Study ID Date Tester Initials

Repeated Chair Stands

1. ***Do you think it would be safe for you to try to stand up from a chair five times without using your arms?***
2. (Demonstrate and explain the procedure): ***Please stand up straight as QUICKLY as you can five times, without stopping in between. After standing up each time, sit down and then stand up again. Keep your arms folded across your chest. I'll be timing you with a stopwatch.***
3. When the participant is properly seated, say: ***"Ready? Stand"*** and begin timing.
4. Count out loud as the participant arises each time, up to five times.
5. Stop if participant becomes tired or short of breath during repeated chair stands.
6. Stop the stopwatch when he/she has straightened up completely for the fifth time.
7. Also stop:
   - ∞ If participant uses his/her arms
   - ∞ After 1 minute, if participant has not completed rises
   - ∞ At your discretion, if concerned for participant's safety
8. If the participant stops and appears to be fatigued before completing the five stands, confirm this by asking ***"Can you continue?"***
9. If participant says "Yes," continue timing. If participant says "No," stop and reset the stopwatch.

SCORING:

Single Chair Stand Test	**YES**	**NO**
A. Safe to stand without help	☐	☐
B. Results:		
Participant stood without using arms	☐	→ **Go to Repeated Chair Stand Test**
Participant used arms to stand	☐	→ End test; score as 0 points
Test not completed	☐	→ End test; score as 0 points
C. If participant did not attempt test or failed, circle why:		
Tried but unable		1
Participant could not stand unassisted		2
Not attempted, you felt unsafe		3
Not attempted, participant felt unsafe		4
Participant unable to understand instructions		5
Other (Specify)		6
Participant refused		7

Repeated Chair Stand Test	**YES**	**NO**
A. Safe to stand five times	☐	☐
B. If five stands done successfully, record time in seconds.		
Time to complete five stands ___ ___. ___ ___ sec		
C. If participant did not attempt test or failed, circle why:		
Tried but unable		1
Participant could not stand unassisted		2
Not attempted, you felt unsafe		3
Not attempted, participant felt unsafe		4

Study ID Date Tester Initials

Participant unable to understand instructions	5
Other (Specify) ______________________	6
Participant refused	7

Scoring the Repeated Chair Test

Participant unable to complete 5 chair stands or completes stands in >60 sec:	☐ 0 points
If chair stand time is 16.70 sec or more:	☐ 1 points
If chair stand time is 13.70 to 16.69 sec:	☐ 2 points
If chair stand time is 11.20 to 13.69 sec:	☐ 3 points
If chair stand time is 11.19 sec or less:	☐ 4 points

SCORING FOR COMPLETE SHORT PHYSICAL PERFORMANCE BATTERY

Test Scores

Total Balance Test score	_____ **points**
Gait Speed Test score	_____ **points**
Chair Stand Test score	_____ **points**
Total Score	_____ **points (sum of points above)**

INDEX